REHABILITATION RESEARCH

REHABILITATION RESEARCH

Principles and Applications

THIRD EDITION

Elizabeth Domholdt, PT, EdD, FAPTA
Professor and Dean
Krannert School of Physical Therapy
University of Indianapolis
Indianapolis, Indiana

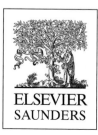

ELSEVIER
SAUNDERS

ELSEVIER
SAUNDERS

11830 Westline Industrial Drive
St. Louis, Missouri 63146

NOTICE

Rehabilitation is an ever-changing field. Standard safety precautions must be followed, but as new research and clinical experience broaden our knowledge, changes in treatment and drug therapy may become necessary or appropriate. Readers are advised to check the most current product information provided by the manufacturer of each drug to be administered to verify the recommended dose, the method and duration of administration, and contraindications. It is the responsibility of the licensed prescriber, relying on experience and knowledge of the patient, to determine dosages and the best treatment for each individual patient. Neither the publisher nor the author assumes any liability for any injury and/or damage to persons or property arising from this publication.

Previous editions copyrighted 1993, 2000

Library of Congress Cataloging-in-Publication Data

Domholdt, Elizabeth, 1958-
  Rehabilitation research: principles and applications/Elizabeth Domholdt.–3rd ed.
     p. ; cm.
  Rev. ed. of: Physical therapy research/Elizabeth Domholdt. c2000.
  Includes bibliographical references and index.
  ISBN 0-7216-0029-8
   1. Medical rehabilitation–Research. I. Domholdt, Elizabeth, 1958-Physical therapy research. II. Title.
  [DNLM: 1. Rehabilitation. 2. Data Interpretation, Statistical. 3. Research–methods. 4. Treatment Outcome.
WB 320 D668r 2005]
  RM930.D66 2005
  617′.03–dc22   2004050696

Acquisitions Editor: *Marion Waldman*
Developmental Editor: *Marjory Fraser*
Publishing Services Manager: *Patricia Tannian*
Senior Project Manager: *Anne Altepeter*
Book Designer: *Amy Buxton*

Printed in the United States of America

Last digit is the print number: 9 8 7 6 5 4 3 2

For Gary L. Shoemaker
Husband and friend
1952-2004

Consultants

Craig R. Denegar, PhD, PT, ATC
Associate Professor
Department of Orthopaedics and Rehabilitation
  and Kinesiology
Pennsylvania State University
University Park, Pennsylvania

Virginia A. Hinton, MA, PhD, CCC-SLP
Associate Professor
Department of Communication Sciences
  and Disorders
School of Health and Human Performance
The University of North Carolina—Greensboro
Greensboro, North Carolina

Penelope A. Moyers, EdD, OTR, FAOTA
Professor and Chair
Department of Occupational Therapy
The University of Alabama—Birmingham
Birmingham, Alabama

Preface

Rehabilitation professionals share a deeply held belief that the exercise of our professional expertise, in partnership with the patients or clients with whom we work, makes a difference in their lives. This deeply held belief is a positive force when it leads to the high levels of professionalism and commitment that are demonstrated daily by rehabilitation professionals around the globe. This belief, however, can also serve as a negative force when it leads practitioners to the uncritical acceptance of all of rehabilitation practice.

The purpose of research, then, is not to justify what we do. Rather, research is needed to determine which of the many things we do as rehabilitation professionals can be justified. This is an important distinction. The former leads to a search for weak evidence that supports our current practices; the latter leads to a search for strong evidence that can help us change and improve our practices based on the evidence.

Evidence-based practice in rehabilitation can be realized only by a joint effort of the producers and consumers of research. This is a textbook that will serve most of the needs of research consumers and can serve many of the foundational needs of research producers. It does so by using straightforward language and relevant examples to capture the diversity and complexity of research that is of interest to rehabilitation professionals. In addition, consumers and producers of research who require more detail on a given topic will find that each chapter is well referenced with a mix of contemporary and classic citations.

The text is divided into two parts: principles and applications. The first 23 chapters present the principles of research that both consumers and producers of research need to know. The final five chapters are designed to help consumers and producers of research apply these principles as they evaluate the literature, design and implement projects, and disseminate results.

The first edition of this text provided a solid grounding in traditional research design and analysis, as well as an introduction to emerging research topics such as qualitative and single-system designs, all in the context of physical therapy research. The second edition maintained the solid grounding in traditional research topics and the context of physical therapy and provided expanded coverage of a number of topics such as outcomes research, epidemiology, qualitative design, single-system design, case reports, survey research, and the data analysis techniques used with these research approaches. For this third edition, I took an important leap—with the assistance of colleagues—from the context of physical therapy research to the broader context of rehabilitation research. The addition of research examples and research approaches used by occupational therapists, speech-language pathologists and audiologists, physiatrists, athletic trainers, and prosthetists and orthotists has added a richness to the text that was missing in the past. This richness is expressed in the wide array of ways in which different authors conceptualize function across the studies cited in this edition, in the addition of more social science and educational research techniques and tools, and in the enhanced emphasis on randomized controlled trials and evidence-based practice.

Successful completion of this edition required the assistance of many individuals. Three colleagues served as interdisciplinary consultants to the third edition: Dr. Craig Denegar, Dr. Virginia A. Hinton, and Dr. Penelope A. Moyers. Representing physical therapy and athletic training, speech-language pathology, and occupational therapy, respectively, they each made unique contributions to the text by either reviewing the second edition and recommending changes or providing feedback to drafts of third-edition chapters. Dr. Denegar challenged some of the ways that I had presented information in the past and pointed me in the direction of many excellent citations from the athletic training and orthopedic surgery literature. Dr. Moyers, a colleague at the University of Indianapolis while I was working on the third edition, helped me weave qualitative research principles better throughout the text and presented me with stacks (stacks!) of occupational therapy research related to each chapter. Dr. Hinton gave me feedback to revised chapters, reminding me when my "physical therapy" voice was overly strong and helping me use unfamiliar terms from the communication disorders literature more accurately. As helpful as these colleagues were during the revision process, I take full responsibility for those times when my physical therapist's perspective prevails or when the way I describe a cited study makes it clear that I'm out of my element!

University of Indianapolis President Jerry Israel and Provost Everette Freeman have supported my desire to remain an active scholar while I fulfilled my administrative and teaching duties for the university. The faculty and staff of the Krannert School of Physical Therapy carried on just fine despite the many days that I blocked out to work on "the book." Stacie Fruth, PT, a doctoral student, was instrumental in the addition of more than 150 new words to the glossary. Jenny Miller, a physical therapy student, and Bina Victor, PT, a graduate student, helped check the accuracy of book and journal references, respectively. Christine Guyonneau and Shirley Bigna, librarians at the University of Indianapolis, provided valuable feedback to the chapter on locating the literature—an area that has undergone and continues to undergo rapid change.

Finally, it is with great love and a profound sense of loss that I thank my late husband, Gary Shoemaker, for the love that he brought to my life and for the memories he will continue to bring as I move past these early months of grief following his unexpected death in January 2004. He was always a steady guy with an understated sense of humor that grabbed you when you least expected it. He was my daily anchor for the 20 years of our marriage, and I miss him deeply.

Elizabeth Domholdt, PT, EdD, FAPTA
Indianapolis, Indiana
March 2004

Contents

SECTION 7   Being a Consumer

SECTION 8   **Implementing Research**

Appendices

Research Fundamentals

Rehabilitation Research

Rehabilitation professionals believe that the work we do makes a difference in the lives of the people we serve. Rehabilitation research is the means by which we test that belief. In the rapidly changing and increasingly accountable world of health care it is no longer enough to say that we do good work. It is no longer enough to casually note that patients or clients feel better after we've intervened. Rather, we must be willing to search for evidence about the value of our practices and then modify those practices in response to the evidence. Rehabilitation professionals who embrace evidence-based practice also embrace the challenge of learning about rehabilitation research. A working knowledge of research

design, methodology, and analysis is a prerequisite to evaluating existing evidence and producing new evidence.

This book provides clinicians and researchers with a framework for understanding and applying the systematic processes of research. As with other fields of study, research is ever-changing and a text can only represent research thought at a particular point in time. This text does, however, present both traditional research methods as well as emerging approaches. Just as evidence-based clinicians regularly challenge their beliefs about rehabilitation practice, researchers must regularly consider new ways of generating research-based evidence.

Learning about rehabilitation research is not easy. First, it involves developing a diverse set of knowledge and skills in research methodologies, research design, statistical and qualitative analysis, presentation, and writing. At the same time a practitioner is acquiring these new skills, he or she is forced to reexamine the status quo, the conventional wisdom of the rehabilitation professions. This combination of trying to learn new material while challenging previously held beliefs can engender frustration with the new material and doubt about previous learning. Some clinicians, unable to cope with such uncertainty, retreat to anecdotes and intuition as the basis for their work in rehabilitation. Others delight in the intellectual stimulation of research and commit themselves to developing an evidence-based practice. Such clinicians balance the use of existing but unsubstantiated practices with critical evaluation of those same practices through regular review of the professional literature and thoughtful discussion with colleagues. Furthermore, these professionals may participate in clinical research to test the assumptions under which they practice.

This introductory chapter defines research, examines reasons for and barriers to implementing rehabilitation research, and considers the current status of rehabilitation research. Based on this foundation, the rest of the book presents the principles needed to understand research and suggests guidelines for the application of those principles to rehabilitation research.

■ DEFINITIONS OF RESEARCH

Research has been defined by almost every person who has written about it. Kettering, an engineer and philanthropist, had this to say:

> "Research" is a high-hat word that scares a lot of people. It needn't;...it is nothing but a state of mind—a friendly, welcoming attitude toward change. ... It is the problem-solving mind as contrasted with the let-well-enough-alone mind. It is the composer mind instead of the fiddler mind. It is the "tomorrow" mind instead of the "yesterday" mind.[1(p91)]

Payton, a physical therapist who has written widely about research, indicates that "research should begin with an intellectual itch that needs scratching."[2(p8)] Kazdin, a psychologist, speaks about various research methods, noting that "they have in common careful observation and systematic evaluation of the subject matter."[3(p2)] Portney and Watkins,[4] Polit and Hungler,[5] Stein and Cutler,[6] and Maxwell and Satake,[7] who have written texts on clinical, nursing, occupational therapy, and communication disorders research, respectively, all emphasize the organized, systematic nature of research. Three important characteristics about research emerge from these different authors: first, research challenges the status quo; second, it is creative; and third, it is systematic.

Research Challenges the Status Quo

The first characteristic is that research challenges the status quo. Sometimes the results of research may support current clinical practices; other times the results point to treatment techniques that are not effective. But whether research does or does not lead to a revision of currently accepted principles, the guiding philosophy of research is one of challenge. Does this treatment work? Is it more effective than another treatment? Would this person recover as quickly without intervention? The status quo can be challenged in several ways, as illustrated in the three examples that follow.

One way of challenging the status quo is to identify gaps in our knowledge—to identify common practices about which we know very little. Because much of our practice as clinicians is based on the collective wisdom of past professionals, we forget that much of this practice has not been verified in a systematic way. In 2001, a group of health care practitioners, the Philadelphia Panel, developed evidence-based clinical practice guidelines for a number of rehabilitation interventions for low back pain.[8] This panel evaluated the clinical literature related to care of acute, subacute, chronic, and post-surgery low back pain and identified which of a variety of interventions were supported by evidence. Figure 1–1 shows a modified version of the summary grid of their findings. The dark shaded areas represent interventions that are supported by scientific evidence, in the judgment of the panel. The unshaded areas represent interventions for which the panel found insufficient or no data. The remaining lightly shaded boxes show the interventions for which the findings supported neither the treatment in question nor the studied alternatives. The panel findings, therefore, should challenge rehabilitation professionals to rethink their use of many standard interventions for low back pain. Furthermore, these findings suggest a powerful research agenda for rehabilitation providers interested in low back pain.

Having identified many rehabilitation practices about which little, if any, data exist, a second approach to challenging the status quo is to systematically test the effects of these practices. Delitto and colleagues[9] did this when they designed a randomized clinical trial to determine whether patients with a certain pattern of low back signs and symptoms benefited more from a treatment approach designed to match their signs and symptoms than they did from a general, unmatched treatment. The patients within their study all had signs and symptoms that would lead many therapists to adopt a treatment approach combining sacroiliac joint mobilization, extension exercises, and avoidance of flexed postures. Their challenge to the status quo could be restated as follows:

Therapists classify patients with low back pain according to signs and symptoms and differentiate their treatments based on these classifications. However, there is really no evidence to show that a specific match between classification and treatment leads to better results than offering nonspecific treatments. Therefore, let's see if patients who receive a specific treatment that is matched to their classification actually have better outcomes than those who receive nonspecific, unmatched treatment.

Patients with low back syndrome who fit an extension-mobilization category were treated with either a matched mobilization and extension routine or with an unmatched program of flexion exercises. Delitto and colleagues found that the patients in the matched group improved faster than the unmatched group, as measured

Intervention	Acute LBP	Subacute LBP	Chronic LBP	Post-surgery LBP
Exercise				
Continue normal activities				
Traction				
Therapeutic ultrasound				
Transcutaneous electrical nerve stimulation				
Massage				
Thermotherapy				
Electrical stimulation				
Electromyographic biofeedback				
Combined rehabilitation interventions				

FIGURE 1–1. Modified summary grid of the Philadelphia Panel findings. The dark shaded areas represent interventions that are supported by scientific evidence, in the judgment of the panel. The unshaded areas represent interventions for which the panel found insufficient or no data. The remaining lightly shaded boxes show the interventions for which the findings supported neither the treatment in question nor the studied alternatives.
Modified from Philadelphia Panel. Evidence-based clinical practice guidelines on selected rehabilitation interventions for low back pain. *Phys Ther.* 2001;81: 1641-1674.

by scores on a standardized functional outcome test.[9] Thus, this challenge to a common set of clinical procedures yielded support for those procedures.

A third way of challenging the status quo is to test novel or traditionally avoided treatments. A long-held and only recently challenged assumption is that traditional resistive muscle strengthening is inappropriate for individuals with upper motor neuron pathology. Damiano and Abel[10] challenged this in their study of lower extremity muscle strengthening in children with spastic cerebral palsy. They found that the children demonstrated increased muscle strength and increased gait velocity after a 6-week lower extremity muscle strength training program. Thus, the results of their challenge to this commonly held belief suggest that clinicians should reexamine their beliefs about the value of strength training for children with spastic muscles and modify their treatment approaches to reflect any change in their beliefs.

These three examples of challenges to the status quo identified gaps in knowledge about rehabilitation practice, provided support for one set of clinical practices, and suggested a need for review of another set of clinical beliefs. Research is about embracing these kinds of challenges. It is about the willingness to test our assumptions, to use what works, and to change our practices in light of new evidence.

Research Is Creative

The second characteristic of research is that it is creative. Rothstein, in an editorial, chastised physical therapists for their willingness to accept authoritarian views of their profession: "Our teachers and our texts tell us how it should be, and we accept this in our eagerness to proceed with patient care."[11(p895)] Researchers are creative individuals who move past the authoritarian teachings of others and look at rehabilitation in a different way.

For example, rehabilitation professionals working with patients who have had strokes or amputations often strive for their patients to exhibit as symmetric a gait pattern as possible. Winter, a biomechanist, was creative enough to ask whether a symmetric gait is the most efficient gait for an individual with unilateral dysfunction:

> At the outset, the author would be cautious about gait retraining protocols which are aimed at improved symmetry based on nothing more than an idea that it would automatically be an improvement. It is safe to say that any human system with major structural asymmetries in the neuromuscular skeletal system cannot be optimal when the gait is symmetrical.[12(p362)]

Clark and colleagues[13] were creative when they designed a randomized controlled trial to determine the impact of preventive occupational therapy on physical and social function of multiethnic, independent-living older adults. They took a creative leap from thinking about occupational therapy intervention for individuals who already have impairments or disabilities to testing its impact as a hedge against impairment or disability in a group thought to be at risk of becoming disabled.

Researchers thrive on the creative intellectual processes that lead to the development of new ways of conceptualizing their disciplines. Creative aspects of rehabilitation research are emphasized in Chapter 2, which presents information about the use of theory in practice and research, and Chapter 4, which provides a framework for the development of research problems.

Research Is Systematic

The third characteristic of research is that it is systematic. In contrast, much of our clinical knowledge is anecdotal, or is passed on through "ecclesiastical succession"[14(p3)] from prominent practitioners who teach a particular treatment to eager colleagues or students. Anecdotal claims for the effectiveness of treatments are colored by the relationship between the clinician and patient and do not control for factors, other than the treatment, that may account for changes in the condition of the patient or client. The systematic nature of some research methodologies attempts to isolate treatment effects from other influences not ordinarily controlled in the clinic setting. Other methodologies focus on systematic description of the phenomenon of interest, rather than control of the research setting. Much of this text presents the systematic principles that underlie research methods: Sections 2 through 4 (Chapters 4 through 16) cover research design, Section 5 (Chapters 17 and 18) discusses measurement tools, and Section 6 (Chapters 19 through 23) introduces data analysis.

■ REASONS FOR DEVELOPING REHABILITATION RESEARCH

There are at least three reasons for conducting rehabilitation research: (1) to develop a body of knowledge for the rehabilitation professions, (2) to determine whether interventions work, and (3) to improve patient and client care. Each of these reasons is examined in the sections that follow.

Develop Body of Knowledge

The "body of knowledge" rationale for rehabilitation research is related to the concept of a profession. The characteristics of a profession have been described by many authors, but include several common elements. Houle[15] divided the characteristics of a profession into three broad groups: conceptual, performance, and collective identity characteristics (Box 1–1). One of the critical performance characteristics is mastery of the theoretical knowledge that forms the basis for the profession.

The theoretical foundations of the rehabilitation professions, discussed further in Chapter 2, include concepts such as occupation, disablement, and movement science. Parham, an occupational therapist, expressed concern that "the understanding of occupation has not progressed much since the founding days of the profession largely because

---

BOX 1–1
Characteristics of a Profession
CONCEPTUAL CHARACTERISTIC
Establishment of a central mission
PERFORMANCE CHARACTERISTICS
Mastery of theoretical knowledge
Capacity to solve problems
Use of practical knowledge
Self-enhancement
COLLECTIVE IDENTITY CHARACTERISTICS
Formal training
Credentialing
Creation of a subculture
Legal reinforcement
Public acceptance
Ethical practice
Penalties
Relations to other vocations
Relations to users of service

List developed from Houle CO. *Continuing Learning in the Professions.* San Francisco, Calif: Jossey-Bass; 1981.

---

we in the field have not made a concerted effort to study it."[16(p486)] In doing so, she made a case for the study of "occupation," a concept that many believe is central to the body of knowledge of occupational therapy. In rehabilitation practice in general, the disablement model is often used for studying and understanding practice. Disablement is a "global term that reflects all the diverse consequences that disease, injury, or congenital abnormalities may have on human functioning."[17(p380)] As such, it relates to the "impact that chronic and acute conditions have on the functioning of specific body systems and on people's abilities to act in necessary, usual, expected and personally desired ways in their society."[18(p3)] It is through research that we can systematically develop a body of knowledge about the rehabilitation professions and their central concepts.

Determine Whether Interventions Work

The second major rationale for performing rehabilitation research relates to determining whether interventions work. When discussing this reason for doing research, clinicians must be careful not to fall into an all-too-common line of reasoning identified by Hayes:

> Too often I hear [clinicians] say that we need to do research to demonstrate that what we do works. This logic concerns me, because it is not the right attitude to carry into clinical research. We must study *whether* what we do works.[19(p12)]

The need for research on the effectiveness of rehabilitation interventions was highlighted by Brummel-Smith when he summarized the research recommendations of a National Institutes of Health Task Force on Medical Rehabilitation Research and applied them to rehabilitation of older adults.[20] He noted four major areas in need of study: the natural history of disability, functional assessment and performance evaluation, intervention issues, and rehabilitation service delivery. In discussing intervention issues, he identified a need to both "evaluate effectiveness of existing interventions and to develop novel approaches to care,"[20(p895)] noting that "current interventions have not received the type of careful scrutiny that is now expected of medical interventions."[20(p895)]

Improve Patient and Client Care

The third reason for rehabilitation research is perhaps the most important one, that of improving patient and client care. Research can improve care by helping clinicians make good decisions about the use of existing practices or by providing systematic evaluation of the effectiveness of new practices.

When we know what has or has not been supported by research, we can make intelligent, evidence-based decisions about which clinical procedures to use with our clients. Within medicine, rates of surgeries such as hysterectomy, prostatectomy, and tonsillectomy have been found to vary widely from community to community.[21] This variation is thought, in part, to result from "conflicting information about whether a particular procedure will improve a patient's health or the quality of his life."[21(p126)] Clinical research about these procedures could provide additional evidence that would help practitioners make informed decisions about recommending the procedures.

Although there are many areas of rehabilitation practice for which evidence is thin, there are other areas where clinicians who are committed to evidence-based practice can find a rich body of evidence on which to base their work. For example, two independent research groups recently synthesized the evidence about the effectiveness of occupational therapy and physical therapy for treating persons with Parkinson's disease.[22,23] Nineteen articles on occupational therapy for Parkinson's disease were reviewed and positive effects were identified for outcomes related to capacities and abilities as well as function during activities and tasks.[22] Twelve articles on physical therapy for Parkinson's disease were reviewed and positive effects were identified for activities of daily living, walking speed, and stride length.[23] Clearly, clinicians working with patients with Parkinson's disease can use these results to set goals and plan interventions.

In addition to helping clinicians make judgments about the use of existing treatments, research can be used to test new procedures so that clinicians can make evidence-based decisions about whether to add them to their clinical arsenal. For example, body-weight–supported treadmill ambulation is one relatively new treatment in need of such testing. In theory, body-weight–supported treadmill ambulation should enable patients to improve their ambulation function by training in a way that ensures safety, does not require handheld assistive devices, uses relatively normal gait patterns, and has reduced energy demands when compared with unsupported walking. A recent study by

Miller[24] evaluated the use of this technique for ambulation training for patients after stroke. Clinicians with a good knowledge base in research will be able to critically evaluate this article to determine whether they can apply the results to the clinical situations in which they work. Chapters 25 and 26 present guidelines for evaluating research literature.

■ BARRIERS TO REHABILITATION RESEARCH

In 1975, Hislop, a physical therapist, articulated one major philosophical barrier to research in the profession:

> A great difficulty in developing the clinical science of physical therapy is that we treat individual persons, each of whom is made up of situations which are unique and, therefore, appear incompatible with the generalizations demanded by science.[25(p1076)]

Although this conceptual barrier may still loom large for some practitioners, many more concrete obstacles to rehabilitation research have been documented.[26-28] These obstacles include lack of familiarity with research methodology, lack of statistical support, lack of funding, lack of a mentor, and lack of time. An additional obstacle is concern for ethical use of humans or animals in research activities.

Lack of Familiarity with the Research Process

Clinicians sometimes view rehabilitation research as a mysterious process that occupies the time of an elite group of professionals, far removed from patient or client care, who develop projects of little relevance to everyday practice. Although this characterization is a caricature, even the most clinically grounded research uses the specialized language of research design and data analysis, and those who have not acquired the vocabulary are understandably intimidated when it is spoken. The goal of this book is to demystify the research process by clearly articulating the knowledge base needed to understand it.

Lack of Statistical Support

The second major barrier to research is lack of statistical support. Section 6 (Chapters 19 through 23) of this book provides the conceptual background needed to understand most of the statistics reported in the rehabilitation research literature.[29,30] A conceptual background does not, however, provide an adequate theoretical and mathematical basis for selection and computation of a given statistic on a particular occasion, particularly for complex research designs. Thus, many researchers will require the services of a statistician at some point in the research process. Guidelines for working with statisticians are provided in Chapter 27.

Lack of Funds

A third barrier to research is lack of funding opportunities, which has been described as a "serious impediment to the development of clinical research in allied health."[31(p207)] Research has many direct costs: the time of researchers or clinicians, or both, that is needed to develop and implement projects, equipment and software, statistical and engineering consultants, clerical time, travel for presentation of the research at conferences, and figure and photographic production costs for presentation and publication of the research. Indirect costs include administrator time related to the project and other institutional costs, such as maintaining an Institutional Review Board to protect the rights of human participants in research studies. Without external funding for research, many administrators find it difficult to justify research activities that take clinicians or faculty members away from practice and teaching activities. Funding sources for rehabilitation research are discussed in Chapter 27.

Lack of Mentors

A fourth barrier to rehabilitation research is lack of mentors. Contemporary research is rarely performed by a single researcher in isolation. Rather, researchers work in teams that, in the aggregate, have the design, analysis, grant writing, and technical writing skills needed to design and implement research projects and disseminate the results. Ideally, novice researchers would be invited by experienced researchers to become members of working research teams with ongoing projects, external funding, and access to a network of colleagues engaged in similar work. The notion that completion of a research-focused doctoral degree prepares a professional for an independent research career is outdated, and many believe that a broad network of post-doctoral opportunities—both formal fellowships and informal mentoring—are needed to encourage the development and retention of rehabilitation researchers.[31] The importance of research mentors—and the difficulty in finding them in the rehabilitation professions—has been discussed for physical medicine and rehabilitation residents,[32] for occupational therapists,[33] and for physiotherapists, occupational therapists, and speech and language therapists in the United Kingdom.[34]

Lack of Time

A fifth barrier to rehabilitation research is lack of time. In a paper advancing the need for outcomes assessment in speech-language pathology, Testa[35] outlined six major factors that influence the completion of research. Two of the six factors referred to "time" directly and two more (complexity and funding) are indirectly related to the time that a researcher has available to devote to the task. Indeed, it is difficult to separate the "time" issue from the "funding" issue, as a lack of external funding generally limits the time available for research. In the absence of external funding, tasks with firm deadlines are given higher priority than research and the

immediate time pressures of the clinic and classroom may lead clinicians and academicians alike to postpone or abandon research ideas. One solution is to design studies that are relatively easy to integrate into the daily routine of a practice. Chapters 10, 12, and 15 present a variety of research designs particularly suitable for implementation in a clinical setting.

Ethical Concerns About Use of Human Participants and Animal Subjects

The sixth barrier to research implementation is ethical concerns related to the use of either human participants or animal subjects in research. Those who choose to study animal models should follow appropriate guidelines for the use, care, and humane destruction of animal subjects. Clinicians who use human participants in their research must pay close attention to balancing the risks of the research with potential benefits from the results. Chapter 3 examines ethical considerations in detail; Chapter 27 provides guidelines for working with the committees that oversee researchers to ensure that they protect the rights of research participants.

Overcoming Barriers

Overcoming these barriers depends on leaders who are willing to commit time and money to research efforts, individuals who are willing to devote time and effort to improving their research knowledge and skills, and improved systems for training researchers and funding research. Cusick's qualitative study of clinician-researchers underscores the importance of making an individual commitment to becoming a researcher, accepting responsibility for driving the research process, and learning to negotiate the administrative and social systems that make clinical research possible.[36] Research is, however, rarely an individual effort. Therefore, one key to overcoming barriers to research is to develop productive research teams composed of individuals who, together, have all the diverse skills needed to plan, implement, analyze, and report research. The different rehabilitation professions are working to develop such teams in different ways: the Foundation for Physical Therapy in 2002 funded its first Clinical Research Network, designed to increase research capacity in physical therapy through collaborative arrangements between academic and clinical sites[37]; the Accreditation Council for Graduate Medical Education recently added a research education requirement to physical medicine and rehabilitation residencies[32]; and building research capacity in the allied health professions has been of interest to policy-making bodies in the United States[31] and the United Kingdom.[34]

■ STATUS OF REHABILITATION RESEARCH

The rehabilitation professions are relative newcomers to the health care arena, as the "conflagrations of World War I and II provided the impetus for the development and growth of the field of rehabilitation."[38(p1)] Mindful of the way in which new professions grow, in 1952 Du Vall, an occupational therapist, wrote about the development of the health care professions into research:

> A study of the growth and development of any well established profession will show that, as it emerged from the swaddling clothes of infancy and approached maturity, research appeared.[39(p97)]

Research has indeed appeared across the rehabilitation professions. A great deal can be learned about the current status of rehabilitation research by examining the role of research in the professional associations of the various rehabilitation disciplines, by reviewing the development of research publication vehicles, by examining the educational standards for the different rehabilitation professions, and by reviewing research funding opportunities for rehabilitation and related research.

Professional Association Goals

All of the major professional associations that promote the rehabilitation professions take a leading role in advancing rehabilitation research. The American Occupational Therapy Association works "through standard-setting, advocacy, education, and research on behalf of its members and the public."[40] The International Society for Prosthetics and Orthotics "promotes and guides research, development, and evaluation activities."[41] The American Physical Therapy Association has developed a clinical research agenda designed to "support, explain, and enhance physical therapy clinical practice by facilitating research that is useful primarily to clinicians."[42(p499)] The American Academy of Physical Medicine and Rehabilitation disseminates "research information needed to provide quality patient care."[43] The National Athletic Trainers' Association has the goal of "advancing the profession of athletic training through education and research."[44] Furthermore, these associations do not simply make empty statements about their roles in research, they follow through with actions to promote research in their respective professions. For example, the American Speech-Language-Hearing Association's commitment to research is shown by its development of a national outcomes measurement system that by 2002 had a database of 50,000 patients.[45]

Research Publication Vehicles

Dissemination of rehabilitation research findings in peer-reviewed journals is an important indicator of the status of rehabilitation research. Over the past several decades, the number of journals with a primary mission to publish research related to rehabilitation has increased dramatically, as shown in Table 1–1, which lists many such journals and the year in which they were founded. In some instances the journal has changed names one or more times; when it could be verified, the date listed is the initial publication date under the original title. In the

TABLE 1-1 Rehabilitation Journals	
Journal	**Founding Year**
Physiotherapy	1914
Archives of Physical Medicine and Rehabilitation	1919
American Journal of Physical Medicine and Rehabilitation	1921
Physical Therapy	1921
Canadian Journal of Occupational Therapy	1933
American Journal of Occupational Therapy	1947
Physiotherapy Canada	1948
Australian Journal of Physiotherapy	1954
Journal of Speech, Language, and Hearing Research	1957
Developmental Medicine and Child Neurology	1958
Language and Speech	1958
Journal of Rehabilitation Research and Development	1963
British Journal of Sports Medicine	1965
Journal of Athletic Training	1965
Medicine and Science in Sports and Exercise	1968
Language, Speech, and Hearing Services in Schools	1971
American Journal of Sports Medicine	1972
Journal of Allied Health	1972
Australian Journal of Human Communication Disorders	1973
Physician and Sportsmedicine	1973
Journal of Child Language	1974
Spine	1976
Prosthetics and Orthotics International	1977
Journal of Orthopaedic and Sports Physical Therapy	1979
Physical and Occupational Therapy in Geriatrics	1980
Physical and Occupational Therapy in Pediatrics	1980
Language and Communication	1981
Occupational Therapy Journal of Research	1981
Clinics in Sports Medicine	1982
Journal of Musculoskeletal Medicine	1983
Clinical Biomechanics	1986
Journal of Hand Therapy	1987
Journal of Physical Therapy Education	1987
Journal of Prosthetics and Orthotics	1988
Journal of Pediatric Physical Therapy	1989
Physical Medicine and Rehabilitation Clinics of North America	1990
WORK: A Journal of Prevention, Assessment, and Rehabilitation	1990
American Journal of Audiology	1991
American Journal of Speech-Language Pathology	1991
Journal of Occupational Rehabilitation	1991
Orthopaedic Physical Therapy Clinics of North America	1992
Occupational Therapy International	1994
Physiotherapy Research International	1996
International Journal of Language and Communication Disorders	1998

early years, available publications were typically the official journals of the professional associations, providing broad coverage across the scope of each respective profession. The increased importance of rehabilitation research across time is apparent both in the ability of the professions to sustain these new journals and in the emergence of new types of publications: specialty journals (e.g., *Journal of Pediatric Physical Therapy*), interdisciplinary journals (e.g., *Journal of Occupational Rehabilitation*), and international journals (e.g., *International Journal of Language and Communication Disorders*).

Educational Standards

As research becomes more important to a profession, the standards against which education programs that prepare new practitioners are evaluated can be expected to reflect this emphasis. A review of educational program requirements for the various rehabilitation professions shows that this is indeed the case, with requirements for research content, research activities, or both. The American Speech and Hearing Association requires that "scientific and research foundations of the professions"[46(p11)] be evident in curriculums to prepare speech-language pathologists and audiologists. The Commission on Accreditation in Physical Therapy Education requires that curriculums include activities designed to promote "critical inquiry," to enable graduates to "evaluate published studies," and to have students "participate in scholarly activities to contribute to the body of physical therapy knowledge."[47(pB-24)] The American Council on Occupational Therapy Education requires that graduates have the "ability to read and understand current research" and be able to "design and implement beginning-level research studies."[48(pp16-17)] The Commission on Accreditation of Allied Health Education Programs, the umbrella agency that accredits many health professions programs, including those that prepare athletic trainers and orthotists and prosthetists, required formal instruction in "statistics and research

design"[49(p11)] for athletic trainers and in "research methods"[50(p7)] for orthotists and prosthetists. Finally, the Accreditation Council for Graduate Medical Education recently enhanced its physical medicine and rehabilitation residency guidelines to include both formal curricular elements related to research design and methodology as well as opportunities to participate in research projects and conferences.[32]

Research Funding

The creation of a vast government-funded medical research enterprise began in earnest in the United States in the 1940s after World War II. One symbol of this expansion of the research enterprise was the transformation in 1948 of the National Institute for Health, formerly a "tiny public health laboratory"[51(p141)] into the plural National Institutes for Health (NIH) that conducts and supports research through many specialized institutes focusing on particular branches of medicine and health care. It was not until the 1980s, however, that NIH, as well as the Centers for Disease Control, became important sources of funding for rehabilitation research.[52] Today, the NIH's National Institute of Child Health and Human Development, National Center for Medical Rehabilitation Research, National Institute on Aging, National Institute of Arthritis and Musculoskeletal and Skin Diseases, National Cancer Institute, National Institute of Mental Health, National Institute of Neurological Disorders and Stroke, and National Institute of Deafness and Other Communication Disorders are important sources of funding for rehabilitation researchers.[31,52] The National Institute for Disability and Rehabilitation Research, an arm of the U.S. Department of Education, is another important source of funding for rehabilitation research.[52] In addition, private foundations associated with the various rehabilitation professions, such as the American Occupational Therapy Foundation, the Foundation for Physical Therapy, and the American-Speech-Language-Hearing Foundation, provide nonfederal sources of research funding.[31] Thus, even though a lack of funding for rehabilitation research has been identified as a serious problem for rehabilitation and the rehabilitation professions, a broad set of government and private sources of funding are available to rehabilitation researchers who choose to compete for external funding of their research efforts.

Although the refrains to increase and improve rehabilitation research do not seem to change from one generation of providers to the next, this review of the status of rehabilitation research shows that, in the early 2000s, professional associations for the rehabilitation disciplines include the development of research among their stated goals, that there is a wide variety of established and emerging journals in which to publish rehabilitation research, that educational standards for rehabilitation providers include criteria related to research, and that external funds for rehabilitation research are available from several sources. These signs of the recent strength of rehabilitation research must be tempered by evidence of declines in research for the system as a whole[51(pp370-399)] and for research related to rehabilitation[53] in response to cost-containment efforts in the health system of the United States.

Yes, the barriers to research are significant. Yes, identifying and using available resources takes initiative and energy. Yes, making research a priority in a cost-containment environment is difficult. However, the incentives to overcome these barriers are substantial, in that the future of rehabilitation within the health care system and society requires that we establish a firm base of evidence on which to build our practices.

■ SUMMARY

Research is the creative process by which professionals systematically challenge their everyday practices. Developing a body of rehabilitation knowledge, determining whether rehabilitation interventions work, and improving patient and client care are reasons for conducting rehabilitation research. Barriers to research are lack of familiarity with the research process, lack of statistical support, lack of funds, lack of mentors, lack of time, and concern for the ethics of using humans and animals in research. The importance of research to the rehabilitation professions is illustrated by professional association goals, publication vehicles for rehabilitation research, educational standards, and funding for rehabilitation research.

REFERENCES

1. Kettering CF. In: Boyd TA, ed. *Prophet of Progress*. New York, NY: EP Dutton; 1961.
2. Payton OD. *Research: The Validation of Clinical Practice*. 3rd ed. Philadelphia, Pa: FA Davis Co; 1994.
3. Kazdin AE. *Research Design in Clinical Psychology*. 4th ed. Boston, Mass: Allyn & Bacon; 2003.
4. Portney LG, Watkins MP. *Foundations of Clinical Research: Applications to Practice*. 2nd ed. Upper Saddle River, NJ: Prentice Hall; 2000.
5. Polit DF, Hungler BP. *Nursing Research: Principles and Methods*. 6th ed. Philadelphia, Pa: Lippincott Williams & Wilkins; 2002.
6. Stein F, Cutler SK. *Clinical Research in Occupational Therapy*. 4th ed. San Diego, Calif: Singular Publishing Group; 2000.
7. Maxwell DL, Satake E. *Research and Statistical Methods in Communication Disorders*. Baltimore, Md: Williams & Wilkins; 1997.
8. Philadelphia Panel. Evidence-based clinical practice guidelines on selected rehabilitation interventions for low back pain. *Phys Ther*. 2001;81:1641-1674.
9. Delitto A, Cibulka MT, Erhard RE, Bowling RW, Tenhula JA. Evidence for use of an extension-mobilization category in acute low back syndrome: a prescriptive validation pilot study. *Phys Ther*. 1993;73: 216-222.
10. Damiano DL, Abel MF. Functional outcomes of strength training in spastic cerebral palsy. *Arch Phys Med Rehabil*. 1998;79:126-133.
11. Rothstein JM. Clinical literature [Editor's Note]. *Phys Ther*. 1989;69:895.
12. Winter DA, Sienko SE. Biomechanics of below-knee amputee gait. *J Biomech*. 1988;21:361-367.
13. Clark F, Azen SP, Zemke R, et al. Occupational therapy for independent-living older adults. *JAMA*. 1997;278: 1321-1326.
14. Currier DP. *Elements of Research in Physical Therapy*. 3rd ed. Baltimore, Md: Williams & Wilkins; 1990.

15. Houle CO. *Continuing Learning in the Professions.* San Francisco, Calif: Jossey-Bass; 1981.

16. Parham DL. What is the proper domain of occupational therapy research? *Am J Occup Ther.* 1998;52: 485-489.

17. Jette AM. Physical disablement concepts for physical therapy research and practice. *Phys Ther.* 1994;74: 380-386.

18. Verbrugge LM, Jette AM. The disablement process. *Soc Sci Med.* 1994;38:1-14.

19. Hayes KW. Rose Excellence in Research Award recipient acceptance speech—February 11, 1995. *Orthop Pract.* 1995;7:12-13.

20. Brummel-Smith K. Research in rehabilitation. *Clin Geriatr Med.* 1993;9:895-904.

21. Wennberg J, Gittelsohn A. Variations in medical care among small areas. *Sci Am.* 1982;246:120-134.

22. Murphy S, Tickle-Degnen L. The effectiveness of occupational therapy-related treatments for persons with Parkinson's disease: a meta-analytic review. *Am J Occup Ther.* 2001;55:385-392.

23. de Goede CJT, Keus SHJ, Kwakkel G, Wagenaar RC. The effects of physical therapy in Parkinson's disease: a research synthesis. *Arch Phys Med Rehabil.* 2001;82: 509-515.

24. Miller EW. Body weight supported treadmill and overground training in a patient post cerebrovascular accident. *Neurorehabilitation.* 2001;16:155-163.

25. Hislop HJ. Tenth Mary McMillan lecture: the not-so-impossible dream. *Phys Ther.* 1975;55:1069-1080.

26. Ballin AJ, Breslin WH, Wierenga KAS, Shepard KF. Research in physical therapy: philosophy, barriers to involvement, and use among California physical therapists. *Phys Ther.* 1980;60:888-895.

27. Taylor E, Mitchell M. Research attitudes and activities of occupational therapy clinicians. *Am J Occup Ther.* 1990; 44:350-355.

28. MacDermid JC, Fess EE, Bell-Krotoski J, et al. A research agenda for hand therapy. *J Hand Ther.* 2002;15: 3-15.

29. Zito M, Bohannon RW. Inferential statistics in physical therapy research: a recommended core. *J Phys Ther Educ.* 1990;4:13-16.

30. Schwartz S, Sturr M, Goldberg G. Statistical methods in rehabilitation literature: a survey of recent publications. *Arch Phys Med Rehabil.* 1996;77:497-500.

31. Selker LG. Clinical research in allied health. *J Allied Health.* 1994;23:201-228.

32. Boninger ML, Chan L, Harvey R, et al. Resident research education in physical medicine and rehabilitation: a practical approach. *Am J Phys Med Rehabil.* 2001;80: 706-712.

33. Case-Smith J. Developing a research career: advice from occupational therapy researchers. *Am J Occup Ther.* 1999;53:44-50.

34. Ilott I, Bury T. Research capacity: a challenge for the therapy professions. *Physiotherapy.* 2002;88:194-200.

35. Testa MH. The nature of outcomes assessment in speech-language pathology. *J Allied Health.* 1995;24: 41-55.

36. Cusick A. The experience of clinician-researchers in occupational therapy. *Am J Occup Ther.* 2001;55: 9-18.

37. Foundation news: CRN to explore effects of muscle strengthening exercises. *PT Magazine.* 2002;10(11):12.

38. Dillingham TR. Physiatry, physical medicine, and rehabilitation: historical development and military roles. *Milit Trauma Rehabil.* 2002;13:1-16.

39. Du Vall EN. Research. *Am J Occup Ther.* 1952;6: 97-99,132.

40. American Occupational Therapy Association. *AOTA Mission Statement.* Available at: *www.aota.org/general/about.asp.* Accessed October 24, 2003.

41. International Society for Prosthetics and Orthotics. *ISPO Aims and Objectives.* Available at: *www.ispo.ws.* Accessed October 24, 2003.

42. Clinical Research Agenda for Physical Therapy. *Phys Ther.* 2000;80:499-513.

43. American Academy of Physical Medicine and Rehabilitation. *AAPM&R Vision Statement.* Available at: *www.aapmr.org/academy/mission.htm.* Accessed October 24, 2003.

44. National Athletic Trainers' Association. *NATA Mission.* Available at: *www.nata.org.* Accessed October 24, 2003.

45. Wolksi CA. Proof positive. *Rehab Manag.* 2002;15(7): 16,18-19,66.

46. Council on Academic Accreditation in Audiology and Speech-Language Pathology. *Standards for Accreditation of Graduate Education Programs.* Available at: *http://professional.asha.org/academic/standards.cfm.* Accessed October 24, 2003.

47. Commission on Accreditation in Physical Therapy Education. *Evaluative Criteria for Accreditation of Educational Programs for the Preparation of Physical Therapists.* Alexandria, Va; Author; 1996.

48. Accreditation Council for Occupational Therapy Education. *Standards for an Accredited Educational Program for the Occupational Therapist.* Available at: *www.aota.org/nonmembers/area13/links/LINK31.asp.* Accessed October 24, 2003.

49. Commission on Accreditation of Allied Health Education Programs. *Standards and Guidelines for an Accredited Educational Program for the Athletic Trainer.* Available at: *www.caahep.org/standards/at_01.htm.* Accessed October 24, 2003.

50. Commission on Accreditation of Allied Health Education Programs. *Standards and Guidelines for an Accredited Program for the Orthotist and Prosthetist.* Available at: *www.caahep.org/standards/op.htm.* Accessed October 24, 2003.

51. Ludmerer KM. *Time to Heal: American Medical Education from the Turn of the Century to the Era of Managed Care.* New York, NY: Oxford University Press; 1999.

52. Cole TM. The 25th Walter J Zeiter lecture: the greening of physiatry in a golden era of rehabilitation. *Arch Phys Med Rehabil.* 1993;74:231-237.

53. Smith QW, Holcomb JD, Galvin J, Roberts JK. The effect of changes in the U.S. health care system on rehabilitation research: the results of a survey of rehabilitation health professionals. *J Allied Health.* 2001;30: 207-214.

Theory in Rehabilitation Research

Relationships Among Theory, Research, and Practice

Definitions of Theory
Level of Restrictiveness
Least Restrictive Definition
Moderately Restrictive Definition
Most Restrictive Definition
Tentativeness of Theory
Testability of Theory

Scope of Theory
Metatheory
Grand Theory
General, or Middle-Range, Theory
Specific, or Practice, Theory
Evaluating Theory
Summary

All of us have ideas about how the world operates. We may even dub some of our ideas "theories." Think of the kind of banter that goes back and forth among a group of friends sharing a meal. "I have this theory that my car is designed to break down the week before payday." "The theory was that my mom and her sisters would rotate who cooks Christmas dinner." "Here's my theory—the electronics manufacturers wait until I buy a new gadget and then they come out with a new, improved model."

When do ideas about the nature of the world become theories? What distinguishes theory from other modes of thought? Is theory important to the applied disciplines of rehabilitation practitioners? The purpose of this chapter is to answer these questions by examining the relationships among theory, practice, and research; by defining theory and some closely related terms, by presenting examples of theories categorized based on scope; and by suggesting a general approach to evaluating theory.

■ RELATIONSHIPS AMONG THEORY, RESEARCH, AND PRACTICE

Theory is important because it holds the promise of guiding both practice and research. Figure 2–1 presents a schematic drawing showing the expected relationships among theory, research, and clinical practice. Theory is generally developed through reflection upon experience (e.g., "It seems to me that patients who pay for their own therapy follow home exercise instructions better than those whose insurance companies cover the cost") or from logical speculation (e.g., "If pain is related to the accumulation of metabolic byproducts in the tissues, then

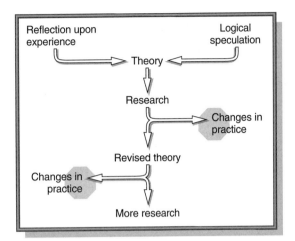

FIGURE 2–1. Relationships among theory, research, and practice.

modalities that increase local blood flow should help reduce pain").[1] Theories developed by reflections upon experience may draw on the careful observations of clinicians in practice or may flow from qualitative research studies that develop theories grounded in qualitative data (see Chapters 5 and 13 for more information). Theory, however it is generated, is then formally tested through research. Based on research results, the theory is confirmed or modified, as are clinical practices based on the theory. Unfortunately, theory and practice are often disconnected from one another, leading Kielhofner to "underscore the need for better ways to connect theoretical explanation and practical action"[2(p13)] by "developing knowledge in ways that make explicit the relationship between theoretical explanation and practical action."[2(p14)]

If research is conducted with animals, with normal human participants, or with techniques that differ from typical clinical practice, then the results are not directly applicable to the clinical setting. However, such research results may lead to modification of theory, and modification of theory may in turn lead clinicians to rethink the ways in which they treat their patients or clients. In contrast, if research is conducted with a clinical population and types of interventions that can be easily implemented in actual practice,

then clinicians may be able to change their practices based on research results themselves. It is incumbent upon the authors of research reports to help readers connect theory and practice through thoughtful discussion of the practical implications—both applicability and limitations—of their work.

■ DEFINITIONS OF THEORY

Theories are, by nature, abstractions. Thus, the language of theory is abstract, and there are divergent definitions of theory and its components. Instead of presenting a single definition of theory, this section of the chapter examines three elements of various definitions of theory: level of restrictiveness, tentativeness, and testability.

Level of Restrictiveness

Definitions of theory differ in their level of restrictiveness, and the level of restrictiveness of the definition then has an impact on the purposes for which a theory can be used. Table 2–1 summarizes the distinctions between the definitions and purposes of theories with different levels of restrictiveness. Different types of theory may be appropriate to different points in the development of a profession and its body of knowledge, with descriptive theory emerging first, predictive theory next, and finally explanatory theory.

To illustrate the differences between various levels of restrictiveness and their corresponding purposes, a simple example about hemiplegia is developed throughout this section of the chapter. This example is not meant to be a well-developed theory; it is merely an illustration based on a clinical entity that many rehabilitation professionals should have encountered at some point in their professional education or practice.

LEAST RESTRICTIVE DEFINITION

The least restrictive form of theory, *descriptive theory*, requires only that a phenomenon be

TABLE 2-1	**Level of Restrictiveness in Theory Definitions**		
	Level of Restrictiveness		
	Least	*Moderate*	*Most*
Definition	Account for or characterize phenomena	Specify relationships between constructs	Specify relationships and form a deductive system
Purpose	Description	Prediction	Explanation
Comments	Subdivided into ad hoc and categorical theories	Sometimes referred to as conceptual frameworks or models	Can take the form of if-then statements

described—and not predicted or explained—in some way, as in Fawcett's permissive definition: "a theory is a set of relatively concrete and specific concepts and the propositions that describe or link those concepts."[3(p4)] Thus, using this least restrictive definition, the statement "Individuals with hemiplegia have difficulty ambulating, eating, and speaking" is a simple form of theory because it describes (difficulty ambulating, eating, and speaking) a phenomenon (individuals with hemiplegia).

Descriptive theories may be further classified as either *ad hoc theories* or *categorical theories*. The statement "Individuals with hemiplegia have difficulty ambulating, eating, and speaking" presents an ad hoc collection of characteristics of individuals with hemiplegia. An ad hoc list is not exhaustive; it is merely a list of possible characteristics. The statement about difficulty ambulating, eating, and speaking in no way implies that these traits are the only difficulties experienced by individuals with hemiplegia. Contrast the ad hoc list with the statement "The deficits experienced by individuals with hemiplegia are motor, sensory, or functional." This is an example of a categorical descriptive theory in that it implies that all the deficits experienced by an individual with hemiplegia can be classified into one of these three categories. In the ad hoc example, discovery of another type of difficulty (e.g., reading) would not invalidate the theoretical statement because the list was not meant to be exhaustive. In the categorical example, discovery of another classification of deficits (e.g., cognitive)

would require revision of the theory because the categories were supposed to be exhaustive.

MODERATELY RESTRICTIVE DEFINITION

Kerlinger and Lee have advanced a more restrictive definition of theory: "A theory is a set of interrelated constructs (concepts), definitions, and propositions that present a systematic view of phenomena by specifying relations among variables, with the purpose of explaining and predicting the phenomena."[4(p9)] Several terms used by Kerlinger and Lee to define theory need definition themselves.

First, although the definition implies that constructs and concepts are similar, Kerlinger and Lee and others distinguish between the two. A *concept* has been defined as a "word or phrase that summarizes the essential characteristics or properties of a phenomenon." [3(p1)] Concepts are generally thought to be observable. Thus, "joint range of motion" is a concept that can be observed by measuring joint motion with a goniometer. A *construct* refers to "a phenomenon that is neither directly nor indirectly observed"[3(p34)] and has been "deliberately and consciously invented or adopted for a special scientific purpose."[4(p27)] Thus, according to this definition, constructs are more abstract than concepts. "Motivation" and "social support" are examples of constructs; direct measurement of the constructs themselves is impossible because levels of motivation and social support can only be inferred from individual and family behaviors.

Although the aforementioned authors recognize a distinction between concepts and constructs, many others use the terms interchangeably. Even those who make the distinction recognize that the boundaries between concept and construct are not clear. Given the blurred distinction between them, the two terms are used interchangeably in this text.

Second, a *proposition* is "a statement about a concept or the relation between concepts."[3(p1)] The term *hypothesis* is sometimes used nearly interchangeably with proposition, as in Kerlinger and Lee's definition that a hypothesis is "a conjectural statement of the relation between two or more variables."[4(p17)] The hallmark of Kerlinger and Lee's definition of theory, then, is that it must specify relationships between concepts.

The earlier statement about individuals with hemiplegia would need to be developed considerably before Kerlinger and Lee would consider it to be theory. Such a developed theory might read like this: "The extent to which individuals with hemiplegia will have difficulty ambulating is directly related to the presence of flaccid paralysis, cognitive deficits, and balance deficits and inversely related to prior ambulation status." This is no longer a simple description of several characteristics of hemiplegia; it is a statement of relationships between concepts.

Researchers who prefer the most restrictive definition of theory may consider descriptions at this moderately restrictive level to be *conceptual frameworks* or *models*. Polit and Hungler,[5] for example, are careful to distinguish between theory and less well articulated conceptual frameworks in nursing.

Theory that meets Kerlinger and Lee's definition is known as *predictive theory* because it can be used to make predictions based on the relationships between variables. If the four factors in this hypothetical theory about hemiplegic gait were found to be good predictors of eventual ambulation outcome, rehabilitation professionals might be able to use information gathered at admission to predict long-term ambulation status.

MOST RESTRICTIVE DEFINITION

The most restrictive view of theory is that "theories involve a series of propositions regarding the interrelationships among concepts, from which a large number of empirical observations can be deduced."[5(p96)] This is the most restrictive definition because it requires both relationships between variables and a deductive system.

Deductive reasoning goes from the general to the specific and can take the form of if-then statements. To make the hypothetical theory of hemiplegic gait meet this definition, we would need to add a general gait component to the theory. This general statement might read "Human gait characteristics are dependent on muscle power, skeletal stability, proprioceptive feedback, balance, motor planning, and learned patterns." The specific deduction from this general theory of gait is the statement "In individuals with hemiplegia, the critical components that lead to difficulty ambulating independently are presence of flaccidity (muscle power), impaired sensation (proprioceptive feedback), impaired perception of verticality (balance), and processing difficulties (motor planning). In an if-then format, this theory might read as follows:

1. *If* normal gait depends on intact muscle power, skeletal stability, proprioceptive feedback, balance, motor planning, and learned patterns, and
2. *If* hemiplegic gait is not normal,
3. *Then* individuals with hemiplegia must have deficits in one or more of the following areas: muscle power, skeletal stability, proprioceptive feedback, balance, motor planning, and learned patterns.

This theory, then, forms a deductive system by advancing a general theory for the performance of normal gait activities, then examining the elements that are affected in individuals with hemiplegia. Figure 2–2 presents this theory schematically. The six elements in the theory are central to the figure. In the absence of pathology, normal gait occurs, as shown above the central

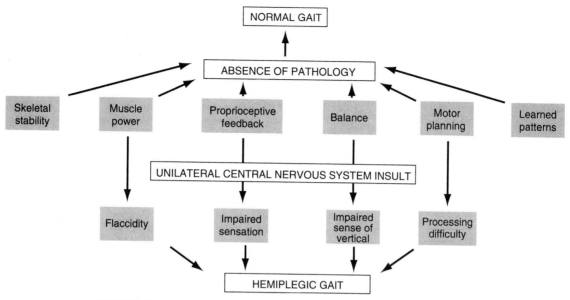

FIGURE 2–2. Diagram of the theory of gait in individuals with hemiplegia.

elements; in the presence of pathology, the elements are altered and an abnormal gait results, as shown below the gait elements.

With a deductive system in place, theory can begin to be used to explain natural phenomena. *Explanatory theory* looks at the why and how questions that undergird a problem, generally in more explicit terms than illustrated in Figure 2–3. The hypothetical explanatory theory about gait begins to explain ambulation difficulty in terms of six elements needed for normal gait.

Tentativeness of Theory

The second element of the definition of theory is its tentativeness. The tentative nature of theory is emphasized by Portney and Watkins:

> Theories reflect the present state of knowledge and must adapt to changes in that knowledge as technology and scientific evidence improve. Therefore, a theory is only a tentative explanation of phenomena....Many theories that are accepted today will be discarded tomorrow.[6(p27)]

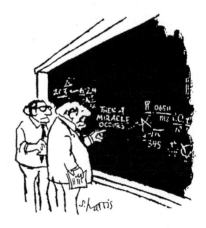

"I THINK YOU SHOULD BE MORE EXPLICIT HERE IN STEP TWO."

FIGURE 2–3. Then a miracle occurs...
Courtesy Sidney Harris, with permission.

Thus, theory is not absolute; rather, it is a view that is acceptable, at the time, to the scientists studying the phenomenon. For example, the idea that the sun revolved around the earth (geocentric theory) suited its time. It was also a useful theory:

> It described the heavens precisely as they looked and fitted the observations and calculations made with the naked eye; ...it fitted the available facts, was a reasonably satisfactory device for prediction, and harmonized with the accepted view of the rest of nature....Even for the adventurous sailor and the navigator it served well enough.[7(p295)]

However, the small discrepancies between the geocentric theory and the yearly calendar were troublesome to Renaissance astronomers and led to the development of the heliocentric theory, the one we still believe, that the earth revolves around the sun. Perhaps a later generation of scientists will develop different models of the universe that better explain the natural phenomena of the changing of days and seasons. Natural scientists do not assume an unchangeable objective reality that will ultimately be explained by the perfect theory; there is no reason for rehabilitation researchers to assume that their world is any more certain or ultimately explainable than the natural world.

Testability of Theory

Testability has been described as a sine qua non (an indispensable condition) of theory.[8] If so, then theory needs to be formulated in ways that allow the theory to be tested. However, theories cannot be proved true because one can never test them under all the conditions under which they might be applied. Even if testing shows that the world behaves in the manner predicted by a theory, this testing does not prove that the theory is true; other rival theories might provide equally accurate predictions. Theories can, however, be proved false by instances in which the predictions of the theory are not borne out.

For example, if one can accurately predict the discharge ambulation status of individuals with hemiplegia based on tone, sensation, vertical sense, and processing difficulty then the theory is consistent with the data. However, rival theories might predict discharge ambulation status just as well. A behaviorally oriented practitioner might develop a theory that predicts discharge ambulation status as a function of the level of motivation of the patient and the extent to which the staff provide immediate rewards for gait activities. If the behavioral theory accurately predicts discharge ambulation status of individuals with hemiplegia as well as the other theory does, it would also be consistent with the data. Neither theory can be proved in the sense that it is true and all others are false; both theories can, however, be shown to be consistent with available information.

■ SCOPE OF THEORY

Theories have been classified by different researchers in terms of their scope, often with four levels: metatheory, grand theory, general (or middle-range) theory, and specific, or practice, theory.[9,10]

Metatheory

Metatheory literally means "theorizing about theory." Therefore, metatheory is highly abstract, focusing on how knowledge is created and organized. The development of occupational science as a broad, organizing framework for occupational therapy has been described as metatheory.[9] In addition, the intellectual process of linking various theories to one another is a form of metatheory. For example, work that examines intersections, commonalities, and differences among the three grand theories described in the following paragraphs would be metatheoretical.

Grand Theory

Grand theories provide broad conceptualizations of phenomena. The World Health Organization's International Classification of Functioning, Disability, and Health (ICF) is a grand theory of importance to all rehabilitation practitioners

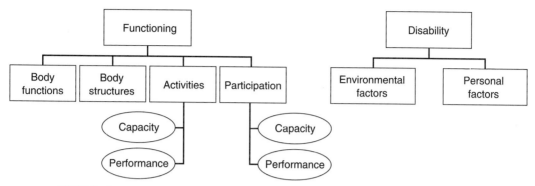

FIGURE 2–4. Schematic diagram of the International Classification of Functioning, Disability, and Health.

(Figure 2–4). A form of descriptive theory, it "provides a description of situations with regard to human functioning and its restrictions and serves as a framework to organize this information."[11(p7)] The ICF is divided into two parts: (1) functioning and disability and (2) contextual factors. Functioning and disability are further divided into body functions (physiology), body structures (anatomy), activities (individual functioning), and participation (societal functioning). The activities and participation classifications are further divided into capacity (what someone can do) and performance (what they actually do) constructs. The contextual factors are divided into environmental and personal factors. Stephens and colleagues[12] used the ICF as a framework for studying the problems experienced by hearing-impaired older adults. They designed a new clinical questionnaire, built around the ICF framework, for use by older adults to identify problems associated with their hearing impairments. When older adults completed the new clinical questionnaire, they identified more participation limitations than they did with previous questionnaires. In this case, then, the link between theory and practice is that using the theoretical model of the ICF facilitated the development of more complete problem lists for use in treatment planning.

Hislop's[13] conceptual model of pathokinesiology and movement dysfunction is a grand theory related to physical therapy. This model looks at physical therapy using the overarching phenomena of movement disorders (others have modified the term from *disorders* to *dysfunction*) and pathokinesiology (the application of anatomy and physiology to the study of abnormal human movement). Figure 2–5 is an interpretation of Hislop's formulation of the pathokinesiological basis for physical therapy. Physical therapy is viewed as a triangle with a base of service values supplemented by science, focusing on treatment of motion disorders through therapeutic exercise based on the principles of pathokinesiology. In this theory, physical therapy is viewed as affecting motion disorders related to four of six components of a hierarchy of systems ranging from the family to the cellular level of the body. The goals of physical therapy are either to restore motion homeostasis or to enhance adaptation to permanent impairment. This theory, presented in 1975, was ground-breaking in that no one before Hislop had advanced a coherent, comprehensive view of the work of physical therapists. This theory challenged physical therapists to think of themselves not as technicians who applied external physical agents to their patients, but as movement specialists who used a variety of tools to effect changes in troublesome movement patterns.

The model of human occupation (MOHO) is an example of grand theory that comes

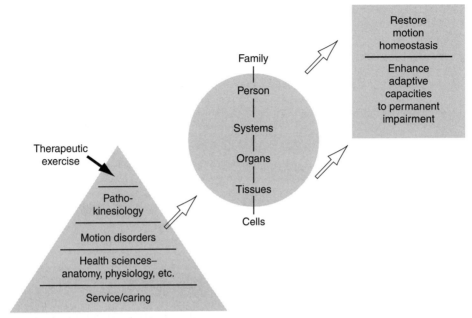

FIGURE 2–5. Interpretation of Hislop's pathokinesiological framework for physical therapy. The triangle represents the structure of physical therapy, the circle a hierarchy of systems affected by physical therapy, and the square the goals of physical therapy.
Modified from Hislop HJ. Tenth Mary McMillan lecture: the not-so-impossible dream. *Phys Ther.* 1975;55:1073, 1075. Reprinted from *Physical Therapy* with the permission of the American Physical Therapy Association.

from the profession of occupational therapy. In the MOHO, people are viewed as having three subsystems (volitional, habituation, and mind-brain-body performance) that interact with the environment to produce occupational behavior (Figure 2–6).[14] The MOHO has been used in clinical practice to organize assessment and treatment activities, as in Pizzi's case report of his work with an individual with acquired immunodeficiency syndrome.[15] In addition, it has been used to structure research activities, as in Chen and colleagues' work on factors influencing adherence to home exercise programs.[16]

General, or Middle-Range, Theory

General, or *middle-range,* theories provide general frameworks for action, but do not purport to

address large ideas (e.g., human functioning) or entire disciplines (e.g., physical therapy or occupational therapy) with a single theoretical context. Three examples of general theories illustrate the wide range of phenomena that can be viewed through a middle-range scope.

The gate control theory of pain, first presented in 1965 by Melzack and Wall, is an important general theory about the way that pain works. Before this theory was advanced, it was assumed that pain was largely a peripheral phenomenon, and treatments aimed at reducing or eliminating pain focused on peripheral solutions. In the words of Melzack himself, "the gate control theory's most important contribution to the biological and medical sciences…was the emphasis on [central nervous system] CNS mechanisms. Never again, after 1965, could anyone try to explain pain exclusively in terms of peripheral factors. The theory forced the medical

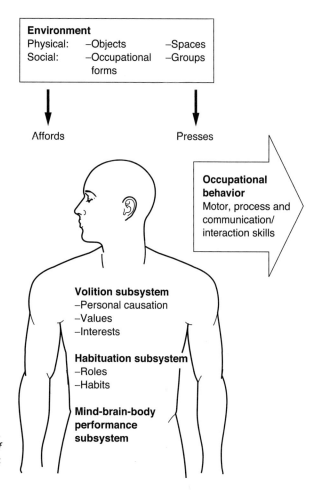

FIGURE 2–6. The model of human occupation. From Kielhofner G. The model of human occupation. In: Kielhofner G, ed. *Conceptual Foundations of Occupational Therapy.* Philadelphia, Pa: FA Davis; 1997:189.

and biological sciences to accept the brain as an active system that filters, selects, and modulates inputs."[17(pS123)] This theory led to the development of new physical modalities such as transcutaneous electrical nerve stimulation (TENS) and to a new emphasis on stress management and multidisciplinary approaches to modulating pain and pain behaviors.

The sensory integration model advanced by Ayres in the 1970s is a middle-range theory that hypothesizes a relationship between motor and learning difficulties and sensory processing problems. Concerned with how people integrate more than one source of sensory information, the sensory integration model focuses on tactile, vestibular, and proprioceptive information.[18] This theory is linked to practice by the development of assessment procedures designed to diagnose and classify sensory integration disorders[19] and by the development of treatment programs designed to have an impact on sensory processing.[20] The effectiveness of sensory integration programs has been studied in different groups of patients, including those with autism,[21] cerebral palsy,[22] and dementia.[23]

Recently, Mueller and Maluf[24] proposed the physical stress theory (PST) as a general theory with broad application to physical therapist practice, education, and research. In this theory, there is one basic premise: changes in the relative level of physical stress cause a predictable adaptive response in all biological tissues.[24(p385)] There are 12 fundamental principles, such as "physical stress levels that exceed the maintenance range (i.e., overload) result in increased tolerance of tissues to subsequent stresses (e.g., hypertrophy)" and "individual stresses combine in complex ways to contribute to the overall level of stress exposure."[24(p385)] And, there are four categories of factors that affect the level of tissue stress or the adaptive response to stress: movement and alignment, extrinsic, psychosocial, and physiological factors. This theory will link to practice if therapists use it as a framework for determining factors contributing to excessive stress and for modifying stresses to permit tissue healing, and if researchers use it as a framework for studying the effectiveness of interventions.

Specific, or Practice, Theory

Specific, or practice, theories can be described as particular applications of grand or general theories. For example, current practice theory supports the early use of powered mobility for some children with disabilities.[25] This contemporary view is consistent with some key ideas put forward in the ICF: that disability exists within an environmental context and that social participation—not just individual activity—are important goals for most people. Using this framework, powered mobility becomes a tool that enables a child to explore his or her environment independently and to participate more fully in family and school activities. In this framework, children with disabilities may work on traditional motor development tasks during portions of their days, but they use powered mobility when they want to go long distances or keep up with a group. This is in sharp contrast to traditional neurodevelopmental approaches that assumed that even part-time use of powered mobility would interfere with acquisition of motor skills. The grand theory advanced by the ICF is

linked to practice through specific theory that conceptualizes powered mobility as a way of modifying the environment to promote participation.

The general gate control theory of pain is linked to practice through the specific theoretical propositions that led to the development of TENS as a treatment for pain.[26] The body of research that tests the effectiveness of TENS for different patient populations provides an indirect way of evaluating the gate control theory of pain.[26,27]

■ EVALUATING THEORY

Researchers and practitioners who use theory to guide their work should critically evaluate those theories. In doing so, there may be a temptation to determine which of several competing theories is "correct." The answer is that none needs to be correct but each must be useful. The purpose of any theory is to organize constructs in ways that help us describe, predict, or explain phenomena of interest. Each theory—regardless of whether it meets restrictive or permissive definitions of theory and regardless of the scope of the theory—should be critically evaluated in terms of the extent to which it accurately describes the phenomenon, provides a framework for the study of the phenomenon, and influences practice. Different researchers will find that one or another theory provides a better framework for the questions they wish to ask, and different readers will simply find that some theories are more appealing to them than others. Stevens articulates her view of the folly of looking for one true theory in any discipline:

> Imagine what we would think of the field of psychology were it to dictate that each of its practitioners be Freudian. Indeed, it is the conflict and diversity among theories that account for much of the progress in any discipline. A search for conformity is an attempt to stultify the growth of a profession.[28(ppxii–xiii)]

Rehabilitation practitioners need not choose a single framework to guide their actions. What they must do is develop, analyze, and use a rich set of different theories to enhance their understanding of the rehabilitation process they undertake with their patients and clients.

■ SUMMARY

Theory, research, and practice are related through theories that are developed through reflection on experience or logical speculation, through research that tests theories, and through revisions of theory and clinical practice based on research results. Theory can be defined according to levels of restrictiveness, tentativeness, and testability. The different levels of theory are used for description, prediction, and explanation. Theories are also differentiated based on scope. Metatheory focuses on how knowledge is created and organized, as in the development of occupational science. Grand theories provide broad conceptualizations of phenomena, as in the World Health Organization's ICF,[11] Hislop's pathokinesiological framework for physical therapy,[13] and Kielhofner's MOHO.[14] General, or middle-range, theories provide general frameworks for action, as in the gate control theory of pain,[17] the sensory integration model,[18] and the PST.[24] Specific, or practice, theories are particular applications of grand or general theories, as in the application of ICF concepts to support the use of powered mobility for children with disabilities[25] and the role of the gate control theory of pain in the development of TENS.[26]

REFERENCES

1. Tammivaara J, Shepard KF. Theory: the guide to clinical practice and research. *Phys Ther.* 1990;70:578-582.
2. Kielhofner G. The organization and use of knowledge. In: Kielhofner G, ed. *Conceptual Foundations of Occupational Therapy.* 3rd ed. Philadelphia, Pa: FA Davis Co; 2004.
3. Fawcett J. *The Relationship of Theory and Research.* 3rd ed. Philadelphia, Pa: FA Davis; 1999.
4. Kerlinger FN, Lee HB. *Foundations of Behavioral Research.* 4th ed. Fort Worth, Texas: Harcourt College Publishers; 2000.
5. Polit DF, Hungler BP. *Nursing Research: Principles and Methods.* 6th ed. Philadelphia, Pa: Lippincott Williams & Wilkins; 2002.
6. Portney LG, Watkins MP. *Foundations of Clinical Research: Applications to Practice.* 2nd ed. Upper Saddle River, NJ: Prentice Hall; 2000.
7. Boorstin DJ. *The Discoverers: A History of Man's Search to Know His World and Himself.* New York, NY: Vintage Books; 1985.
8. Krebs DE, Harris SR. Elements of theory presentations in *Physical Therapy. Phys Ther.* 1988;68:690-693.
9. Reed KL. Theory and frame of reference. In: Neistadt ME, Crepeau EB, eds. *Willard and Spackman's Occupational Therapy.* Philadelphia, Pa: JB Lippincott; 1998:521-524.
10. Hagstrom F. Using and building theory in clinical action. *J Commun Disord.* 2001;34:371-384.
11. World Health Organization. *International Classification of Functioning, Disability, and Health.* Available at: *www.who.int/classification/icf.* Accessed October 27, 2003.
12. Stephens D, Gianopoulos I, Kerr P. Determination and classification of the problems experienced by hearing-impaired elderly people. *Audiology.* 2001;40:294-300.
13. Hislop HJ. Tenth Mary McMillan lecture: the not-so-impossible dream. *Phys Ther.* 1975;55:1069-1080.
14. Kielhofner G. The model of human occupation. In: Kielhofner G, ed. *Conceptual Foundations of Occupational Therapy.* 3rd ed. Philadelphia, Pa: FA Davis; 2004.
15. Pizzi M. The Model of Human Occupation and adults with HIV infection and AIDS. *Am J Occup Ther.* 1990; 44:257-264.
16. Chen C-Y, Neufeld PS, Feely CA, Skinner CS. Factors influencing compliance with home exercise programs among patients with upper-extremity impairment. *Am J Occup Ther.* 1999;53:171-180.
17. Melzack R. From the gate to the neuromatrix. *Pain.* 1999;6:S121-S126.
18. Kielhofner G. The sensory integration model. In: Kielhofner G, ed. *Conceptual Foundations of Occupational Therapy.* 3rd ed. Philadelphia, Pa: FA Davis; 2004.
19. Ayres AJ, Marr DB. Sensory integration and praxis tests. In: Bundy AC, Lane SJ, Murray EA, eds. *Sensory Integration: Theory and Practice.* 2nd ed. Philadelphia, Pa: FA Davis; 2002.
20. Bundy AC. The process of planning and implementing intervention. In: Bundy AC, Lane SJ, Murray EA, eds. *Sensory Integration: Theory and Practice.* 2nd ed. Philadelphia, Pa: FA Davis; 2002.
21. Dawson G, Watling R. Interventions to facilitate auditory, visual, and motor integration in autism: a review of the evidence. *J Autism Dev Disord.* 2000;30:415-421.
22. Bumin G, Kayihan H. Effectiveness of two different sensory-integration programmes for children with spastic diplegic cerebral palsy. *Disabil Rehabil.* 2001;23:394-399.
23. Robichaud L, Hebert R, Desrosiers J. Efficacy of a sensory integration program on behaviors of inpatients with dementia. *Am J Occup Ther.* 1994;48:355-360.

24. Mueller MJ, Maluf KS. Tissue adaptation to physical stress: a proposed "physical stress theory" to guide physical therapist practice, education, and research. *Phys Ther.* 2002;82:383-403.

25. Wiart L, Darrah J. Changing philosophical perspectives on the management of children with physical disabilities—their effect on the use of powered mobility. *Disabil Rehabil.* 2002;24:492-498.

26. Rushton DN. Electrical stimulation in the treatment of pain. *Disabil Rehabil.* 2002;24:407-415.

27. Osiri M, Welch V, Brosseau L, et al. Transcutaneous electrical nerve stimulation for knee osteoarthritis (Cochrane Review). *The Cochrane Library, Issue 1, 2003.* Oxford: Update Software.

28. Stevens B. *Nursing Theory: Analysis, Application, Evaluation.* 2nd ed. Boston, Mass: Little, Brown; 1984.

Research Ethics

Jesse Gelsinger, an 18-year-old with a mild form of a nitrogen metabolism disorder that could be managed with diet and medication, died in September 1999, four days after participating in a gene therapy research trial at the Institute for Human Gene Therapy at the University of Pennsylvania. His death, which triggered a number of events including an independent investigation, a wrongful death lawsuit, suspension of all research trials at the center where the research was conducted, and a U.S. Senate subcommittee investigation, raised a number of issues related to the conduct of the research: Did he even meet the eligibility criteria specified in the approved research protocol? Were there undisclosed conflicts of interest between the researchers and biotechnology companies? Did consent forms improperly omit information about deaths in monkeys receiving the gene therapy? Were coercive appeals used to recruit participants for the study?[1]

The same kind of complex ethical issues raised by Jesse Gelsinger's death should be raised every time researchers ask others to assume the risks of their research—even seemingly low-risk research. The purpose of this chapter is to articulate ethical principles of importance to the conduct of research. First, attention is given to determining the boundaries between practice and research. Second, basic moral principles of action are presented. Examples of these moral principles in action are given for occurrences in everyday life, for treatment situations, and for research settings. Third, a special case of the moral principle of autonomy—informed consent—is examined in detail. Fourth, the application of the moral principles to research is illustrated through analysis of several widely used research codes of ethics. Finally, a categorization of research risks is presented.

A note on terminology is required before moving into the content of the chapter. Contemporary usage favors the term research "participant" rather than "subject," emphasizing the active role played by individuals who consent to participate in research studies. However, this usage is sometimes confusing when writing about researchers and subjects, as both are participants in the research process. In addition, in a chapter like this in which practice and research are contrasted, it is useful to sharpen the differences between patients or clients seeking services for their own benefit and subjects or research participants who should not expect benefits from their participation. Therefore, the term "subject" is used when "participant" would be confusing or would not set up the desired contrast.

■ BOUNDARIES BETWEEN PRACTICE AND RESEARCH

Every provider–patient relationship is predicated on the principle that the provider can render services that are likely to benefit the patient or client. The roles, relationships, and goals found in the treatment milieu are, however, vastly different from those in the research setting. In the research setting, the health care professional becomes an investigator rather than a practitioner; the patient becomes a participant or subject. The patient seeks out a practitioner who may or may not decide to accept the patient for treatment; the investigator seeks out potential subjects who may or may not agree to participate in the proposed research. The patient's goal is improvement; the investigator's goal is development of knowledge.

When standard health care is delivered in the context of provider–patient interaction, it is clear that the intent of the episode is therapeutic.

When an innovative treatment technique is tested on a group of normal volunteers, it is clear that the intent of the episode is knowledge development. However, when a new technique is administered to a clinical population, the distinction between treatment and research becomes blurred. If the health care professional views each participant as a patient, then individualized treatment modifications based on each patient's response would be expected. Alternatively, if the clinician views each participant as a subject, then standardization of treatment protocols is often desirable. Protecting subjects from the risks of participating in research requires that one be able to distinguish research from practice. The National Commission for the Protection of Human Subjects of Biomedical and Behavioral Research, in its historic *Belmont Report,* developed a definition of research that makes such a distinction:

> Research (involving humans) is any manipulation, observation, or other study of a human being…done with the intent of developing new knowledge and which differs in any way from customary medical (or other professional) practice….Research may usually be identified by virtue of the fact that [it] is conducted according to a plan.[2(pp6,7)]

Three main elements of this definition warrant careful consideration: intent, innovation, and plan.

The Belmont definition recognizes that a fundamental difference between practice and research is that the two entities have different intents. Practice goals relate to individual patients; research goals relate to the development of new knowledge. Because of these disparate goals, different levels of protection from risk are needed for patients and subjects.

Health care rendered to an individual is always presumed to have some probability of benefit. When deciding whether to undergo a particular treatment, a patient will evaluate its risks against its potential benefits. In contrast, research on human participants is often of no benefit to the individual who assumes the risk of participation; rather, subsequent patients benefit from the application of the new knowledge.

Some projects fall in a gray zone between research and practice. In this zone, innovative therapies with potential benefits are tested, providing both potential individual benefits and new knowledge.[2]

The second element of the Belmont definition is that the procedure differs in some way from customary practice. Simply reporting the treatment results of a series of patients who have undergone standard shoulder reconstruction rehabilitation would not be considered research. Because the treatment given is not innovative, the patients do not need special protection; the risk of being a patient whose results happen to be reported is no different than the risk associated with the treatment. Note, however, that if standard treatment calls for formal strength testing every 4 weeks, but the group in the series is tested every week, this should now be considered research. The risks of repeated formal strength testing, however minimal, are different than the risks of standard treatment alone. An implication of this component of the Belmont definition is that innovative therapies should be considered research and be conducted with appropriate research safeguards, until they can be shown to be effective and are adopted as accepted or customary practice.

The third element of the Belmont definition distinguishing research from practice is that research generally is conducted according to a plan. This implies a level of control and uniformity that is usually absent from clinical practice.

■ MORAL PRINCIPLES OF ACTION

All professionals deal with complex, specialized issues for which the correct course of action may not be clear. Thus, professionals tend to be guided not by a rigid set of rules, but by general principles that demand that each practitioner assess a given situation in light of those principles and make decisions accordingly.

Although the content of the decisions one makes as a professional differs from one's personal decisions, the underlying principles that should guide these decisions are the same. This is also the case whether one is acting as a practitioner seeing a patient or as an investigator studying a research participant: the content of practice and research decisions may differ, but the underlying principles remain the same. Before presenting ethical principles for the conduct of research, it is therefore appropriate to lay a common groundwork of moral principles of action. Four major principles are discussed: nonmaleficence, beneficence, utility, and autonomy. Examples from daily life, practice, and research are used to illustrate these principles.

The Principle of Nonmaleficence

The principle of nonmaleficence states that "we ought to act in ways that do not cause needless harm or injury to others."[3(p32)] In addition, the principle implies that we should not expose others to unnecessary risk. In daily life this means that one should not rob people at knifepoint in the subway nor should one drive while intoxicated. People with backyard pools need to have them fenced properly to protect curious children from accidental drowning. Society levels civil and criminal penalties against members who violate the principle of nonmaleficence.

For health care providers nonmaleficence means that one should neither intentionally harm one's patients nor cause unintentional harm through carelessness. Suppose that a therapist is seeing a frustrating patient—one who demands much but does not appear to follow through with a suggested home program of exercise. The therapist decides to "teach the patient a lesson," being deliberately vigorous in mobilization techniques to make the patient "pay" for not following directions. This action would violate the principle of nonmaleficence because the regimen was intentionally sadistic, not therapeutic.

The practice of any of the rehabilitation professions does, however, require that we expose patients to various risks in order to achieve treatment goals. We cannot guarantee that no harm will come to patients in the course of treatment: they may fall, they may become frustrated, they may become sore, their skin may become irritated, they may experience adverse effects of medications. However, fulfilling the principle of nonmaleficence means exercising due care in the practice of one's profession. Due care requires the availability of adequate personnel during transfers and functional activities, planned progression of exercise intensity, monitoring of skin condition during procedures, screening for drug allergies and interactions, and considering the patient's or client's readiness to change.

In the conduct of research we also must avoid exposing participants to unnecessary risk. Detailed delineation of the risks of research is presented later in this chapter. In general, though, the principle of nonmaleficence requires that we refrain from research that uses techniques we know to be harmful and that research be terminated if harm becomes evident. Although the risks of harm as a consequence of research can be great, there is also harm associated with *not* conducting research. If research is not performed to assess the effects of rehabilitation procedures, then patients may be exposed to time-consuming, expensive, or painful treatments that may be ineffective or harmful. If researchers are to systematically assess the effects of treatments of unknown effectiveness, then doing so will necessarily place someone at risk. The researcher must work carefully to minimize these risks.

The Principle of Beneficence

The principle of beneficence states that "we should act in ways that promote the welfare of other people."[3(p34)] Not only should we not harm them, but we should also attempt to help them. A daily example of the principle of beneficence is the person who goes grocery shopping for a homebound neighbor.

The professional–client relationship is based on the principle of beneficence. Patients would not come to health care professionals unless the patients believed that the professionals could

help them. The extent of beneficence required is not always clear, however. Occasionally holding a family conference outside of usual clinic or office hours to accommodate family members who cannot attend during usual hours is a reasonable expectation of a professional. Never taking a vacation out of a sense of duty to one's patients is an unreasonable expectation.

The principle of beneficence presents conflicts for researchers. As noted previously, the individual participants who assume the risks of the research may not receive any benefits from the research project. Individuals who agree to be in a clinical trial to assess the effectiveness of a new drug to manage spasticity accept the risk that the drug may produce serious, unanticipated side effects. They may or may not experience any improvement in their spasticity as a result of participating in the trial. The researcher–subject relationship puts immediate beneficence aside for the sake of new knowledge that may eventually translate into benefits for future patients.

The Principle of Utility

The principle of utility states that "we should act in such a way as to bring about the greatest benefit and the least harm."[3(p36)] If a family has limited financial resources, they need to make utility decisions. Should funds be spent on health insurance or life insurance? Which is potentially more devastating financially, an enormous hospital bill or loss of the primary earner's income? The answer that would bring about the most potential benefit and the least risk of harm would vary from family to family. If a practice cannot accommodate all the patients who desire appointments on a given day, decisions about who receives an appointment should focus on who will benefit most from immediate treatment, and who will be harmed least by delayed treatment. Health services researchers may frame health care funding debates in terms of utility. For example, what will bring about the greatest benefit and the least harm: funding for prenatal care or funding for neonatal intensive care treatment for premature infants?

In the conduct of research the principle of utility can guide the development of research agendas. Which projects will contribute most to the advancement of patient care in rehabilitation? Which projects involve risks that are disproportional to the amount of beneficial information that can be gained? Should a funding agency support a project that would assess the effects of different stretching techniques on prevention of injury in recreational athletes or a project that would provide augmented communication equipment for individuals with amyotrophic lateral sclerosis? The former project has the potential to reduce lost workdays for large numbers of full-time employees; the latter has potential to improve quality of life and employability of small numbers of patients with the disease. Knowing about the principle of utility does not make allocation decisions easy!

The Principle of Autonomy

The principle of autonomy states that "rational individuals should be permitted to be self-determining."[3(p40)] Suppose that your elderly mother owns and lives alone in a house that badly needs a new roof. She indicates that it doesn't rain often, that it only leaks in the formal dining room, and that she won't live long enough to get her money's worth out of a new roof. The principle of autonomy indicates that you should respect her decision to determine whether her roof will be repaired. However, you may believe that since the house is your mother's primary financial asset and may be used to pay for her long-term care in the future, she will benefit from the preservation of that asset, even if you must violate her autonomy by hiring a roofer yourself. This violation of the principle of autonomy "for someone's own good" is known as *paternalism.*

Autonomy issues in patient treatment and research revolve around the concept of informed consent. Informed consent is an essential

component of the research process and is therefore discussed in detail in the following section.

■ INFORMED CONSENT

Informed consent requires that patients or subjects give permission for treatment or testing, and that they be given adequate information in order to make educated decisions about undergoing the treatment or test. Four components are required for true autonomy in making either health care or research participation decisions: disclosure, comprehension, voluntariness, and competence.[4] In addition, as recommended by the 2001 Institute of Medicine's Committee on Assessing the System for Protecting Human Research Participants, informed consent should be viewed as an ongoing process within research, not as the isolated event of signing a consent form:

> The informed consent process should be an ongoing, interactive dialogue between research staff and research participants involving the disclosure and exchange of relevant information, discussion of that information, and assessment of the individual's understanding of the discussion.[5(p120)]

Information about treatment or research is needed before a patient or subject can make an informed decision from among several treatment options. Disclosure of treatment details should include the nature of the condition, the long-term effects of the condition, the effects of not treating the condition, the nature of available treatment procedures, anticipated benefits of any procedures, the probability of actually achieving these benefits, and potential risks of undergoing the procedure. Time commitments related to the treatment should be detailed, as should cost of the treatment. For patients undergoing routine, low-risk procedures, providing this information may be verbal or written. The practitioner explains the evaluative procedures to the patient, proceeds with an evaluation if the patient agrees, and then outlines the planned course of treatment to the patient. The patient then determines whether the time, risks, and expense associated with the treatment is worth the anticipated benefit.

Disclosure of research details involves many of the same information items, depending on the nature of the research. Because research is usually not for the immediate benefit of the participant, more formal protection of the research subject is required than is needed for the patient. Thus, information about research risks and potential benefits must be written. If the research involves deception (e.g., disguising the true purpose of the study when full knowledge would likely alter participant responses), it is generally accepted that a "debriefing" procedure after completion of the study is important to fully inform participants about the true nature of the experiment.[6] Other instances in which debriefing may be appropriate are to "unmask" the assignment of participants to different placebo or treatment groups, to communicate research findings to interested subjects, or to bring closure to a research process that has required extended interactions of researchers and subjects (as in some qualitative research studies).

However, disclosing information is not enough. The practitioner or researcher must ensure that the patient or subject comprehends the information given. Practitioners who are sensitive to the comprehension issue describe procedures in lay language, prepare written materials that are visually appealing, provide ample time for explanation of procedures and for answering questions, and allow ample time before requiring a participation decision. Unfortunately, informed consent documents often are written at a level that may exceed the reading skills of the intended sample,[7] although research with participants in a set of 14 different trials showed that they believed they received an appropriate amount of information and that they understood the information presented to them.[8]

The clinician or researcher also needs to ensure the voluntariness, or freedom from coercion, of consent. If free health care is offered in exchange for participation in a research study, will a poor family's decision to participate be truly voluntary? When a clinician requests that a man who is a patient participate in a study, and ensures him that his care will not suffer if he chooses not to participate, is it unreasonable for the patient to feel coerced based on the presumption that there might be subtle consequences of not participating? Practitioners and researchers need to be sensitive to real or perceived coercive influences faced by their patients or subjects.

Competence is the final component of informed consent. One must determine whether potential patients or research participants are legally empowered to make decisions for themselves. Consent from a legal guardian must be sought for minor children. If a legal guardian has been appointed for individuals who are mentally ill, mentally retarded, or incompetent, then consent must be sought from this party. When conducting research with populations in whom "proxy" consent is required, the researcher should also consider whether the subjects themselves "assent" or "dissent" to participation.[9] Suppose that an occupational therapist wishes to study the differences between in-class and out-of-class therapy for public school children with cerebral palsy. If out-of-class therapy has been the norm, a boy who voices a preference for out-of-class treatment should not be required to be a member of the in-class group even though his parents have given permission for him to be assigned to either group. Unfortunately, knowledge of legislation governing proxy consent has been shown to be low, raising concerns about whether these individuals are adequately protected.[10]

A related problem occurs when a group is legally empowered to make decisions, but the characteristics of the group make informed consent difficult or impossible. For example, at state institutions for developmentally disabled adults, many of the residents may be their own legal guardians, with the legal ability to make their own decisions about participation in many activities. They might, however, be unable to comprehend the risks and potential benefits of participation in a research project, and therefore any consent they gave would not be informed.

It is clear that informed consent is required when experimental research that exposes participants to harm is undertaken, but what about research in which existing health care records are used to examine the outcomes of care that has already been delivered? In the recent past, individual consent to use personal health information in such studies was rarely sought, as long as researchers had reasonable procedures in place to maintain the anonymity of the records. In the United States, the newly implemented Health Insurance Portability and Accountability Act (HIPAA) requires dramatic change in this practice. In general, HIPAA requires specific authorization whenever protected health information (PHI) is disclosed. However, institutional review boards may authorize the research use of PHI under some circumstances even without individual consent. Six provisions of HIPAA have been described as "transformative" with respect to the conduct of research using medical records and insurance databases: (1) the need to track disclosures of PHI, (2) the need to assure that research collaborators comply with the privacy rules, (3) the relationship between HIPAA and regulations for institutional review boards (IRBs), (4) the principle that researchers should have access to only the minimum data necessary to carry out their work, (5) the requirement to de-identify data, and (6) the imposition of civil and criminal penalties for unlawful disclosure of PHI.[11] Similar issues have been raised in the United Kingdom with the implementation of a new Data Protection Act.[12]

■ RESEARCH CODES OF ETHICS

The general moral principles of action discussed earlier become formalized when they are developed into codes of ethics to guide the practice of various professionals. There are three general codes of ethics that can provide rehabilitation researchers with guidance on ethical issues. The first of these is the Nuremberg Code developed in 1949 as a reaction to Nazi atrocities in the name of research.[13] The second is the World Medical Association's Declaration of Helsinki developed in 1964, most recently modified in 2000 and then clarified in 2002.[14] The third is the U.S. Department of Health and Human Services (DHHS) regulations that govern research conducted or funded by the department, revised most recently in 1991.[15] All are available on-line, either at the Internet addresses noted in the reference list or by doing an Internet search. In addition, they are reproduced in whole or in part in various texts related to research ethics.[5,16] Furthermore, readers wishing to solidify their knowledge of research ethics are encouraged to complete an on-line education program, prepared by the DHHS, through its National Institutes of Health, which reviews the history of human participant protections and the principles promulgated for the protection of human research subjects.[17]

Seven distinct ethical themes can be gleaned from these resources; most are present in more than one of the documents. The themes are informed consent, whether the research design justifies the study, avoidance of suffering and injury, risks commensurate with potential benefit, independent review of research protocols, integrity in publication, and explicit attention to ethics.

Informed Consent

One common principle is that of voluntary consent of the individual participating in the research. The responsibility for ensuring the quality of consent is with the individual who "initiates, directs, or engages in"[13(p1)] the experiment. This means that the very important issues of consent should be handled by an involved researcher. Using clerical staff to distribute and collect informed consent forms does not meet this requirement. In addition to securing the consent of their human research participants, researchers should treat animal subjects humanely and respect the environment[14] in the course of their research. Box 3–1 highlights the Tuskegee

BOX 3-1

Tuskegee Syphilis Study[18]

The Tuskegee Syphilis Study, spanning 40 years from 1932 to 1972, is one of the most infamous cases of ethical abuses in health care research within the United States. The study was conducted by the U.S. Public Health Service in cooperation with a variety of other agencies, including the Alabama State Department of Health, the Macon County Health Department, and the Tuskegee Institute. The basic fact of the case is that approximately 400 black men with syphilis were left untreated for 40 years to study the "natural history" of the disease. Participants did not realize that they were being studied, did not know that they were being tested for syphilis, were not informed of the results of testing, and were not aware that treatment was being withheld.

Miss Eunice Rivers, a young black nurse, coordinated data collection within the study. She played a critical role by establishing credibility with participants and providing continuity throughout the extended study. The study itself involved physical examination of the men, radiographs, lumbar punctures, minimal treatment for the syphilis, and a variety of "perks" for participants, including free aspirin and tonics, burial funds, and some health care for their families. Therefore, Nurse Rivers both coordinated the nontreatment study and played an important public health role within the rural black community in Macon County.

There were several points at which it might have been "natural" to discontinue the study. The first was in the early 1940s when penicillin became available. If the researchers could justify the early years of the study because of the equivocal effectiveness of the then-available treatments for syphilis, they could no longer use this justification once penicillin became a known treatment. A second natural opportunity to stop the study and provide treatment to participants also occurred during the early 1940s when many participants received draft notices for World War II. If a man who was drafted was found to have syphilis, protocol indicated that he should receive treatment for the disease. However, special exceptions to this protocol were made for members of the Tuskegee study, who were neither inducted into service nor treated for their syphilis.

The problems with the study were exposed in 1972, nearly 40 years after its initiation. Hearings about the study resulted in the development of revised procedures for federally sponsored human experimentation. Contemporary guidelines under which most institutional review boards operate today are based on these post-Tuskegee regulations. Ultimately, surviving participants were provided with comprehensive medical care and cash settlements and the heirs of deceased participants received cash settlements.

The Tuskegee experiment inspired the play *Miss Evers' Boys*,[19] which reminds us that responsible scientific inquiry rests on the moral choices of individual researchers:

Miss Evers [representing Nurse Rivers]: There was no treatment. Nothing to my mind that would have helped more than it hurt.

Caleb [representing a participant]: Maybe not in '33. But what about '46 and that penicillin? That leaves every year, every month, every day, every second right up to today to make a choice. It only takes a second to make a choice.

Syphilis Study, an important historical example documented in a book,[18] a play,[19] and a film based on the play,[20] in which the principles of informed consent were violated in particularly egregious ways by the U.S. Public Health Service in its study of syphilis in African-American men.

Design Justifies Study

A link exists between research methodology and research ethics: "The experiment should be so designed...that the anticipated results will justify the performance of the experiment."[13(p1)] The implication is that it is not appropriate to expose humans to risks for a study that is so poorly designed that the stated purposes of the research cannot be achieved. This, then, is essentially a utility issue: Why expose people to risk if the probability of benefit is low? Recent recommendations in the United States call for the development of separate scientific and ethical reviews of research proposals to ensure that the appropriate level of expertise is brought to bear on each review process.[5(pp72-82)]

Although this principle would seem to call for methodological rigor in the design of research studies, finding a balance between methodological and ethical rigor is complex. For example, consider the question of whether to use a placebo-controlled design versus an active-controlled design. In a placebo-controlled design, the control group receives a sham treatment, the experimental group receives the new treatment, and an effective treatment should show markedly different results than the placebo group. In an active-controlled design, the control group receives currently accepted treatment, the experimental group receives the new treatment, and an effective new treatment should be at least marginally better than the accepted current treatment. Researchers considering which design to use need to balance factors such as the number of participants needed to demonstrate a statistically significant effect (placebo-controlled studies typically require fewer participants than active-controlled studies because

differences between groups are expected to be larger in the placebo-controlled studies), the impact of withholding currently accepted treatments, and the risks of both the current and new treatments.[21]

Avoidance of Suffering and Injury

Avoidance of suffering and injury is a nonmaleficence concern. Risks can be avoided through careful consideration during the design of a study, and by careful protection of physical safety and avoidance of mental duress during the implementation of the study. A safety concern in the design phase of a study might occur for researchers deciding how to quantify the effects of exercise on the biceps brachii muscle. They might consider using various histologic, strength, radiologic, or girth measures to document change. The final decision about which measures to use would depend both on the specific research questions and on which measures are likely to cause the least amount of suffering or injury.

Safety issues during research implementation should be addressed as needed. For example, a speech-language pathologist implementing a study of techniques to improve swallowing for individuals with dysphagia would need to select appropriate food and drink for treatment sessions and attend to positioning to minimize the risk of aspiration during treatment or testing.

Privacy during evaluation and treatment, as well as confidentiality of results can also be considered here as an issue of prevention of mental suffering. Seemingly innocuous portions of the research protocol may be stressful to the participant. For example, a protocol that requires documentation of body weight may be acceptable to a participant if the measure is taken and recorded by only one researcher. The same participant may be extremely uncomfortable with a protocol in which the body weight is recorded on a data sheet that accompanies the participant to five different measurement stations for viewing by five separate researchers.

In some qualitative research studies, participants may recall and explore upsetting events within their lives. For example, consider an occupational therapist using qualitative methods to explore the experiences of young adults with substance abuse problems. In the course of such a study, a research participant may share information about past sexual abuse or current suicidal ideation. Minimizing suffering requires that researchers implementing such studies plan for referral to appropriate mental health professionals. Even questionnaire-based research may be worrisome to participants or lead to expectations that cannot be met by the researchers, as in a recent report of participant reactions to a mailed questionnaire study of breast disease management.[22]

A final component of the safety issue relates to the issue of how a researcher should decide when to terminate a study prematurely. One end point is when injury or harm becomes apparent. A drug trial in the 1990s was halted after five patients died of liver failure and two patients survived only after receiving liver transplants after taking long-term doses of the drug fialuridine to treat hepatitis B.[23] Although the injury or harm that may occur in much of rehabilitation research is less dramatic than liver failure and death, researchers must still conduct their trials in ways that allow them to identify safety concerns in a timely fashion. Another end point is when a new procedure is found to be superior to the comparison procedure. In opposing viewpoints about the ethical issues involved in premature termination of clinical trials, one set of authors reviewed a study they believed should have been stopped earlier than it was in order to permit new patients to take advantage of a treatment that proved to be superior to the control in reducing in-hospital deaths in patients being treated for acute myocardial infarction.[24] Another set of authors came to the very different conclusion that the statistical trends were not strong enough to justify a premature termination of the study and that 6-month survival data gave a different picture of the relative effectiveness of the techniques, justifying the continuation of the study to its original end point.[25] This point-counterpoint illustrates the complexity of putting research ethics into action.

Risk Is Commensurate with Potential Benefit

High-risk activities can only be justified if the potential for benefit is also great. Levine noted that researchers are usually quick to identify potential benefits of their research, without always considering carefully all the potential risks to participants.[2] Because of the subtle nature of many risks, and the duty of researchers to minimize and consider all risks, the last section of this chapter presents an analysis of risks associated with research.

Independent Review

Adequate protection of human participants requires that a body independent of the researcher review the protocol and assess the level of protection afforded to the human participants. The generic name for such an independent body in the United States is an *institutional review board* (IRB); in other countries it may be referred to as a research ethics committee, a research ethics board, or an independent ethics committee.[5,26] By whatever name, the research ethics committee's charge is to examine research proposals to ensure that there is adequate protection of human participants in terms of safety and confidentiality, that the elements of informed consent are present, and that the risks of the study are commensurate with the potential benefits. Specific information about the nature of these committees and the procedures for putting the principles of informed consent into action are discussed in Chapter 27.

Publication Integrity

Researchers need to ensure the accuracy of reports of their work, should not present another's work as their own, and should acknowledge any financial support or other assistance received during the conduct of a research study. Chapter 28 provides specific guidelines for determining who should be listed as a study author and how to acknowledge the participation of those who are not authors.

Explicit Attention to Ethics

Researchers need to give explicit attention to ethical principles when they design, implement, and report their research. Researchers should act to change research projects for which they are responsible if ethical problems arise or should dissociate themselves from projects if they have no control over unethical acts. For example, assume that a prosthetist is collecting data in a study that is being conducted by a different primary investigator. If the prosthetist believes that patient consent is being coerced, he or she should seek to change the consent procedure with the primary investigator, discuss his or her concerns with the research ethics committee that approved the study, or refuse to participate further if no change occurs.

■ RESEARCH RISKS

Much of the discussion in this chapter is related in some way to risk–benefit analysis. The risks of research can be categorized as physical, psychological, social, and economic.[2] Each category is described and examples from the rehabilitation literature are presented.

Physical Risks

The physical risk associated with some research is well known. When a particular risk is known, participants should be informed of its likelihood, severity, duration, and reversibility. Methods for treating the physical harm should also be discussed if appropriate. If a strengthening study provides an eccentric overload stimulus to hamstring musculature, participants need to know that almost all will develop delayed muscle soreness, that it appears within 2 days after exercise, and typically lasts up to 8 days.[27] Higher-risk procedures, such as an invasive muscle biopsy or fine-wire electromyography, might include the risk of infection. Participants in such studies would need to receive information about signs and symptoms of infection, and procedures to follow if infection occurs.

A different form of physical risk is the impact of *not* receiving treatment. A controversial aspect of the most recent revision of the Declaration of Helsinki is its Clause 29, which states that

> The benefits, risks, burdens, and effectiveness of a new method should be tested against those of the best current prophylactic, diagnostic, and therapeutic methods. This does not exclude the use of placebo, or no treatment, in studies where no proven prophylactic, diagnostic or therapeutic method exists.[14(p4)]

This principle is controversial enough that the World Medical Association added a note of clarification, reaffirming that "extreme care must be taken in making use of a placebo-controlled trial" but clarifying that placebo-controlled trials may be acceptable even if proven therapies are available when there are "compelling and scientifically sound methodological reasons" for using the placebo-controlled trials or when the therapy being investigated is for a minor condition "and the patients who receive placebo will not be subject to an additional risk of serious or irreversible harm."[14(p4)] The related Clause 30 states that

> At the conclusion of the study, every patient entered into the study should be assured of access to the best proven prophylactic, diagnostic and therapeutic methods identified in the study.[14(p4)]

Some critics believe that strict adherence to these principles, while appropriate for research in developed nations where resources exist to provide the kind of care described in Clauses 29 and 30, would severely limit research in developing nations by "imposing demands on local and national health systems that, without massive additional investments, simply cannot be met."[28] The international research community needs to strike a balance between research that exploits individuals in developing nations by exposing them to all of the risks of research and few of the benefits of contemporary best health care practices and research that provides at least some care to communities that would not otherwise receive it.

Because rehabilitation research is often concerned with matters of long-term quality of life rather than immediate matters of life and death, it is often possible to delay treatments to some groups without additional risk of serious harm. However, even research on seemingly minor conditions requires careful consideration of both the risks of receiving and not receiving treatment. For example, Green and colleagues performed a randomized controlled trial of passive joint mobilization for the treatment of acute ankle sprains.[29] Even though serious, irreversible harm may not come to individuals who receive no treatment for acute ankle sprains, they nevertheless chose to compare their treatment group (which received passive joint mobilization in addition to rest, ice, compression, and elevation) to an active control group receiving rest, ice, compression, and elevation.

Risks of research may be population specific. For example, treatments such as the use of ultrasound over epiphyseal plates are relatively low risk in adults but may have high risks for children.[30] When delineating the risks of participation in a given study, researchers must consider whether the procedures they are using pose special risks to the population they are studying. In addition, physical risks of an intervention are not always known or may not become apparent for long periods of time. Researchers must always consider whether the potential benefit of a study is proportional to its long-term or hidden risks.

Psychological Risks

Although rehabilitation researchers may focus on the physical risks of their research, they must also consider psychological risks. Participant selection that requires normality can cause psychological harm to those identified as abnormal. Those receiving an experimental treatment may lie awake nights wondering what untoward effects they may experience. Or participants in a placebo-controlled study may be anxious about whether their condition is being undertreated with a placebo. Qualitative researchers must guard against psychological risks that arise from the interactions among researchers and participants that occur across time.[31] Participants in studies that investigate sensitive topics may have emotional reactions to data collection efforts.[32] Regardless of the type or topic of a study, researchers must carefully consider ways to minimize the psychological risks to participants in their studies.

Social Risks

The major social risk to individual research participants is the breach of confidentiality. As discussed earlier, recent legislation in both the United States and the United Kingdom provides new protections to individuals relative to the privacy of their health information. These new laws require that researchers be more vigilant than ever in protecting the privacy of research participants, including both those who are active participants receiving experimental measures or interventions as well as those who are more passive participants whose medical records or health insurance data are used to evaluate care that has already been delivered.

Economic Risks

When research has a combined knowledge and treatment effect, at least some portion of the payment for the research will generally be the responsibility of participants or the participants' health care insurers. Even if the treatment in question is not experimental, the participant may incur additional costs through lost work hours, baby-sitting fees while undergoing treatment, and transportation costs to and from the research facility.

A major source of economic risk associated with research involves the cost of care related to negative outcomes of research. Levine indicates that current ethical thought is that researchers should provide compensation for untoward effects of their research. He notes, though, that few centers have taken the initiative to develop a system for accomplishing this compensation.[16]

■ SUMMARY

The differences between practice and research demand that the participants in research receive special protection from the risks associated with research. The general moral principles of non-maleficence, beneficence, utility, and autonomy form the base on which research codes of ethics are built. Informed consent requires that participation be a voluntary action taken by a competent individual who comprehends the risks and benefits of research participation as disclosed by the researcher. In addition to securing the informed consent of their participants, researchers must ensure that the design of a study justifies its conduct, that procedures are designed to minimize risk, that risk is commensurate with potential benefits, that an independent review body has approved the conduct of the research, that integrity is maintained in publication of the research, and that careful consideration is given to all ethical concerns related to the study. The risks associated with research may be physical, psychological, social, and economic.

REFERENCES

1. Savulescu J. Harm, ethics committees and the gene therapy death. Editorial. *J Med Ethics.* 2001;27:148-150.
2. Levine RJ. The boundaries between biomedical or behavioral research and the accepted and routine practice of medicine. In: The National Commission for the Protection of Human Subjects of Biomedical and Behavioral Research, ed. *The Belmont Report: Ethical Principles and Guidelines for the Protection of Human Subjects of Research, Appendix*

Volume I. DHEW Publication OS 78-0013. Washington, DC: US Government Printing Office; 1975.
3. Munson R. *Intervention and Reflection: Basic Issues in Medical Ethics.* 6th ed. Belmont, Calif: Wadsworth/ Thomson Learning; 2000.
4. Sim J. Informed consent: ethical implications for physiotherapy. *Physiotherapy.* 1986;72:584-587.
5. Federman DD, Hanna KE, Rodriguez LL, Institute of Medicine (US) Committee on Assessing the System for Protecting Human Research Participants. *Responsible Research: A Systems Approach to Protecting Research Participants.* Washington, DC: National Academies Press; 2003.
6. Kazdin AE. Ethical issues and guidelines for research. In: Kazdin AE, ed. *Research Design in Clinical Psychology.* 4th ed. Boston, Mass: Allyn & Bacon; 2003:497-544.
7. Paasche-Orlow MK, Taylor HA, Brancati FL. Readability standards for informed-consent forms as compared with actual readability. *N Engl J Med.* 2003;348:721-726.
8. Ferguson PR. Patients' perceptions of information provided in clinical trials. *J Med Ethics.* 2002;28:45-48.
9. Allmark P. The ethics of research with children. *Nurs Res.* 2002;10:7-19.
10. Bravo G, Pâquet M, Dubois M-F. Knowledge of the legislation governing proxy consent to treatment and research. *J Med Ethics.* 2003;29:44-50.
11. Durham ML. How research will adapt to HIPAA: a view from within the healthcare delivery system. *Am J Law Med.* 2002;28:491-502.
12. Cassell J, Young A. Why we should not seek individual informed consent for participation in health services research. *J Med Ethics.* 2002;28:313-317.
13. *Nuremberg Code.* Available at: *http://ohsr.od.nih.gov/ nuremberg.php3.* Accessed March 3, 2003.
14. World Medical Association. *World Medical Association Declaration of Helsinki.* 2002 clarification. Available at: *http://www.wma.net/e/policy/17-c_e.html.* Accessed October 27, 2003.
15. US Department of Health and Human Services. *Title 45 CFR Part 46 Protection of Human Subjects.* Available at: *http://ohsr.od.nih.gov/mpa/45cfr46.php3.* Accessed October 30, 2003.
16. Levine RJ. *Ethics and Regulation of Clinical Research.* 2nd ed. New Haven, Conn: Yale University Press; 1988.
17. US Department of Health and Human Services National Institutes of Health. *Human Participant Protections Education for Research Teams.* Available at: *http://cme. cancer.gov/c01/.* Accessed October 30, 2003.
18. Jones JH. *Bad Blood: The Tuskegee Syphilis Experiment.* New and expanded ed. New York, NY: Maxwell McMillan International; 1993.
19. Feldshuh D. *Miss Evers' Boys.* Acting ed. New York, NY: Dramatists Play Service; 1995.
20. Miss Evers' Boys [videotape]. Distributed by: Home Box Office; 1997.

21. Miller FG, Shorr AF. Unnecessary use of placebo controls: the case of asthma clinical trials. Commentary. *Arch Intern Med*. 2002;162:1673-1677.

22. Evans M, Robling M, Maggs Rapport F, Houston H, Kinnersley P, Wilkinson C. It doesn't cost anything to ask, does it? The ethics of questionnaire-based research. *J Med Ethics*. 2002;28:41-44.

23. Thompson L. The cure that killed. *Discover*. 1994;15:56, 58, 60-62.

24. Verdú-Pascual F, Castelló-Ponce A. Randomised clinical trials: a source of ethical dilemmas. *J Med Ethics*. 2001; 27:177-178.

25. Hilden J, Gammelgaard A. Premature stopping and informed consent in AMI trials. *J Med Ethics*. 2002;28: 188-189.

26. Shaul RZ. Reviewing the reviewers: the vague accountability of research ethics committees. *Critical Care*. 2002; 6:121-122.

27. Kellis E, Baltzopoulos V. Isokinetic eccentric exercise. *Sports Med*. 1995;19:202-222.

28. Tollman SM. Fair partnerships support ethical research. *BMJ*. 2001;323:1417-1423.

29. Green T, Refshauge K, Crosbie J, Adams R. A randomized controlled trial of a passive accessory joint mobilization on acute ankle inversion sprains. *Phys Ther*. 2001;81:984-993.

30. McDiarmid T, Ziskin MC, Michlovitz SL. Therapeutic US. In: Michlovitz SL, ed. *Thermal Agents in Rehabilitation*. Philadelphia, Pa: FA Davis; 1996:168-212.

31. Glesne C. *Becoming Qualitative Researchers: An Introduction*. 2nd ed. New York, NY: Addison Wesley Longman; 1999:113-129.

32. Cowles KV. Issues in qualitative research on sensitive topics. *West J Nurs Res*. 1988;10:163-179.

Research Design

Research Problems, Questions, and Hypotheses

Developing Answerable Research Questions
Topic Identification and Selection
Problem Identification and Selection
Action-Knowledge Conflict
Knowledge-Knowledge Conflict
Policy-Action Conflict
Knowledge Void
Theoretical Framework Identification and Selection
Question Identification and Selection

Research Methods Identification and Selection
Criteria for Evaluating Research Problems
Study Is Feasible
Problem Is Interesting
Problem Is Novel
Problem Can Be Studied Ethically
Question Is Relevant
Summary

The challenge in searching for a research question is not a shortage of uncertainties in the universe; it is the difficulty of finding an important one that can be transformed into a feasible and valid study plan."[1(p17)]

The first step in any research venture is to define the problem that is to be studied. The clarity with which a researcher views the problem at hand will greatly influence each subsequent step of the research process. Researchers should therefore devote a great deal of intellectual energy to developing their research problems. The purpose of this chapter is to present strategies to facilitate problem and question development

and to advance criteria for determining whether a question has promise as a basis for research.

■ DEVELOPING ANSWERABLE RESEARCH QUESTIONS

Novice researchers usually have little difficulty identifying a general topic of interest: "I want to do something with the knee" or "My interest is in children with cerebral palsy." From these general statements of interest, novice researchers often take a giant leap directly into asking research questions: "What is the relationship between hamstring strength and knee stability in patients with anterior cruciate ligament tears?" "Which individuals with spinal cord injury respond best to intrathecal baclofen for management of spasticity?"

The answers to these questions may well be important to advancing the body of knowledge in rehabilitation. Moving directly from topic to question, however, does not establish that the questions are relevant to problems within the field. This leap also fails to place the research question in a theoretical context. At the inception of a research project, researchers need to focus on broad *problems* within the profession, rather than on narrow questions they would like to answer. By focusing on problems, researchers are more likely to develop relevant questions, and their research is more likely to advance the practice of rehabilitation. The process of moving from a general topic to a specific research question involves four sets of ideas: topic identification and selection, problem identification and selection, theoretical framework identification and selection, and question identification and selection. A fifth step, determining the research methods, flows from the development of the ideas in the previous four steps. For each step in the process, researchers must first be creative enough to generate many ideas, and then must be selective enough to focus on a limited number of ideas for further study. Figure 4–1 shows this process. Each diamond represents an expansion and contraction of ideas; the ovals represent the idea selected for further development, and each row of the figure represents one expansion-contraction cycle. The background of the figure (shaded rectangle) is the professional literature, which guides the entire problem development process.

Topic Identification and Selection

As noted earlier, selection of a general topic is usually not a problem for researchers. For those who cannot identify a general area of interest, direction should come from reading widely in the literature and discussing problems with colleagues until a spark of interest is found. From all the

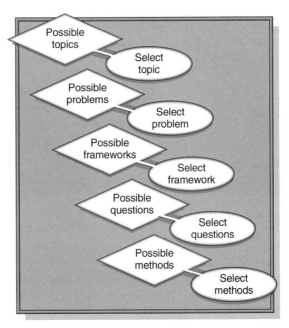

FIGURE 4–1. Research problem development. The diamonds represent the expansion and contraction of ideas; the ovals represent selection of an idea for further development, and the shaded rectangle in the background represents the professional literature that is the foundation on which all problems are built.

possible topics considered by a researcher, one is selected for further study. For example, a practitioner who begins a new job at a work conditioning center might quickly identify several areas of possible study: the role of cardiovascular conditioning in return to work, the use of back belts on the job, or the concept of injury legitimacy. Note that while focused on one area of practice, all of the topics are relatively broad because the practitioner does not yet know what is and is not known about each topic. Finding out more about each will allow the practitioner to determine which topics seem most likely to yield interesting and feasible research possibilities. The practitioner in this example chooses to study the use of back belts on the job, thereby completing the first of the four cycles of expansion (identification of many possible topics) and contraction (selection of a single topic from the many) of ideas that takes place during the development of a research question.

Problem Identification and Selection

After a topic is selected, it is the job of the researcher to articulate important problems related to that topic area. Problems, whether in daily life or in research, are perplexing situations without clear solutions. The purpose of rehabilitation research is to shed light on perplexing situations in rehabilitation practice.

One way of articulating research problems is to develop a series of logical statements that can be thought of as "givens," "howevers," and "therefores." The "given" is a statement of information that is generally accepted as true. The "however" contradicts or casts doubt on the "given." The conflict between the "givens" and the "howevers" creates the perplexing situation that is the research problem. The perplexing situation leads, "therefore," to the development of a research question. The conflicts that lead to research questions may be between actions, policies, or knowledge, as articulated by Clark.[2] In the following quotes from published research studies, the terms "given," "however," and "therefore" are inserted to allow the reader to see how the authors have used this logical process to identify their problems of interest.

ACTION-KNOWLEDGE CONFLICT

These conflicts arise when practitioners act in ways that are not consistent with the formal knowledge of the profession:

> [GIVEN:] Back supports or back belts recently have been marketed as a significant aid in the prevention of low back pain. [HOWEVER,] the scientific literature does not confirm their benefit. [THEREFORE,] more substantial work in this area is needed before the approach can be considered acceptable.[3(p1271)]
>
> [GIVEN:] According to conventional...practice, therapeutic ultrasound (US) should not be used on patients with cancer because of the possibility of exacerbating tumor growth. [HOWEVER,] this contention is not adequately supported in the scientific literature.... [THEREFORE,] the purpose of our study was to determine whether the

application of continuous therapeutic US would alter the growth or metastasis of [a sarcoma] in mice.[4(pp3,5)]

KNOWLEDGE-KNOWLEDGE CONFLICT

The conflict here is between different types of knowledge, in this example, between general knowledge and scientifically based knowledge:

> [GIVEN:] General descriptions of Huntington's disease (HD) and Parkinson's disease (PD) have traditionally stated that these diseases are not associated with language deterioration....[HOWEVER,] an increasing number of studies have identified language deficits in patients with HD or PD, even when they are in early stages of their disease.... [THEREFORE,] the purpose of this study was to identify and characterize spoken language deficits associated with HD and PD.[5(pp350-1351)]

POLICY-ACTION CONFLICT

This type of conflict examines the relationship between professional actions and internal or external rules:

> [GIVEN:] [There are] reports of widespread use of physical therapy aides to deliver patient treatment.... [HOWEVER,] controversy surround[s] this practice. [THEREFORE,] we wished to obtain a baseline of information about the practices and opinions of physical therapists within our state relative to utilization of on-the-job-trained support personnel.[6(p422)]

KNOWLEDGE VOID

This type of problem is generated because of a void, rather than a conflict:

> [GIVEN:] Handwriting constitutes the primary way that elementary school students demonstrate their knowledge in all academic areas.... Academic failure can result from... problems associated with poor handwriting. [HOWEVER,] empirically based evidence documenting handwriting intervention effectiveness is minimal. [THEREFORE,] the purpose of this study was to examine the effects of school-based occupational therapy on children's handwriting and associated school functions.[7(p17-18)]

[GIVEN:] The most common complications after hip arthroplasty surgery are dislocation of the prosthesis, local infection, and loosening.... Many studies have reported on the rate of hip dislocation in acute hospitals. [HOWEVER,] there have been no studies reporting on the incidence of dislocation in rehabilitation hospitals.... [THEREFORE,] this study was undertaken as a first step toward understanding hip dislocation in the rehabilitation setting."[8(p444)]

As shown by the examples just presented, a problem cannot be defined until the researcher understands what is or is not known (the "givens" and "howevers") about the topic area of interest. Any given topic will yield many potentially researchable conflicts. Identifying and then selecting from among these potential problems is the second of the series of expansion and contraction of ideas that must occur before a research study is designed. The conflicts and voids that form the basis for research problems can be identified through a review of the professional literature. Table 4–1, based on the work of Kazdin,[9] shows how to develop ideas for rehabilitation research by adding novel "twists" to existing work found during the review of the literature. Details about finding relevant literature and synthesizing the results are presented in Chapters 24 to 26.

Theoretical Framework Identification and Selection

Once a problem is selected, it needs to be placed into a theoretical framework that will allow it to be viewed in relation to other research. The literature review that was conducted to establish the problem was likely to be fairly narrowly focused on the topic at hand. In contrast, the theoretical grounding provides a much broader perspective from which to view the problem. Defining and selecting a theoretical framework for the study is the third cycle of expansion (identification of possible frameworks) and contraction (selection of a framework) of ideas within the problem development process. Sometimes a researcher will be drawn to a particular framework based on

previous interests or education; other times the researcher will need to read widely in several areas to settle on a framework that seems most promising for further study.

One of the example problems presented earlier was based on the conflict between the popular use of back supports to prevent low back pain and the lack of scientific evidence of their effectiveness.[3] One theoretical framework for thinking about the use and effectiveness of back supports might be thought of as a biomechanical framework, presented schematically in Figure 4–2. In this framework, back supports are viewed as biomechanical devices that increase intraabdominal pressure and decrease compressive load on the spine. Studying back supports from this biomechanical perspective would involve defining variables related to the framework. For example, if back supports decrease compressive loads on the spine, then demands on back extensor muscles should be reduced. If demands on back extensors are reduced when wearing a back support, then endurance of back extensors should be enhanced. This approach to the study of the effect of back supports was used by Ciriello and Snook.[3] Choosing a biomechanical framework had several implications for their study. First, the back support they studied needed to be a rigid enclosure belt that would provide the type of abdominal compression indicated in the model. Flexible supports that provide a reminder to lift carefully, but do not offer a great deal of abdominal compression, would not be appropriate for study using this biomechanical framework. Second, the measured variables within the study needed to represent back extensor endurance. Variables such as injury rates and time lost to back injuries when using back supports may be interesting, but they are not relevant when viewing back supports from this biomechanical framework.

This biomechanical approach to the study of the use and effectiveness of back supports is not, however, the only way to conceptualize this topic. For example, other researchers might prefer to work from a health promotion framework, shown in Figure 4–3. In such a framework,

TABLE 4-1 Using Existing Research to Develop New Research Problems	
General Form of Problem	**Specific Hypothetical Question**
Studying a well-known clinical phenomenon in the context of a new population	How does clinical depression present itself in individuals with acquired spinal cord injury?
Studying subgroups of clinical populations	What distinguishes adolescents with myelomeningocele who remain community ambulators from those who do not?
Developing research problems that apply basic research findings to clinical populations	Can the findings from animal research on tissue responses to overload stimuli from electrical stimulation be replicated in humans?
Extending previous work by modifying aspects of the independent variable	Would the same results have been achieved if speech therapy sessions were conducted more frequently?
Extending previous work by adding new dependent variables	Does aquatic therapy for individuals with knee osteoarthritis improve participation levels and health-related quality of life, in addition to its established impact on impairment measures such as strength and range of motion?
Extending previous work by studying new clinical populations or new health care settings	Can preschool-aged children with disabilities benefit from powered mobility to the same extent as the school-aged children who have been the subject of previous studies?
Studying the impact of covariates on the clinical phenomena	Do individuals from different cultures and from different socioeconomic strata perform differently on tests of aphasia?

use of back supports would be viewed through a lens that looks at health promotion behaviors in the workplace as the result of the convergence of a complex set of cognitive factors (e.g., the perceived level of control that workers have over health in the workplace) and modifying factors (e.g., situational factors such as the consequences of violating company policies about the use of safety equipment on the job).[10]

Researchers who use this framework for thinking about the use and effectiveness of back supports would likely measure worker behaviors and beliefs, rather than physical factors such as endurance of back extensors. Whereas the biomechanical framework may show the physiological effects of the back support, the health promotion model may shed light on factors that would increase usage of the device among workers.

Adopting a theoretical framework, then, is a way of choosing a lens through which one views the problem of interest. The framework helps the researcher define what will and will not be studied and helps the researcher select appropriate variables for study.

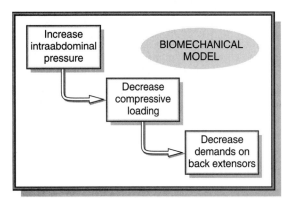

FIGURE 4–2. Biomechanical framework for studying back supports.

Question Identification and Selection

Once the problem is identified and placed in a theoretical perspective, the researcher must develop the specific questions that will be studied. This is done through the fourth cycle of expansion (identification of many possible questions) and contraction (selection of a limited number of questions for study) of ideas within the problem development process. The biomechanical framework for studying the use and effectiveness of back supports might yield the following research questions:

1. Do back supports increase intraabdominal pressure?
2. How well do different back supports unload the spine?
3. Are the strength and endurance characteristics of back extensor muscles different

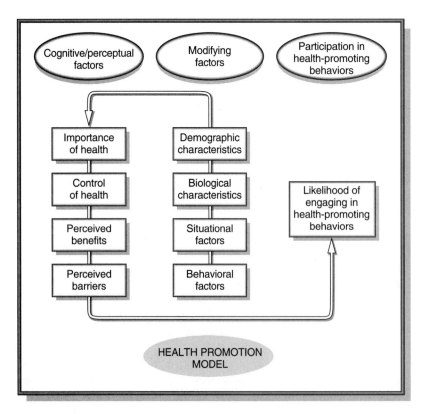

FIGURE 4–3. Health promotion framework for studying back supports.

for workers who do and do not wear back supports on the job?

4. Do back supports preserve the endurance characteristics of back extensor muscles?

Other questions could be generated, but four are enough to demonstrate the types of questions suggested by the framework. Some researchers prefer to state the purpose of their study as a question; others prefer to state their purpose as an objective, which takes the form of a declarative sentence. Ciriello and Snook studied question 3 in the list, but stated their purpose as an objective: "The study investigated whether back supports preserve the endurance characteristics of the back extensors, indirectly indicating decreased loading."[3(p1271)]

After stating their purpose as either a question or an objective, many researchers advance a *research hypothesis*. The research hypothesis is the researchers' educated guess about the outcome of the study. This educated guess is generally based on the theoretical grounding for the study, previous research results, or on the clinical experiences of the researchers. Ciriello and Snook advanced the following hypothesis in their study of back supports: "It was hypothesized that there would be significant differences in the [endurance of back extensor muscles] as a result of wearing the back belt."[3(p1272)] Having such a hypothesis enables researchers to place their results into the context of the theory or experience that led them to conduct the study. Research hypotheses should not be confused with the statistical hypotheses within a study. The statistical hypotheses, subdivided into *null* and *alternate* hypotheses, are essentially given once a particular type of statistical analysis is selected. Statistical hypotheses are discussed in greater detail in Chapters 19 and 20.

Research Methods Identification and Selection

Only after the research question is determined can the investigator begin to consider which

research methods are appropriate to answer the question. Research methods are discussed in detail in Chapters 5 through 16.

■ CRITERIA FOR EVALUATING RESEARCH PROBLEMS

While proceeding through the steps of research problem development, the researcher is faced with several selection decisions. Which topic, problem, or question should be studied? Which research approach to the question should be adopted? Cummings and colleagues[1(p19)] believe that a good research problem is feasible, interesting, novel, ethical, and relevant; the acronym FINER can be used to remember these five characteristics.

Study Is Feasible

Feasibility should be assessed in terms of subjects, equipment and technical expertise, time, and money. For example, if practitioners wish to study differences between two electrical stimulation bicycle ergometry programs for patients with spinal cord injuries, they need to have access to adequate numbers of patients who will be willing to participate in a lengthy study. If the phenomenon of delayed muscle soreness is to be studied, subjects who are willing to experience soreness must be found.

Researchers need to be realistic about the technical resources available to them. If a practitioner wishes to study hindfoot movement when landing from a jump, then motion analysis equipment is required. If the proper equipment is not available, then another problem should be selected for study.

The time needed to complete a research study is often underestimated. As noted in Chapter 1, lack of time is a significant impediment for clinical researchers. Therefore, clinicians need to develop research questions that can be answered within the time constraints of their practices. Chapters on case reports (Chapter 12), single-system designs (Chapter 10), and outcomes research (Chapter 15) introduce research methods that may fit well within the context of a busy clinical practice.

Financial resources needed to conduct research must also be considered. Direct costs such as equipment, postage, and printing must be met. Personnel costs may include salaries and benefits for the primary investigator, data collectors, secretaries, statisticians, engineers, and photographers. If there are no funds for statisticians and engineering consultants, then complex experimental designs with highly technical measures should not be attempted.

Problem Is Interesting

The research question must be of interest to the investigator. Because rehabilitation is practiced by a broad set of professionals who are just beginning to articulate its research base, a wide range of interesting unanswered questions exists. All rehabilitation practitioners should therefore be able to identify several questions that whet their intellectual appetites. The discovery that accompanies research is exciting, but several steps along the way are tedious and time-consuming. Thus, interest in the topic must be high to motivate the researcher to move through the drudgery to reach the discovery.

Problem Is Novel

Good research is novel in that it adds to knowledge. However, novice researchers are often unrealistic in their desire to be totally original in what they do. Novelty can be found in projects that confirm or refute previous findings, extend previous findings, or provide new findings. Because many aspects of rehabilitation are not well documented, novel research ideas abound.

Problem Can Be Studied Ethically

An ethical study is one in which the elements of informed consent can be met and the risks of the research are in proportion to the potential benefits of the research, as described in Chapter 3. In the rehabilitation literature, for example, there are no experimental studies that compare a comprehensive rehabilitation program for patients who have had cerebral vascular accidents to a program consisting of no rehabilitation services. Such a protocol would be considered unethical because a totally untreated control group would be at risk for developing complications of bed rest or requiring extended care. Researchers overcome this ethical concern by comparing different levels of rehabilitation services, rather than completely depriving some patients of such care.

Question Is Relevant

When developing research questions, rehabilitation practitioners need to answer an important relevancy question: "Who cares?" If the first phase of the problem development process was taken seriously, the researcher should be able to provide a ready answer to that question. If the researcher skipped that phase, and generated a research question without knowing how it related to a problem within rehabilitation, then the question may not be relevant to the field. Relevant rehabilitation research questions are grounded in day-to-day problems faced by practitioners.

■ SUMMARY

The research problem development process involves selection of a topic of interest, a problem within the profession, a theoretical framework for the study, and one or more specific questions related to the problem as conceptualized through the theoretical framework. The research hypothesis articulates the researchers' educated guess about the outcome of the study.

Good research problems are feasible, interesting, novel, ethical, and relevant.

REFERENCES

1. Cummings SR, Browner WS, Hulley SB. Conceiving the research question. In: Hulley SB, Cummings SR, Browner WS, Grady D, Hearst N, Newman TB, eds. *Designing Clinical Research: An Epidemiological Approach*. 2nd ed. Philadelphia, Pa: Lippincott Williams & Wilkins; 2001.
2. Clark DL. Worksheet A-Statement of the Problem. Unpublished material. Charlottesville, Va: School of Education, University of Virginia; 1990.
3. Ciriello VM, Snook SH. The effect of back belts on lumbar muscle fatigue. *Spine*. 1995;20:1271-1278.
4. Sicard-Rosenbaum L, Lord D, Danoff JV, Thom AK, Eckhaus MA. Effects of continuous therapeutic ultrasound on growth and metastasis of subcutaneous murine tumors. *Phys Ther*. 1995;75:3-13.
5. Murray LL. Spoken language production in Huntington's and Parkinson's diseases. *J Speech Lang Hearing Res*. 2000;43:1350-1366.
6. Bashi HL, Domholdt E. Use of support personnel for physical therapy treatment. *Phys Ther*. 1993;73: 421-436.
7. Case-Smith J. Effectiveness of school-based occupational therapy intervention on handwriting. *Am J Occup Ther*. 2002;56:17-25.
8. Krotenberg R, Stitik T, Johnston M. Incidence of dislocation following hip arthroplasty for patients in the rehabilitation setting. *Am J Phys Med Rehabil*. 1995;74: 444-447.
9. Kazdin AE. Selection of the research problem and design. In: Kazdin AE, ed. *Research Design in Clinical Psychology*. 4th ed. Boston, Mass: Allyn & Bacon; 2003.
10. Pender NJ, Walker SN, Sechrist KR, Frank-Stromborg M. Predicting health-promoting lifestyles in the workplace. *Nurs Res*. 1990;39:326-332.

Research Paradigms

Knowledge is continually evolving. What was believed to be true yesterday may be doubted today, scorned tomorrow, and resurrected in the future. Just as knowledge itself evolves, beliefs about how to create knowledge also evolve. Our beliefs about the methods of obtaining knowledge constitute *research paradigms*.[1(p15)] The beliefs that constitute a paradigm are often so entrenched that researchers themselves do not question the assumptions that undergird the

research methodology they use. Although the details of various research methods are presented in later chapters, this chapter is presented to provide readers with a broad framework for thinking about the research paradigms that support those methods.

Although differences in the research approaches of the different rehabilitation professions can be seen, the dominant research paradigm across the rehabilitation disciplines is the quantitative paradigm. Two competing paradigms of importance are the qualitative and single-system paradigms. The study of competing research paradigms in rehabilitation is important for two reasons. First, research based on the competing paradigms is reported in the rehabilitation literature, so consumers of the literature need to be familiar with the assumptions that undergird these paradigms. Second, competing research paradigms in any discipline emerge because of the inability of the dominant paradigm to answer all the important questions of the discipline. Researchers therefore need to consider competing paradigm research not only in terms of the specific research questions addressed but also in terms of what the research implies about the limitations of the dominant paradigm.

The purpose of this chapter is to develop these three research paradigms for consideration. This is done by first emphasizing differences between the paradigms (some might say by presenting caricatures of each paradigm) and later examining relationships among the paradigms. The quantitative paradigm is discussed first. This paradigm focuses on the study of groups whose treatment is often manipulated by the investigator. The qualitative paradigm is then discussed. This paradigm focuses on broad description and understanding of phenomena without direct manipulation. The final paradigm to be analyzed is the single-system paradigm, which focuses on individual responses to manipulation.

Deciding on the terminology to use for the different research paradigms is difficult. The paradigms are sometimes described in philosophical terms, sometimes in terms of components of the paradigm, and sometimes in terms of the methods that usually follow from the philosophical underpinnings of the paradigm. Box 5–1 presents the various names that have been used to identify what are being labeled in this chapter as quantitative, qualitative, and single-system paradigms. Accurate use of the different philosophical labels requires a strong background in the history and philosophy of science, backgrounds that most clinicians do not have. To avoid imprecise use of the language of philosophy, the more

---

BOX 5-1

Alternate Names for the Three Research Paradigms

Quantitative Paradigm
  Positivist
  Received view
  Logical positivist
  Nomothetic
  Empiricist
Qualitative Paradigm
  Naturalistic
  Phenomenological
  Ethnographic
  Idiographic
  Postpositivist
  New paradigm
Single-System Paradigm
  Idiographic
  N = 1
  Single-subject
  Single-case experimental design

"methodological" terms are used in this text rather than the more "philosophical" terms. This choice may, however, lead to the misconception that paradigms and methods are interchangeable. They are not. A paradigm is defined by the assumptions and beliefs that guide researchers. A method is defined by the actions taken by investigators as they implement research. Adoption of a paradigm implies the use of certain methods but does not necessarily limit the researcher to those methods. The presentation of the assumptions of each paradigm is followed by general methodological implications of the paradigm. Later chapters present specific designs associated with these paradigms.

■ QUANTITATIVE PARADIGM

The quantitative paradigm is what has become known as the traditional method of science. The term *quantitative* comes from the emphasis on measurement that characterizes this paradigm. The paradigm has its roots in the 1600s with the development of Newtonian physics.[2,3] In the early 1900s, the French philosopher Auguste Comte and a group of scientists in Vienna became proponents of related philosophical positions often labeled *positivism* or *logical positivism*.[4] This positivist philosophy is so labeled because of the central idea that one can only be certain, or positive, of knowledge that is verifiable through measurement and observation.

Assumptions of the Quantitative Paradigm

Just as there are multiple terms for each paradigm, there are multiple views about the critical components of each paradigm. Lincoln and Guba use five basic axioms to differentiate what they refer to as positivist and naturalistic paradigms.[1(p37)] Their five axioms are presented here as the basis of the quantitative paradigm. The qualitative and single-system paradigms are developed by retaining or replacing these with alternate axioms. Table 5–1 summarizes the assumptions of the three paradigms.

ASSUMPTION 1

The first assumption of the quantitative paradigm is that there is a single objective reality. One goal of quantitative research is to determine the nature of this reality through measurement and observation of the phenomena of interest. This

reliance on observation is sometimes termed *empiricism*. A second goal of quantitative research is to predict or control reality. After all, if researchers can empirically determine laws that regulate reality in some predictable way, then they should be able to use this knowledge to attempt to influence that reality in equally predictable ways.

ASSUMPTION 2

The second basic assumption of the quantitative paradigm is that the investigator and subject, or object of inquiry, can be independent of one another. In other words, it is assumed that the investigator can be an unobtrusive observer of a reality that does not change by virtue of the fact that it is being studied. Researchers who adopt the quantitative paradigm do, however, recognize that it is sometimes difficult to achieve this independence. Rosenthal,[5] in his text on experimenter effects in behavioral research, related a classic story about "Clever Hans," a horse who could purportedly tap out the correct response to mathematical problems by tapping his hoof. Hans's skills intrigued a researcher, Pfungst, who tested Hans's abilities under different controlled conditions. Pfungst found that Hans could tap out the correct answer only when his questioner was a literate individual who knew the answer to the question. He found that knowledgeable questioners unconsciously raised their eyebrows, flared their nostrils, or raised their heads as Hans

TABLE 5-1 **Assumptions of the Three Research Paradigms**

	Paradigm		
Assumption	**Quantitative**	**Qualitative**	**Single-System**
Reality	Single, objective	Multiple, constructed	Single, objective
Relationship between investigator and subject	Independent	Dependent	Independent
Generalizability of findings	Desirable and possible	Situation specific	System specific
Cause-and-effect relationships	Causal	Noncausal	Causal
Values	Value free	Value bound	Value free

was coming up to the correct number of taps. Rosenthal notes:

> Hans' amazing talents…serve to illustrate further the power of self-fulfilling prophecy. Hans' questioners, even skeptical ones, expected Hans to give the correct answers to their queries. Their expectation was reflected in their unwitting signal to Hans that the time had come for him to stop his tapping. The signal cued Hans to stop, and the questioner's expectation became the reason for Hans' being, once again, correct.[5(p138)]

Despite the recognition of the difficulty of achieving the independence of the investigator and subject, the assumption of the quantitative paradigm is that it is possible and desirable to do so through a variety of procedures that isolate subjects and researchers from information that might influence their behavior. Ways to maximize this independence are presented in Chapter 6.

ASSUMPTION 3

The third basic assumption of the quantitative paradigm is that the goal of research is to develop generalizable characterizations of reality. The generalizability of a piece of research refers to its applicability to other subjects, times, and settings. The concept of generalizability leads to the classification of qualitative research as *nomothetic,* or relating to general or universal principles. Quantitative researchers recognize the limits of generalizability as threats to the validity (discussed in greater detail in Chapter 7) of a study; however, they believe generalizability is an achievable aim and research that fails to be reasonably generalizable is flawed.

ASSUMPTION 4

The fourth basic assumption of the quantitative paradigm is that causes and effects can be determined and differentiated from one another. Quantitative researchers are careful to differentiate experimental research from nonexperimental research on the basis that causal inferences can only be drawn if the researcher is able to manipulate an independent variable (the "presumed cause") in a controlled fashion while observing the effect of the manipulation on a dependent variable (the "presumed effect"). Quantitative researchers attempt to eliminate or control extraneous factors that might interfere with the relationship between the independent and dependent variables (see Chapters 9 and 11 for more information on experimental and nonexperimental research).

ASSUMPTION 5

The final assumption of the quantitative paradigm is that research is value free. The controlled, objective nature of quantitative research is assumed to eliminate the influence of investigator opinions and societal norms on the facts that are discovered. Inquiry is seen as the objective discovery of truths and the investigator the impartial discoverer of these truths.

Quantitative Methods

The adoption of these quantitative assumptions has major implications for the methods of quantitative research. Five methodological issues are discussed in relation to the assumptions that underlie the quantitative paradigm: theory, selection, measurement, manipulation, and control. These issues are summarized in Table 5–2. Quotes from a single quantitative piece of research are used to illustrate the way in which each of these methodological issues is handled within the quantitative paradigm.

THEORY

The first methodological issue relates to the role of theory within a study. Quantitative researchers are expected to articulate an *a priori* theory, that is, theory developed in advance of the conduct of the research. The purpose of the research is then to determine whether the components of the theory can be confirmed. This

TABLE 5-2	Methods of the Three Research Paradigms		

	Paradigm		
Method	*Quantitative*	*Qualitative*	*Single-System*
Theory	A priori	Grounded	A priori
Number and selection of subjects	Groups, random	Small number, purposive	One, purposive
Measurement tools	Instruments	Human	Instruments
Type of data	Numerical	Language	Numerical
Manipulation	Present	Absent	Present
Control	Maximized	Minimized	Flexible

top-down notion of theory development was presented in Chapter 2 on theory and Chapter 4 on problem development. Klein and colleagues[6] used a quantitative research approach when they compared the effects of exercise and lifestyle modification on the overuse symptoms in polio survivors. As such, an a priori theoretical perspective guided the study:

> Symptoms of upper-extremity overuse are also common among people with mobility impairments. In such cases shoulder disorders result when the arms are used repetitively to compensate for weak leg muscles during weight-bearing tasks such as getting up from a chair or using an assistive device while walking.... If lower-extremity weakness predisposes to upper-extremity overuse, then the relevant lower-extremity muscle groups must be strengthened and/or behavioral patterns leading to overuse must be altered.[6(pp708-709)]

The elements of this theory are (1) if shoulder disorders in polio survivors result from overuse secondary to lower-extremity weakness, (2) then treatment that improves lower-extremity muscle strength or alters the behavioral patterns leading to overuse should improve the overuse symptoms. The purpose of the study, then, was to test this "if-then" hypothesis. A further indication of the importance of theory to this study is seen in the prediction of outcomes based on the theory:

> We predicted that the subjects who received both interventions [exercise and lifestyle modification

instruction] would show the most improvement, and this improvement would be associated with an increase in leg strength.[6(p709)]

SELECTION

The second methodological issue relates to the generalizability of the research. Because quantitative researchers want to be able to generalize their findings to subjects similar to those studied, they often articulate an elaborate set of inclusion and exclusion criteria so that readers can determine the group to which the research can be generalized:

> Subjects were recruited from a pool of 194 polio survivors.... Other inclusion criteria for this study were bilateral knee-extensor and hip-extensor strength ≥ grade 3 but less than a grade 5 on manual muscle testing and shoulder pain with daily activity for at least 30 days. Exclusion criteria included any major disabilities or conditions unrelated to polio that could cause weakness or overuse problems (e.g., stroke, amputation, inflammatory arthritis...), serious illness such as heart or lung disease that could make exertion during a strength test unsafe (e.g., severe emphysema, poorly controlled asthma, recent heart attack), history of shoulder trauma, and recent fracture or surgery.... Subjects with significant upper-extremity weakness who could not use their arms to push out of a chair were also excluded.[6(p709)]

Once individuals are selected for a quantitative study, the way they are placed into treatment groups is also viewed as an important control mechanism, with random assignment to groups being the preferred way to maximize the chances that the groups have similar characteristics at the start of the study.

MEASUREMENT

The third methodological issue relates to a desire for a high level of precision in measurements as an expression of the belief in an objective reality. Klein and colleagues carefully document their measurement procedures and their own reliability in using the measurement tools used within their study:

> The dynamometer was placed proximal to the malleoli on the anterior aspect of the tibia. For each muscle group, the maximum force generated in each of 3 trials was recorded. Subjects had a minimum of 30 seconds to rest between trials. The reliability of these measurements was established previously in a sample of 2 polio survivors and 4 adults with no history of polio.... All [intraclass correlation coefficients] were greater than .910, with the exception of hip extension on the dominant side, which was .787.[6(p709)]

Measurement theory, presented later in this text, is largely based on the concept that researchers use imperfect measurement tools to estimate the "true" characteristics of a phenomenon of interest and that the best measures are those that come closest to this "truth" on a consistent basis.

MANIPULATION

The fourth methodological issue is related to the role of manipulation within a study. Quantitative researchers believe that the best research for documenting the effect of interventions is that which allows one to determine causes and effects in response to controlled manipulations of the experimenter. Klein and colleagues show this preference for experimental evidence when they identify one source of evidence, clinical observation, as insufficient to establish the causal link their study addresses:

> Based on clinical observation, survivors who comply with the recommended changes [muscle strengthening and lifestyle changes] often experience a reduction in their pain and fatigue. To date, however, there have been no published studies that compare the effectiveness of lifestyle modification therapy with exercise in reducing pain and maintaining function in polio survivors. Therefore, this study sought to compare the effectiveness of 2 interventions (exercise and lifestyle modification instruction) alone and in combination in alleviating shoulder overuse symptoms in polio survivors with lower-extremity weakness.[6(p709)]

Quantitative researchers place a great deal of emphasis on this type of controlled manipulation as the only valid source of evidence for the effectiveness of interventions.

CONTROL

The fifth and final methodological issue is related to the control of extraneous factors within the research design. Klein and colleagues included many control elements in their study. Each subject received similar education and educational materials at the beginning of the study: a visit with a therapist, an educational videotape, and printed materials. Intensity, duration, and frequency of exercise were standardized across subjects. In addition, the total time spent with a therapist in follow-up visits across the study was the same across subjects, regardless of group assignment. Because of these controls, the treatments administered within this study likely differed from routine clinical practice, with more initial education and more regular follow-up than might be typical. Researchers who adopt the quantitative paradigm generally believe that control of extraneous variables is critical to establishment of cause-and-effect relationships, even when such control leads to the implementation of experimental procedures that may not be fully representative of typical clinical practices.

These, then, are examples of how five methodological issues—theory, selection, measurement, manipulation, and control—are handled by researchers who work within the framework of the quantitative paradigm.

■ QUALITATIVE PARADIGM

Just as the mechanistic view of Newtonian physics provided the roots for the development of the quantitative paradigm, the relativistic view of quantum mechanics provided the roots for the development of the qualitative paradigm. Zukav contrasted the "old" Newtonian physics with the "new" quantum physics:

> The old physics assumes that there is an external world which exists apart from us. It further assumes that we can observe, measure, and speculate about the external world without changing it. ...The new physics, quantum mechanics, tells us clearly that it is not possible to observe reality without changing it. If we observe a certain particle collision experiment, not only do we have no way of proving that the results would have been the same if we have not been watching it, all that we know indicates that it would not have been the same, because the results that we got were affected by the fact that we were looking for it.[2(pp30-31)]

Because the quantitative paradigm has proved inadequate even for the discipline of physics, a seemingly "hard" science, qualitative researchers argue that there is little justification for continuing to apply it to the "soft" sciences in which human behavior is studied.

Assumptions of the Qualitative Paradigm

The assumptions that form the basis for the qualitative paradigm are antithetical to the assumptions of the quantitative paradigm. Once again Lincoln and Guba's[1] concepts, but not their terminology, form the basis for this section of the chapter. What Lincoln and Guba label the *naturalistic paradigm* is referred to in this text as the *qualitative paradigm*. Table 5–1 provides an overview of the assumptions of the qualitative paradigm.

ASSUMPTION 1

The first assumption of the qualitative paradigm is that the world consists of multiple constructed realities. "Multiple" means that there are always several versions of reality. "Constructed" means that participants attach meaning to events that occur within their lives, and that this meaning is an inseparable component of the events themselves. Refer to Box 5–2 for a simple test of the phenomenon of multiple constructed realities. It is easy to demonstrate how multiple constructed realities may be present within clinician–patient interactions. For example, if one man states that his physician is cold and unfeeling, that is his reality. If a woman states that the same physician is professional and candid, that is her reality. The notion of a single, objective reality is rejected. Researchers who adopt the qualitative paradigm believe that it is fruitless to try to determine the physician's "true" manner because the physician's demeanor does not exist apart from how it is perceived by different patients.

BOX 5-2

Instructions: Count the number of "F"s in the quote below:

"FABULOUS FITNESS FOLLOWS FROM YEARS OF FREQUENT WORKOUTS COMBINED WITH FOCUSED FOOD CHOICES."

See solution on p. 68.

ASSUMPTION 2

The second assumption of the qualitative paradigm is that investigator and subject are interdependent, that is, the process of inquiry itself changes both the investigator and the subject. Whereas quantitative paradigm researchers seek to eliminate what is viewed as undesirable interdependence of investigator and subject, qualitative paradigm researchers accept this interdependence as inevitable and even desirable. For example, a qualitative researcher would recognize that a physician who agrees to participate in a study of clinician demeanor is likely to change, at least in subtle ways, his or her demeanor during the period that he or she is observed.

ASSUMPTION 3

The third assumption of the qualitative paradigm is that knowledge is time and context dependent. Qualitative paradigm researchers reject the nomothetic approach and its concept of generalizability. In this sense, then, qualitative research is *idiographic,* meaning that it pertains to a particular case in a particular time and context. The goal of qualitative research is a deep understanding of the particular. Researchers who adopt the qualitative paradigm hope that this particular understanding may lead to insights about similar situations. Although not generalizable in the quantitative tradition, themes or concepts found consistently in qualitative research with a small number of subjects may represent essential components of phenomena that, with further investigation, would also be found in larger samples.

ASSUMPTION 4

The fourth assumption of the qualitative paradigm is that it is impossible to distinguish causes from effects. The whole notion of cause is tied to the idea of prediction, control, and an objective reality. Researchers who adopt the qualitative paradigm believe it is more useful to describe and interpret events than it is to attempt to control them to establish oversimplified causes and effects. In the physician demeanor example, qualitative researchers believe that it would be impossible to determine whether a certain physician demeanor caused better patient outcomes or whether certain patient outcomes caused different physician demeanors. Because of their belief in the inability to separate causes from effects, qualitative researchers would instead focus on describing the multiple forces that shape physician–patient interactions.

ASSUMPTION 5

The fifth assumption of the qualitative paradigm is that inquiry is value bound. This value-ladenness is exemplified in the type of questions that are asked, the way in which constructs are defined and measured, and the interpretation of the results of research. The traditional view of scientists is that they are capable of "dispassionate judgment and unbiased inquiry."[7(p109)] Qualitative researchers, however, believe that all research is influenced by the values of the scientists who conduct research and the sources that fund research. The status of research about the use of hormone replacement therapy during menopause provides one example of the value-ladenness of the research enterprise. In July 2002, the results of a randomized controlled trial of combined estrogen and progestin versus placebo on coronary heart disease and invasive breast cancer for postmenopausal women were published.[8] The study had been halted in May 2002, approximately 3 years earlier than planned, because increased risks for development of coronary heart disease and invasive breast cancer were found. The results of this trial received widespread publicity and comment, in both the popular media and the health care literature. The following exchange, from a U.S. National Public Radio science program, illustrates some of the ways in which the health care and research environment may be influenced by cultural values and business interests:

Dr. GRADY [physician guest]: I object to the word "replacement" and try never to use it. And that's because a normal postmenopausal woman is not sick. This is a normal transition in life, just like puberty.

FLATOW [program host]: This whole idea of using hormone replacement to create this so-called fountain of youth for women, is this a male-dominated research item made by a man that...

Dr. RICHARDSON [physician guest]: Well, I don't think there's been enough research done on this in general anyway. I mean, we don't know what the physiology of hot flashes is. And one of my fond hopes with all of this publicity is that maybe someone will fund more research so we can figure out what causes hot flashes and fix them.

FLATOW: Well, I was thinking more as a marketing technique to make money on a replacement therapy more than, you know, if men had to do it for them themselves, they wouldn't have been so fast to do it, as they used to talk about men and birth control pills.

Dr. BARRETT-CONNOR [physician guest]: Well, you know, it's very interesting that now that testosterone patches are being developed for men in their older years when their testosterone levels fall—this is a fairly popular treatment, but it's been hard to get trials of it because both the scientists and the people who sponsor studies are worried about prostate cancer.[9]

In this short exchange in the popular media, we hear many value-laden questions: whether male-dominated health care and research interests influenced the widespread adoption of hormone replacement therapy even in the absence of randomized controlled trials, why mechanisms behind menopausal symptoms haven't been studied more fully, whether economic factors related to the profitability of hormone replacement therapy influenced the research agenda, and how safety concerns may be influencing trials for testosterone replacement therapy for men.

Researchers who adopt the qualitative paradigm recognize that they are unable to separate values from inquiry. They do not believe that it is productive to pretend that science is objective, particularly in light of questions such as those raised by the recent hormone replacement therapy controversy.

Qualitative Methods

These five assumptions have an enormous impact on the conduct of qualitative paradigm research. The roles of theory, selection, measurement, manipulation, and control are all vastly different in qualitative research than in quantitative research, as summarized in Table 5–2. Dudgeon and associates[10] used the qualitative paradigm to structure their study of physical disability and the experience of chronic pain. This study is used to provide examples of the methods that flow from adoption of the beliefs of the paradigm.

THEORY

The first methodological issue relates to the role of theory. Because researchers who adopt the qualitative paradigm accept the concept of multiple constructed realities, they do not begin their inquiry with a researcher-developed theoretical framework. They begin the research with an idea of what concepts or constructs may be important to an understanding of a certain phenomenon, but they recognize that the participants in the inquiry will define other versions of what is important. A rigid theoretical framework of the researcher would constrain the direction of the inquiry and might provide a less than full description of the phenomenon of interest. Dudgeon and colleagues express this in the broad, exploratory language of their purpose statement:

> The purpose of this study was to explore the nature of pain that accompanies physical disability, getting an insider's views about experiencing and dealing with pain as part of daily living and communicating.[10(p229)]

In addition, the authors do not advance a set of predictions about their findings, as was the case with the quantitative study example cited earlier in the chapter.

SELECTION

The second methodological issue relates to the way in which subjects are selected. Rather than selecting a randomized group of individuals, qualitative researchers purposely select individuals who they believe will be able to lend insight to the research problem. Dudgeon and colleagues describe just such a method:

> We asked the health care liaisons to identify participants who they regarded as representative of the specific clinical population [spinal cord injury, amputation, or cerebral palsy] and who were particularly fluent in describing their views.[10(p230)]

In this example, purposive sampling procedures led to the selection of only nine individuals, three from each of the diagnostic groups of interest. Most traditional quantitative researchers would find this sample to be insufficient because it would not likely be representative of a larger group and because small samples do not lend themselves to statistical analysis. Because neither representativeness nor statistical analysis are required for a qualitative study to be valid, these issues are not considered to be problematic.

MEASUREMENT

The third methodological issue relates to the primary measurement tool of qualitative research, the "human instrument." Because of the complexity of the multiple realities the qualitative researcher is seeking to describe, a reactive, thinking instrument is needed, as noted by Dudgeon and associates:

> The interviews were open ended and relatively unstructured.... Because we wanted the participants to guide the interviews, the protocol was flexible and the order of discussion often shifted, depending on the direction taken by the individual.[10(p230)]

The data collected in qualitative studies are usually not numerical, but, rather, are verbal and consist of feelings and perceptions rather than presumed facts. Researchers gather a great deal of descriptive data about the particular situation they are studying so that they can provide a "rich" or "thick" description of the situation.

MANIPULATION AND CONTROL

Fourth and fifth, the qualitative researcher does not manipulate or control the research setting. Rather, the setting is manipulated in unpredictable ways by the interaction between the investigator and the participants. The mere fact that the researcher is present or asks certain questions is bound to influence the participants and their perception of the situation.

The natural setting is used for qualitative research. Because everything is time and context dependent, researchers who adopt the qualitative paradigm believe there is little to be gained—and much to be lost—from creating an artificial study situation. Dudgeon and associates, for example, interviewed participants in their homes or in the researchers' offices, whichever was preferred by the participant. Researchers guided by the quantitative paradigm would probably view this as an undesirable source of uncontrolled variation. Being guided by the qualitative paradigm, however, meant that researchers were unconcerned about the location of the interviews and presumably assumed that the location preferred by the participant would yield the richest conversation about their pain experiences.

It is clear from this example that these five methodological issues—theory, selection, measurement, manipulation, and control—are handled very differently within a qualitative framework compared with a quantitative one. Theory unfolds during the study instead of directing the study. Small numbers of participants are selected for their unique ability to contribute to the study. Measurement is done with a "human instrument" who can react and redirect the data gathering process rather than being done with a standardized measurement protocol. The object of the study is observed rather than manipulated. And, finally, the setting for data collection is natural and uncontrolled rather than artificial and tightly controlled.

SINGLE-SYSTEM PARADIGM

The single-system paradigm developed out of a concern that the use of traditional group research methods focused away from the unit of clinical interest: the individual. Assume that a group study of the effectiveness of a particular gait training technique on gait velocity is implemented with 30 patients who have undergone transtibial amputation. If gait velocity improves for 10 patients, remains the same for 10 patients, and declines for 10 patients, then the average velocity for the group does not change very much and the group conclusion is likely to be that the treatment had no effect. This group conclusion ignores the fact that the treatment was effective for 10 patients but detrimental for 10 other patients. A clinically relevant conclusion might be that the treatment has the potential to improve velocity but that clinicians should also recognize that the opposite effect is also seen in some patients. An appropriate focus for future research would be the identification of those types of patients for whom this technique is effective. Unfortunately, this type of subgroup analysis rarely occurs, and practitioners are left with the general group conclusion that the new technique is not effective. Single-system research eliminates the group conclusion and focuses on treatment effects for individuals.

Box 5–1 lists several different names for single-system research. Kazdin[11] uses the term *single-case experimental design* to emphasize the controlled manipulation that is characteristic of this paradigm. Ottenbacher[12(p45)] uses the term *single-system* rather than the more common *single-subject* because there are some instances in which the single unit of interest would itself be a group rather than an individual. For example, a rehabilitation administrator might wish to study departmental productivity before and after a reorganization. If the concern was not with changes in individual therapist productivity, but

only with the productivity of the department as a whole, then the effect of the reorganization could be studied as a single system. Because *single system* is the more inclusive term, it is used throughout this text.

Assumptions of the Single-System Paradigm

The basic assumption of the single-system paradigm is that the effectiveness of treatment is subject and setting dependent. Single-system researchers believe that research should reflect the idiographic nature of practice by focusing on the study of individuals. Except for this focus on individuals rather than groups, the rest of the assumptions of the single-system paradigm are those of the quantitative paradigm, as shown in Table 5–1. In fact, the single-system paradigm focuses exclusively on experimental problems in which there is active manipulation of the individual under study.

The single-system paradigm is sometimes confused with the clinical case report or case study. The two are very different. The case report or case study is a description, very often a retrospective description, of a course of treatment of an individual (see Chapter 12). Single-system research, on the other hand, uses a systematic process of introduction and withdrawal of treatments to allow for controlled assessment of the effects of a treatment (see Chapter 10).

Single-System Methods

Because many assumptions are shared between the quantitative and single-system paradigms, many methods are shared as well, as shown in Table 5–2. Hannah and Hudak's[13] study of splinting for radial nerve palsy is used to illustrate these methods in practice. In this study, three different types of splints were compared for an individual with radial nerve palsy: static volar wrist cock-up splint, dynamic tenodesis suspensio splint, and dorsal wrist cock-up splint with dynamic finger extension splint.

THEORY

First, single-system paradigm research generally operates from an *a priori* theoretical foundation, as illustrated in the introductory material in which the rationale for intervening with splinting is established:

> One of the challenges for hand therapists during this period of nerve regeneration is to fabricate a splint that prevents over-stretching of denervated extensor musculature while maximizing hand function.[13(p195)]

Thus, splints that are consistent with this theoretical framework should include elements that position and protect the hand to prevent over-stretching and elements that address functional use of the hand.

SELECTION

Second, selection of the individual for study is purposive. Single-system researchers would not choose to study someone for whom they did not believe the interventions were uniquely appropriate. This is in contrast to a group approach in which 30 participants who had radial nerve palsy would be studied with a randomly assigned splint. How likely is it that the assigned splint would be uniquely appropriate for each of these 30 subjects? As noted by Hannah and Hudak:

> A randomized controlled trial is not the best way to determine the treatment of choice for a specific patient, since results are based on average improvement scores for all subjects and therefore do not provide information on the performance of individual subjects.[13(pp195-196)]

The single-system paradigm requires that the individual studied have a specific need for the treatment implemented and enables the researcher to observe treatment effects in that individual.

MEASUREMENT

Third, precise measurement is an integral part of the single-system paradigm. Repeated measures taken during baseline and treatment phases are compared. Thus, measurement accuracy and reliability are critical to the ability to draw conclusions about the effects of treatment. This measurement focus is apparent in Hannah and Hudak's study:

> Four established outcomes measures were chosen to assess the following variables—performance of the upper extremity during activities of daily living (Test Evaluant Les Members Superièurs des Personnes Agèes, TEMPA), self-reported level of disability (Disabilities of the Arm, Shoulder and Hand questionnaire, DASH), self-perceived performance in activities or daily living (Canadian Occupational Performance Measure, COPM), and strength of specific muscle groups (manual muscle testing).... High reliability as well as content, face, and preliminary construct validity in this population have been reported [for the TEMPA]. Preliminary results provide evidence of the reliability and convergent validity of the DASH.... Preliminary results provide evidence of test-retest reliability of the COPM as well as of content validity and responsiveness to clinical change.[13(pp197-198)]

This focus on the use of standardized tools with documented reliability and validity is important to most single-system designs.

MANIPULATION AND CONTROL

Experimental manipulation is an essential part of the definition of single-system research. This is illustrated in Hannah and Hudak's[13] study by their manipulation of four phases of the study: baseline without any splint, with the static cock-up splint, with the dynamic tenodesis splint, and with the dynamic finger extension splint.

Finally, control of extraneous factors is important in the conduct of single-system research, as it was with quantitative research. Hannah and Hudak[13] controlled the experimental setting by randomly determining the order in which the patient would test the splints, by having the same therapist fabricate each splint, and by standardizing the instructions for wear and care of each splint. In addition, the patient was asked to keep a log showing the time spent wearing each splint, in part to establish that each splint had received a fair trial during the 3-week period of time assigned for its use. Table 5–2 indicates, however, that the control in single-system paradigm research may be more flexible than that of traditional group designs. In group designs, researchers usually attempt to control the nature of the treatment administered so that all individuals within the group receive approximately the same treatment. With the single-system designs, the treatment can be administered as it would be in the clinic. Thus, the intervention can be tailored to accommodate scheduling changes, status changes, or varying patient moods. Chapter 10 presents several designs that use the general methods associated with the single-system paradigm.

■ RELATIONSHIPS AMONG THE RESEARCH PARADIGMS

There are those who believe that the paradigms are mutually exclusive, that in adopting the assumptions of one paradigm the assumptions of the others must be forsaken. Lincoln and Guba make a case for the separateness of the quantitative and qualitative paradigms:

> Postpositivism is an entirely new paradigm, *not* reconcilable with the old....We are dealing with an entirely new system of ideas based on fundamentally *different*—indeed sharply contrasting—assumptions.... What is needed is a transformation, not an add-on. That the world is round cannot be added to the idea that the world is flat [emphasis in original].[1(p33)]

A more moderate view is that the assumptions underlying the different paradigms are relative rather than absolute. Relative assumptions need not be applied to every situation; they can be applied when appropriate to a given research problem. This text adopts the moderate view

that all forms of study have the potential to add to knowledge and understanding. The contrasting assumptions of the paradigms can be managed as we all manage many belief-action clashes on a daily basis. For example, many people believe that the world is round. However, in daily activities they act as if the world is flat by using flat maps to get from place to place and by visualizing the part of the world they are most familiar with as flat. They hold one belief, but find it useful to suspend that belief in their daily activities.

Likewise, a belief in multiple constructed realities need not prevent one from studying a certain problem from the perspective of a single objective reality. A belief that it is impossible to study any phenomenon without affecting it in some way need not prevent one from attempting to minimize these effects through the design control methods developed in Chapters 6 through 16. The potential contributions of the different research paradigms are best realized when investigators recognize the assumptions that undergird their methods and make explicit the limitations of their methods.

Furthermore, the development of a line of research on a particular topic may benefit from the use of different research paradigms at different points in time. Consider the example of research on constraint-induced movement therapy, a technique that restrains the unaffected upper extremity of a person with hemiplegia to force the use of the hemiparetic limb. Over the past 20 years or so, this technique has been studied through all three research paradigms. In 1981, an early report on the technique used a single-subject experimental design with an adult with hemiplegia.[14] In 1989, a group quantitative paradigm study of the technique was reported with adults with stroke and head injury.[15] By the early 2000s, the technique had been extended to new aspects of stroke rehabilitation (treating aphasia with constraint-induced principles applied to communication, studied through quantitative paradigm methods)[16] and to new patient populations (children with hemiplegia, studied with case report methods).[17]

Basic science research in the quantitative tradition has also been conducted on this treatment technique, both with human participants assessed with magnetic resonance imaging[18] and with rats assessed with skill testing and measurement of tissue losses.[19] Finally, a qualitative study was published in 2003, looking at perceptions and experiences of patients who participated in constraint-induced therapy home programs.[20] This brief, incomplete history of research on constraint-induced therapy demonstrates the complex interplay between what is known and not known about a topic and the ways in which new knowledge about a topic can be developed.

The moderate view adopted in this text also implies that the paradigms can be mixed within a study to address different aspects of a research problem. For example, Bat-Chava's[21] study of the impact of child and family characteristics on sibling relationships of deaf children combined quantitative and qualitative methods. Parents of 37 children who were deaf were interviewed about the quality of sibling relationships. In addition to the identification of themes about sibling relationships from the interview data, as would be expected in a qualitative study, the authors also constructed a scale to measure the quality of sibling relationships. They then used this scale in a quantitative way to search for factors such as birth order, gender, family size, and so forth that could explain differences in sibling relationships in different families.

Patton, in his text on qualitative research methods, offers a contemporary analogy about the mixing of research paradigms:

> Mixing parts of different approaches is a matter of philosophical and methodological controversy.... In practice, it is altogether possible, as we have seen, to combine approaches, and to so do creatively. Just as machines that were originally created for separate functions such as printing, faxing, scanning, and copying have now been combined into a single integrated technological unit, so too methods that were originally created as distinct, stand-alone approaches can now be combined into more sophisticated and multifunctional designs.[22(p252)]

■ SUMMARY

Research paradigms are the beliefs that underlie the conduct of inquiry. The dominant paradigm in rehabilitation research is currently the quantitative paradigm, which emphasizes generalizable measurement of a single objective reality with groups of subjects that are often manipulated by the investigator. The competing qualitative paradigm emphasizes the study of multiple constructed realities through in-depth study of particular settings, with an emphasis on determining underlying meanings within a particular context. The competing single-system paradigm includes many of the beliefs of the quantitative paradigm with the important exception of the concept of generalizability; single-system studies look at changes in individuals, because the individual is the unit of interest within a discipline such as rehabilitation. Some researchers believe that adoption of one paradigm precludes the use of other paradigms; others believe that all three paradigms are useful when applied to appropriate questions.

REFERENCES

1. Lincoln YS, Guba EG. *Naturalistic Inquiry.* Beverly Hills, Calif: Sage Publications; 1985.
2. Zukav G. *The Dancing Wu Li Masters: An Overview of the New Physics.* New York, NY: Bantam Books; 1979.
3. Irby DM. Shifting paradigms of research in medical education. *Acad Med.* 1990;65:622-623.
4. Phillips DC. After the wake: postpositivistic educational thought. *Educ Res.* 1983;12:4-12.
5. Rosenthal R. *Experimenter Effects in Behavioral Research.* Enlarged ed. New York, NY: Irvington Publishers; 1976.
6. Klein MG, Whyte J, Esquenazi A, Keenan MA, Costello R. A comparison of the effects of exercise and lifestyle modification on the resolution of overuse symptoms of the shoulder in polio survivors: a preliminary study. *Arch Phys Med Rehabil.* 2002;83:708-713.
7. Mahoney MJ. *Scientist as Subject: The Psychological Imperative.* Cambridge, Mass: Ballinger Publishing; 1976.
8. Rossouw JE, Anderson GL, Prentice RL, et al. Risks and benefits of estrogen plus progestin in healthy post-menopausal women: principal results from the Women's Health Initiative randomized controlled trial. *JAMA.* 2002;288:321-333.
9. Risks and benefits of hormone replacement therapy. Distributed by: National Public Radio; July 26, 2002.

10. Dudgeon BJ, Gerrard BC, Jensen MP, Rhodes LA, Tyler EJ. Physical disability and the experience of chronic pain. *Arch Phys Med Rehabil.* 2002;83:229-235.

11. Kazdin AE. Observational research: case-control and cohort designs. In: Kazdin AE, ed. *Research Design in Clinical Psychology.* 4th ed. Boston, Mass: Allyn & Bacon; 2003.

12. Ottenbacher KJ. *Evaluating Clinical Change: Strategies for Occupational and Physical Therapists.* Baltimore, Md: Williams & Wilkins; 1986.

13. Hannah SD, Hudak PL. Splinting and radial nerve palsy: a single-subject experiment. *J Hand Ther.* 2001;14:195-201.

14. Ostendorf CG, Wolf SL. Effect of forced use of the upper extremity of a hemiplegic patient on changes in function: a single-case design. *Phys Ther.* 1981;61:1022-1028.

15. Wolf SL, Lecraw DE, Barton L, Jann BB. Forced use of hemiplegic upper extremities to reverse the effect of learned nonuse among chronic stroke and head-injured patients. *Exp Neurol.* 1989;104:125-132.

16. Pulvermuller F, Neininger B, Elbert T, et al. Constraint-induced therapy of chronic aphasia after stroke. *Stroke.* 2001;32:1621-1626.

17. Glover JE, Mateer CA, Yoell C, Speed S. The effectiveness of constraint-induced movement therapy in two young children with hemiplegia. *Pediatr Rehabil.* 2002;5:125-131.

18. Schaechter JD, Kraft E, Hilliard TS, et al. Motor recovery and cortical reorganization after constraint-induced movement therapy in stroke patient: a preliminary study. *Neurorehabil Neural Repair.* 2002;16:326-338.

19. DeBow SB, Davies ML, Clarke HL, Colbourne F. Constraint-induced movement therapy and rehabilitation exercises lessen motor deficits and volume of brain injury after striatal hemorrhagic stroke in rats. *Stroke.* 2003;34:1021-1026.

20. Gillot AJ, Holder-Walls A, Kurtz JR, Varley NC. Perceptions and experiences of two survivors of stroke who participated in constraint-induced movement therapy home programs. *Am J Occup Ther.* 2003;57:168-176.

21. Bat-Chava Y. Sibling relationships of deaf children: the impact of child and family characteristics. *Rehabil Psychol.* 2002;47:73-91.

22. Patton MQ. *Qualitative Research and Evaluation Methods.* 3rd ed. Thousand Oaks, Calif: Sage Publications; 2002.

BOX 5-2 (continued from page 60)

Solution: If you are like most adults, you counted seven "F"s in the sample. Read it again: "FABULOUS FITNESS FOLLOWS FROM YEARS OF FREQUENT WORKOUTS COMBINED WITH FOCUSED FOOD CHOICES."

There are 7 "F" sounds (fabulous, fitness, follows, from, frequent, focused, food), but 8 "F"s (of). People who understand the relationship between letters and sounds intuitively search for the "F" sound when doing this exercise. In doing so, the task that is completed is different than the task that was assigned. If it is possible to interpret even a simple letter-counting exercise in different ways, think of the difficulty in developing "objective" measures that are more complicated! Qualitative researchers believe that such attempts are futile and instead embrace the depth of understanding that accompanies different ways of seeing the world.

Design Overview

Identification of Variables
Analysis of Research Titles
Levels and Types of Independent
Variables
Dependent Variables

Design Dimensions
Research Purposes
Timing of Data Collection
Manipulation
Manipulation Is Retrospective
The Variable Is Nonmanipulable
The Researcher Chooses Not to Manipulate
*The Independent Variable Is a Component of
the Dependent Variable*
*Interpretation Based on Controlled
Manipulation*

Control
Implementation of the
Independent Variable
Selection and Assignment of
Participants
Extraneous Variables in the Setting
Extraneous Variables Related to
Participants
Measurement Variation
Information Received by
Participants and Researchers
Incomplete Information
Masking of Participants
Masking of Researchers

Summary

Research design is a creative process during which the investigators determine how they can best answer their research questions. A prerequisite to understanding research design is the ability to identify the different types of variables within a design. Once the variables are defined, research designs can be analyzed based on three basic dimensions: the purpose of the research, the timing of the data collection, and the extent to which the researcher manipulates participants. Once these dimensions are determined, researchers use a variety of techniques to control various aspects of the research process. This chapter analyzes the variables within research studies, presents a matrix of research types, and outlines ways in which controls are implemented within research designs. Even though this chapter on design is presented separately from earlier chapters on problem development and later chapters on validity and data analysis, recognize that these phases of the research process are, in fact, inseparable. The research problem influences the design, which, in turn, influences the validity of the research and the analysis of the data.

IDENTIFICATION OF VARIABLES

A *variable* is some characteristic that takes different forms within a study. In contrast, a *constant* takes only one form within a study. If differences between range-of-motion values for men and women are studied, then gender is a variable. If range-of-motion values for women only are studied, then gender is a constant. When research is used to describe phenomena or relationships, then researchers do not need to differentiate among different types of variables. When the purpose of research is to analyze differences among groups or treatments, then it is important to differentiate between *independent* and *dependent* variables within the study. According to Kerlinger, "an *independent variable* is the *presumed* cause of the *dependent variable,* the *presumed* effect."[1(p32)] An independent variable is also sometimes called a *factor.* Unfortunately, authors do not always explicitly identify the number and character of the variables within their studies. Three examples are presented here to illustrate a process by which readers can discern the often complicated sets of variables within research studies.

Analysis of Research Titles

The article title of a published research study presents preliminary information about the independent and dependent variables. Preliminary identification of the independent and dependent variables in three research reports is presented in Table 6–1, based solely on the information contained in the title of each article.[2-4]

Levels and Types of Independent Variables

A full description of each independent variable includes the *levels* of the independent variable. The levels of the independent variable are the forms that the independent variable takes within the study. The three articles whose titles are listed in Table 6–1 are used to demonstrate what is meant by levels of the independent variable. The studies are more complex than their titles alone indicate.

Identification of the independent variable in the first example, Carter and associates' research on magnet therapy for treatment of wrist pain, is straightforward.[2] The design is diagrammed in

TABLE 6–1 Independent and Dependent Variables in Three Research Article Titles		
Title	*Independent Variable*	*Dependent Variable*
The effectiveness of magnet therapy for treatment of wrist pain attributed to carpal tunnel syndrome[2]	Magnet therapy	Wrist pain
Effect of high-voltage pulsed current and alternating current on macromolecular leakage in hamster cheek pouch microcirculation[3]	Current	Macromolecular leakage
Effects of positioning and exercise on intracranial pressure in a neurosurgical intensive care unit[4]	Positioning and exercise	Intracranial pressure

Figure 6–1. There was one independent variable, which could be titled "group" or "magnet therapy." There were two levels of group: "true magnet," which was the experimental treatment, and "sham magnet," which was the control treatment. The dependent variable was "wrist pain reduction" as measured on a visual analog scale at the beginning of the study and at various points during and after treatment. Concisely stated, the purpose of the study was to determine whether there was a difference in pain reduction between the true magnet and the sham magnet groups. The levels of the independent variable in this study represent different groups of participants. Therefore, the term for this type of independent variable is a *between-groups* independent variable, or an independent variable with "independent levels."

The second example, a study of the effect of electrical stimulation on the microcirculation of hamster cheek pouches, is more complex than the magnet study. As diagrammed in Figure 6–2, Taylor and associates examined seven different groups of hamsters, each receiving a different form of electrical stimulation, across three different time periods.[3] The first independent variable, therefore, was "group" with seven levels: control, cathodal high-voltage pulsed current (HVPC) at 90% of visible motor threshold (VMT),

cathodal HVPC at 50% of VMT, cathodal HVPC at 10% of VMT, anodal HVPC at 90% of VMT, anodal HVPC at 50% of VMT, and alternating current at 90% of VMT. The dependent variables were derived from histological images that allowed counting of the number of leakage sites in the microcirculation, the area of the leakage, and the brightness of the leakage. The images were collected at 1.5, 3, 4, and 5 minutes after the start of treatment, with the 1.5-minute data being used as a baseline against which to compare the other three times. Thus, time was a second independent variable, with three levels: 3 minutes, 4 minutes, and 5 minutes after treatment. The "group" variable in this study, like that in the magnet study, is a between-groups variable, or a variable with independent levels. With a between-groups independent variable, each participant appears in only one level of the variable. The time variable is a different type of independent variable because each participant appears in each level of the independent variable. This type of independent variable is known as a *within-group* variable, or a variable with "dependent levels."

In the third example, Brimioulle and colleagues examined the effects of positioning and exercise on intracranial pressure in a neurosurgical intensive care unit.[4] Their study design adds

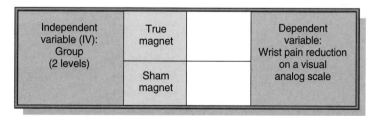

FIGURE 6–1. Study of the effect of magnet therapy on wrist pain. One independent variable, "group," was used. Measures of wrist pain were recorded at the beginning of the study and at various points during and after treatment. For one of the most important comparisons between groups, the authors took the difference between post-treatment and pretreatment pain to form the dependent variable, "wrist pain reduction."
Design presented in Carter R, Hall T, Aspy CB, Mold J. The effectiveness of magnet therapy for treatment of wrist pain attributed to carpal tunnel syndrome. *J Fam Pract*. 2002;51:38-40.

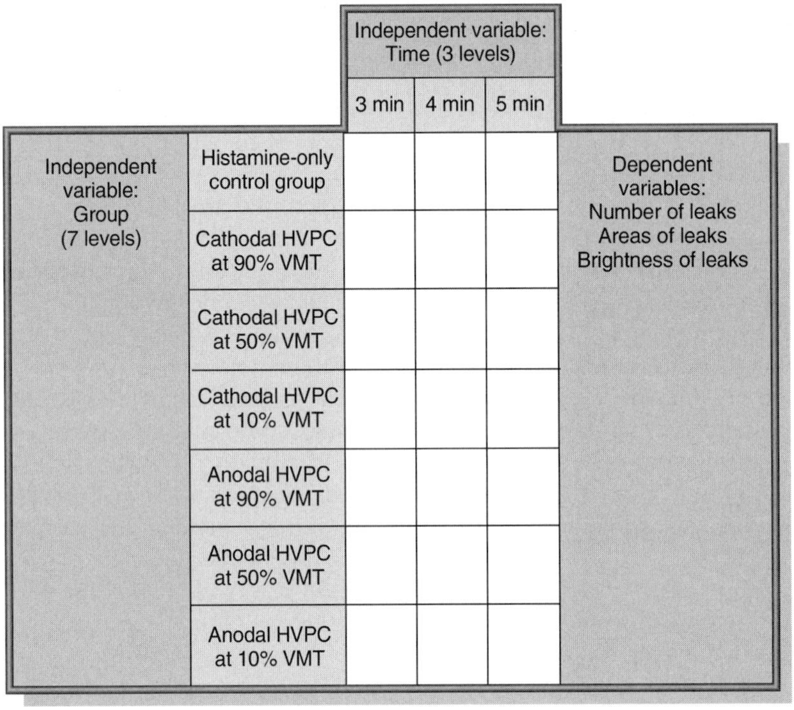

		Independent variable: Time (3 levels)		
		3 min	4 min	5 min
Independent variable: Group (7 levels)	Histamine-only control group			
	Cathodal HVPC at 90% VMT			
	Cathodal HVPC at 50% VMT			
	Cathodal HVPC at 10% VMT			
	Anodal HVPC at 90% VMT			
	Anodal HVPC at 50% VMT			
	Anodal HVPC at 10% VMT			

Dependent variables:
Number of leaks
Areas of leaks
Brightness of leaks

FIGURE 6–2. Study of the effect of current on macromolecular leakage. Two independent variables were used: "group" with seven levels and "time" with three levels. Although the leakage variables were actually measured four times, the first measurement was not directly compared with the other measures; rather, it was used as a baseline that was subtracted from the measures collected at each of the other times. *HVPC,* High-voltage pulsed current; *VMT,* visible motor threshold. Design presented in Taylor K, Mendel FC, Fish DR, Hard R, Burton HW. Effect of high-voltage pulsed current and alternating current on macromolecular leakage in hamster cheek pouch microcirculation. *Phys Ther.* 1997; 77: 1729-1740.

another layer of complexity to the identification of independent variables, as diagrammed in Figure 6–3. Patients with high or low intracranial pressure underwent either passive or active exercise in up to three different positions. The dependent variables of heart rate, systemic arterial pressure, intracranial pressure (ICP), and cerebral perfusion pressure were measured at rest and during various motions. On first analysis, then, it appears that there might be four independent variables within this study: group (high vs. normal intracranial pressure), exercise type (active vs. passive), position (supine, head up 30 degrees, head up 45 degrees), and activity (rest vs. motion). On closer examination of the study, one finds that the authors never compare the high-pressure with the normal-pressure groups, nor do they compare the active with the passive groups. Rather than dealing with these groupings as independent variables, the authors, in effect, conducted four "mini-studies": one with patients with high ICP who received passive exercise, one with patients with normal

ICP who received passive exercise, one with patients with high ICP who received active exercise, and one with patients with normal ICP who received active exercise. This leaves two potential independent variables for each of the mini-studies: position and activity.

For the two mini-studies of patients with normal intracranial pressure, the authors tested each patient at rest and in motion in each of the three positions. Therefore, these studies had two independent variables, position and activity. Each of the variables had dependent levels because each patient was represented at each level of each variable. Thus, both of these independent variables would be considered "within-group" variables.

For the two mini-studies of patients with high ICP, the authors tested each patient at rest and in motion at only one position, the 30-degree head-up position. The position variable was not investigated for these groups because the other positions may be contraindicated for patients with elevated intracranial pressure. Thus, for the patients with high intracranial pressure, the studies

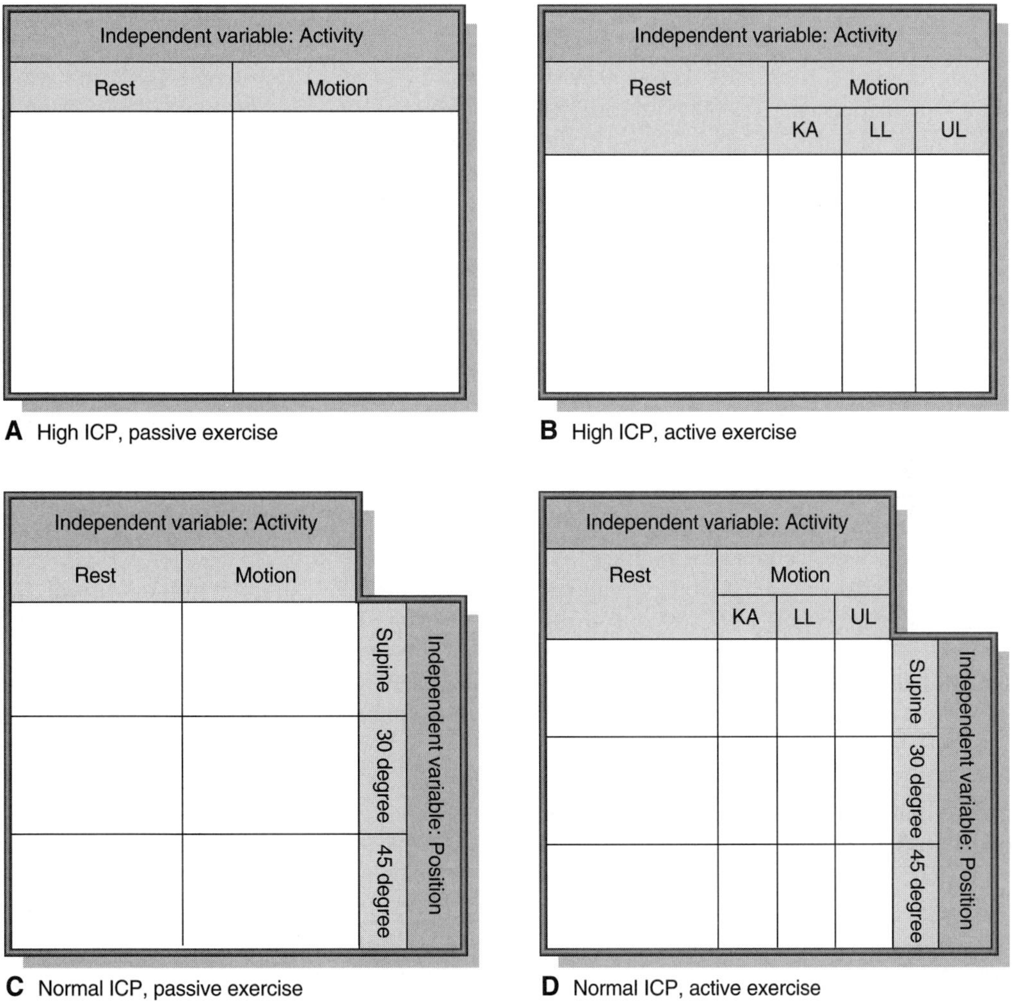

FIGURE 6–3. Study of the effect of exercise and position on intracranial pressure. This article presents a complex design that is actually four mini-studies in one. **A** and **B,** For patients with high intracranial pressure (ICP) only the effect of exercise was examined. **C** and **D,** For patients with normal ICP, the impact of both exercise and position was examined. **A** and **C,** For the passive groups, only rest and motion phases were compared for the activity variable. **B** and **D,** For the active groups, comparisons for the activity variable were made between rest phases and three different motion phases (knee adduction [KA], lower limb activity [LL], and upper limb activity [UL]). **C** and **D,** For the normal ICP groups the position variable was examined at three levels: supine, with the head up 30 degrees, and with the head up 45 degrees.

Design presented in Brimioulle S, Moraine JJ, Norrenberg D, Kahn RJ. Effects of positioning and exercise on intracranial pressure in a neurosurgical intensive care unit. *Phys Ther.* 1997;77:1682-1689.

had only one independent variable, "activity," with dependent levels.

From the examples presented in this section of the chapter, readers should now understand how to identify the names and levels of the independent variables within the studies. This identification process involves making some preliminary judgments about possible variables based on the article title, purpose statement, and methods. Final determination of the variables and their levels depends on determining which comparisons the authors actually make within the study. Sometimes entire variables "disappear" because no comparisons are made. In Brimioulle and associates' study of patients in neurosurgical intensive care units,[4] for example, "pressure" was not a variable because there was no comparison between patients with high and normal ICP. Sometimes entire variables disappear because the levels are combined mathematically for analysis. In Carter and associates' study,[2] the apparent "time" variable was eliminated when posttreatment scores were subtracted from pretreatment scores. Finally, levels of variables sometimes disappear because one level is used to normalize the other levels (e.g., in the electrical stimulation study of Taylor and colleagues,[3] the data collection that occurred at 1.5 minutes into treatment was not a level in and of itself, but was used as a baseline against which to compare the other levels).

Dependent Variables

Dependent variables as the presumed "effects" within a study are "dependent" on the differences in the levels of the independent variables. If the independent variables can be thought of as the "grouping" factors, then the dependent variables can be thought of as the "measured" factors. Unlike independent variables, the different values that dependent variables take within a study are not described as levels.

When identifying dependent variables, it is often useful to differentiate between the "conceptual" dependent variable and the "operational"

dependent variable. In the magnet therapy study of Carter and associates,[2] the conceptual dependent variable is "pain reduction" and the operational dependent variable is "pain reduction as measured on a visual analogue scale." In the electrical stimulation study of Taylor and colleagues,[3] the conceptual dependent variable is "macromolecular leakage" and the operational dependent variables are number of leaks, area of the leakage, and brightness of the leakage as seen through histological analysis. Describing the dependent variables in both conceptual and operational terms provides a framework for analyzing articles from both theoretical and technical viewpoints.

■ DESIGN DIMENSIONS

The interplay among three research design dimensions is shown in a matrix of research types in Figure 6–4. There are three broad purposes of research: *description, analysis of relationships,* and *analysis of differences* between groups or treatments. There are two levels to the time dimension: *retrospective,* in which the researcher uses data collected before the research question was developed, and *prospective,* in which the researcher completes data collection after the

		Timing of data collection	
		Retrospective	Prospective
Purpose of research	Description	Nonexperimental	Nonexperimental
	Analysis of relationships	Nonexperimental	Nonexperimental
	Analysis of differences	Nonexperimental	Nonexperimental Experimental
	Manipulation (experimental or nonexperimental)		

FIGURE 6–4. Matrix of research types showing three design dimensions: purpose of the research (rows), timing of data collection (columns), and manipulation (cells).

research question is developed.[5] There are also two basic levels of the manipulation dimension: *experimental* research involves controlled manipulation of participants; *nonexperimental* research does not.

Research Purposes

To illustrate what is meant by the three different purposes of research, imagine that you are interested in studying the broad topic of functional recovery after total knee arthroplasty (TKA). One purpose for research about this topic would be to *describe* the functional status of patients at various intervals after TKA. A second purpose would be to *analyze the relationships* among various preoperative factors (e.g., gait velocity, medication use, or activities of daily living) and functional status at intervals after TKA surgery. A third purpose would be to *analyze the differences* in functional recovery after TKA between, for example, one group of patients who received individualized postoperative rehabilitation services and another group who participated in group rehabilitation classes after surgery. Although each of these examples presents an approach to studying the topic of functional recovery after TKA, each project serves a very different purpose. Data from the first project would enable clinicians to describe typical recovery patterns to their patients; data from the second study would enable clinicians to predict which patients might be at risk for a poor recovery; and data from the third study would help clinicians determine preferred patterns of care for patients after TKA. One of the projects is not inherently superior to any of the others, in that each of these hypothetical projects fulfills a need for a particular type of information related to the topic.

Timing of Data Collection

The timing of data collection with respect to development of the research problem is the second important dimension of research design.

There are two levels to the time dimension: *retrospective,* in which the researcher uses data collected before the research question was developed, and *prospective,* in which the researcher completes data collection after the research question is developed.[5]

All three of the general research purposes can be accomplished with either prospective or retrospective designs. One could describe the functional status of patients at various intervals after TKA either by extracting functional recovery data from existing medical records (retrospective) or by setting up a data collection protocol to gather systematic functional recovery data at specified intervals after surgery (prospective). One could analyze relationships among preoperative factors and functional status after TKA surgery either by extracting both the preoperative and functional data from the medical records of patients who have completed their rehabilitation after TKA (retrospective) or by collecting both the preoperative and functional data under controlled conditions designed to answer a specific question (prospective). One could also analyze differences in functional recovery after TKA between patients receiving individual or group rehabilitation services either by extracting discharge data from the charts of patients who happened to receive individualized rehabilitation to those who happened to receive group rehabilitation (retrospective) or by randomly assigning new patients to individual or group rehabilitation groups and then tracking their functional progress during recovery (prospective).

There are two notable twists to the use of the terms *retrospective* and *prospective.* First, in practice, research projects may combine retrospective and prospective elements, as previously defined. For example, a researcher might analyze relationships between preoperative factors and postoperative recovery by first extracting preoperative data from the medical record (retrospective) and then collecting new data on functional outcomes after surgery (prospective).

Second, an alternate set of definitions for retrospective and prospective focuses on the sequence of cause-and-effect determinations, rather than on timing of data collection. These definitions are commonly used in epidemiological research, which is covered in more detail in Chapter 14. Imagine that a researcher wishes to determine the effect of activity on development of osteoarthritis of the knee. The alternate definition for retrospective research is research in which the researcher works backward from effect (osteoarthritis) to cause (activity). Doing such a study would first involve identifying groups of older patients with and without osteoarthritis. Next, the researcher would ask those patients to complete a lifelong activity questionnaire that might quantify "activity" through items about physical activity at work, during activities of daily living, and through participation in exercise and sports. Although the activity data are "prospective" according to our original definition (they were collected for the purpose of this particular study), the study involves a "retrospective" look, according to the alternate definition, at possible causes for osteoarthritis.

The alternate definition for prospective research is research in which the researcher works forward from cause to effect. Studying the link between activity and osteoarthritis from such a "prospective" viewpoint would involve identifying a group of young people without osteoarthritis, tracking their activity levels throughout their lives, determining which of the original participants actually developed osteoarthritis, and then analyzing the data to determine whether activity levels are related to the development of osteoarthritis.

The common element of both the original and the alternate definitions relates to the level of control within the study. With either set of definitions, researchers have less control over the variables within retrospective studies than they do the variables in prospective ones. Methods for controlling variables are discussed later in this chapter.

Manipulation

There are two basic levels of the manipulation dimension: *experimental* research involves controlled manipulation of participants; *nonexperimental* research does not. Figure 6–4 illustrates the relationship of the manipulation dimension to the purpose and time dimensions. Research that describes phenomena or analyzes relationships among variables is nonexperimental, regardless of whether the data are collected prospectively or retrospectively. Research that analyzes differences retrospectively is also nonexperimental. Research that analyzes differences prospectively may be either experimental or nonexperimental. Thus, experimental research is but one of many different types of research that a clinician may encounter during a career of reading the literature or participating in research studies.

Many authors divide experimental research into *true experimental* and *quasiexperimental* subcategories based on the level of control present in the study. True experiments are characterized by high levels of control. This control takes the form of at least two separate groups of participants, with random assignment of participants to groups. The terms *randomized clinical trial* or *randomized controlled trial* (both abbreviated as RCT) are often used to describe health care research that is truly experimental in nature. More information on RCTs is included in Chapter 9.

Quasiexperimental research is characterized by less control than true experimental research, and this lesser degree of control of the experimental situation is achieved either with a single participant group, whereby participants act as their own controls, or by using multiple groups to which participants are not randomly assigned. Campbell and Stanley, in their classic text on research design, imply that quasiexperimental studies are inferior designs that should only be used when a true experimental study is not feasible.[6]

There are two problems with such sharp differentiation between true experimental and quasiexperimental research. First, the value of quasiexperimental research designs in which participants are used as their own controls is underestimated. There are many clinical research questions for which single-group, quasiexperimental designs are ideal; several are presented in later chapters. Second, the ability of true experimental designs to capture the complexity of the clinical situation is overestimated. True experiments are often far more controlled than the daily practice of rehabilitation, and the results of such experiments may apply only to similarly controlled situations. In this text, then, the term *experimental research* is used to refer to both truly experimental and quasiexperimental designs.

In this text, the specification that manipulation be controlled is what distinguishes experimental designs from nonexperimental. However, determination of whether controlled manipulation has occurred is more complicated than might be imagined. In some experiments, controlled manipulation is obvious. For example, Carter and associates measured pain levels before and after true magnet therapy or sham magnet therapy in two groups of patients with wrist pain attributed to carpal tunnel syndrome.[2] Treatment with either true or sham magnet therapy was the manipulation. Random assignment to treatment group, standardization of the way in which the device was applied, and standardization of patient activity during the treatment lent a great deal of control to the experiment.

However, some nonexperimental research studies at first appear to be experimental because an independent variable takes several values within the study. Closer examination reveals that although an independent variable is present, it has not been manipulated in a controlled manner by the researcher. There are four general categories of nonmanipulated independent variables: (1) the manipulation was retrospective, (2) the variable is inherently nonmanipulable, (3) the variable could have been manipulated but was not, and (4) the independent variable is an integral part of the measurement of the dependent variable.

MANIPULATION IS RETROSPECTIVE

Consider a case in which a clinician reviews the initial and discharge range-of-motion measurements reported in the clinical records of his or her last 20 patients with low back pain who received heat and exercise. This type of study is retrospective because the researcher seeks to answer a question by examining data that were collected before the question was developed. When the data are collected before the question is developed, the researcher has little or no control over the actual implementation of the treatment, the outside activities of the patients, or the technique of measuring range of motion. Even though the heat and exercise are manipulations, this example does not meet the controlled-manipulation criterion and would be considered a nonexperimental study.

THE VARIABLE IS NONMANIPULABLE

Common examples of nonmanipulable independent variables are participant age, ethnicity, diagnosis, or socioeconomic status. Researchers cannot change these characteristics of participants who present themselves for study; they can only group participants according to these characteristics. For example, Murray compared spoken language production in individuals with Huntington's and Parkinson's diseases, and with age-matched control groups.[7] The independent variable, diagnosis, had four levels: individuals with Huntington's disease, those with Parkinson's disease, a control group matched in age to the Huntington's group, and a control group matched in age to the Parkinson's group. This type of nonmanipulated independent variable is called an *attribute* or a *classification* variable. When a grouping is made based on some attribute, and not through random assignment, it is called a *block*.

THE RESEARCHER CHOOSES NOT TO MANIPULATE

Sometimes a variable could be manipulated but is not. In a nonexperimental study by Klungel and colleagues, drug treatment for hypertension was a nonmanipulated independent variable.[8] It is possible to manipulate drug treatment for hypertension experimentally by identifying individuals with hypertension and then assigning them to different drug treatment groups. Klungel and colleagues, however, did not actually *manipulate* drug treatment for hypertension. Rather, they identified a group of hypertensive individuals and noted which ones were receiving drug treatment and which were untreated. They then compared the risk of stroke between the two groups. Despite the potential for manipulation of the drug treatment variable, the researchers chose to study the problem nonexperimentally, without controlled manipulation. In fact, the question that prompted their study—to determine whether drug treatment as it occurs in regular clinical practice can reduce the risk of stroke as much as it does in more highly controlled, randomized clinical trials—required this nonexperimental approach.

THE INDEPENDENT VARIABLE IS A COMPONENT OF THE DEPENDENT VARIABLE

Sometimes an inherent part of the measurement of a dependent variable is treated as an independent variable. With the increasing sophistication of measurement tools in rehabilitation comes the ability to vary aspects of the measurement itself.

An example of this form of nonmanipulation of an independent variable is found in Ninos and colleagues' study of electromyographic (EMG) analysis of the squat performed in two different foot positions.[9] The data analysis procedure for this study included four different independent variables: knee flexion angle (five levels between 10 and 60 degrees of knee flexion), direction of movement (two levels, ascending and descending phases of the squat), muscle (four levels: vastus medialis, vastus lateralis, semimembranosus and semitendinosus, and biceps femoris), and foot placement (neutral and 30 degrees turned out).

The first three of these variables are inherent components of doing a squat. The knees move through different angles, there are ascending and descending phases, and muscles on both sides

of the knees are active. Certainly the researchers "manipulated" the participants by having them do squats. However, the three variables that are inherent in doing any squat would be part of any descriptive study of EMG activity during squats. The final variable, foot placement, appears to be the only element of this study that can be considered experimental. The varied foot placement represents the researchers' manipulation of the way in which squats are done.

When the only manipulation that occurs is an inherent part of the measurement of the dependent variable, the research should be considered nonexperimental. However, an important distinction must be made between testing versus training. Knee flexion angle in the Ninos and associates' study was a nonmanipulated component of doing the squats within the study. If they had done a study in which they compared knee extensor strength following "deep-squat" versus "shallow-squat" exercise programs, then the independent variable would become knee angle. Manipulating the knee angle in this way during a squat would be an experimental approach; recording EMG activity during the angles normally occurring during a squat is a nonexperimental, descriptive approach.

INTERPRETATION BASED ON CONTROLLED MANIPULATION

Experimental research occurs when the researcher manipulates a variable or variables in a controlled fashion. Nonexperimental research describes existing phenomena, without alteration through manipulation. Although one type of research is not inherently superior to the other, interpretation of research results differs depending on the methods of study. Thus, it is important that readers of the literature be able to distinguish between experimental and nonexperimental studies.

In particular, the presence of controlled manipulation enables researchers to draw *causal conclusions* about the variable under study. For example, Wolfson and associates studied the effects of balance and strength training on various functional measures in older adults.[10] In one component of this complex study, they assigned each participant to one of four groups (control, balance training, strength training, and combined balance and strength training). The training proceeded for 3 months, after which balance, strength, and gait measures were taken. They found, in part, that the groups that received balance training exhibited significant improvements in some of the balance variables. The controlled manipulation of the training program allowed them to conclude that the balance activities caused the changes in balance performance.

In contrast, Lynn and coworkers implemented a nonexperimental study comparing balance characteristics of women with and without osteoporosis.[11] They found that the women with osteoporosis exhibited different balance strategies than the women without osteoporosis. Because there was no controlled manipulation of the bone density variable, it cannot be said that the presence or absence of osteoporosis *caused* the balance changes any more than it can be said that different balance strategies *caused* the osteoporosis.

■ CONTROL

In any type of study, some level of control must be present. Six types of control are common: control of implementation of the independent variable, control of participant selection and assignment, control of extraneous variables related to the setting, control of extraneous variables related to the participants, control of measurement of the dependent variable, and control of information given to participants and researchers.

Implementation of the Independent Variable

In controlling the independent variable, the investigator must develop a rationale to govern the implementation of the variable and a mechanism to monitor the implementation. In a study of the effect of pre-season conditioning on injury rates of collegiate athletes, the implementation of pre-season conditioning would need to be systematized in some way. Does "pre-season" conditioning mean aerobic conditioning, strength training, flexibility training, skills training, or some combination of two or more components? If aerobic conditioning is a component of the training, should all athletes undergo conditioning at a similar intensity and duration? Or should the conditioning be tailored by sport, or by positions within a sport, or individualized completely?

Feinstein[12] described two general research philosophies that influence how these implementation decisions are made: fastidiousness and pragmatism. Fastidious researchers seek precise control over all aspects of implementation, believing that the ability to draw causal conclusions is jeopardized by variations in treatment implementation. Pragmatic researchers seek closer simulation of clinical environments, believing that research results are most useful when the setting reflects the vagaries of the clinical setting. Both approaches are acceptable, but the limitations of both approaches need to be acknowledged by researchers. Fastidious researchers must acknowledge the limited clinical applicability of their work; pragmatic researchers must acknowledge their limited ability to draw causal conclusions from their work. In Chapter 7, the limitations of both fastidious and pragmatic designs are analyzed in detail when the concepts of internal and external validity are introduced.

Selection and Assignment of Participants

The second control component is control over the selection of participants for the study and assignment of participants to groups within the study. First, criteria for selection of individuals to be included in the study must be determined. In our hypothetical study of pre-season conditioning, many participant selection questions would arise. Should both men and women be studied? What sports should be included? Does it make any difference if an athlete has been injured in a previous season? Those who prefer fastidious designs tend to define selection criteria narrowly and therefore study relatively homogeneous groups. Those who prefer pragmatic designs develop broader selection criteria and therefore study relatively heterogeneous groups.

Once the criteria for admission to the study are determined, actual admission of individuals to the study must proceed. Random selection of a limited number of participants from a larger participant pool is generally considered the best way to control for a variety of participant factors by maximizing the probability that any extraneous factors in the sample are present in the proportions actually found in the overall population. An in-depth discussion of sampling is presented in Chapter 8.

Extraneous Variables in the Setting

The third component of control is control over the setting. *Extraneous,* or *confounding,* variables are factors other than the independent variables that may influence the dependent variables. Control of extraneous variables includes, for example, keeping the temperature, lighting, time of day of testing, and the like constant to rule out differences in these factors as possible explanations for any changes in the dependent variable. In the hypothetical study of the effect of pre-season conditioning on injury rates for collegiate athletes, an extraneous factor in the "setting" (i.e., a factor that is related to something outside of individual player characteristics) might be whether one or more teams in the study competed in post-season tournaments. The researchers would need to decide whether to count post-season tournament injuries when computing injury rates.

Extraneous Variables Related to Participants

Control of extraneous variables related to the participant is the fourth means of control within research design. Researchers usually attempt to hold factors other than the independent variable constant for all participants or groups. In this way, extraneous variables are controlled because they will affect all participants or groups equally. In our hypothetical study of pre-season conditioning, one extraneous variable might be recreational athletic activities. A fastidious approach to the research problem would require tight control over activities other than the pre-season conditioning program (e.g., researchers might restrict participants from playing recreational sports such as racquetball); a pragmatic approach would permit each athlete to participate in recreational athletic pursuits of their choosing.

The use of a randomly assigned control group, in and of itself, is a powerful tool that balances extraneous variables throughout the groups. If a randomly assigned, untreated control group is used in the study of pre-season conditioning, controlling the recreational athletic activities of participants may not be necessary. The process of randomization increases the chance (but does not guarantee) that the effects of any recreational athletic activities will be balanced across the treatment and control groups.

In studies with only one group, control of extraneous variables must be achieved through means other than a control group. If one were to study a single group of patients after cerebral vascular accident to determine the effect of body-weight–supported ambulation on gait velocity, it would be important to establish that changes were the result of treatment and not the normal healing process (maturation). One way to control for the effect of maturation would be to take weekly velocity measurements of all patients and admit into the study only those who had several weeks of stable velocity measures.

A second common way to control extraneous variables is to use the same participants for all levels of the independent variable. This only works when the effect that the researcher is measuring is thought to be short-lived. Szabo and colleagues studied the effects of slow- and fast-rhythm classical music on the maximum workload achieved during progressive cycling.[13] They used a control condition without music and four different treatment conditions with different music tempos. Because exercising to maximal workload on only five occasions is not expected to provide a substantial training effect in individuals with a relatively high starting fitness level, an ideal way to control extraneous participant factors is to use a *repeated measures,* or *repeated treatment,* design, whereby participants act as their own controls and receive all experimental conditions. In addition, repeated treatment designs require fewer participants and may require less time for setup and preparation because the number of participants is reduced.

The repeated measures design, however, introduces its own set of extraneous variables related to the administration of multiple treatments. If one of the music tempos is always given last, familiarity with the testing setup, combined with any training effect of the repeated testing, may increase the maximum workload at which the participants are able to cycle. Conversely, if the testing sessions have been close together, fatigue may reduce the maximum workload demonstrated during the last condition. One way to control the effects of familiarization with equipment or procedures for any design is to schedule one or more training sessions with participants before actual data collection begins.

Another way to control fatigue and learning in a repeated treatment design is by randomizing, or *counterbalancing,* the order of presentation of the experimental conditions (i.e., some of the participants get slow music during the first test, others get fast music during the first test). This becomes problematic when more than two levels of treatment are present. If there are three levels (A, B, and C) of the independent variable, there are six possible presentation orders (3!— i.e., 3 factorial, or $3 \times 2 \times 1 = 6$): ABC, ACB, BAC, BCA, CAB, and CBA. With four levels, the number of permutations increases to 24 (4!—$4 \times 3 \times 2 \times 1 = 24$). With six levels, there are 720 possible orders (6!—$6 \times 5 \times 4 \times 3 \times 2 \times 1 = 720$). Random assignment of participants to all available orders in a study with six levels of an independent variable would require a minimum of 720 participants. To obviate the need for so many participants, a sampling of orders can be used.

There are two basic strategies for selecting treatment orders in a repeated measures design with several levels of the independent variable. These two strategies can be illustrated by a hypothetical study of gait characteristics with four different foot units in a transtibial prosthesis: a solid-ankle-cushion-heel foot (SC), a single-axis foot (SA), a multiaxial foot (MA), and a dynamic response foot (DR). The first strategy is to randomly select an order and then rotate the starting position, as shown in Figure 6–5, *A*. In a *random start with rotation,* each condition appears at each position in the rotation equally often. One fourth of the participants would be randomly assigned the order in the first row; one fourth, the order in the second row; and so on.

The second strategy is to use a *Latin square* technique. The Latin square technique ensures not only that each condition appears at each position equally often, but also that each condition precedes and follows every other condition equally often. Thus, a Latin square has a greater level of randomization than does a random start with rotation. A sample Latin square is shown in Figure 6–5, *B*. Rules for the formation of a Latin square can be found in several texts and on the Internet.[14-17]

Measurement Variation

The fifth component of control is control of the measurement techniques used to provide data for the experiment. Reliability and validity of measurements used in experiments are critical to the ability to draw conclusions from the data. Sound design includes pilot testing of the measures to be used to ensure that each measure is reproducible. If multiple raters are used in the study, standardized instructions to testers, training sessions for testers, and a pilot study to ensure the interrater reliability of measures are essential. Chapters 17 and 18 are devoted to measurement

A Random order with rotation			
Presentation position			
1st	2nd	3rd	4th
SC	SA	MA	(DR)
SA	MA	(DR)	SC
MA	(DR)	SC	SA
(DR)	SC	SA	MA

B Latin square			
Presentation position			
1st	2nd	3rd	4th
SC	SA	MA	(DR)
SA	(DR)	SC	MA
(DR)	MA	SA	SC
MA	SC	(DR)	SA

FIGURE 6–5. Selection of presentation orders from many possibilities. With four levels of the independent variable (SC = solid ankle cushion heel; SA = single axis; MA = multiaxial; DR = dynamic response), there are 24 (4!) possible orders. **A,** Selection of four orders through random ordering of the first row, and through rotation of orders for the remaining rows. The highlighted condition, DR, illustrates that each level is represented at each presentation position in a systematic way through rotation. **B,** Selection of four orders through generation of a Latin square. The highlighted condition, DR, illustrates that each level is represented at each presentation position in a random way that also ensures that each condition precedes and follows each other condition only once.

theory, and examination of research designs that evaluate reliability and validity of measurement tools.

Information Received by Participants and Researchers

The final means of control in designs is control of the information given to the participant and the researcher during the course of the study. Placebo effects, participant expectations, and researcher expectations may all result in changes in the dependent variable that are unrelated to the implementation of the independent variable. Three means of information control are commonly used to limit these effects: incomplete information, blinding or masking of participants, and blinding or masking of researchers.

INCOMPLETE INFORMATION

Sometimes participants are given incomplete information about the purpose of the study to control any effects that their expectations about the results would cause. For example, Gahimer studied patient education behaviors of therapists in outpatient orthopedic settings, but did not want the therapists in the study to know the specific variable of interest.[18] She assumed that if therapists knew the specific purpose of the study they might change their teaching behaviors during the observation period. When Gahimer obtained informed consent from participants, she stated only that she wished to study patient–therapist interaction. In this way she was truthful, but incomplete, in that the specific measure of interest was disguised from the therapists.

With an innocuous study involving patient education behaviors of therapists during the provision of routine care, there are few ethical concerns about withholding the specific purpose of the study. However, the use of an incomplete information strategy is clearly not appropriate for the study of higher-risk procedures, which require complete disclosure of purposes and risks so that eligible participants can make an informed decision about participation.

MASKING OF PARTICIPANTS

A second means of controlling information is to withhold information about which of several treatments a research participant is receiving. In the past, this was referred to as "blinding participants." Today, the term "masking" is often preferred to "blinding." Alternatively, researchers may refer to participants being "naive" to the treatment being given. In many procedures in rehabilitation, participant masking is not possible because of the nature of the procedures themselves. Participants in the pre-season conditioning study would obviously be able to determine whether they were in the conditioning or the control group based on the activities that were required or permitted during the pre-season period.

When the treatment is a physical modality, participants may be kept partially naive to which physical modalities they are receiving. For example, participants may be told that they may or may not feel a sensation with electrical stimulation; the control group may then receive placebo or sham electrical stimulation, whereby the machine is not plugged in or the intensity is not turned on. This approach was used by Peters and associates in their study of the use of electrical stimulation as an adjunct treatment for diabetic foot ulcers.[19] The electrical stimulators were modified for the placebo group so that they appeared to turn on and deliver current, even though no current was actually delivered. Ethical treatment of research participants requires that they be informed of the possibility of receiving a placebo treatment.

MASKING OF RESEARCHERS

A third means of controlling information is to mask the researchers to the group membership of, or treatment received by, the participants. In this way any expectations that the experimenter may have about the outcome of the study are not inadvertently communicated to participants.

Researcher masking was implemented in the Peters and associates study.[19] An assistant set up the electrical stimulation units as real or placebo, based on the predetermined group assignments. The investigators treating the patients and taking wound measurements did not know whether true or sham electrical stimulation was being given. If the treatment is such that the clinician cannot be masked to the treatment (e.g., a study of two different forms of manual therapy), then a different investigator would need to take the measures of interest in the study, without knowing which patients had received which treatment.

A study in which either the participant or the researcher is naive to the treatment administered is termed a *single-blind* study. A study in which both participant and researcher are masked is termed a *double-blind* study. Studies may also be referred to as *triple-blind* if the participant, the person who implements treatment, and the person who collects data are all unaware of group assignment. If in addition, the person who does the data analysis for the study does not know which group is which, the study may be called a *quadruple-blinded* study. Unfortunately, research designs that attempt to mask either researchers or participants may not be as effective as hoped. Deyo and associates studied the effectiveness of masking techniques with transcutaneous electrical nerve stimulation.[20] After completion of a double-blind study, they asked participants to indicate whether they believed their units were working properly and asked researchers to indicate which participants they believed had functioning units. They found that both participants and researchers guessed correctly more often than would have been predicted by chance, indicating only partial success of the masking procedure. They hypothesized that the lack of full masking was due to sensory differences between real and sham therapy and to unintended communication between the participants and researchers.

Implementation of the treatment, extraneous variables in the setting, extraneous participant variables, selection and assignment of participants, measurement techniques, and information given to participants and researchers must all be controlled in an experimental design. These control elements are elaborated on in the next two chapters of this text. In Chapter 7, a detailed look at how these control elements influence the validity of research is presented. In Chapter 8, more detailed information on selection and assignment of participants is given. Then, Sections 3 and 4 (Chapters 9 through 16) provide a more detailed look at different types of experimental and nonexperimental designs.

■ SUMMARY

Variables within studies are often classified as independent (the "grouping" variable) or dependent (the "measured" variable). Independent variables, in turn, have levels that are compared with one another with respect to the dependent variables. Research types can be defined according to three dimensions: purpose (description, analysis of relationships, analysis of differences), timing (retrospective or prospective data collection), and manipulation (experimental, nonexperimental). Researchers can achieve control by uniformly implementing the independent variable, selecting and assigning participants randomly, eliminating extraneous variables from the setting, limiting extraneous variables related to participants, ensuring the reliability of measurements of the dependent variable, and limiting the information provided to themselves and to participants.

REFERENCES

1. Kerlinger FN, Lee HB. *Foundations of Behavioral Research*. 4th ed. Fort Worth, Tex: Harcourt College Publishers; 2000.
2. Carter R, Hall T, Aspy CB, Mold J. The effectiveness of magnet therapy for treatment of wrist pain attributed to carpal tunnel syndrome. *J Fam Pract*. 2002;51:38-40.
3. Taylor K, Mendel FC, Fish DR, Hard R, Burton HW. Effect of high-voltage pulsed current and alternating current on macromolecular leakage in hamster cheek pouch microcirculation. *Phys Ther*. 1997;77:1729-1740.
4. Brimioulle S, Moraine JJ, Norrenberg D, Kahn RJ. Effects of positioning and exercise on intracranial pressure in a neurosurgical intensive care unit. *Phys Ther*. 1997;77:1682-1689.
5. Tietjen GL. *A Topical Dictionary of Statistics*. New York, NY: Chapman & Hall; 1986:125.
6. Campbell DT, Stanley JC. *Experimental and Quasi-Experimental Designs for Research*. Chicago, Ill: Rand McNally College Publishing; 1963.
7. Murray LL. Spoken language production in Huntington's and Parkinson's diseases. *J Speech Lang Hearing Res*. 2000;43:1350-1366.
8. Klungel OH, Stricker BH, Breteler MM, Seidell JC, Psaty BM, de Boer A. Is drug treatment of hypertension in clinical practice as effective as in randomized controlled trials with regard to the incidence of stroke? *Epidemiology*. 2001;12:339-344.
9. Ninos JC, Irrgang JJ, Burdett R, Weiss JR. Electromyographic analysis of the squat performed in self-selected lower extremity neutral rotation and 30 degrees of lower extremity turn-out from the self-selected neutral position. *J Orthop Sports Phys Ther*. 1997;25:307-315.
10. Wolfson L, Whipple R, Derby C, et al. Balance and strength training in older adults: intervention gains and Tai Chi maintenance. *J Am Geriatr Soc*. 1996;44:497-506.
11. Lynn SG, Sinaki M, Westerlind KC. Balance characteristics of persons with osteoporosis. *Arch Phys Med Rehabil*. 1997;78:273-277.
12. Feinstein AR. An additional basic science for clinical medicine, II: limitations of randomized trials. *Ann Intern Med*. 1983;99:544-550.
13. Szabo A, Small A, Leigh M. The effects of slow- and fast-rhythm classical music on progressive cycling to voluntary physical exhaustion. *J Sports Med Phys Fitness*. 1999;39:220-225.
14. Shaughnessy JJ, Zechmeister EB. *Research Methods in Psychology*. 6th ed. New York, NY: McGraw-Hill; 2002.
15. Winer BJ. *Statistical Principles in Experimental Design*. 2nd ed. New York, NY: McGraw-Hill; 1971:685-691.
16. Kirk RE. *Experimental Design: Procedures for the Behavioral Sciences*. Belmont, Calif: Wadsworth Publishing Co; 1968.
17. *Latin squares*. Available at: *http://www.cut-the-knot.org/arithmetic/latin.shtml*. Accessed October 27, 2003.
18. Gahimer JE, Domholdt E. Amount of perceived education in physical therapy practice and perceived effects. *Phys Ther*. 1996;76:1089-1096.
19. Peters EJ, Lavery LA, Armstrong DG, Fleischli JG. Electrical stimulation as an adjunct to heal diabetic foot ulcers: a randomized controlled trial. *Arch Phys Med Rehabil*. 2001;82:721-725.
20. Deyo RA, Walsh NE, Schoenfeld LS, Ramamurthy S. Can trials of physical treatments be blinded? The example of transcutaneous electrical nerve stimulation for chronic pain. *Am J Phys Med Rehabil*. 1990;69:6-10.

Research Validity

The validity of a piece of research is the extent to which the conclusions of that research are believable and useful. Cook and Campbell[1] have outlined four types of validity and this chapter relies to a great extent on their work. When determining the value of a piece of research, readers need to ask four basic questions:

1. Is the research designed so that there are few alternative explanations for changes in the dependent variable other than the effect of the independent variable? Factors other than the independent variables that could be related to changes in

the dependent variable are threats to *internal validity*.

2. Are the research constructs defined and used in such a way that the research can be placed in the framework of other research within the field of study? Poor definition of constructs or inconsistent use of constructs is a threat to *construct validity*.

3. To whom can the results of this research be applied? Sampling and design factors that lead to limited generalizability are threats to *external validity*.

4. Are statistical tools used correctly to analyze the data? Irregularities in the use of

statistics are threats to *statistical conclusion validity*.

The purpose of this chapter is to provide a discussion of the first three types of validity. Because understanding statistical conclusion validity requires a background in statistical reasoning, its threats are discussed in Chapter 19 after statistical reasoning is introduced. Each of the remaining three types of validity has several identifiable threats that can be illustrated either in examples from the rehabilitation literature or in examples of hypothetical rehabilitation research. For each of these threats, at least one example is presented and mechanisms for controlling the threat are suggested. The chapter ends with an examination of the interrelationships among the types of validity.

■ INTERNAL VALIDITY

Internal validity is the extent to which the results of a study demonstrate that a causal relationship exists between the independent and dependent variables. In experimental research, the central question about internal validity is whether the treatments (or the various levels of the independent variable) caused the observed changes in the dependent variable. The classic randomized controlled trial, with random assignment to experimental and control groups, is considered the best way to control threats to internal validity when studying interventions. In nonexperimental research designed to delineate differences between groups in the absence of controlled manipulation by the researcher, the question becomes less "causal" and instead focuses on whether the independent variable is a plausible explanation of group differences on the dependent variable. In nonexperimental research designed to describe a phenomenon or establish relationships among variables, internal validity is not an issue in that no comparisons between levels of the independent variable are being made.

The general strategy that researchers use to increase internal validity is to maximize their control over all aspects of the research project, as first described in Chapter 6. The researcher carefully monitors the control and experimental groups to ensure that experimental groups receive the intervention as designed and that control groups do not inadvertently receive components of the intervention. Randomized assignment of participants to treatment groups maximizes the probability that extraneous participant characteristics will be evenly distributed across groups. To check randomization, the researcher can collect information about participant characteristics that threaten internal validity to determine whether the characteristics in question were equally represented across groups. Eliminating extraneous variables through control of the experimental setting removes them as plausible causes of changes in the dependent variable. Research assistants are carefully trained to collect and record information accurately and reliably. Information about which participants are receiving which treatment is concealed, when possible, from both the participants as well as the researchers who collect data and interact with participants.

When developing research proposals, investigators should carefully consider each threat to internal validity to determine whether their design is vulnerable to that threat. If it is, the researchers must decide whether to institute additional controls to minimize the threat, collect additional information to document whether the threat materialized, or accept the threat as an unavoidable design flaw. There is no perfect research design, and high levels of internal validity may compromise construct or external validity, as discussed at the end of the chapter. Eleven of Cook and Campbell's[1] threats to internal validity are important for rehabilitation researchers and are discussed below.

History

History is a threat to internal validity when events unrelated to the treatment of interest occur during the course of the study and may plausibly change the dependent variable. Case-Smith[2] studied the effect of an occupational therapy intervention on handwriting skills in children with poor handwriting legibility. She used a non-random method to assign participants to the intervention and control groups. The intervention group was made up of 31 second-, third-, and fourth-grade students who were receiving school-based occupational therapy services for poor handwriting. The control group was made up of 13 children in the same schools who had poor handwriting but did not receive occupational therapy services. Several historical events could reduce the internal validity of this, or any, study. Consider the effect on the study if the elementary schools involved in the study adopted a "back to basics" curriculum initiative in the same year as the study, placing much more emphasis on handwriting than had been typical in past years. This hypothetical historical event, not under the researchers' control, would introduce additional handwriting practice into the study. In the absence of control, researchers should gather information to help them determine how much of an effect this additional practice may have had on the results of the study.

Researchers could ask teachers to estimate how much writing was required of students in and out of class compared with the previous year. If intervention and control groups participated in the "back to basics" handwriting activities equally, then the effect of this additional practice would be uniform across the two groups, and some separation of the effects of general handwriting practice versus the effects of the occupational therapy handwriting program could be accomplished, as shown in Figure 7–1. The hypothetical data in this figure show that the groups began the study with the same handwriting legibility, that the control group improved slightly, and that the intervention group improved markedly. The conclusion drawn from these hypothetical data might be written in a journal article as follows:

The control group improved legibility by 5 percentage points over starting legibility of 75%, perhaps related to the intensive handwriting practice that was a part of the "back-to-basics" curriculum adopted by the school for the academic year. The intervention group, who received occupational therapy as well as the intensive handwriting practice of the "back-to-basics" curriculum, showed 3 times the legibility improvement of the control group, improving by approximately 15 percentage points from their starting point of 75%. We assume that the intervention group results represent an approximately 5-point improvement related to the "back-to-basics" handwriting practice and a 10-point improvement attributable to the occupational therapy program.

Researchers can use three strategies to minimize the effects of history: planning, use of a randomly selected control group, and description of unavoidable historical events. In experimental studies, careful planning by the researcher can minimize the chances that historical events will influence the study. If a geographical region is usually snowed in during February, a study that requires participant attendance at treatment sessions 5 days per week should probably be scheduled at another time of year. If testing of participants requires a full day with half-hour rests between measurements, it might be wise to isolate participants and researchers from radios and televisions so that news that happens to occur on the day of testing does not influence participant or researcher performance.

Use of a control group provides the researcher with some ability to separate the effects of history from the effects of the treatment. Use of a control group in this manner is illustrated by the hypothetical example of the "back-to-basics" curriculum, in which the effect of intensive handwriting practice by the control group was separated from the combined effect of intensive handwriting practice and occupational therapy in the intervention group. Random assignment of participants to groups is the best way to minimize the effects of history, because the different groups will likely be affected equally by the historical event.

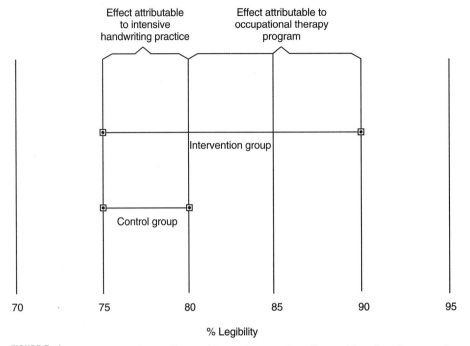

FIGURE 7–1. Separation of the effects of intensive, teacher-directed handwriting practice (control) from the effects of an occupational therapy handwriting intervention (intervention). Both the control and intervention groups participated in intensive handwriting practice; only the intervention group participated in occupational therapy. Both groups had mean pretest scores of 75% legibility; the control group had a mean posttest score of 80% legibility, and the intervention group had a mean posttest score of 90% legibility. For the control group, changes in legibility can be attributed to the intensive, teacher-directed handwriting practice. For the intervention group, part of the change seen can be attributed to the intensive, teacher-directed handwriting practice; the change above that seen in the control group can be attributed to added effect of the occupational therapy program.

In some instances, historical events that cannot be avoided may occur. In retrospective nonexperimental studies, control of history is impossible because the historical events have already occurred. If an uncontrolled historical event that may cause changes in the dependent variable does occur, it is important to collect and present information about the event. Emery[3] did a retrospective study of the impact of the implementation of Medicare's prospective payment system on physical therapy practice and clinical education in teaching hospitals. Since the number and degree level of physical therapy education programs was changing during the time period

he studied, it is difficult to know which of the clinical education changes might be related to changes in the payment system versus changes in the educational system. When unable to control a threat, researchers have a responsibility to present information about the threat so that readers may form an opinion about its seriousness.

Maturation

Maturation, that is, changes within a participant due to the passage of time, is a threat to internal validity when it occurs during the course of a study and may plausibly cause changes in the dependent variable. Participants get older, more experienced, or bored during the course of a study. Patients with neurological deficits may experience spontaneous improvement in their conditions; participants with orthopedic injuries may become less edematous, have less pain, and be able to bear more weight with time.

As was the case with historical threats to internal validity, single-group studies do not provide a basis from which the researcher may separate the effects of maturation from the effects of treatment. Yarkony and associates[4] used a single-group design to document the functional improvement of patients with paraplegia completing an inpatient rehabilitation program. The maturation threat in this study is that, with experience, young people with paraplegia may demonstrate increased skill in managing their injury even in the absence of a formal rehabilitation program.

Maturation effects can be controlled in several ways. The first is through use of a control group, preferably with random assignment of participants to either the control or the experimental group. Use of the control group allows the effects of maturation alone to be observed in the control group. The treatment effects are then evaluated in terms of how much the treatment group improved in comparison with the control group.

A second way to control for the effects of maturation is to take multiple baseline measures of participants before implementing the treatment. Suppose that you have a group of patients with ankle sprains who have persistent edema despite protected weight bearing, compression bandage wrap, elevation when possible, and use of ice packs three times daily. Documentation of baseline volume over a period of several days or weeks would provide appropriate comparison measures against which the effects of a compression and cryotherapy pump regimen could be evaluated. Figure 7–2 shows three patterns of baseline measurements: stable, irregular, and steadily progressing. Results after the intervention are interpreted in light of the baseline pattern documented before the intervention. Patients in Figure 7–2, *A,* had no change in the weeks before

intervention but showed dramatic improvements after treatment. Patients in Figure 7–2, *B,* had weekly fluctuations in edema before treatment and marked improvement after treatment. Patients in Figure 7–2, *C,* showed consistent, but slow, improvement in the weeks before treatment and more rapid improvement after treatment.

Maturation effects may be seen in repeated treatment research designs. Any time participants receive more than one treatment, they may respond differently to later treatments than to earlier treatments. Performance on the dependent variable may improve for later treatments because of increased experience with the treatment, or performance may decline because of fatigue or boredom. For example, Collier and Thomas[5] conducted a repeated treatment study of range of motion at the wrist during basketball shooting when wearing four different wrist extension orthoses. Participants may have felt more accustomed to orthotic wear over time, giving a more relaxed performance with greater range of motion at the wrist during later trials. Conversely, they may have fatigued during the course of the study, demonstrating decreased energy and wrist motion during later trials. The authors controlled for these possible effects by randomizing the order in which they presented the treatments to participants.

Testing

Testing is a threat to internal validity when repeated testing itself is likely to result in changes in the dependent variable. For example, on the first day of speech therapy, a child who has a speech delay may feel uncomfortable in the surroundings and intimidated by the speech-language pathologist, giving worse than normal responses to testing. Improved measurements on subsequent days may reflect familiarization with the testing procedure and the therapist rather than effectiveness of the treatment.

Three basic design strategies can be used to minimize testing effects. The first is to use randomly selected experimental and control groups

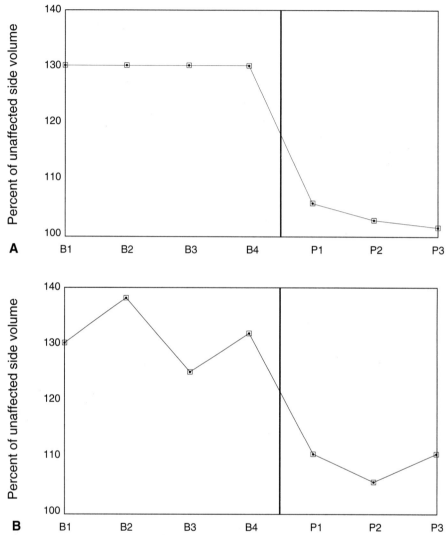

FIGURE 7–2. Patterns of baseline (B) measurements in relation to posttreatment (P) measurements. **A,** Stable baseline. **B,** Irregular baseline.

Continued

so that the effects of testing in the control group can be removed by comparison with the effects of testing and treatment in the experimental group. This is analogous to the removal of the effects of history and maturation through use of a control group.

The second strategy is to eliminate multiple testing through use of a posttest-only design. However, in the absence of a pretest to establish that control and experimental groups were the same at the start of the experiment, posttest-only studies must have effective random assignment of participants to groups.

The third design strategy is to conduct familiarization sessions with the testing personnel or equipment so that the effects of learning are

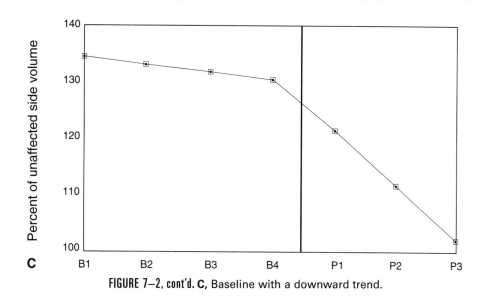

FIGURE 7–2, cont'd. C, Baseline with a downward trend.

accounted for before the independent variable is manipulated. To determine the extent of familiarization needed, the researcher should conduct a pilot study to determine how much time or how many sessions are needed before performance is stable. One drawback of multiple testing is the possibility that the familiarization process will itself constitute a "treatment." For example, if participants familiarize themselves with a strength-testing protocol once a week for 4 weeks, they may have exercised enough during familiarization to show a training response.

Instrumentation

Instrumentation is a threat to internal validity when changes in measuring tools themselves are responsible for observed changes in the dependent variable. Many tools that record physical measurements need to be calibrated with each testing session. Calibration is a process by which the measuring tool is compared with standard measures to determine its accuracy. If inaccurate, some tools can be adjusted until they are accurate. If a tool has limited adjustability, the researcher may need to apply a mathematical correction

factor to convert inaccurate raw scores into accurate transformed scores. If temperature or humidity influences measurement, these factors must be controlled, preferably through testing under constant conditions or, alternatively, through mathematical adjustment for the differences in physical environment.

Researchers themselves are measuring tools ("human instruments"). An example of the variability in the human instrument has surely been felt by almost any student: It is almost impossible for an instructor to apply exactly the same criteria to each paper in a large stack. Maybe the instructor starts out grading leniently but "cracks down" as he or she proceeds through the stack of papers. Maybe the instructor who is a stickler at first adopts a more permissive attitude when the end of the stack is in sight. Maybe a middling paper is graded harshly if it follows an exemplary paper; the same paper might be graded favorably if it follows an abysmal example. A variety of observational clinical measures, such as perception of voice characteristics, identification of gait deviations, functional levels, or abnormal tone, may suffer from similar problems. Measurement issues in rehabilitation research are addressed in detail in Section 5.

Statistical Regression to the Mean

Statistical regression is a threat to internal validity when participants are selected based on extreme scores on a single administration of a test. A hypothetical example illustrates the mathematical principle behind statistical regression to the mean: We have three recreational runners, each of whom has completed ten 10-km runs in an average time of 50 minutes, and a range of times from 40 to 60 minutes. The distribution in Figure 7–3, *A*, represents the race times of the three runners.

Suppose we wish to test a new training regimen designed to decrease race times to see whether the regimen is equally effective with runners at different skill levels. We place runners into categories based on a single qualifying race time, have them try the training regimen for 1 month, and record their times at an evaluation race completed at the end of the 1-month training period. At the qualifying race, we place runners into one of three speed categories based on their time in that race: Participants in the fast group finished in less than 45 minutes, participants in the average group finished between and including 45 and 55 minutes, and participants in the slow group finished in greater than 55 minutes.

The times marked with a Q in Figure 7–3, *B*, show that Runner 1 performed much better than average on the day of the qualifying race (40 minutes), Runner 2 performed much worse than usual on the qualifying day (60 minutes), and Runner 3 gave an average performance (49 minutes). Runners 1 and 2 gave atypical performances on the qualifying day and in subsequent races would be expected to perform closer to their "true" running speed. Thus, even without intervention, Runner 1 would likely run the next race slower and Runner 2 would likely run the next race faster. Runner 3, who gave a typical performance, is likely to give another typical performance at the next race. In other words, the extreme scores tend to "regress toward the mean." This regression toward the mean for the evaluation race is represented by the times marked with an E in Figure 7–3, *B*. If we do not consider the effects of statistical regression, we might conclude

that the training program has no effect on average runners, speeds up the slow runners, and slows down the fast runners.

In general, the way to control for statistical regression toward the mean is to select participants for groups based on reliable, stable measures. If the measures used to form groups are inherently variable, then participants are best assigned to groups based on a distribution of scores collected over time, rather than by a single score that might not reflect true ability.

Assignment

Assignment to groups is a threat to internal validity when groups of participants are different from one another on some variable that is related to the dependent variable of interest. Cook and Campbell labeled this particular threat "selection."[1] The term *assignment* is more precise and differentiates between this internal validity threat related to group assignment and the external validity threat, presented later, of participant selection.

Assignment threatens internal validity most often in designs in which participants are not randomly assigned to groups or in nonexperimental designs in which study group membership cannot be manipulated by the investigator. For example, Mäenpää and Lehto[6] used a retrospective nonexperimental design to determine the relative success of three different nonoperative ways to manage patellar dislocation. The three different groups were immobilized as follows: plaster cast, posterior splint, and bandage/brace. Because the treatment received was based on physician preference, there is no way to determine why individual participants were treated with a particular immobilization method, and no randomization process to increase the likelihood that the groups would be similar on important extraneous variables. For example, the bandage/brace group consisted of proportionately more women than the other groups. Because women may have more predisposing anatomical factors for patellar dislocation than men, perhaps

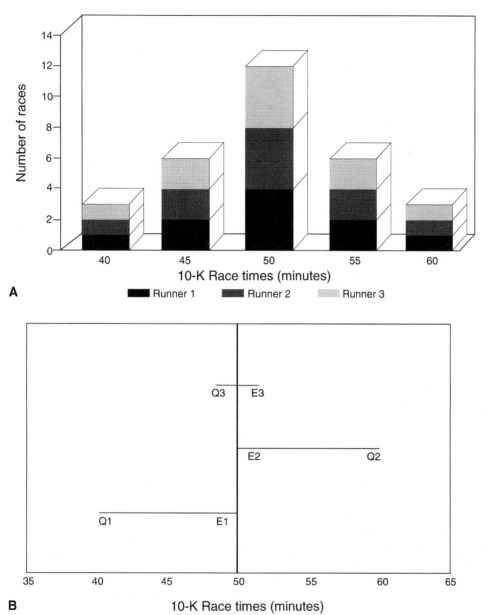

A

B   10-K Race times (minutes)

FIGURE 7-3. Statistical regression toward the mean. **A,** The distribution of race times for three runners, as shown by the different shading patterns on the bars. All three runners have an average race time of 50 minutes. **B,** The effect of statistical regression toward the mean if the runners are placed into different groups based on qualifying times at a single race. *Q* represents qualifying times for each runner; *E* represents the runners' evaluation times at a subsequent race. Runner 1 appears to have slowed from 40 to 50 minutes, Runner 2 appears to have speeded up from 60 to 50 minutes, and Runner 3 stayed approximately the same.

the higher redislocation rate for the bandage/brace group is related to the higher proportion of women, rather than to the type of immobilization.

Control of assignment threats is most effectively accomplished through random assignment to groups within a study (see Chapter 8). When random assignment to groups is not possible, researchers may use statistical methods to "equalize" groups (see Chapter 21).

Mortality

Mortality is a threat to internal validity when participants are lost from the different study groups at different rates or for different reasons. Despite the best efforts of the researcher to begin the study with randomly assigned groups who are equivalent on all important factors, differential mortality can leave the researcher with very different groups by the end of the study. Assume that a researcher has designed a strengthening study in which one group of 50 participants participates in a combined concentric and eccentric program of moderate intensity and another group of 50 participates in a largely eccentric program of higher intensity. Forty-five of the participants in the moderate group complete the program, with an average increase in strength of 20%. Fifteen of the participants in the high-intensity group complete the program, with an average increase in strength of 40%. Concluding that the high-intensity program was superior to the moderate-intensity program would ignore the differential mortality of participants from the two groups. This problem of mortality might be written up as follows in a journal article:

Participants who completed the high-intensity program showed greater strength increases than did participants who completed the moderate-intensity program. There was, however, differential loss of participants from the two groups. Ninety percent of the moderate-intensity group completed the program. The five participants who dropped out did so because of time constraints that prevented regular participation in the exercise program. Only 30% of the high-intensity group completed the program. Of the 35 participants who dropped out of the study, five did so because of time constraints and 30 did so because they were unable to tolerate the delayed muscle soreness associated with this exercise program. We conclude that the moderate-intensity program provides moderate strength gains and is tolerated by a majority of participants. The high-intensity program provides impressive strength gains for the few who can tolerate the discomfort associated with the program.

Researchers can control experimental mortality by planning to minimize possible mortality and collecting information about the lost participants and about reasons for the loss of participants.

Researchers need to make adherence to an experimental routine as easy as possible for participants while maintaining the intent of the experiment. Administering treatments at a place of work or at a clinic where participants are already being treated will likely lead to better attendance than if patients have to drive across town to participate in the study. Developing protocols that minimize discomfort are likely to lead to higher levels of retention within a study. Testing and treating on a single day avoids the loss of participants that inevitably accompanies a protocol that requires several days of participation.

When answering the research question requires longer-term participation and its attendant loss of participants, researchers should document the characteristics of the participants who drop out of the study to determine whether they are similar to those who remain in the study. If the dropouts have characteristics similar to those of participants who remain in the study, and if the rate and character of dropouts are similar across study groups, then differential mortality has not occurred. Such a loss of participants is random and affects the study groups equally.

Interactions Between Assignment and Maturation, History, or Instrumentation

Assignment effects can interact with maturation, history, or instrumentation to either obscure or exaggerate treatment effects. These interactions occur when maturation, history, or instrumentation effects act differently on treatment and control groups.

A hypothetical example of an Assignment × History interaction would be seen in Case-Smith's[2] study if only one of the groups of children was affected by a "back to basics" curriculum with intensive handwriting practice. Assume that members of the control group attended a school that added a "back to basics" curriculum and that members of the experimental group attended a school that did not add such a component to their curriculum. In this scenario, the historical event of the "back to basics" curriculum changed the study from a comparison of a control group versus an occupational therapy group to a comparison of intensive handwriting practice versus an occupational therapy handwriting intervention. This problem might be described as follows in a journal article:

During the course of the study, a "back to basics" curriculum that included intensive handwriting practice was implemented in the school attended by control group members but not in the school attended by the occupational therapy group members. Rather than comparing an experimental group receiving occupational therapy with an untreated control group as originally planned, the comparison was between a group who participated in an occupational therapy handwriting intervention and a group who participated in teacher-directed, intensive handwriting practice.

In this scenario, the hypothetical threat of an Assignment × History interaction to internal validity was uncontrollable but explainable. Such threats can be explained only if researchers remain alert to possible threats and collect information about the extent to which participants were affected by the threat.

An interaction between assignment and maturation occurs when different groups are maturing at different rates. If a study of the effectiveness of a rehabilitation program for patients who have had a cerebral vascular accident (CVA) compared one group of patients 6 months after their CVA with another group 2 months after their CVA, the group with the more recent CVA would be expected to show greater spontaneous improvement.

An Assignment × Instrumentation interaction occurs when an instrument is more or less sensitive to change in the range at which one of the treatment groups is located. For example, assume that a researcher seeks to determine which of two methods of instruction, lecture or Web-based, results in superior student achievement in pharmacology. The students in the different instructional groups take a pretest that has a maximum score of 100 points. The group being taught by the lecture method has an average pretest score of 60; the group being taught via the Web-based approach has an average pretest score of 20. The traditional group can improve only 40 points; the Web-based group can improve up to 80 points. Thus, the interaction between assignment and instrumentation exaggerates the differences in gain scores between the two groups by suppressing the gain of the group who started at 60 points. When scores "top out" and an instrument cannot register greater gains, this is termed a *ceiling effect*; when scores "bottom out" and an instrument cannot register greater declines, this is termed a *basement* or *floor effect*.

Control of interactions with assignment is accomplished through the same means that assignment, history, maturation, and instrumentation are controlled individually: random assignment to groups, careful planning, and collection of relevant information when uncontrolled threats occur. As is the case with assignment threats alone, mathematical equalization of groups can sometimes compensate for interactions between assignment and history, maturation, or instrumentation.

Diffusion or Imitation of Treatments

Diffusion of treatments is a threat to internal validity when participants in treatment and control groups share information about their respective treatments. Assume that an experiment evaluates the relative effectiveness of plyometrics versus traditional resistive exercise in restoring quadriceps torque in patients who have undergone anterior cruciate ligament reconstruction in a single clinic. Can you picture a member of the plyometrics group and a member of the traditional group discussing their respective programs while icing their knees down after treatment? Perhaps a man in the traditional group decides that low-intensity jumping is just the thing he needs to speed his rehabilitation program along and a man in the plyometric group decides to buy a cuff weight and add some leg lifts to his program. If this treatment diffusion occurs, the difference between the intended treatments will be blurred.

Researchers can control treatment diffusion by minimizing contact between participants in the different groups, masking participants when possible, and orienting participants to the importance of adhering to the rehabilitation program to which they are assigned. Sometimes researchers offer participants the opportunity to participate in the alternate treatment after the study is completed if it proves to be the more effective treatment. This offer should make participants less tempted to try the alternate treatment during the study period.

Compensatory Equalization of Treatments

Compensatory equalization of treatment is a threat to internal validity when a researcher with preconceived notions about which treatment is more desirable showers attention on participants who are receiving the treatment the researcher perceives to be less desirable. This extra attention may alter scores on the dependent variable if the attention leads to increased adherence to treatment instructions, increased effort during testing, or even increased self-esteem leading to a general sense of well-being.

Researchers should control compensatory equalization of treatment by avoiding topics about which they are biased or by designing studies in which their bias is controlled through researcher masking. In addition, if there is strong existing evidence that one treatment is more desirable than the other, researchers need to consider whether it is ethical to contrast the two treatments in another experimental setting.

Compensatory Rivalry or Resentful Demoralization

Rivalry and demoralization are threats to internal validity when members of one group react to the perception that they are receiving a less desirable treatment than other groups. This reaction can take two forms: compensatory rivalry (a "we'll show them" attitude) and resentful demoralization (a "why bother" attitude). Compensatory rivalry tends to mask differences between control and treatment groups; resentful demoralization tends to exaggerate differences between control and experimental groups. Researchers can control rivalry and resentment by controlling the information given to participants, masking themselves and participants to group membership, and having a positive attitude toward all groups.

■ CONSTRUCT VALIDITY

Construct validity is concerned with the meaning of variables within a study. In contrast to internal validity, which is only relevant when researchers are looking for explanations for differences between groups within a study, construct validity is an issue in all research studies. One of the central questions related to construct validity is whether the researcher is studying a "construct as labeled" or a "construct as implemented." An example of the difference between these two constructs is illustrated by a hypothetical example wherein a researcher uses active range of motion as a dependent measure of shoulder function. The construct as labeled is "function"; the construct as implemented is "active range of motion." Some readers might consider active range of motion to be a good indicator of function, but others might consider it an incomplete indicator of function. Those who are critical of the use of active range of motion as a functional indicator are questioning the construct validity of the dependent variable.

Cook and Campbell[1] described 10 separate threats to construct validity. Their list is collapsed into the four threats described in the following sections. The general strategy for controlling threats to construct validity is to develop research problems and designs through a thoughtful process that draws on the literature and theory of the discipline.

Construct Underrepresentation

Construct underrepresentation is a threat to construct validity when constructs are not fully developed within a study. In Manfroy and associates' study of the effect of exercise, prewrap, and athletic tape on resistance to ankle inversion, the independent variable construct "exercise" was not developed fully.[7] This variable had two levels: "before exercise" and "after 40 minutes of exercise." As the authors note,

> A point of practical interest concerns the time point when the tape lost its effectiveness: was it after 5, 10, 20, or 30 minutes of exercise? … Because the two measurement points were more than 40 minutes apart in the present study, we could not resolve the time course of any short-term changes in resistance.[7(p161)]

Fuller explication of the construct of exercise would require more than two measures across time—perhaps at 5, 10, 20, and 40 minutes of exercise.

Construct underrepresentation may also be a concern related to the dependent variables within a study. For example, Powers and associates[8] studied the locomotor function of individuals with patellofemoral pain (PFP). Each participant's gait was analyzed during free-speed and fast walking, ascending and descending stairs, and ascending and descending ramps. McClay, in an invited commentary to the article, noted that

> The activities tested…may not have been painful for these subjects.…The authors' assumption was that the subjects with PFP would exhibit a compensatory pattern. However, if the activity does not cause pain, mechanics are not likely to be altered.[9(p1076)]

In this example, the concern is that the construct of "locomotion" has been underrepresented by selecting low-level activities that do not elicit pain.

Construct underrepresentation can also apply to the intensity of a construct. Kluzik and colleagues studied the effect of a neurodevelopmental treatment on reaching in children with spastic cerebral palsy.[10] They analyzed reaching motions before and after a single neurodevelopmental treatment. In an invited commentary accompanying publication of Kluzik and associates' article, Scholz noted the following:

> Something, albeit subtle, has resulted from the intervention. Expecting a more dramatic improvement in the reaching performance of this population following only one treatment is probably too much to ask in the first place. Future work should focus on the evaluation of long-term effects.[11(p77)]

Scholz thus recognized that the construct has been underrepresented because it was applied only once and recommended future work with a more intense representation of the construct. It should be noted that two of the original authors, Fetters and Kluzik, have now published follow-up work that addresses this concern by comparing the impact of 5 days of neurodevelopmental treatment with 5 days of practice of reaching tasks.[12]

Experimenter Expectancies

Experimenter expectancy is a threat to construct validity when the participants are able to guess the ways in which the experimenter wishes them to respond. In Chapter 5, "Clever Hans" was introduced during the discussion of whether it is possible to have independence of the investigator and participant. Recall that Clever Hans was a horse who could provide the correct response to mathematical problems by tapping his foot the correct number of times. His talents could be explained by the fact that questioners apparently unconsciously raised their eyebrows, flared their nostrils, or raised their heads as Hans was coming up to the correct number of taps. Rosenthal, who wrote about Hans, framed the issue in terms of the expectation of the examiner:

> Hans' questioners, even skeptical ones, expected Hans to give the correct answers to their queries. Their expectation was reflected in their unwitting signal to Hans that the time had come for him to stop his tapping. The signal cued Hans to stop, and the questioner's expectation became the reason for Hans' being, once again, correct.[13(p138)]

In the story of Clever Hans, the construct as labeled was "ability to do mathematics." The construct as implemented, however, was "ability to respond to experimenter cues."

Morgan and associates' work on children's willingness to share activities with a peer with a physical disability is an example of a study in which experimenter expectancy may have been a threat to construct validity.[14] In this study, elementary school children were assigned to view a videotape of a child who was ambulatory or the same child using a wheelchair. They then rated their own willingness, as well as their perception of the willingness of classmates, to interact with the child in the videotape. They found that the children expressed very positive personal intentions toward the child using the wheelchair, but less positive perceptions of the intentions of classmates toward the same child. If even elementary school-aged children understand that the adults around them would like them to interact freely with a child using a wheelchair, their responses may reflect their knowledge of the social desirability of positive attitudes toward children using wheelchairs. The construct as labeled was "attitudes about peers with disabilities"; however, the construct as implemented

probably was "expressed attitudes about peers with disabilities by children who know that positive attitudes are socially desirable."

Researchers can control experimenter expectancy effects by limiting information given to participants and themselves, by having different researchers who bring different expectations to the experimental setting replicate their study, and by selecting topics from which they can maintain an objective distance.

Interaction Between Different Treatments

Interaction between different treatments is a threat to construct validity when treatments other than the one of interest are administered to participants. McIntosh and colleagues[15] studied facilitation of gait patterns in patients with Parkinson's disease with different forms of rhythmic auditory stimulation. Some of the patients with Parkinson's disease were taking dopaminergic medications on their regular dosing schedule and some had discontinued their medication 24 hours in advance of the study. If the authors had put all of the patients with Parkinson's disease into a single group, it would have been impossible for them to separate the effects of the stimulation from the effect of being on medication. In fact, the authors had a specific theoretical reason for examining patients on and off of medication (to determine the contribution of the basal ganglia in responding to rhythmic stimulation) and therefore analyzed each group separately.

In some instances, control of interaction between different treatments is often difficult to achieve because of ethical considerations in clinical research. For example, if it would be unsafe for patients with Parkinson's disease to be off their medication temporarily, then McIntosh and colleagues would have had no choice but to study the combined impact of stimulation and medication. However, researchers can document who receives additional treatment and can analyze data by subgroups if not all participants are exposed to the additional treatments. If all participants are exposed to multiple treatments, then researchers need to carefully label the treatments to make this obvious.

Interaction Between Testing and Treatment

Interaction between testing and treatment is a threat to construct validity when a test itself can be considered an additional treatment. As discussed in the section on testing as a threat to internal validity, controlling for the threat to internal validity made by familiarization with the test may sometimes constitute an additional treatment. In the case of strength testing, repeated familiarization sessions with the equipment may constitute a training stimulus. The treatment as labeled may be "nine strength training sessions"; the treatment as implemented may be "nine strength training sessions and three strength testing sessions."

One way to control for interaction between testing and treatment is to compare a treatment group who was pretested, a treatment group who was not pretested, a control group who was pretested, and a control group who was not pretested. This allows the researcher to compare the effects of the test and treatment combined with the effects of treatment alone, the test alone, and neither the test nor the treatment. Few examples of this design (known as a *Solomon four-group design*) can be found in the rehabilitation literature, presumably because of the large number of participants that would be required to form all four groups. One example of such a design is Knaus and colleagues' work on use of the "AIDS quilt" as a health communication intervention.[16] In addition, researchers can control for interaction between testing and treatment by limiting testing to the end of the study.

■ EXTERNAL VALIDITY

External validity is concerned with to whom, in what settings, and at what times the results of research can be generalized. Cook and Campbell distinguished between generalizing *across*

groups, settings, or times and generalizing *to* particular persons, settings, or times.[1] One can generalize to groups, settings, or times similar to the one studied. One can generalize across groups, settings, or times if one has studied multiple subgroups of people, settings, or times. If researchers study the effect of a progressive resistive exercise technique on the biceps strength of elderly women, they can generalize their results only to elderly women. If they study the same question with a diverse group of men and women with an average age of 35 years, they can generalize their results to other diverse groups with an average age of 35. Even though the researchers have tested men and women of different age groups in the second example, they cannot generalize across age groups or sexes unless they analyze the diverse group according to subgroups. In this example, the overall group might show an increase in strength even if the elderly individuals in the group showed no change.

As was the case with construct validity, the question of generalizability of research results is equally applicable to descriptive research, relationship analysis, or difference analysis. Unlike internal validity and construct validity, both of which depend a great deal on the design of the study, external validity is influenced by the design of the study as well as by the research consumer who hopes to use the study findings. From a design perspective, controlling the threats to external validity requires thoughtful consideration of the population to whom the results of the study can be applied, combined with practical considerations of the availability of participants for study and with attention to how closely the research resembles clinical practice. From a consumer perspective, external validity will relate to how closely the research participants and settings match the patients or clients to whom, and settings to which, the reader will apply the findings.

Selection

Selection is a threat to external validity when the selection process is biased in that it yields participants who are in some manner different from the population to which the researchers or readers hope to generalize the results. Individuals who are willing to serve as research participants may differ from the general population. As stated by Cook and Campbell, "Even when respondents belong to a target class of interest, systematic recruitment factors lead to findings that are only applicable to volunteers, exhibitionists, hypochondriacs, scientific do-gooders, those who have nothing else to do, and so forth."[1(p73)]

For example, consider a hypothetical experimental study in which a speech-language pathologist seeks volunteers to participate in a program to reduce foreign language accents among nonnative speakers of English. The program, which proves to be successful with the initial volunteer group, is considered for implementation by several corporations seeking to improve English language skills of their workers who are nonnative speakers. One consideration for these corporations must be how well the results from volunteers could be generalized to nonvolunteers. Volunteers who have a personal goal to reduce their accents would likely adhere to recommendations for practice outside the therapy environment. Contrast these volunteers with employees participating in a mandatory program imposed by their employers. If the employees in the imposed program do not practice recommended speech activities outside the therapy environment, their results could be substantially different from those found with the volunteers who do.

The threat of selection to external validity in a descriptive research report is illustrated in a study by Hanke and colleagues.[17] The purpose of the study was to determine the reliability of measurements of body center-of-mass momentum of healthy adults while rising from sitting to standing. Participants were 19 healthy adults between the ages of 25 and 38 years. In an invited commentary accompanying the research article, DiFabio noted that:

> the use of subjects without known impairments to establish criterion standards for evaluating clinical impairment must be analyzed carefully. Measures

of motor performance in nondisabled subjects do not have automatic validity, and studies done exclusively with nondisabled subjects need to establish the relevancy and usefulness of the measure intended for clinical use.[18(p115)]

The authors responded to this concern by noting that:

> If the expertise of a physical therapist resides in the evaluation and enhancement of human movement function, then knowledge of how movement is generated by healthy persons across the lifespan should equip the practitioner with valuable tools and insights for solving problems displayed by persons with disorders of movement function.[17(p117)]

This useful intellectual exchange illustrates how different readers may approach the issue of external validity differently, depending on how they plan to use the research results.

Researchers can control selection as a threat to external validity by carefully considering the target population to whom they wish to generalize results, selecting participants accordingly, and carefully writing their research conclusions to avoid making inferences to groups or across subgroups who have not been studied. A selection issue receiving increased attention today is the need to ensure racial, ethnic, age, and gender representativeness of research participants to maximize generalizability across and to these groups.

Setting

Setting is a threat to external validity when peculiarities of the setting in which the research was conducted make it difficult to generalize the results to other settings. In a study of leg movements of preterm infants, Heriza videotaped leg movements in an effort to sample spontaneous leg movements of each infant.[19] To meet the requirements of her data analysis system, she had to stabilize the infants in some way during taping; she did so by using one hand to support the head and the other hand to maintain the trunk in a midline position. This level of interference with the child is certainly less than, for example, using a pinprick as a stimulus to begin kicking. However, the researcher and the reader still must consider the possibility that an infant's kicking behavior while he or she is supported by a human touch may differ from the infant's kicking behavior in the absence of support. In a later study, Heriza and her colleagues were able to reduce this threat to external validity by using a taping system that recorded spontaneous kicks without physical support from the investigators.[20]

Control of threats to external validity posed by setting requires that researchers simulate as closely as possible the setting to which they hope to generalize their results. Researchers who hope their studies will have clinical applicability must try to duplicate the complexities of the clinical setting within their studies. Researchers who wish to describe participants or settings as they exist naturally must make the research process as unobtrusive as possible.

Time

Time is a threat to external validity when the results of a study are applicable to limited time frames. For example, conclusions that can be drawn from Domholdt and colleagues' study of the spring 2000 status of the profession's transition to the Doctor of Physical Therapy (DPT) degree are time limited.[21] The data were collected in spring 2000, analyzed in late 2000, submitted for publication in 2001, and published in 2002. Even though publication of these results was fairly timely, changes toward the DPT degree continued to move rapidly after data collection. Someone reading the article on the day it was published—much less a year or more after publication—would need to take into account these changes when determining the usefulness of Domholdt and colleagues' data to their setting.

Time threats to external validity can be managed by authors through timely submission of research results for publication and by description of known changes that make the research results less applicable than when the data were collected.

In addition, when articles are used some years after their publication date, readers have the responsibility to incorporate contemporary knowledge into their own review of the usefulness of the results to current practice.

■ RELATIONSHIPS AMONG TYPES OF VALIDITY

Eighteen different threats to validity have been presented. These threats are not, however, independent entities that can be controlled one by one until the perfect research design is created. The relationship between the validity threats can be either cumulative or reciprocal.

Cumulative relationships occur when a change that influences one of the threats influences other threats in the same way. For example, researchers may initially think to use a randomly assigned control group in a study because they want to control for the effects of maturation. By controlling for maturation in this way they also control for history, assignment, testing, and so on.

Reciprocal threats occur when controlling a threat to one type of validity leads to realization of a different threat to validity. For instance, if a researcher wants to achieve the highest level of internal validity possible, he or she will standardize the experimental treatment so that there are few extraneous variables that could account for changes in the dependent measures. However, this standardization compromises external validity because the results can be applied only to settings in which the treatment would be equally well controlled. These reciprocal threats form the basis for the differentiation between research to test the efficacy of an intervention (testing biological effects under tightly controlled conditions with high internal validity) and effectiveness of an intervention (testing clinical usefulness under clinic-like conditions with high external validity). These concepts are explored further in Chapter 15 on outcomes research.

The reciprocal relationship between validity threats is illustrated in Mäenpää and Lehto's study of conservative care of patients with patellar dislocation.[6] As noted earlier, one of the groups of patients seemed to have a higher proportion of women patients than the other two groups. This represents an assignment threat to internal validity. To eliminate this threat from this retrospective study, the authors could have chosen to study only men or only women. In doing so, they would have reduced external validity by narrowing the group to whom the results of the study could be generalized. Mäenpää and Lehto couldn't win. If they studied men and women, they had to cope with a possible threat to internal validity. Conversely, if they studied only men, they would have limited external validity.

■ SUMMARY

Threats to the believability and utility of research can be classified as threats to internal, construct, or external validity. Internal validity concerns whether the treatment caused the effect; construct validity concerns the meaning attached to concepts used within the study; and external validity concerns the persons, settings, or times to which or across which the results can be generalized. Many of the threats to validity are reciprocal because controlling one leads to problems with another.

REFERENCES

1. Cook T, Campbell D. *Quasi-Experimentation: Design and Analysis Issues for Field Settings.* Chicago, Ill: Rand McNally; 1979.
2. Case-Smith J. Effectiveness of school-based occupational therapy intervention on handwriting. *Am J Occup Ther.* 2002;56:17-25.
3. Emery MJ. The impact of the prospective payment system: perceived changes in the nature of practice and clinical education. *Phys Ther.* 1993;73:18-29.
4. Yarkony GM, Roth EJ, Meyer PR, Lovell LL, Heinemann AW. Rehabilitation outcomes in patients with complete thoracic spinal cord injury. *Am J Phys Med Rehabil.* 1990;69:23-27.
5. Collier SE, Thomas JJ. Range of motion at the wrist: a comparison study of four wrist extension orthoses and the free hand. *Am J Occup Ther.* 2002;56:180-184.
6. Mäenpää H, Lehto M. Patellar dislocation: the long-term results of nonoperative management in 100 patients. *Am J Sports Med.* 1997;25:213-217.
7. Manfroy PP, Ashton-Miller JA, Wojtys EM. The effect of exercise, prewrap, and athletic tape on the maximal active and passive ankle resistance to ankle inversion. *Am J Sports Med.* 1997;25:156-163.
8. Powers CM, Perry J, Hsu A, Hislop HJ. Are patellofemoral pain and quadriceps femoris muscle torque associated with locomotor function? *Phys Ther.* 1997;77:1063-1078.
9. McClay IS. Invited commentary. *Phys Ther.* 1997;77:1075-1076.
10. Kluzik J, Fetters L, Coryell J. Quantification of control: a preliminary study of effects of neurodevelopmental treatment on reaching in children with spastic cerebral palsy. *Phys Ther.* 1990;70:65-76.
11. Scholz JP. Commentary. *Phys Ther.* 1990;70:76-78.
12. Fetters L, Kluzik J. The effects of neurodevelopmental treatment versus practice on the reaching of children with spastic cerebral palsy. *Phys Ther.* 1996;76:346-358.
13. Rosenthal R. *Experimenter Effects in Behavioral Research.* Enlarged ed. New York, NY: Irvington Publishers; 1976.
14. Morgan SB, Bieberich AA, Walker M, Schwerdtfeger H. Children's willingness to share activities with a physically disabled peer: Am I more willing than my classmates? *J Pediatr Psychol.* 1998;23:367-375.
15. McIntosh GC, Brown SH, Rice RR, Thaut MH. Rhythmic auditory-motor facilitation of gait patterns in patients with Parkinson's disease. *J Neurol Neurosurg Psychiatry.* 1997;62:22-26.
16. Knaus CS, Pinkleton BE, Austin EW. The ability of the AIDS quilt to motivate information seeking, personal discussion, and preventative behavior as a health communication intervention. *Health Commun.* 2000;12:301-316.
17. Hanke TA, Pai Y-C, Rogers MW. Reliability of measurements of body center-of-mass momentum during sit-to-stand in healthy adults. *Phys Ther.* 1995;75:105-118.
18. DiFabio RP. Invited commentary. *Phys Ther.* 1995;75:113-115.
19. Heriza CB. Organization of leg movements in preterm infants. *Phys Ther.* 1988;68:1340-1346.
20. Geerdink JJ, Hopkins B, Beek WJ, Heriza CB. The organization of leg movements in preterm and full-term infants after term age. *Dev Psychobiol.* 1996;29:335-351.
21. Domholdt E, Stewart JC, Barr JO, Melzer BA. Entry-level doctoral degrees in physical therapy: status as of spring 2000. *J Phys Ther Educ.* 2002;16(1):60-68.

Selection and Assignment of Participants

Researchers rarely have the opportunity to study all the individuals who possess the characteristics of interest within a study. Fiscal and time constraints often limit researchers' ability to study large groups of participants. In addition, the study of very large groups may be undesirable because it takes time and resources away from improving other components of the research design.[1(p3)] *Sampling* is the process by which a subgroup of participants is selected for study from a larger group of potential participants. *Assignment* is the process by which participants in the sample are assigned to groups within the study. This chapter acquaints readers with the major methods of selecting participants and assigning them to groups.

■ SIGNIFICANCE OF SAMPLING AND ASSIGNMENT

If a rehabilitation team is interested in studying, for example, rehabilitation outcomes in patients who have undergone total knee arthroplasty (TKA), they must somehow determine which of thousands of possible participants will be studied. The way in which participants are identified for study, and for groups within the study, profoundly affects the validity of the study.

Sampling methods influence the characteristics of the sample, which, in turn, influence the generalizability, or external validity, of a piece of research. If, for example, a sample of patients with TKA includes only participants older than 75 years, then the research results cannot be generalized to younger patient groups.

The method by which participants are assigned to groups within the study influences the characteristics of participants within each group, which in turn influences the internal validity of the study. Assume that we design an experiment on the effect of postoperative femoral nerve block (FNB) on early knee range of motion after TKA. We use a design that includes one experimental group (routine rehabilitation plus FNB) and one control group (routine rehabilitation only). The threats to internal validity posed by history, maturation, testing, and assignment can all be controlled by assignment procedures that yield groups of patients with similar ages, medical problems, preoperative ambulation status, and the like.

■ POPULATIONS AND SAMPLES

The distinction between a population and a sample is an important one. A *population* is the total group of interest. A *sample* is a subgroup of the group of interest. *Sampling* is the procedure by which a sample of *units* or *elements* is selected from a population. In clinical research, the sampling unit may be the individual or a group of related individuals, such as graduating classes of practitioners or patients treated at particular clinics.

Defining the population of interest is not a simple matter. There are generally two types of populations who are considered in research—the target population and the accessible population. The *target population* is the group to whom researchers hope to generalize their findings. The *accessible population* is the group of potential research participants who are actually available for a given study.

Hulley and colleagues listed four types of characteristics that define populations: clinical, demographic, geographical, and temporal.[2(p28)] Clinical and demographic characteristics define the target population. The target population for our TKA study might be defined as individuals who have undergone a unilateral TKA and were at least 60 years of age at the time of the surgery. Geographical and temporal characteristics define the accessible population. The accessible population for our TKA study might consist of individuals with the aforementioned clinical and demographic characteristics who underwent surgery in any one of eight Indianapolis hospitals during the 5-year period from 1999 to 2003. Table 8–1 presents a hypothetical distribution of patients at the eight hospitals during this time period. This accessible population of 3000 patients provides the basis for many of the examples in this chapter.

TABLE 8-1 **Hypothetical Sample of Patients Who Underwent Total Knee Arthroplasty by Hospital and Year**

Hospital	1999	2000	2001	2002	2003	Total
A	22	25	28	26	24	125
B	50	55	60	40	45	250
C	48	49	52	51	50	250
D	80	78	75	71	71	375
E	72	72	77	77	77	375
F	95	107	98	97	103	500
G	100	103	95	100	102	500
H	120	130	130	122	123	625
Total	587	619	615	584	595	3000

Once the researcher has defined the accessible population in a general way, he or she needs to develop more specific *inclusion* and *exclusion* characteristics. We already know that patients aged 60 years or older who underwent unilateral TKA at one of eight hospitals from 1999 to 2003 are included in our accessible population. Some patients who fit this description should, nevertheless, be excluded from participation in the study. For example, we need to decide whether to exclude patients who experienced postoperative infection, surgical revision, or rehospitalization soon after the TKA.

The decision to include or exclude participants with certain characteristics must be made in light of the purpose of the research. If the purpose of our study is to provide a description of functional outcomes after TKA, then excluding cases with complications would artificially improve group outcomes by eliminating those likely to have a poor outcome. In contrast, if the purpose of a study is to describe the functional outcomes that can be expected after completion of a particular rehabilitation regimen, then exclusion of patients who could not complete therapy seems reasonable.

After the researcher specifies inclusion and exclusion criteria, he or she needs a sampling frame from which to select participants. A *sampling frame* is a listing of the elements in the accessible population. In our TKA study, we would ask that someone in the medical records department in each of the eight hospitals create a sampling frame by developing a list of patients aged 60 years or older who underwent a TKA from 1999 to 2003.

Existing sampling frames are available for some populations. If we wish to study occupational and physical therapists' opinions on the use of assistants in delivering rehabilitation services, we could use either a professional association membership list or a professional licensing board list as our sampling frame. Use of an existing sampling frame necessarily defines the target population for the research. If we use the professional association membership list, we can generalize only to other professional association members; if we use the licensing board list, we can generalize to licensed occupational and physical therapists regardless of whether they belong to the professional association.

The most basic distinction between sampling methods is between *probabilistic* and *nonprobabilistic* methods. Generation of probability samples involves randomization at some point in the process; generation of nonprobability samples does not. Probability samples are preferable when the researcher hopes to generalize from an accessible population to a target population. This is because probability samples tend to have less sampling error than nonprobability samples. *Sampling error* "refers to the fact that the vagaries of chance will nearly always ensure that one sample will differ from another, even if the two samples are drawn from exactly the same target population in exactly the same random way."[3(pp45,46)] Probability samples tend to be less variable and better approximations of the population than nonprobability samples.

■ PROBABILITY SAMPLING

Four types of probability sampling are presented in this section. As required by definition, all involve randomization at some point in the sampling process. The extent of randomization, however, differs from technique to technique.

Simple Random Sampling

Simple random sampling is a procedure in which each member of the population has an equal chance of being selected for the sample, and selection of each subject is independent of selection of other participants. Assume that we wish to draw a random sample of 300 participants from the accessible population of 3000 patients in Table 8–1. To literally "draw" the sample, we would write each patient's name on a slip of paper, put the 3000 slips of paper in a rotating cage, mix the slips thoroughly, and draw out 300 of the slips. This is an example of sampling *without replacement,* because each slip of paper is not replaced in the cage after it is drawn. It is also possible to sample with replacement, in which case the selected unit is placed back in the population so that it may be drawn again. In clinical research it is not feasible to use the same person more than once for a sample, so sampling without replacement is the norm.

Drawing a sample from a cage, or even from a hat, may work fairly well when the accessible population is small. With larger populations, it becomes difficult to mix the units thoroughly. This apparently happened in the 1970 U.S. draft lottery, when troops were being deployed to Vietnam. Capsules representing days of the year were placed in a cage for selection to determine the order in which young men would be drafted into the armed forces. Days from the later months of the year were selected considerably earlier than days from months earlier in the year. Presumably, the capsules were not mixed well, leading to a higher rate of induction among men with birthdays later in the year.[3(pp5-7)]

The preferred method for generating a simple random sample is to use random numbers that are provided in a table or generated by a computer. Table 8–2 shows a portion of the random numbers table reproduced in Appendix A.[4] Internet sites for random number generation are also available.[5] Before consulting the table, the researcher numbers the units in the sampling frame. In our TKA study, the patients would be numbered from 0001 to 3000. Starting in a random place on the table, and moving in either a horizontal or vertical direction, we would include in our sample any four-digit numbers from 0001 to 3000 that we encounter. Any four-digit numbers greater than 3000 are ignored, as are duplicate numbers. The process is continued until the required number of units is selected. From within the boldface portion of Table 8–2 in column 7, rows 76 through 80, the following numbers, which correspond to individual participants, would be selected for our TKA sample: 1945, 2757, and 2305.

Simple random sampling is easy to comprehend, but it is sometimes difficult to implement.

If the population is large, the process of assigning a number to each population unit becomes extremely time-consuming. The other probability sampling techniques are easier to implement than simple random sampling and may control sampling error as well as simple random sampling. Therefore, the following three probability sampling procedures are used more frequently than simple random sampling.

Systematic Sampling

Systematic sampling is a process by which the researcher selects every nth person on a list. To generate a systematic sample of 300 participants from the TKA population of 3000, we would select every 10th person. The list of 3000 patients might be ordered by patient number, social security number, date of surgery, or birth date. To begin the systematic sampling procedure, a random start within the list of 3000 patients is necessary. To get a random start we can, for example, point to a number on a random numbers table, observe four digits of the license plate number on a car in the parking lot, reverse the last four digits of the accession number of a library book, or ask four different people to select numbers between zero and nine and combine them to form a starting number. There are endless ways to select the random starting number for a systematic sample. If the random starting number for a systematic sample of our TKA population is 1786, and the sampling interval is 10, then the first four participants selected would be the 1786th, 1796th, 1806th, and 1816th individuals on the list.

Systematic sampling is an efficient alternative to simple random sampling, and it often generates samples that are as representative of their populations as simple random sampling.[6] The exception to this is if the ordering system used somehow introduces a systematic error into the sample. Assume that we use dates of surgery to order our TKA sample and that for most weeks during the 5-year period there were 10 surgeries performed. Because the sampling interval is 10,

TABLE 8–2 Segment of a Random Numbers Table*

Row	1	2	3	4	5	6	7	8	9	10	11	12	13	14
71	9122*7*	21199	31935	270*22*	84067	05462	352*16*	14486	29891	686*07*	41867	14951	91696	85065
72	500*01*	38140	66321	199*24*	72163	09538	12151	06878	919*03*	18749	344*05*	56087	82790	70*925*
73	65390	05224	72958	286*09*	814*06*	39147	25549	48542	42627	45233	572*02*	946*17*	23772	07896
74	275*04*	961*31*	83944	41575	10573	086*19*	64482	739*23*	36152	05184	94142	25299	84347	34925
75	37169	94851	39177	896*32*	00959	16487	65536	49071	39782	17095	023*30*	74301	00275	48280
76	115*08*	70225	511*11*	38351	19444	66499	71*945*	05442	13442	78675	48081	66938	93654	59894
77	37449	30362	06694	54690	04052	531*15*	62*757*	95348	78662	11163	81651	50245	34971	52924
78	46515	70331	85922	38379	57015	15765	97161	17869	45349	61796	66345	81073	49106	79860
79	30986	81223	42416	58353	21532	30502	32*305*	86482	05174	07901	54339	58861	78*418*	46942
80	63798	64995	46583	09765	44160	78128	83991	42865	92520	83531	80377	35909	81250	54238

From Beyer WH, ed. *Standard Mathematical Tables*. 27th ed. Boca Raton, Fla:CRC Press; 1984.
*Complete table appears in Appendix A.

and there were usually 10 surgeries performed per week, systematic sampling would tend to overrepresent patients who had surgery on a certain day of the week. Table 8–3 shows an example of how patients with surgery on Monday might be overrepresented in the systematic sample; the boldface entries indicate the units chosen for the sample. If certain surgeons usually perform their TKAs on Tuesday, their patients would be underrepresented in the sample. If patients who are scheduled for surgery on Monday typically have fewer medical complications than those scheduled for surgery later in the week, this will also bias the sample. It is unlikely that the assumptions made to produce this hypothetical bias would operate so systematically in real life—the number of cases per week is likely more variable than presented here, and surgeons likely perform TKAs on more than one day of the week. However, possible systematic biases such as this should be considered when one is deciding how to order the population for systematic sampling.

TABLE 8-3	Systematic Bias in a Systematic Sample	
Subject	**Date of Surgery**	**Surgeon**
1786	**1-6-2003 (Monday)**	**A***
1787	1-6-2003 (Monday)	A
1788	1-7-2003 (Tuesday)	B
1789	1-7-2003 (Tuesday)	B
1790	1-8-2003 (Wednesday)	C
1791	1-8-2003 (Wednesday)	C
1792	1-9-2003 (Thursday)	D
1793	1-9-2003 (Thursday)	D
1794	1-10-2003 (Friday)	E
1795	1-10-2003 (Friday)	E
1796	**1-11-2003 (Monday)**	**A**
1797	1-11-2003 (Monday)	A

*Boldface rows indicate the patients selected for the study. If the sampling interval is 10, and approximately 10 surgeries are performed per week, patients of Surgeon A, who usually performs total knee arthroplasties on Monday, will be overrepresented in the sample.

Stratified Sampling

Stratified sampling is used when certain subgroups must be represented in adequate numbers within the sample or when it is important to preserve the proportions of subgroups in the population within the sample. In our TKA study, if we hope to make generalizations across the eight hospitals within the study, we need to be sure there are enough patients from each hospital in the sample to provide a reasonable basis for making statements about the outcomes of TKA at each hospital. On the other hand, if we want to generalize results to the "average" patient undergoing a TKA, then we need to have proportional representation of participants from the eight hospitals.

Table 8–4 contrasts *proportional* and *nonproportional* stratified sampling. In proportional sampling, the percentage of participants from each hospital is the same in the population and the sample (with minor deviations because participants cannot be divided in half; compare columns 3 and 5). However, the actual number of participants from each hospital in the sample ranges from 12 to 62 (column 4). In nonproportional sampling, the percentage of participants from each hospital is different for the population and the sample (compare columns 3 and 7). However, the actual number of participants from each hospital is the same (column 6, with minor deviations because participants cannot be divided in half).

Stratified sampling from the accessible population is implemented in several steps. First, all units in the accessible population are identified according to the stratification criteria. Second, the appropriate number of participants is selected from each stratum. Participants may be selected from each stratum through simple random sampling or systematic sampling. More than one stratum may be identified. For instance, we might want to ensure that each of the eight hospitals and each of the 5 years of the study period are equally represented in the sample. In this case, we first stratify the accessible population into eight groups by hospital, then stratify each

| TABLE 8-4 | Proportional and Nonproportional Stratified Sampling of Patients at Eight Hospitals |

Hospital	Population Distribution		Proportional Sample		Nonproportional Sample	
	N	%	N	%	N	%
A	125	4.1	12	4.0	37	12.3
B	250	8.3	25	8.3	37	12.3
C	250	8.3	25	8.3	37	12.3
D	375	12.5	38	12.7	37	12.3
E	375	12.5	38	12.7	38	12.7
F	500	16.7	50	16.7	38	12.7
G	500	16.7	50	16.7	38	12.7
H	625	20.8	62	20.6	38	12.7
Total	3000	100.0	300	100.0	300	100.0

hospital into five groups by year, and finally draw a random sample from each of the 40 Hospital × Year subgroups.

Stratified sampling is easy to accomplish if the stratifying characteristic is known for each sampling unit. In our TKA study, both the hospital and year of surgery are known for all elements in the sampling frame. In fact, those characteristics were required for placement of participants into the accessible population. A much different situation exists, however, if we decide that it is important to ensure that certain knee replacement models are represented in the sample in adequate numbers. Stratifying according to this characteristic would require that someone read all 3000 medical charts to determine which knee model was used for each subject. Because of the inordinate amount of time it would take to determine the knee model for each potential subject, we should consider whether simple random or systematic sampling would likely result in a good representation of each knee model.

Another difficulty with stratification is that some strata require that the researcher set classification boundaries. The strata discussed so far (hospital, year, and knee model) are discrete categories of items. Consider, though, the dilemma that would occur if we wanted to stratify on a variable such as "amount of inpatient rehabilitation."

If we wanted to ensure that differing levels of rehabilitation are represented in the sample, we would need to decide what constitutes low, medium, and high amounts of inpatient rehabilitation. Not only would we have to determine the boundaries between groups, we would also have to obtain the information on all 3000 individuals in the accessible population. Once again, we should consider whether random or systematic sampling would likely result in an adequate distribution of the amount of rehabilitation received by patients in the sample.

In summary, stratified sampling is useful when a researcher believes it is imperative to ensure that certain characteristics are represented in a sample in specified numbers. Stratifying on some variables will prove to be too costly and must therefore be left to chance. In many cases, simple random or systematic sampling will result in an adequate distribution of the variable in question.

Cluster Sampling

Cluster sampling is the use of naturally occurring groups as the sampling units. It is used when an appropriate sampling frame does not exist or when logistical constraints limit the researcher's ability to travel widely. There are often several stages to a cluster sampling procedure. For example, if we wanted to conduct a nationwide study on outcomes after TKA, we could not use simple random sampling because the entire population of patients with TKA is not enumerated—that is, a nationwide sampling frame does not exist. In addition, we do not have the funds to travel to all the states and cities that would be represented if a nationwide random sample were selected. To generate a nationwide cluster sample of patients who have undergone a TKA, therefore, we could first sample states, then cities within each selected state, then hospitals within each selected city, and then patients within each selected hospital. Sampling frames for all of these clusters exist: The 50 states are known, various references list cities and populations within each state,[7] and other references list hospitals by city and size.[8]

Each step of the cluster sampling procedure can be implemented through simple random, systematic, or stratified sampling. Assume that we have the money and time to study patients in six states. To select these six states, we might stratify according to region and then randomly select one state from each region. From each of the six states selected, we might develop a list of all cities with populations greater than 50,000 and randomly select two cities from this list. The selection could be random or could be stratified according to city size so that one larger and one smaller city within each state are selected. From each city, we might select two hospitals for study. Within each hospital, patients who underwent TKA in the appropriate time frame would be selected randomly, systematically, or according to specified strata. Figure 8–1 shows the cluster sampling procedure with all steps illustrated for one state, city, and hospital. The same process would occur in the other selected states, cities, and hospitals.

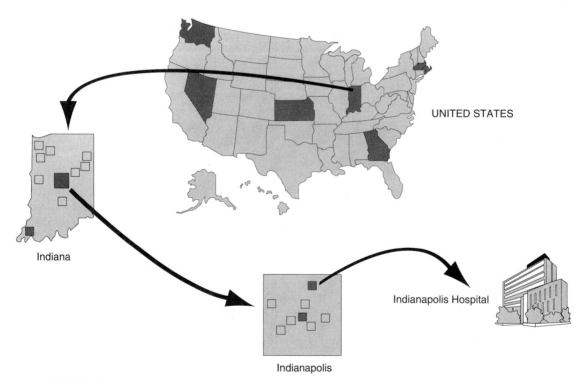

FIGURE 8–1. Partial example of cluster sampling. Six of 50 states are selected, two cities are selected in each state, and two hospitals are selected from each city. Selected units are shaded; only one state, city, and hospital is illustrated.

Cluster sampling can save time and money compared with simple random sampling because participants are clustered in locations. A simple random sample of patients after TKA would likely take us into 50 states and hundreds of cities. The cluster sampling procedure just described would limit the study to 12 cities in six states.

Cluster sampling can occur on a smaller scale as well. Assume that some researchers wish to study the effectiveness of a speech therapy approach for children who stutter, and the accessible population consists of children who seek treatment for stuttering in a single city. This example is well suited to cluster sampling because a sampling frame of this population does not exist. In addition, it would be difficult to train all speech-language pathologists within the city to use the new approach with their clients. Cluster sampling of a few speech therapy departments or practices, and then a few therapists within each department or practice, would be efficient use of the researcher's time for both identifying appropriate children and training therapists with the new modality.

Cluster sampling may also be necessitated by administrative constraints. Assume that researchers wish to determine the relative effectiveness of two educational approaches to third graders' developing awareness of individuals with physical disabilities: In one approach, children simulate disabilities themselves and, in the other approach, individuals with disabilities make presentations to the students. A superintendent is unlikely to allow the study to take place if it requires a random sampling of third graders across the school system with disruption of classrooms. Because third graders exist in clusters, it seems natural to use schools or classrooms as the sampling unit, rather than the individual pupil.

■ NONPROBABILITY SAMPLING

Nonprobability sampling is widely used in rehabilitation research and is distinguished from probability sampling by the absence of randomization. One reason for the predominance of nonprobability sampling in rehabilitation research is limited funding. Because many studies are self-funded, subject selection is confined to a single setting with a limited number of available patients, so the researcher often chooses to study the entire accessible population. Three forms of nonprobability sampling are discussed: convenience, snowball, and purposive sampling.

Samples of Convenience

Samples of convenience involve the use of readily available participants. Rehabilitation researchers commonly use samples of convenience of patients in certain diagnostic categories at a single clinic. If we conducted our study of patients after TKA by using all patients who underwent the surgery from 1999 to 2003 at a given hospital, this would represent a sample of convenience. If patients who undergo TKA at this hospital are different in some way from the overall population of patients who have this surgery, then our study would have little generalizability beyond that facility.

The term "sample of convenience" seems to give the negative implication that the researcher has not worked hard enough at the task of sampling. In addition, we already know that probability samples tend to have less sampling error than nonprobability samples. But before one totally discounts the validity of samples of convenience, it should be pointed out that the accessible populations discussed earlier in the chapter can also be viewed as large samples of convenience. An accessible population that consists of "patients post-TKA who are 60 years old or older and had the surgery at one of eight hospitals in Indianapolis from 1999 to 2003" is technically a large sample of convenience from the population of all the individuals in the world who have undergone TKA. Figure 8–2 shows the distinctions among a target population, an accessible population, a random sample, and a sample of convenience.

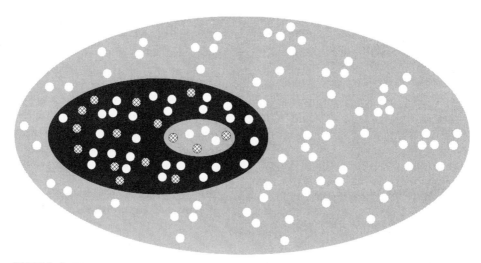

FIGURE 8–2. Distinctions among target populations, accessible populations, samples of convenience, and random samples. The white dots represent elements within the population. The large gray ellipse represents the target population. The black ellipse represents the accessible population. The small gray ellipse represents a sample of convenience. The cross-hatched dots represent a random sample from the accessible population.

Consecutive sampling is a form of convenience sampling. Consecutive samples are used in a prospective study in which the population does not exist at the beginning of the study; in other words, a sampling frame does not exist. If researchers plan a 2-year prospective study of the outcomes of TKA at a particular hospital beginning January 1, 2003, the population of interest does not begin to exist until the first patient has surgery in 2003. In a consecutive sample, all patients who meet the criteria are placed into the study as they are identified. This continues until a specified number of patients is collected, a specified time frame has passed, or certain statistical outcomes are seen.

Snowball Sampling

A snowball sample may be used when the potential members of the sample are difficult to identify. In a snowball sample researchers identify a few participants who are then asked to identify other potential members of the sample. If a team of researchers wishes to study patients who return to sports activities earlier than recommended after ligament reconstruction surgery, snowball sampling is one way to generate a sufficient sample. The investigators will neither be able to purchase a mailing list of such patients, nor will they be able to determine return-to-sport dates reliably from medical records since many patients will not disclose their early return to the health care providers who advised against it. However, if the researchers can use personal contacts to identify a few participants who returned early, it is likely that those participants will be able to identify other potential participants from among their teammates or workout partners.

Purposive Sampling

Purposive sampling is a specialized form of nonprobability sampling that is typically used for qualitative research. Purposive sampling is used when a researcher has a specific reason for selecting particular participants for study. Whereas convenience sampling uses whatever units are readily available, purposive sampling uses handpicked units that meet the researcher's needs. Random, convenience, and purposive samples can be distinguished if we return to the hypothetical study of different educational modes for teaching children about physical disabilities. If there are 40 elementary schools in a district and the researchers randomly select two of them for study, this is clearly a random sample of schools from the accessible population of a single school district. For a sample of convenience, the researchers might select two schools in close proximity. For a purposive sample, the researchers might pick one school because it is large and students are from families with high median incomes and pick a second school because it is small and draws students from families with modest median incomes. Rather than selecting for a representative group of participants, the researchers deliberately pick participants who illustrate different levels of variables they believe may be important to the question at hand. Patton succinctly contrasts random sampling with purposive sampling:

> The logic and power of random sampling derive from statistical probability theory. A random and statistically representative sample permits confident generalization from a sample to a larger population.

The logic and power of purposeful sampling lie in selecting *information-rich cases* for study in depth. Information-rich cases are those from which one can learn a great deal about issues of central importance to the purpose of the inquiry.[9(p230)]

Purposive sampling was used by Pizzari and associates[10] in their study of adherence to anterior cruciate ligament rehabilitation. Because the purpose of their study was to "identify variables that influence adherence to rehabilitation after ACL reconstruction,"[10(p91)] they wanted to sample in a way that ensured that their participants reflected a full range of adherence to rehabilitation recommendations. To do so, they selected five participants whose self-report diaries indicated completion of more than 80% of recommended

home exercises, one participant who reported completion of 60% to 70% of exercises, and five participants who reported completion of less than 60% exercises. This purposive sampling strategy is known as a "maximum variability" or "heterogeneity" sampling, 1 of 16 purposive sampling strategies delineated by Patton.[9(pp230-242)] Further information on qualitative research methods can be found in Chapter 13.

■ ASSIGNMENT TO GROUPS

When a study requires more than one group, the researchers need a method for assigning participants to groups. Random assignment to groups is preferred and is appropriate even when the original selection procedure was nonrandom. Thus, many studies in the rehabilitation literature use a sample of convenience combined with random assignment to groups. The goal of group assignment is to create groups that are equally representative of the entire sample. Because many statistical techniques require equal group sizes, a secondary goal of the assignment process is often to develop groups of equal size.

There are four basic ways to randomly assign participants to groups within a study. These methods can be illustrated by a hypothetical sample of 32 patients who have undergone TKA; age and sex are listed for each patient in Table 8–5. The sample has a mean age of 68 years and consists of 50% women and 50% men. Each of the four assignment techniques was applied to this sample; the processes are described in the following four sections, and the results are presented in Tables 8–6 to 8–9.

The design of our hypothetical study calls for four groups of patients, each undergoing a different post-TKA management. The four programs are variations based on whether or not the patient receives continuous passive motion (CPM or no-CPM) or a femoral nerve block (FNB or no-FNB) after surgery. CPM is one independent variable and FNB is the second independent variable. One group receives CPM and FNB, one group receives CPM but no-FNB, one group receives FNB but no-CPM, and the final group receives no-CPM and no-FNB.

Random Assignment by Individual

The first method of random assignment is to randomly assign each individual in the sample to one of the four groups. This could be done with a roll of a die, ignoring rolls of 5 and 6. When this assignment technique was applied to the

hypothetical sample in Table 8–5, the CPM/FNB condition was represented by a roll of 1, the CPM/no-FNB condition by a roll of 2, the no-CPM/FNB condition by a roll of 3, and the no-CPM, no-FNB condition by a roll of 4. The results of the procedure are shown in Table 8–6. Note that the group sizes range from 4 to 12 participants.

The advantage of assignment by individual is that it is easy to do. The main disadvantage is that with a small sample size, the resulting group sizes are not likely to be equal. With a larger sample size, the probability that group sizes will be nearly equal is greater.

Random Assignment by Block

The second assignment method uses blocks of participants to ensure equal group sizes. Say that in our sample of patients who underwent TKA, we wish to have four groups of eight participants. To assign by block, we can use a random numbers table to select eight numbers for the

| TABLE 8–5 | Existing Sample Characteristics: Case Number, Sex, and Age* |

1. F, 70	9. F, 62	17. M, 70	25. M, 76
2. M, 60	10. F, 78	18. F, 63	26. F, 72
3. M, 71	11. F, 68	19. M, 71	27. F, 77
4. F, 64	12. M, 81	20. F, 76	28. F, 67
5. F, 65	13. F, 69	21. F, 61	29. F, 69
6. F, 68	14. F, 60	22. M, 67	30. M, 67
7. M, 68	15. M, 66	23. M, 65	31. M, 65
8. M, 69	16. M, 66	24. M, 63	32. M, 62

*Mean age is 68 years; 50% of sample is female.
F, Female; M, male.

| TABLE 8–6 | Random Assignment by Individual |

Group 1*: CPM/FNB	Group 2[†]: CPM/No–FNB	Group 3[‡]: No–CPM/FNB	Group 4[§]: No–CPM/No–FNB
5. F, 65	4. F, 64	1. F, 70	6. F, 68
9. F, 62	14. F, 60	2. M, 60	7. M, 68
17. M, 70	15. M, 66	3. M, 71	8. M, 69
21. F, 61	20. F, 76	10. F, 78	14. F, 60
	24. M, 63	12. M, 81	18. F, 63
	28. F, 67	13. F, 69	19. M, 71
	30. M, 67	16. M, 66	22. M, 67
	31. M, 65		23. M, 65
	32. M, 62		25, M, 76
			26. F, 72
			27. F, 77
			29. F, 69

*n = 4, mean age = 64.5 years, women = 75.0%.
[†]n = 9, mean age = 65.5 years, women = 44.4%.
[‡]n = 7, mean age = 70.7 years, women = 42.8%.
[§]n = 12, mean age = 68.8 years, women = 50.0%.
CPM, Continuous passive motion; FNB, femoral nerve block; F, female; M, male.

first group, eight for the second group, and so on. Looking at the last two digits in each column and proceeding from left to right beginning in column 1 of row 71 of the random numbers table (see Table 8–2), the numbers between 01 and 32 are bold and italic, skipping any duplicates. The first eight participants who correspond to the first eight numbers constitute the first group. The next eight numbers constitute the second group, and so on. The complete results of this assignment procedure are shown in Table 8–7. Random assignment to groups by block can become time-consuming with large samples.

Systematic Assignment

The process of systematic assignment is familiar to anyone who has taken a physical education class where teams were formed by "counting off." Researchers count off by using a list of the

TABLE 8–7 **Random Assignment by Block**

Group 1*: CPM/FNB	Group 2†: CPM/No–FNB	Group 3‡: No–CPM/FNB	Group 4§: No–CPM/No–FNB
1. F, 70	2. M, 60	8. M, 69	10. F, 78
3. M, 71	4. F, 64	11. F, 68	12. M, 81
7. M, 68	5. F, 65	15. M, 66	13. F, 69
16. M, 66	6. F, 68	18. F, 63	14. F, 60
21. F, 61	9. F, 62	19. M, 71	20. F, 76
22. M, 67	17. M, 70	23. M, 65	26. F, 72
24. M, 63	25. M, 76	30, M, 67	28. F, 67
27. F, 77	31. M, 65	32. M, 62	29. F, 69

*Mean age = 67.9 years, women = 37.5%.
†Mean age = 66.3 years, women = 50.0%.
‡Mean age = 66.3 years, women = 25.0%.
§Mean age = 71.5 years, women = 87.5%.
CPM, Continuous passive motion; FNB, femoral nerve block; F, female; M, male.

TABLE 8–8 **Systematic Assignment**

Group 1*: CPM/FNB	Group 2†: CPM/No–FNB	Group 3‡: No–CPM/FNB	Group 4§: No–CPM/No–FNB
1. F, 70	2. M, 60	3. M, 71	4. F, 64
5. F, 65	6. F, 68	7. M, 68	8. M, 69
9. F,62	10. F, 78	11. F, 68	12. M, 81
13. F, 69	14. F, 60	15. M, 66	16. M, 66
17. M, 70	18. F, 63	19. M, 71	20. F, 76
21. F, 61	22. M, 67	23. M, 65	24. M, 63
25. M, 76	26. F, 72	27. F, 77	28. F, 67
29. F, 67	30. M, 67	31. M, 65	32. M, 62

*Mean age = 67.5 years, women = 75.0%.
†Mean age = 66.9 years, women = 62.5%.
‡Mean age = 68.9 years, women = 25.0%.
§Mean age = 68.5 years, women = 37.5%.
CPM, Continuous passive motion; FNB, femoral nerve block; F, female; M, male.

TABLE 8-9 Matched Assignment			
Group 1*: **CPM/FNB**	**Group 2†:** **CPM/No–FNB**	**Group 3‡:** **No–CPM/FNB**	**Group 4§:** **No–CPM/No–FNB**
14. F, 60	21. F, 61	9. F, 62	18. F, 63
31. M, 65	24. M, 63	32. M, 62	2. M, 60
28. F, 67	4. F, 64	5. F, 65	6. F, 68
15. M, 66	22. M, 67	16. M, 66	23. M, 65
1. F, 70	29. F, 69	11. F, 68	13. F, 69
30. M, 67	7. M, 68	17. M, 70	8. M, 69
10. F, 78	27. F, 77	20. F, 76	26. F, 72
3. M, 71	19. M, 71	25. M, 76	12. M, 81

*Mean age = 68.0 years, women = 50.0%.
†Mean age = 67.5 years, women = 50.0%.
‡Mean age = 68.1 years, women = 50.0%.
§Mean age = 68.4 years, women = 50.0%.
CPM, Continuous passive motion; FNB, femoral nerve block; F, female; M, male.

sample and systematically placing subsequent participants into subsequent groups. Table 8–8 shows the groups generated by systematic assignment for this example. The first person was assigned to the CPM/FNB group, the second person to the CPM/no-FNB group, the third person to the no-CPM/FNB group, the fourth person to the no-CPM/no-FNB group, the fifth person to the CPM/FNB group, and so on.

Matched Assignment

In matched assignment, participants are matched on important characteristics and these subgroups are randomly assigned to study groups. In our sample of TKA patients, participants were matched on both age and sex. The four youngest women in the sample were placed in a subgroup and then were randomly assigned to study groups. To randomly assign the matched participants to groups, four different-colored poker chips, each representing a study group, were placed into a container. As shown in Table 8–9, the first chip drawn placed the youngest woman into the CPM/FNB group; the second chip drawn placed the next youngest woman into the CPM/no-FNB group, and so on. The four youngest men were then placed into a subgroup

and were assigned randomly to study groups. This procedure continued for the next youngest subgroups until all participants were assigned to groups.

The matched assignment procedure is somewhat analogous to stratified sampling and has some of the same disadvantages as stratified sampling. First, it ensures relatively equal distributions only on the variables that are matched. The possibility that other characteristics may not be evenly distributed across the groups may be forgotten in light of the homogeneity on the matched variables. In addition, the information needed for matching on some variables is difficult and expensive to obtain. If we wanted to match groups according to range of motion and knee function before surgery, we would have had to collect these data ourselves or depend on potentially unreliable retrospective data.

Consecutive Assignment

The four assignment methods presented thus far are used when an existing sample is available for assignment to groups. This is not the case when consecutive sampling is being used, for example, to identify patients as they undergo surgery or enter a health care facility. When a consecutive sample is used, then assignment to groups needs to be consecutive as well. The basic strategy used for consecutive assignment is the development of an ordered list with group assignments made in advance. As participants enter the study, they are given consecutive numbers and assigned to the group indicated for each number.

Deciding on an Assignment Method

The best assignment method ensures that group sizes are equal, group characteristics are similar, and group characteristics approximate the overall sample characteristics. Assignment by individuals leads to a situation in which group sizes are not necessarily equal; this is more of a problem with small group studies than with large group studies. Matched assignment obviously often leads to the least variability between groups on the matched variables, but it may not randomize other extraneous factors. In addition, it may be expensive and time-consuming to collect the information on which participants will be matched. The difference in assignment outcomes between block assignment and systematic assignment is often minimal, unless the researcher suspects some regularly recurring pattern in participants that would suggest that block assignment would be more appropriate. However, because random allocation of participants to groups is seen as critical to the quality of many trials, block assignment is usually preferred to systematic assignment because it introduces random elements as each block is allocated.

■ SAMPLE SIZE

The preceding discussion of sampling and assignment was based on one major assumption—that the researcher knows how many participants should be in the sample and in each group. In the real world, researchers must make decisions about sample size, and these decisions have a great deal of impact on the validity of the statistical conclusions of a piece of research.

A complete discussion of the determination of sample size is deferred until the statistical foundation of the text is laid, but one general principle of sample size determination is presented here.

This general principle is that larger samples tend to be more representative of their parent populations than smaller samples. To illustrate this principle, consider our hypothetical sample of 32 patients who underwent TKA as an accessible population from which we shall draw even smaller samples. From the population of 32 participants, four independent samples of two participants and four independent samples of eight participants are selected. An independent sample is drawn, recorded, and replaced into the population before the next sample is drawn.

Tables 8–10 and 8–11 show the results of the sampling, and Figure 8–3 plots the distribution of the average age of participants in the different-sized samples. Note that average ages for the samples of eight participants are clustered more closely around the actual population age than are the average ages for the smaller samples. This, then, is a visual demonstration of the principle that large samples tend to be more representative of their parent populations. In addition, this clustering of sample characteristics close to the population characteristics means that there is less variability from sample to sample with the larger sample sizes.

For experimental research, group sizes of about 30 participants are often considered the minimum size needed to make valid generalizations to a larger population and to meet the

TABLE 8-10 Characteristic with Sample Sizes of Two			
Sample 1	*Sample 2*	*Sample 3*	*Sample 4*
7. M, 68	27. F, 77	21. F, 61	10. F, 78
17. M, 70	11, F, 68	4. F, 64	25. F, 76

Note: In samples 1 though 4, the mean ages are 69.0, 72.5, 62.5, and 77.0 years, respectively. The percentage of women in each sample ranges from 0.0% to 100.0%.
F, Female; *M,* male.

assumptions of certain statistical tests.[1,11] For descriptive research, the precision of the description depends on the size of the sample. For example, a survey of 100 respondents shows that 60% prefer Brand X handheld dynamometer and 40% prefer Brand Y. Without going into any of the statistical theories underlying how researchers determine the precision of their results, with this result with 100 participants we could be 95% certain that the true preference for Brand X is between 50.2% and 69.8%. With 1000 participants, we could be 95% certain that the true preference for Brand X is between 56.9% and 63.1%. With 2000 participants we could be 95% certain that the true preference for Brand X is between 57.8% and 62.2%. As a researcher, one has to determine whether the increase in precision from 100 to 1000 to 2000 participants is worth the additional time and money associated with the larger samples.

When deciding on sample size, researchers should always account for anticipated experimental mortality. If a subject's participation is required on only 1 day, then retention of selected participants should be relatively high. If participation requires a commitment of a great deal of time, over a longer time period, researchers should expect that experimental mortality will be high.

Sometimes researchers are glibly advised to "get as many participants as you can." If only 20 participants are available, it is good advice—the researcher should try to use them all. However, if several hundred participants are available, such advice may be inappropriate. First, recommending that sample sizes be as large as possible is ethically questionable, because this means large numbers of individuals are exposed to procedures with unknown benefits. Second, very large samples can create administrative problems that detract from other aspects of the research process. Third, sometimes the results of research on very large groups produce statistical distinctions that are trivial in practice, as is discussed in greater detail in Chapter 19.

TABLE 8–11	Characteristic with Sample Sizes of Eight		
Sample 1	*Sample 2*	*Sample 3*	*Sample 4*
1. F, 70	1. F, 70	3. M, 71	3. M, 71
3. M, 71	6. F, 68	4. F, 64	5. F, 65
6. F, 68	7. M, 68	5. F, 65	6. F, 68
14. F, 60	17. M, 70	6. F, 68	9. F, 62
15. M, 66	22. M, 67	7. M, 68	16. M, 66
29. F, 69	25. M, 76	14. F, 60	17. M, 70
30. M, 67	27. F, 77	24. M, 63	26. F, 72
32. M, 62	30. M, 67	27. F, 77	32. M, 72

Note: In Samples 1 though 4, the mean ages are 66.6, 70.4, 67.0, and 68.3 years, respectively. The percentage of women in each sample ranges from 37.5% to 68.3%.
F, Female; *M,* male.

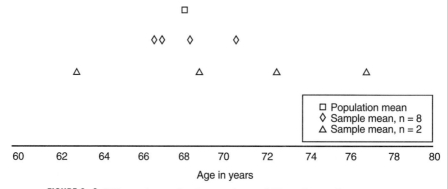

FIGURE 8–3. Effect of sample size on the stability of sample mean age.

■ SUMMARY

Selection and assignment of participants influence the internal, external, and statistical conclusion validity of research. Populations are total groups of interest; samples are subgroups of populations. Probability samples use some degree of randomization to select participants from the population. Common methods of probability sampling are simple random, systematic, stratified, and cluster sampling. Nonprobability samples do not rely on randomization. Common methods of nonprobability sampling are convenience, snowball, and purposive sampling. Assignment to groups within a study can be accomplished randomly regardless of whether or not the method used to select the sample was random. Common forms of assignment are individual, block, systematic, and matched assignment. A general principle in determining an appropriate sample size is that larger samples tend to be more representative of their parent populations than smaller samples.

REFERENCES

1. Fink A. *How to Sample in Surveys*. 2nd ed. Thousand Oaks, Calif: Sage Publications; 2002.

2. Hulley SB, Newman TB, Cummings SR. Choosing the study subjects: specification, sampling, and recruitment. In: Hulley SB, Cummings SR, Browner WS, Grady D, Hearst N, Newman TB, eds. *Designing Clinical Research*. 2nd ed. Philadelphia, Pa: Lippincott Williams & Wilkins; 2001.

3. Williams B. *A Sampler on Sampling*. New York, NY: John Wiley & Sons; 1978.

4. Beyer WH, ed. *Standard Mathematical Tables*. 27th ed. Boca Raton, Fla: CRC Press; 1984.

5. *True Random Number Service*. Available at: *www. random.org*. Accessed December 19, 2003.

6. Floyd JA. Systematic sampling: theory and clinical methods. *Nurs Res*. 1993;42:290-293.

7. *Rand McNally 2003 Commercial Atlas and Marketing Guide*. Chicago, Ill: Rand McNally; 2003.

8. *American Hospital Association Guide to the Health Care Field, 2002-2003*. Chicago, Ill: American Hospital Association; 2002.

9. Patton MQ. *Qualitative Research and Evaluation Methods*. 3rd ed. Thousand Oaks, Calif: Sage Publications; 2002.

10. Pizzari T, McBurney H, Taylor NF, Feller JA. Adherence to anterior cruciate ligament rehabilitation: a qualitative analysis. *J Sport Rehabil*. 2002;11:90-102.

11. Kraemer HC, Thiemann S. *How Many Subjects? Statistical Power Analysis in Research*. Newbury Park, Calif: Sage Publications; 1987:27.

Experimental Designs

9

Group Designs

Randomized Controlled Trials

Single-Factor Experimental
  Designs
    Pretest–Posttest Control-Group
      Design
    Posttest-Only Control-Group
      Design
    Single-Group Pretest–Posttest
      Design
    Nonequivalent Control-Group
      Design
    Time Series Design

    Repeated Measures or Repeated
      Treatment Designs

Multiple-Factor Experimental
  Designs
    Questions That Lead to a Multiple-
      Factor Design
    Factorial Versus Nested Designs
    Completely Randomized Versus
      Randomized-Block Designs
    Between-Groups, Within-Group,
      and Mixed Designs

Summary

Experimental research, as defined in Chapter 6, is characterized by controlled manipulation of an independent variable or variables by researchers. This controlled manipulation can be used with groups of participants or with individuals. In this chapter, experimental designs for groups of participants are described in detail. First, the randomized controlled trial is presented. Then, a variety of different single-factor and multiple-factor research designs are outlined.

The purpose of this chapter is to introduce readers to the terminology and information necessary to understand how experimental group designs are structured. There is, however, much more to designing valid experiments than just arranging for group allocation, measurement, and intervention, as noted in the many designs presented in this chapter. The control elements presented in Chapter 6 and the selection and assignment procedures presented in Chapter 8 must be implemented carefully to control the threats to validity outlined in Chapter 7. Chapter 27 presents implementation ideas for group experiments as well as other types of research. In addition, statistical tools, presented in Chapters 19 through 23, must be used correctly. Finally, the report of the experiment in the literature (Chapter 28) must present readers with the information needed to assess the quality of the trial.

■ RANDOMIZED CONTROLLED TRIALS

This textbook presents a broad view of research, acknowledging the value of different research paradigms (quantitative, qualitative, and single-system paradigms), different research purposes (description, relationship analysis, and difference analysis), and both experimental and nonexperimental designs. Notwithstanding the value of these diverse types of research, there is strong consensus that one particular type of research—the *randomized controlled trial* or *randomized clinical trial* (RCT)—can provide the strongest evidence for one particular research purpose—determining whether clinical interventions work.

RCTs are prospective and experimental, meaning that (1) the independent (treatment) variable is subject to the controlled manipulation of the investigator and (2) the dependent (measurement or outcome) variables are collected under controlled conditions. The independent variable consists of at least two levels, including a treatment group and some form of comparison, or control, group. The "randomized" component of the RCT refers to random allocation of participants to treatment and control groups. RCTs may take many forms, but all contain the elements noted above. By definition then, all RCTs are experimental designs. However, not all experimental designs are RCTs, in that there are many nonrandom ways of placing participants into groups.

Although the RCT is considered the strongest form of evidence about the effect of an intervention, RCTs are not appropriate to answer all questions, nor is every topic of study ready for RCTs. For example, if one wanted the strongest possible evidence about whether cigarette smoking causes lung cancer, one would design and implement an RCT comparing a smoking group to a nonsmoking group. Given the strength of evidence from nonrandomized trials, would it be ethical to randomly assign a large group of adolescents to smoking and nonsmoking groups and follow them throughout their lives to determine the relative rates at which they develop lung cancer? Clearly not.

In the development of new pharmacological agents, researchers conduct a well-established sequence of trials on humans, termed *phase I, II, and III trials*.[1] A phase I drug trial, usually conducted on a single group of healthy volunteers, is the initial trial to establish the safety of a new drug at different doses in humans. A phase II drug trial, usually conducted on a small group of patients expected to benefit from the drug, is done to "establish the efficacy of different doses and frequencies of administration."[1(Chapter 2, p4)] Depending on the type of outcome expected from the drug, phase II trials may be nonrandomized (if the outcomes are expected to be clear-cut and objective) or randomized (if the outcomes are expected to be subjective and more susceptible to placebo effects). Only after demonstrating safety in a phase I trial and promising treatment effects in a phase II trial do drugs move into phase III RCTs. In these RCTs, the new drug is compared with either a placebo or with the accepted standard treatment. Rehabilitation research does not have this tradition of a standardized, named, progression of increasingly rigorous research about our interventions. However, the same type of progression is appropriate to the study of many rehabilitation interventions. For example, this progression can be seen in the literature related to the technique of body-weight–supported treadmill training for individuals with locomotor disabilities. Some of the earliest literature about this technique documented the responses in men without locomotor disabilities, similar in concept to a phase I drug study.[2] Next, researchers published the results of nonrandomized trials of small numbers of individuals with spastic paretic gait that determined the impact of treadmill training with or without body weight support on gait patterns, similar in concept to phase II trials.[3,4] More recently, RCTs comparing body-weight–supported treadmill training to traditional gait training have been published, similar to phase III trials.[5,6] Finally, we see the emergence of the review article to help summarize the growing body of evidence about body-weight–supported tread-mill training.[7]

Yes, rehabilitation researchers should be working toward the implementation of high-quality RCTs to test the effectiveness of our interventions. Every study of treatment effectiveness that is not an RCT, however, should not be dismissed simply because it uses a less rigorous design. Instead, these studies should be examined in the light of related literature to determine whether they are important, either in their own right or as building blocks toward RCTs.

■ SINGLE-FACTOR EXPERIMENTAL DESIGNS

Single-factor experimental designs have one independent variable. Although multiple-factor experimental designs, which have more than one independent variable, are becoming increasingly common, single-factor designs remain an important part of the rehabilitation literature. In 1963, Campbell and Stanley published what was to become a classic work on single-factor experimental design: *Experimental and Quasi-Experimental Designs for Research.*[8] Their slim volume diagrammed 16 different experimental designs and outlined the strengths and weaknesses of each. Such a comprehensive catalogue of single-factor designs cannot be repeated here, but several of the more commonly observed designs are illustrated by studies from the rehabilitation literature. It should be noted that some of the studies presented included secondary purposes that involved an additional independent variable. If readers go to the research reports themselves, they will find that some of the studies are more complex than would be assumed from reading this chapter.

Pretest–Posttest Control-Group Design

The first design example is the pretest–posttest control-group design, one of the classic RCT designs. The pretest–posttest control group design is represented by the following notation, from Campbell and Stanley[8(p13)]:

R   O   X   O

R   O   O

The Os represent observation, or measurement. The X represents an intervention, or manipulation. The blank in the second row represents the control group. The intervention and the control, therefore, constitute the two levels of the independent variable. The R indicates that participants were assigned randomly to the two groups. Another term for this type of design is a *between-subjects design* or a *between-groups design* because the differences of interest are those differences that occur between subject groups. This may also be referred to as a *parallel group design,* wherein each group receives only one of the levels of the independent variable. The control group in this design may be referred to as a *passive control group* because it receives no treatment at all or else receives a sham or placebo treatment.

Runeson and Haker[9] used the classic pretest–posttest control-group design to study the effect of iontophoresis with cortisone on the treatment of lateral epicondylitis, or tennis elbow. They compared two groups: a treatment group that received cortisone iontophoresis and a passive control group that received sham iontophoresis. They were treated four times over 2 weeks and were measured at the conclusion of the treatment and at 3 and 6 months following the completion of the treatment. Both groups improved during the study and follow-up period and there was no significant difference in the response between the two groups, leading the authors to question the use of cortisone iontophoresis in the treatment of tennis elbow.

In clinical research, the pretest–posttest control-group design is often altered slightly, as follows:

R   O X_1 O

R   O X_2 O

This alteration is made when the researcher does not believe it is ethical to withhold treatment altogether. In this version of the RCT, one group receives a typical treatment and the other group receives the experimental treatment. A control group receiving a standard treatment can be referred to as an *active control group.*

Pulvermuller and colleagues[10] used a pretest–posttest control-group design with an active control group in their study of constraint-induced therapy for chronic aphasia after stroke. The treatment group received constraint-induced therapy with intense practice over 10 days. The control group received conventional therapy for aphasia over 4 weeks. The constraint-induced aphasia therapy group showed significant improvement in a number of communication variables compared with the conventional group.

Additional variations on the classic pretest–posttest control-group design include taking more than two measurements and using more than two treatment groups. The general notation for this design would be as follows, with the appropriate number of groups and measurement periods:

R   O   O   X$_1$ O   O
R   O   O   X$_2$ O   O
R   O   O   O   O

Clark and associates' study[11] of occupational therapy for independent-living older adults follows this variation on the pretest–posttest control-group design. They randomly assigned participants to one of three groups: the intervention group, which received preventive occupational therapy services; an active control group, which received a social activity program; and a passive control group, which received no services. Outcomes were based on self-report questionnaires that assessed physical and social function, health-related quality of life, life satisfaction, and depressive symptoms. Testing was done at baseline and after 9 months of treatment.

Ten of 15 outcome measures showed significant favorable changes in the group receiving occupational therapy compared with the control groups. In a follow-up phase of the study, significant differences that favored the occupational therapy group persisted 6 months after the conclusion of the treatment.[12]

Posttest-Only Control-Group Design

A second design is the posttest-only control-group design. Researchers use this design when they are not able to take pretest measurements. Therefore, the posttest is the only basis on which to make judgments about the effect of the independent variable on the dependent variable. Like the pretest–posttest control-group design, this design is an RCT and a between-groups design. The Campbell and Stanley notation for this design is as follows[8(p25)]:

R   X   O
R   O

An example of this design is found in Arciero and colleagues' study[13] of tourniquet use in anterior cruciate ligament (ACL) surgery. They compared a variety of measures—including quadriceps and hamstring muscle strength and hopping tests—between a group of patients who had a tourniquet during ACL reconstruction surgery and a group that did not have a tourniquet during the procedure. In this study, preoperative and immediate postoperative measures of strength and hopping ability would not be accurate because of the pain and dysfunction associated with either an injured or acutely reconstructed knee. Therefore, only postsurgical measures were taken. Because participants were randomly assigned to groups, it is assumed (but not guaranteed) that the randomization procedure balanced any extraneous variables across the two groups.

Single-Group Pretest–Posttest Design

The Campbell and Stanley notation for the single-group pretest–posttest design is as follows[8(p7)]:

O   X   O

Unlike the pretest–posttest control-group design and the posttest-only control-group design, the single-group design is neither an RCT nor a between-groups design. Because there is only one group, there is no opportunity for random allocation of participants into groups, nor is there any between-group comparison to be made. Instead, comparisons are made within the single experimental group, making this a *within-group design*.

Damiano and Abel used a single-group pretest–posttest design to study the functional outcomes of strength training in children with spastic cerebral palsy.[14] In this study, 11 children with spastic cerebral palsy participated in a 6-week strength training program. The independent variable was strength training, with two levels: pretreatment and posttreatment. The dependent variables were muscle strength, gross motor function, gait velocity and cadence, and energy expenditure during walking. Participants showed significant improvements in strength, gait velocity and cadence, and gross motor function, but no change in energy expenditure during walking. This design does not control for the possibility that these children would have made similar gains without a formal strength training program. Based on the promising results from this single-group pretest–posttest design, a useful next step might be to conduct an RCT of a strength training group compared with an active or passive control group.

Nonequivalent Control-Group Design

The nonequivalent control-group design is used when a nonrandom control group is available for comparison. The Campbell and Stanley notation for this design is as follows[8(p47)]:

O   X   O
- - - - - - - - - - -
O   O

The dotted line between groups indicates that participants were not randomly assigned to groups. Thus, this design is not considered a randomized controlled design. It is, however, a between-groups design because the comparison of interest is between the nonrandom groups.

Case-Smith's study of the effectiveness of a school-based occupational therapy intervention on handwriting is an example of a nonequivalent control-group design.[15] In this study, occupational therapists in five school districts identified potential participants for the intervention group from among those who had been referred to them for occupational therapy to improve handwriting skills. Then, teachers in those same districts identified potential participants for the comparison group from among students with poor handwriting who had not been referred to occupational therapy. There were some differences between the two groups that probably resulted from this nonrandom allocation to groups: several children in the occupational therapy group but none in the comparison group were receiving speech therapy and physical therapy and higher proportions of children in the occupational therapy group were diagnosed with learning or developmental disabilities.

Another approach to the nonequivalent control-group design is the use of cohorts for the experimental groups. The term *cohort* is generally used to refer to any group; a more specific use of the term refers to groups of individuals who follow each other in time. A cohort approach is often used in educational research because of the naturally occurring cohorts that follow one another in time. An example of this design is Lake's work comparing traditional lecture methods (used in a fall quarter) with active learning methods (used in a winter quarter) to teach physiology to physical therapy students.[16]

Time Series Design

The time series design is used to establish a baseline of measurements before initiation of treatment to either a group or an individual. When a comparison group is not available, it becomes important to either establish the stability of a measure before implementation of treatment or document the extent to which the measure is changing solely as a function of time. The Campbell and Stanley notation for the time series design is as follows[8(p37)]:

O   O   O   O   X   O   O   O   O

The number of measurements taken before, after, or even during the intervention varies depending on the nature of the study. If it is important to assess changes over many time intervals, any of the two or more group designs can be modified by use of additional measurements before or after treatment.

Ulione used a time series approach to study the impact of a health promotion and injury prevention program at a child development center.[17] Data on the upper respiratory illnesses, diarrhea, and injuries of the children in the development center were collected once a week for 4 weeks before and after the health promotion program. The four measurements taken before and after the intervention provide a fuller picture of the health status of the children than would single pretest and posttest measures. Although the time series approach can be applied to group designs, as it was in Ulione's work, in rehabilitation research it is commonly used with a single-system approach, which is considered in detail in Chapter 10.

Repeated Measures or Repeated Treatment Designs

Repeated measures designs are widely used in health science research. The term *repeated measures* means that the same participants are measured under all the levels of the independent variable. In this sense, any of the pretest–posttest designs can be considered a repeated measures design because each participant is measured at both levels (before and after treatment) of a possible independent variable. The *repeated treatment* design is a type of repeated measures design in which each participant receives more than one actual treatment. The repeated measures designs are also referred to as *within-subjects* or *within-group* designs because the effect of the independent variable is seen within participants in a single group rather than between the groups. When the order in which participants receive the interventions is randomized, this design is considered an RCT with a *cross-over design*.

Collier and Thomas studied the impact of four different wrist orthoses on range of motion at the wrist during a basketball shot.[18] The independent variable, "orthosis," had five levels: three different manufactured orthoses, one custom-fabricated orthosis, and no orthosis. The 40 participants each took three basketball shots under each condition, with brief rests between conditions. Although repeated treatment designs ensure that participant characteristics such as age, height, and weight, remain constant across the levels of the independent variable, they create a new set of extraneous factors related to familiarization with the experimental procedures. These factors should be controlled by random assignment to different orders, which Collier and Thomas did in their study. Chapter 6 includes additional details about methods to counterbalance the order in which repeated treatments are presented to participants.

■ MULTIPLE-FACTOR EXPERIMENTAL DESIGNS

Multiple-factor experimental designs are used frequently in rehabilitation research. Because of their widespread use, it is essential that rehabilitation professionals have command of the language and concepts related to multiple-factor designs. This section of the chapter is divided into several subsections. After a discussion of the basic research questions that would prompt a researcher to develop a multiple-factor design, some common multiple-factor designs are presented.

Questions That Lead to a Multiple-Factor Design

Researchers usually design multiple-factor experiments because they are interested not only in the individual effects of the multiple factors on the dependent variable, but also in the effects of the interaction between the multiple factors on the dependent variable. For example, say we wanted to conduct a study to determine the effects of different rehabilitation programs on swallowing function after cerebral vascular accident. We could start by selecting 60 patients for study and randomly assigning them to one of the three groups (posture program, oral-motor program, and a feeding cues program). The first independent variable would therefore be type of treatment, or group. Then assume that two different therapists—perhaps a speech-language pathologist and an occupational therapist—are going to provide the treatments. We might wonder whether one therapist might simply get better results than the other therapist, regardless of the type of treatment provided. A second independent variable, then, is therapist. If therapist is added as a second independent variable, a third question must also be asked in this design: Is one therapist more effective with one type of treatment and the other therapist more effective with another type of treatment? In other words, is there an interaction between type of treatment and therapist? It is the study of interaction that clearly differentiates a multiple-factor experimental design from a single-factor design.

Factorial Versus Nested Designs

The Type of Treatment × Therapist design developed previously is a factorial design. In a *factorial design,* the factors are crossed, meaning that each level of one factor is combined with each level of each other factor. This simply means that

each treatment group has members who are exposed to each therapist, and each therapist is exposed to members of each treatment group. This design is diagrammed in Figure 9–1. "Group" is one variable, with three levels: posture, oral-motor, and feeding cues. "Therapist" is the second variable, with two levels: A and B. There are six cells in the design, formed by crossing the two factors. In this example, assume there is an equal number, say 20, of participants in each cell. Swallowing function is measured at the beginning of the program, the appropriate program is administered to each participant, and swallowing function is measured again at the conclusion of the program. The dependent variable is the change in swallowing function from pretest to posttest.

Figure 9–2 shows a hypothetical set of data and a graph of the data. Figure 9–2, *A,* shows that Therapist A is superior overall to Therapist B (the overall mean for Therapist A is a 40-percentage point improvement in swallowing function; the overall mean for Therapist B is a 30-percentage point improvement), regardless of the type of treatment being delivered. The feeding cues program (overall improvement of 45 percentage points) is superior overall to the posture and

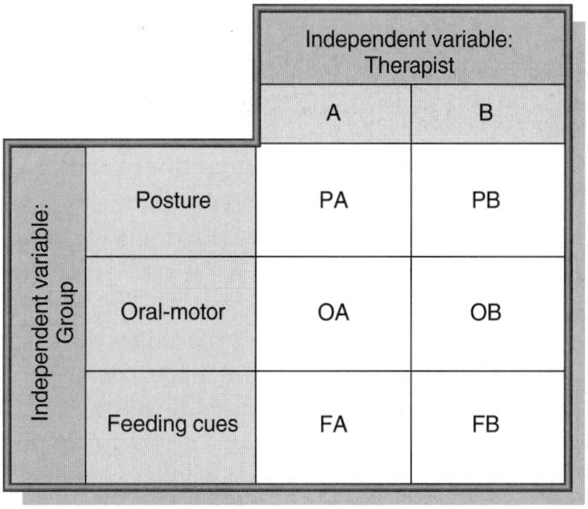

FIGURE 9–1. Two-factor, 3 × 2 factorial design. The notation within each cell shows the combination of the two independent variables. For example, PA indicates that individuals within this cell received the posture program from Therapist A.

Independent variable: Group	Independent variable: Therapist A	Independent variable: Therapist B	
Posture	$\bar{X}_{PA} = 30$	$\bar{X}_{PB} = 20$	$\bar{X}_P = 25$
Oral-motor	$\bar{X}_{OA} = 40$	$\bar{X}_{OB} = 30$	$\bar{X}_O = 35$
Feeding cues	$\bar{X}_{FA} = 50$	$\bar{X}_{FB} = 40$	$\bar{X}_F = 45$
	$\bar{X}_A = 40$	$\bar{X}_B = 30$	

A

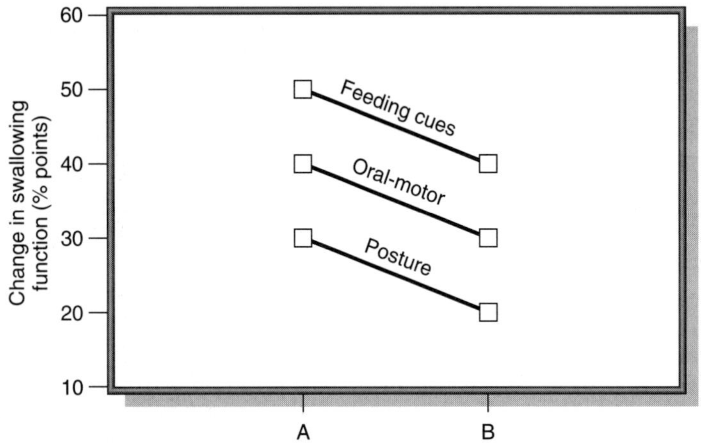

B

FIGURE 9–2. Example with no interaction. **A,** Sample data. The notations within the cells represent the mean ($\bar{X}$) scores for participants for each combination. The means in the margins are the overall means for the column or row. **B,** Graph of sample data. Parallel lines indicate that there is no interaction between therapist and treatment.

oral-motor programs (overall improvement of 25 and 35 percentage points, respectively), regardless of which therapist was delivering the treatment. In this example, there is no interaction between treatment and therapist. The feeding cues stimulation program is the superior treatment, regardless of therapist, and Therapist A gets superior results, regardless of the treatment given. This lack of interaction is shown graphically by the parallel lines in Figure 9–2, *B,* between therapists for the three treatments. A concise way to summarize these results is to say that there are *main effects* for both type of treatment and therapist, but no interaction between type of treatment and therapist.

Figure 9–3 presents a different set of data. In this instance, Figure 9–3, *A,* shows that there are no overall differences in treatment (mean improvement for each treatment, regardless of therapist, is 30 percentage points) and no overall differences in therapist results (mean improvement for each therapist, regardless of treatment, is 30 percentage points). However, there is a significant interaction between treatment and therapist. In Figure 9–3, *B,* Therapist A achieved better results using a feeding cues program and Therapist B achieved better results using a posture program. Both obtained intermediate results using the oral-motor approach. A concise way of summarizing these results is to

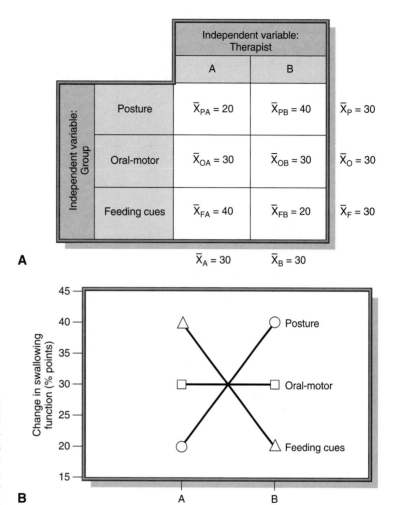

FIGURE 9–3. Example with interaction. **A,** Sample data. The notations within the cells represent the mean ($\bar{X}$) scores for participants for each combination. The means in the margins are the overall means for the column or row. **B,** Graph of sample data. Nonparallel lines indicate an interaction between therapist and treatment.

say there are no main effects for either type of treatment or therapist, but there is an interaction between type of treatment and therapist. If we had studied only the different treatment types without examining the second factor, therapists, we would have concluded that there were no differences between these treatments. The two-factor study allows us to come to a more sophisticated conclusion: Even though there are no overall differences between the treatments and therapists studied, certain therapists are considerably more effective when using certain treatments.

Nested designs occur when all the factors do not cross one another. For example, we could make the earlier example more complex by

adding some additional therapists and an additional clinic. The treatment variable remains the same: It has three levels—posture, oral-motor, and feeding cues. Perhaps there are two competing rehabilitation hospitals in town—one attracts patients with varied diagnoses, and the other specializes in neurological disorders. This is a second independent variable, with two levels: general and specialty rehabilitation hospitals. One research question might be whether patient outcomes at the two hospitals are different. The research question of whether different therapists achieve different results remains. This could be studied by using three different therapists at each hospital. Because there are different therapists at

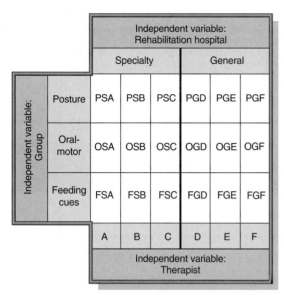

FIGURE 9–4. Schematic diagram of three-factor, nested design. Treatment (P, O, F) and rehabilitation hospital (S, G) are crossed factors. Therapist (A-F) is nested within hospital.

each hospital, the therapist variable is nested within the hospital variable. Figure 9–4 presents a schematic view of this hypothetical design in which treatment and hospital are crossed and therapist is nested within hospital.

Completely Randomized Versus Randomized-Block Designs

The Treatment × Therapist example just presented could also be termed a *completely randomized design* because type of treatment and therapist assignment were both manipulable variables and participants were assigned randomly to both treatment group and therapist.

Sometimes a *randomized-block design* is used, in which one of the factors of interest is not manipulable. If, for example, we had wanted to look at the factors of patient gender and treatment, then gender would have been a classification or attribute variable. Participants would be placed into blocks based on gender and then randomly assigned to treatments.

Between-Groups, Within-Group, and Mixed Designs

The Treatment × Therapist example could also be termed a *between-groups* design for both factors. Different participants were placed into each of the six cells of the design. The research questions relate to the interaction between treatment and therapist, to differences between groups who received different treatments, and to differences between groups who had different therapists.

An example of a two-factor between-groups design from the literature is Chin A Paw and colleagues' work on the use of physical exercise and enriched foods for functional improvement in frail older adults.[19] One factor was exercise program with two levels: exercise and no exercise. One factor was an enriched food regimen with two levels: enriched food and no enriched food. These two levels were crossed to yield four cells for the design, each with different participants: 39 participants exercised but did not eat enriched foods, 39 participants ate enriched foods but did not exercise, 42 participants exercised and ate enriched foods, and 37 participants served as controls who neither exercised nor ate enriched foods. There was no interaction between exercise and eating enriched foods; the exercisers demonstrated significant improvements in functional performance compared with nonexercisers; and there were no significant differences between those who did and did not eat enriched foods.

In a *within-group* design, one group of participants receives all levels of the independent variable. Moore and colleagues used a fully within-group design to study the biophysical effects of ultrasound on median nerve distal latencies.[20] There were two independent variables: treatment (five levels: 1-MHz continuous ultrasound, 1-MHz pulsed ultrasound, 3-MHz continuous ultrasound, 3-MHz pulsed ultrasound, and placebo ultrasound) and time (five levels: pretreatment, 2, 4, and 6 minutes into treatment, and posttreatment). All 15 participants received all five ultrasound treatments (in counterbalanced orders) and were measured at all five times for

FIGURE 9–5. One- and two- factor approaches to the pretest—posttest control-group design. The one-factor approach on the right uses group as the independent variable and range-of-motion difference scores as the dependent variable. The two-factor approach on the left uses group and time as independent variables and range-of-motion scores as the dependent variable.
Sample data, with cell and margin means, are included from Bandy WD, Irion JM. The effect of time on static stretch on the flexibility of the hamstring muscles. *Phys Ther.* 1994;74:845-852.

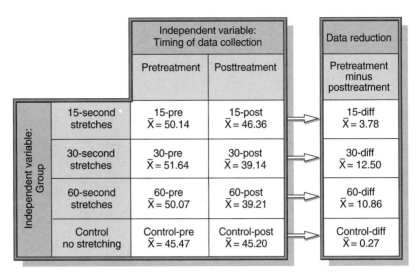

| | | Independent variable: Timing of data collection | | Data reduction |
		Pretreatment	Posttreatment	Pretreatment minus posttreatment
Independent variable: Group	15-second stretches	15-pre $\overline{X} = 50.14$	15-post $\overline{X} = 46.36$	15-diff $\overline{X} = 3.78$
	30-second stretches	30-pre $\overline{X} = 51.64$	30-post $\overline{X} = 39.14$	30-diff $\overline{X} = 12.50$
	60-second stretches	60-pre $\overline{X} = 50.07$	60-post $\overline{X} = 39.21$	60-diff $\overline{X} = 10.86$
	Control no stretching	Control-pre $\overline{X} = 45.47$	Control-post $\overline{X} = 45.20$	Control-diff $\overline{X} = 0.27$

each treatment. Thus, both independent variables in this study were repeated measures factors, making this a fully within-subject design.

A *mixed*, or *split-plot*, design contains a combination of between-subjects and within-subject factors. Bandy and Irion[21] studied hamstring stretching with such a design. Participants were randomly assigned to one of four stretching groups (group with four levels: 15-second stretches, 30-second stretches, 60-second stretches, and a control group that did not stretch) and measured before and after 6 weeks of stretching (time with two levels: pretreatment and posttreatment). In this study, a common mixed design, the familiar single-factor, pretest–posttest, control-group design is treated as a two-factor design. However, readers should realize that this type of study can also be treated as a one-factor design. Figure 9–5 shows the two different ways of treating this design. The left-hand grid shows the two-factor approach, with "group" as one independent variable and "time" as the second independent variable. Analyzing the design as a two-factor study requires that one determine whether the pattern of change across time is consistent between the groups. Figure 9–6 graphs eight average data points (four groups at two times), clearly showing that the control group has a different pattern than the other

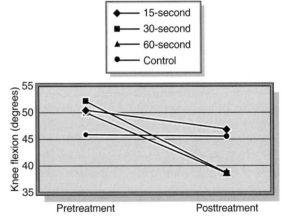

FIGURE 9–6. Interaction with two-factor approach. Nonparallel lines between treatment and control groups indicate a group × time interaction.
Data from Bandy WD, Irion JM. The effect of time on static stretch on the flexibility of the hamstring muscles. *Phys Ther.* 1994;74:845-852.

groups, and that the 30- and 60-second groups have very similar patterns of change across time.

The right-hand grid of Figure 9–5 shows how the "time" variable can be eliminated by reducing each group's average from two data points (pretreatment and posttreatment) to one data point (pretreatment–posttreatment difference). Analyzing the design as a one-factor study would involve comparing the four average differences to determine whether they are different from one another. Whether a study is analyzed as a one-factor or a two-factor design depends on a variety of mathematical assumptions that are discussed later (see Chapters 19 through 21).

■ SUMMARY

Experimental research is characterized by controlled manipulation of variables by the researcher. Although RCTs provide the best evidence for determining whether a clinical intervention works, some questions related to interventions cannot be answered with RCTs and some rehabilitation topics are not yet ready for rigorous testing with RCTs. Single-factor experimental designs are those in which the researcher manipulates only one variable. Common single-factor designs include the pretest–posttest control-group design, the posttest-only control-group design, the single-group pretest–posttest design, the nonequivalent control-group design, the time series design, and the repeated treatment design. Multiple-factor research designs are those in which the researcher studies more than one variable and is interested in the interactions among variables. Common forms of multiple-factor designs include factorial and nested designs; completely randomized and randomized-block designs; and between-groups, within-group, and mixed designs.

REFERENCES

1. Jadad AR. *Randomised Controlled Trials*. Available at: *www.bmjpg.com/rct*. Accessed October 24, 2003.
2. Finch L, Barbeau H, Arsenault B. Influence of body weight support on normal human gait: development of a gait retraining strategy. *Phys Ther*. 1991;71:842-855.
3. Visintin M, Barbeau H. The effects of parallel bars, body weight support and speed on the modulation of the locomotor pattern of spastic paretic gait: a preliminary communication. *Paraplegia*. 1994;32:540-553.
4. Waagfjord J, Levangie P, Certo CM. Effects of treadmill training on gait in a hemiparetic patient. *Phys Ther*. 1990;70:549-558.
5. Visintin M, Barbeau H, Korner-Bitensky N, Mayo N. A new approach to retrain gait in stroke patients through body weight support and treadmill stimulation. *Stroke*. 1998;29:1122-1128.

6. Nilsson L, Carlsson J, Danielsson A, et al. Walking training of patients with hemiparesis at an early stage after stroke: a comparison of walking training on a treadmill with body weight support and walking training on the ground. *Clin Rehabil*. 2001;15:515-527.
7. Hesse S, Werner C, von Frankenberg S, Bardeleben A. Treadmill training with partial body weight support after stroke. *Phys Med Rehabil Clin N Am*. 2003;14:S111-S123.
8. Campbell DT, Stanley JC. *Experimental and Quasi-Experimental Designs for Research*. Chicago, Ill: Rand McNally College Publishing; 1963.
9. Runeson L, Haker E. Iontophoresis with cortisone in the treatment of lateral epicondylalgia (tennis elbow)—a double-blind study. *Scand J Med Sci Sports*. 2002;12:136-142.
10. Pulvermuller F, Neininger B, Elbert T, et al. Constraint-induced therapy of chronic aphasia after stroke. *Stroke*. 2001;32:1621-1626.
11. Clark F, Azen SP, Zemke R, et al. Occupational therapy for independent-living older adults: a randomized controlled trial. *JAMA*. 1997;278:1321-1326.
12. Clark F, Azen SP, Carlson M, et al. Embedding health-promoting changes into the daily lives of independent-living older adults: long-term follow-up of occupational therapy intervention. *J Gerontol B Psychol Sci Soc Sci*. 2001;56:P60-P63.
13. Arciero RA, Scoville CR, Hayda RA, Snyder RJ. The effect of tourniquet use in anterior cruciate ligament reconstruction: a prospective, randomized study. *Am J Sports Med*. 1996;24:758-764.
14. Damiano DL, Abel MF. Functional outcomes of strength training in spastic cerebral palsy. *Arch Phys Med Rehabil*. 1998;79:126-133.
15. Case-Smith J. Effectiveness of school-based occupational therapy intervention on handwriting. *Am J Occup Ther*. 2002;56:17-25.
16. Lake DA. Student performance and perceptions of a lecture-based course compared with the same course utilizing group discussion. *Phys Ther*. 2001;81:896-902.
17. Ulione MS. Health promotion and injury prevention in a child development center. *J Pediatr Nurs*. 1997;12:148-154.
18. Collier SE, Thomas JJ. Range of motion at the wrist: a comparison study of four wrist extension orthoses and the free hand. *Am J Occup Ther*. 2002;56:180-184.
19. Chin A Paw MJM, de Jong N, Schouten EG, Hiddink GJ, Kok FJ. Physical exercise and/or enriched foods for functional improvement in frail, independently living elderly: a randomized controlled trial. *Arch Phys Med Rehabil*. 2001;82:811-817.
20. Moore JH, Gieck JH, Saliba EN, Perrin DH, Ball DW, McCue FC. The biophysical effects of ultrasound on median nerve distal latencies. *Electromyogr Clin Neurophysiol*. 2000;40:169-180.
21. Bandy WD, Irion JM. The effect of time on static stretch on the flexibility of the hamstring muscles. *Phys Ther*. 1994;74:845-852.

10

Single-System Design

Problems with Group Designs	Multiple-Baseline Designs
Characteristics of Single-System	Alternating-Treatment Designs
Designs	Interaction Designs
Single-System Designs	**Limitations of Single-System**
A-B Designs	**Designs**
Withdrawal Designs	**Summary**

A great difficulty in developing...clinical science...is that we treat individual persons, each of whom is made up of situations which are unique and, therefore, appear incompatible with the generalizations demanded of science.[1(p1076)]

This quote elegantly frames the basic argument in favor of studying individuals rather than groups. As noted in Chapter 5, the limitations of traditional group designs have led to the creation of a new research paradigm—the single-system paradigm—that focuses on the effectiveness of treatment in the context of a specific person in a specific setting. In addition to this basic philosophical argument in favor of single-system designs, advocates of this paradigm also cite many practical disadvantages of group designs in rehabilitation research.

■ PROBLEMS WITH GROUP DESIGNS

First, it is often difficult to structure powerful group designs in rehabilitation settings. Although a complete discussion of statistical power is deferred until Chapter 19, for now it is enough to know that powerful designs are those in which the data have the mathematical characteristics that make it likely that any true differences between groups will be detected by the statistical tools used to analyze the data. These mathematical characteristics include large sample sizes, participants who have similar values on the dependent variable at the beginning of the study, and large differences between groups at the conclusion of the study. Imagine that you are

135

a prosthetist who wishes to compare a number of gait variables between individuals with trans-femoral amputation who use a traditional hydraulic knee and those who use a computer-controlled knee. To create a powerful design, you should probably have 30 people in each group, you should specify that each participant who enters the study must have certain baseline gait characteristics, and you need to follow each person for the length of time required for accom-modation and adjustment to the alternate knee. If your practice sees one new client with a trans-femoral amputation each week, and if half of those meet your other eligibility criteria, it would take 120 weeks to recruit the 60 participants needed to implement a powerful group design! Because most practices do not have the resources needed to mount a 2-year study, the result is that many group studies without ade-quate power are implemented. Such studies often have few participants in each group, include heterogeneous participants who vary greatly on the dependent variable at the begin-ning of the study, and study participants for short periods of time. When a study lacks power and no difference between groups is identified, it is difficult to determine whether there is, in fact, no benefit to the experimental treatment or whether there is, in fact, a real benefit that was not detected because the design did not create the mathematical conditions needed to identify a difference. Advocates of single-system research believe that carefully crafted single-system designs provide clinicians with more useful information than do poorly crafted group designs.

Second, group designs typically only call for measurement of participants a few times within the study. When participants are only measured at the beginning and end of a study, the researcher is unable to determine the typical pat-tern of fluctuation in the dependent variable in the absence of an experimental manipulation. A difference from pretest to posttest may be part of a pattern of natural fluctuation, rather than a dif-ference related to the independent variable. As is shown later in the chapter, single-system designs

are characterized by extended baselines that establish the extent of natural fluctuation on the variables of interest within the study.

Third, group designs often have problems with external validity. Because of the need to standardize treatment across participants within the study, there may be a mismatch between some participants and the intervention that is planned. On average, the treatment may be appropriate for the participants within the group, but it may not be ideal for each participant. In addition, the standardization that is typical of group designs means that treatment is controlled in ways that may not be typical of clinical prac-tice. When a statistical advantage is found in an experimental group compared with a control group, clinicians know that the treatment, when applied to groups similar to the one that was studied, is likely to be effective for the group as a whole. The group design, however, usually provides little information about which sub-groups responded best—or did not respond at all. This means that the results of group designs often provide clinicians little guidance on whether a treatment is likely to be effective with a particular individual with particular char-acteristics. The generalizability of results from group studies can be described as "sample-to-population" generalizability.

In contrast, single-system designs are charac-terized by experimental treatments that are tai-lored to the needs of the specific participant being studied. In addition, the participant is usu-ally described in detail. This means that clini-cians can determine the similarity of one of their patients to the single participant under study and make an educated clinical judgment about the applicability of the treatment to their patient. Sim refers to this as "case-to-case generalizability," and believes that this kind of generalizability is important to clinicians trying to make evidence-based treatment decisions.[2] Generalizability of single-system designs can be enhanced by the replication of the design across several individu-als. In a replicated single-system design, the unit of analysis remains the single case. However, the researchers then discuss the case-to-case generalizability of the replicated results: consistent results across cases provide generalized evidence about the intervention, while inconsistent results point to the need for further research to determine which subgroups of patients are most likely to benefit from a certain intervention.

■ CHARACTERISTICS OF SINGLE-SYSTEM DESIGNS

Single-system designs are often confused with clinical case reports or case studies. The two are very different. The case report or case study is a description, very often a retrospective description, of a course of treatment of an individual. The case report is therefore a nonexperimental form of inquiry, which is covered in more detail in Chapter 12. Single-system designs, in contrast, include controlled manipulation of an independent variable and are conducted prospectively. Sim defines single-system research as:

> A quasiexperimental, prospective design utilising a sample of one, involving the sequential introduction and withdrawal (or modification) of an intervention (the predictor variable), to determine its effect on one or more outcome variables, through repeated measurement.[2(p263)]

The important elements of this definition are that single-system designs are experimental, involve repeated measurements, and are prospective. Kazdin articulates four key characteristics of single-system experimental designs, most of which are either explicit or implied in the definition above: continuous assessment, baseline assessment, stability of performance, and use of different phases.[3]

The experimental nature of single-system designs is shown by the controlled way in which the independent variable is implemented and the dependent variables are measured. All single-system designs have at least two levels of the independent variable, typically a baseline phase and an intervention phase. The participant serves as his or her own control through the collection of an extended series of baseline measurements,

which are contrasted to a series of measurements obtained during the intervention phase. Interpretation of single-system design results is simplified if stable performance during the baseline phase is documented.

The prospective nature of single-system designs is illustrated by the deliberate, planned intervention. Even though the researcher may deviate from the original treatment plan to accommodate the specific needs of the patient, these changes are carefully documented and recorded. Because of the planned nature of the study, researchers go through standard institutional review board processes to obtain approval to do the study, and they seek formal informed consent from the individuals who participate in the research.

■ SINGLE-SYSTEM DESIGNS

Several authors have categorized single-system designs in different ways.[4-6] For the purpose of this chapter, a slight modification of Backman and associates' classification is used.[5] To their scheme of four basic variations (A-B designs, withdrawal designs, multiple-baseline designs, and alternating-treatment designs) is added a fifth (interaction designs). Each of these designs is described in this chapter. Readers who wish a more complete enumeration of examples of the different designs should consult the review article of Backman and associates,[5] which describes 40 single-system designs related to rehabilitation that were published between 1985 and 1995.

A-B Designs

A-B designs have been described as the foundation of single-system research. By convention, A represents baseline phases, and B represents treatment phases. An A-B design represents a baseline phase followed by a treatment phase. The researcher collects multiple measures over time during the baseline phase to document the patient's status before implementation of the treatment. When the treatment is initiated, the measurements continue, and the pattern of change during the treatment phase is compared with the pattern established during the baseline. One weakness of the design is that it does not control for events or extraneous factors that might act simultaneously with the implementation of the treatment. If present, such factors, rather than the treatment, might be the cause of any changes seen in the dependent variables.

Cadenhead and colleagues[7] used an A-B design to evaluate the effect of passive range of motion on lower extremity range of motion of adults with cerebral palsy. For one case, baseline measurements of range of motion were obtained weekly during an 8-week A phase when passive range of motion was not provided. Then during the 8-week B phase, range-of-motion exercises were initiated and range-of-motion measurements continued to be obtained weekly. If differences in range of motion were seen during the B phase, a simple A-B design would not control for historical influences, such as a change in spasticity medications, that might influence lower extremity range of motion during the study. As is seen when this study is discussed again later, additional design elements were present that allowed the researchers to draw stronger conclusions than they might have if the single case described here was the full extent of their study.

A slight variation on the A-B design was used by Mulcahey and colleagues[8] to evaluate outcomes of tendon transfer surgery and occupational therapy in a child with tetraplegia secondary to spinal cord injury. Ten or more measures of various hand function tests were obtained during the A phase, before surgery. After surgery, the patient participated in standard postoperative care, including occupational therapy, for 4 weeks. Thus, the intervention for this study was the combination of the surgery and the postoperative care. The B phase in this study was subdivided into three follow-up phases at $2\frac{1}{2}$ months, 6 months, and 12 months after surgery. During each of the three follow-up phases, at least nine measures of each variable were obtained over a 2-week period. This extended follow-up phase permits the researchers to draw conclusions about both the short-term and long-term impact of the tendon transfer surgery.

Withdrawal Designs

Withdrawal designs, sometimes referred to generically as A-B-A designs, are characterized by implementation and withdrawal of treatment over the course of the study. In an A-B-A design, a baseline is followed by treatment and then by another baseline. Other variants either reverse the order of treatments and baselines (B-A-B) or have multiple cycles of application and withdrawal of treatment (A-B-A-B). When studying a phenomenon that is expected to change as the intervention is implemented and withdrawn, these designs provide good control of extraneous factors by enabling the researcher to determine whether the hypothesized change occurs each time the treatment is applied or withdrawn.

One potential difficulty with withdrawal designs is that the researcher must consider the ethical implications of withdrawing a treatment that appears to be successful. A second potential difficulty with withdrawal designs is that the expected pattern of change in the dependent variable with each new phase of the study will occur only if the changes are reversible. For example, if one is studying aerobic performance with different ankle-foot orthoses, as Bean and colleagues[9] did in their study of the impact of brace modification on aerobic performance of an individual with Charcot-Marie-Tooth disease, aerobic performance would be expected to change with the application and withdrawal of each orthosis. If this happens, this is considered good evidence that the treatment, and not some extraneous factor, is the cause of the changes in the dependent variable. On the other hand, if one is studying the effect of a particular program on gait characteristics of a patient using a prosthesis after transfemoral amputation, one hopes that improvements are maintained after the therapy has ended. If the second baseline phase remains the same as the treatment phase, some might interpret this to mean that some factor other than the treatment might have caused the sustained change. Others might argue that such a pattern of evidence, rather than providing weak evidence of treatment effectiveness, provides strong support for the long-term impact of the treatment. Thus, it is difficult to interpret the results of A-B-A designs with variables that are not expected to change when the intervention is removed.

Deitz and colleagues[10] conducted an A-B-A single-system design to study the effect of powered mobility on child-initiated movement, contact with others, and affect for two children with complex developmental delays. First, the dependent variables were collected during gym class or outdoor recess during the A1 phase when the children did not have powered mobility. Then the children were trained in the use of a powered riding toy car. Then data were collected during the B phase when the children used the car for mobility during gym class or outdoor recess activities. This B phase with the car was followed by an A2 phase during which the car was not available. For both children, self-initiated movements increased markedly with the introduction of the car in the B phase, and decreased markedly with the withdrawal of the car in the A2 phase, thereby providing strong evidence that the car was the cause of the change in mobility.

In contrast to this classic use of an A-B-A design with a variable that is expected to return to baseline upon withdrawal of the treatment, Miller used an A-B-A design to study the impact of body-weight–supported treatment and over-ground training in a woman who was 19 months post-stroke.[11] In this situation, an effective treatment would be reflected by improvements during the intervention phase and retention of those improvements after the treatment was completed. Measures of gait and balance were collected 10 times during the A1 baseline phase. During the B intervention phase, gait training with the partial body-weight–support system was implemented three times per week for 8 weeks, with collection of gait and balance data twice a week. The gait and balance measures were then collected another 10 times during the A2 withdrawal phase after treatment was complete. In general, improvements were seen from phase A1 to B and performance remained stable from B to A2. For a study such as this, then, the benefit of an A-B-A design is that is allows for documentation of carry-over effects after intervention is concluded. This is in contrast to the original use of the A-B-A design to control for history and maturation effects by looking for patterns of change at both the initiation and withdrawal of an intervention with a short-lived effect.

Multiple-Baseline Designs

There are several variations of the multiple-baseline designs. However, they all share the same purpose, to control for threats to internal validity without requiring that treatment be withdrawn.[5] The general format for the multiple-baseline study is to conduct several single-system studies, with baselines at different times or for different durations. An example of this design is Dekker and associates' study of the effects of intraarticular triamcinolone acetonide on pain, range of motion, and function of the painful shoulders of patients with hemiplegia.[12] Nine inpatients from the same rehabilitation center were identified over the course of a 12-month period and were randomly assigned to baselines of either 2 weeks or 3 weeks. Thus, this design included both ways of varying the baselines—by having baselines occur at different times and for different durations. To illustrate the benefit of having baselines at different times, assume that a historical threat to internal validity occurred during the second half of the 12-month period. For example, if the nursing staff implemented a protected positioning and transfer program during months 6 through 12 of the study, decreases in pain for the last several patients might be because of this program, rather than because of the effect of the steroid injections. If only one case was used, it would be impossible to separate the effects of the staffing change from the effect of the injections.

To illustrate the benefit of having baselines of different durations, assume that shoulder dysfunction in hemiplegia remits as patients experience less inadvertent shoulder trauma as they require less assistance with transfers, gait, and activities of daily living. If this recovery pattern tends to kick in after about 2 weeks of inpatient rehabilitation, and if the baseline is 2 weeks long for all patients, then changes in the dependent variables might be because of this natural progression rather than because of the effects of the injections. By having varied baselines of 2 and 3 weeks, any natural improvement at 2 weeks would be observable in those patients with the longer baseline. Figure 10–1 shows hypothetical scores that assume that pain decreases are related to natural history and not to the effect of the injections. The addition of the other patients allows the researcher to see that all participants had stable baselines for the first 2 weeks and all

participants had decreases in pain after 2 weeks, regardless of when the injections were started.

Multiple baselines were used by Cadenhead and associates[7] to strengthen the conclusions that they could draw from their A-B study of the effect of passive range of motion on lower extremity mobility of adults with cerebral palsy. Three different individuals received no-treatment baseline periods of 4, 8, and 11 weeks' duration. In addition, three more individuals participated with the treatment and baseline phases reversed: they first participated in treatment periods of 5, 8, and 11 weeks' duration followed by no-treatment withdrawal of passive range of motion. This complex multiple-baseline design enabled the researchers to accomplish several things. First, by using baselines of different lengths they were able to control for extraneous factors, other than the initiation or withdrawal of range of motion exercises, which might be advanced as alternative explanations for any changes in range-of-motion measurements. Second, the combined A-B and B-A designs enabled them to

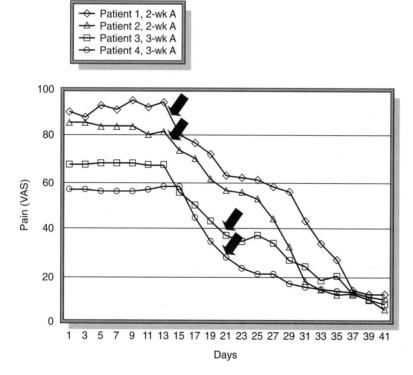

FIGURE 10–1. Hypothetical data presentation for a multiple-baseline study. Note that all baselines are stable until approximately 2 weeks and show a decreasing trend thereafter, regardless of the beginning of treatment *(arrows)*. *VAS,* Visual analog scale.

implement the study in a fairly nonobtrusive way—in particular this benefited individuals who were already receiving range-of-motion exercises when the study was initiated, because they could continue their usual routine during the first phase of the study.

Alternating-Treatment Designs

Alternating-treatment designs include the use of different treatments, each administered independently of the other. In describing such designs, the letters B, C, D, E, and so on are used to represent the different treatments; A continues to represent the baseline phase or phases. This design is well-suited to treatments that are expected to have short-lived effects. For example, a straightforward study of gait velocity of a patient wearing different ankle-foot orthoses might be represented by the notation A-B-A-C-A. This would mean that a baseline with no orthosis was established (A); this baseline phase was followed by gait assessments while the patient wore one orthosis, perhaps a solid-ankle plastic ankle-foot orthosis (B); followed by a second baseline phase (A); followed by gait assessments while the patient wore the second orthosis, perhaps an articulating-ankle plastic ankle-foot orthosis (C); and the study concluded with a final baseline phase (A). In this hypothetical case, the alternate treatments are administered in different phases of the study.

Washington and associates[13] used a different variation of the alternating-treatment design to study the impact of a contoured foam seat on sitting alignment and upper extremity function of infants with neuromotor impairments. Alignment and upper extremity function were measured with the children seated in a standard highchair during the baseline phase. During the intervention phase, two different interventions were presented each day: use of a thin foam liner within the highchair and use of a contoured foam seat within the highchair. Notation for this study might be "A-B,C" with the comma indicating that the two conditions (B and C) were alternated within a single phase.

Another interesting design element of this particular study was the random reintroduction of the standard highchair at some point during the intervention phase for all children, to determine whether maturation could be an explanation for any changes in status. Figure 10–2 shows these various elements for all four infants with whom the single-system design was replicated. The alternating treatment design works particularly well when the status of an individual is expected to fluctuate from day to day, as may be the case with infants who can be cranky and distracted on one day and cheery and focused on another day, without any true change in status. The alternating design lets the researcher evaluate each condition in light of the performance exhibited on a given day. Thus, day-to-day variability is controlled because the measure of interest is not absolute performance, but rather the difference in performance between conditions for a given day.

One specific form of an alternating-treatment design is sometimes referred to as an N of 1 randomized controlled trial (RCT).[14] In such a trial, two different treatments are randomly implemented during different phases of a study. The usual purpose of an N of 1 RCT is to determine which of two or more competing treatments is more effective for a given patient.

Interaction Designs

Interaction designs are used to evaluate the effect of different combinations of treatments. Assume that a multimodal speech therapy program, such as that documented by Murray and Ray,[15] has been designed for individuals with aphasia. Two important components of this program are traditional syntax stimulation (B) and nontraditional relaxation training (C). Researchers might wish to differentiate the effects of these components to determine whether a single component or the combination of components is most effective. The following design could separate these effects A-B-A-C-A-BC-A. That is, baseline phases separate a syntax stimulation phase, a relaxation phase, and a combined-treatment phase.

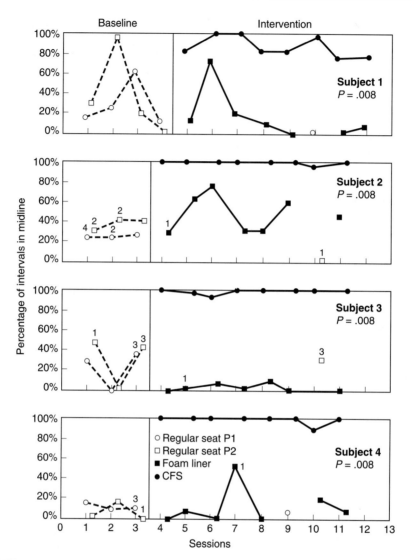

FIGURE 10–2. Example of data presentation for an alternating-treatment study. The authors tested the postural alignment of infants with neuromotor impairments under one baseline condition in a standard highchair and two alternating conditions (a thin foam liner in a standard highchair and a contoured foam seat in the highchair). From Washington K, Deitz JC, White OR, Schwartz IS. The effects of a contoured foam seat on postural alignment and upper-extremity function in infants with neuromotor impairments. *Phys Ther.* 2002;82:1064-1076.

An example of this design is Embrey and associates' examination of the effects of neurodevelopmental treatment and orthoses on knee flexion during gait.[16] The design of this study is A-B-A-BC-A, with neurodevelopmental treatment as the B intervention and orthoses as the C treatment. In this study, the researchers apparently were not interested in the effect of the orthoses alone, hence the absence of an isolated C treatment.

■ LIMITATIONS OF SINGLE-SYSTEM DESIGNS

Although many authors and researchers are enthusiastic about the information that can be gleaned from carefully constructed single-system designs, others are sharply critical of this form of inquiry for at least four reasons.[17,18] First, the designs may create ethical dilemmas because the need for an extended baseline leads to a delay in treatment, because researchers may withdraw effective treatments during the course of the study, and because of the increased cost of care related to data collection during baseline and withdrawal phases.

Second, the weaker single-system designs are subject to internal validity threats because they do not adequately control for extraneous factors, such as history or maturation, that might be responsible for changes in the dependent variables. In addition, there is the possibility that apparent improvements may reflect either familiarity with, or a treatment effect from, the repeated testing.

Third, generalizability may be low. Because the interventions may change during the course of the study to meet the individual needs of the patient, these designs are difficult to replicate. Because patients and interventions are carefully matched, therapists may have difficulty determining whether patients they are seeing are good matches for the treatments described in the study. Researchers who advance these generalizability concerns are not persuaded that case-to-case generalizability, as described by Sim,[2] is as valid as the sample-to-population generalizability that characterizes group designs.

Fourth, the theory and practice of statistical analysis of single-system designs is in its infancy. Some authors believe that the common methods of analysis that are reported in the literature frequently violate a variety of statistical tenets. A more complete discussion of statistical analysis of single-system designs is presented in Chapter 21.

■ SUMMARY

Group research designs are often limited because too few participants are available for powerful statistical analysis and because the impact of the treatment on individuals is obscured by the group results. Single-system designs overcome these limitations with controlled initiation and withdrawal of individualized treatments for a single participant, with repeated measurements of the dependent variables across time, and by analysis methods designed for use with data from only one participant. Broad categories of single-system designs include A-B designs, withdrawal designs, multiple-baseline designs, alternating-treatment designs, and interaction designs. Despite the advantages of single-system designs, some find them to be limited because of ethical concerns, lack of control of extraneous variables, limited generalizability, and violation of statistical assumptions.

REFERENCES

1. Hislop HJ. Tenth Mary McMillan lecture: the not-so-impossible dream. *Phys Ther.* 1975;55:1069-1080.
2. Sim J. The external validity of group comparative and single system studies. *Physiotherapy.* 1995;81:263-270.
3. Kazdin AE. The case study and single-case research designs. In: Kazdin AE, ed. *Research Design in Clinical Psychology.* 4th ed. Boston, Mass: Allyn & Bacon; 2003.
4. Ottenbacher KJ. *Evaluating Clinical Change: Strategies for Occupational and Physical Therapists.* Baltimore, Md: Williams & Wilkins; 1986.
5. Backman CL, Harris SR, Chisholm J-AM, Monette AD. Single-subject research in rehabilitation: a review of studies using AB, withdrawal, multiple baseline, and alternating treatments designs. *Arch Phys Med Rehabil.* 1997;78:1145-1153.
6. Zhan S, Ottenbacher K. Single subject research designs for disability research. *Disabil Rehabil.* 2001;23:1-8.

7. Cadenhead SL, McEwen IR, Thompson DM. Effect of passive range of motion exercise on lower-extremity goniometric measurement of adults with cerebral palsy: a single-subject design. *Phys Ther*. 2002;82:658-669.

8. Mulcahey MJ, Smith BT, Betz RR, Weiss AA. Outcomes of tendon transfer surgery and occupational therapy in a child with tetraplegia secondary to spinal cord injury. *Am J Occup Ther*. 1995;49:607-617.

9. Bean J, Walsh A, Frontera W. Brace modification improves aerobic performance in Charcot-Marie-Tooth disease: a single-subject design. *Am J Phys Med Rehabil*. 2001;80:578-582.

10. Deitz J, Swinth Y, White O. Powered mobility and preschoolers with complex developmental delays. *Am J Occup Ther*. 2002;56:86-96.

11. Miller EW. Body weight supported treadmill and overground training in a patient post cerebrovascular accident. *Neurorehabilitation*. 2001;16:155-163.

12. Dekker JHM, Wagenaar RC, Lankhorst GJ, de Jong BA. The painful hemiplegic shoulder: effects of intra-articular triamcinolone acetonide. *Am J Phys Med Rehabil*. 1997;76:43-48.

13. Washington K, Deitz JC, White OR, Schwartz IS. The effects of a contoured foam seat on postural alignment and upper-extremity function in infants with neuromotor impairments. *Phys Ther*. 2002;82:1064-1076.

14. Backman CL, Harris SR. Case studies, single subject research, and N of 1 randomized trials: comparisons and contrasts. *Am J Phys Med Rehabil*. 1999;78:170-176.

15. Murray LL, Ray AH. A comparison of relaxation training and syntax stimulation for chronic nonfluent aphasia. *J Commun Disord*. 2001;34:87-113.

16. Embrey DG, Yates L, Mott DH. Effects of neuro-developmental treatment and orthoses on knee flexion during gait: a single-subject design. *Phys Ther*. 1990; 70:626-637.

17. Bithell C. Single subject experimental design: a case for concern? *Physiotherapy*. 1994;80:85-87.

18. Reboussin DM, Morgan TM. Statistical considerations in the use and analysis of single-subject designs. *Med Sci Sports Exerc*. 1996;28:639-644.

Nonexperimental Research

Overview of Nonexperimental Research

In contrast to experimental research, nonexperimental research does not involve manipulation of variables. Instead, "in the nonexperimental research situation...control of the independent variables is not possible. Investigators must take things as they are and try to disentangle them."[1(p349)] In nonexperimental studies, then, the researcher examines records of past phenomena, documents existing phenomena, or observes new phenomena unfolding. The label "*non*experimental" may imply an unfavorable comparison with research that meets the controlled-manipulation criterion for "experimental" research. This is an unfortunate implication, in that nonexperimental research is exceedingly important within the rehabilitation literature. Law and colleagues articulate four situations in

which more exploratory, generally nonexperimental, designs may be appropriate: (1) when little is known about the topic, (2) when outcomes are not easily quantified, (3) when ethical issues preclude experimental approaches, and (4) when the purpose of the research is something other than determination of treatment effectiveness.[2]

The purpose of this chapter is to provide the reader with an overview of the diversity of nonexperimental research designs. Because nonexperimental research does not have to fit a rigid definition of controlled manipulation, the variety of nonexperimental designs is greater than that of experimental designs. In fact, there are nonexperimental research designs to fit every research type in the design matrix introduced in

147

Purpose of research	Timing of data collection: Retrospective	Timing of data collection: Prospective
Description	Nonexperimental	Nonexperimental
Analysis of relationships	Nonexperimental	Nonexperimental
Analysis of differences	Nonexperimental	Nonexperimental Experimental
	Manipulation (experimental or nonexperimental)	

FIGURE 11–1. Matrix of research types showing three design dimensions: purpose of the research (rows), timing of data collection (columns), and manipulation (cells).

Chapter 6 and reproduced here as Figure 11–1. Therefore, this chapter is organized by providing examples of nonexperimental research articles that fit into each of the six cells of the matrix of research types. As in earlier chapters, the pertinent portion of each study is reviewed; readers who go to the literature will find that some of the articles are more involved than would be assumed just from reading this chapter. A factor that complicates discussion of nonexperimental research is that there are many different terms that are used to describe certain types of nonexperimental studies. Table 11–1 provides a brief description of these forms of research. Because some of these forms of nonexperimental research are extremely important within the rehabilitation literature, they are presented in more detail in later chapters: case reports (Chapter 12), qualitative research (Chapter 13), epidemiological research (Chapter 14), outcomes research (Chapter 15), survey research (Chapter 16), and methodological research (Chapters 17 and 18).

DESCRIPTION

The purpose of descriptive research is to document the nature of a phenomenon through the systematic collection of data. In this text, a study is considered descriptive if it either provides a snapshot view of a single sample measured once or involves measurement and description of a sample several times over an extended period of time. The former approach is said to be *cross-sectional;* the latter is referred to as *longitudinal.*

In a typical descriptive study, many different variables are documented. For the most part, though, there is no presumption of cause or effect. Thus the distinction between independent and dependent variables is not usually made in reports of descriptive research. As is the case with all three research purposes that make up the matrix of research types, a distinction can be made between prospective and retrospective descriptive research designs.

Retrospective Descriptive Research

The purpose of retrospective descriptive research is to document the past. The description of the past may be of inherent interest, may be used to evaluate the present against the past, or may be used to make decisions in the present based on information from the past. The common denominator among research studies of this type is the reliance on archival data. *Archives* are "records of documents recounting the activities of individuals or of institutions, governments, and other groups."[3(p130)] Archival data may be found in medical records, voter registration rosters, newspapers and magazines, telephone directories, meeting minutes, television news programs, and a host of other sources. The information found in archival records must be systematically analyzed by the researcher for its relevance. *Content analysis* is the painstaking process that involves applying operational definitions and decision rules to the records to extract the data of interest.

Examples of the decisions that might need to be made can be seen in Schatz and associates' study in which they used data from rehabilitation records to determine rehabilitation outcome after traumatic brain injury.[4] One criterion for

TABLE 11-1 **Types of Nonexperimental Research**	
Case report	Systematic documentation of a well-defined unit; usually a description of an episode of care for an individual, but sometimes an administrative, educational, or other unit
Case-control design	An epidemiological research design in which groups of individuals with and without a certain condition or characteristic (the "effect") are compared to determine whether they have been differentially exposed to presumed causes of the condition or characteristic
Cohort design	An epidemiological research design that works forward from cause to effect, identifying groups of participants thought to have differing risks for developing a condition or characteristic and observing them over time to determine which group of participants are more likely to develop the condition or characteristic
Correlational research	Research conducted for the purpose of determining the interrelationships among variables
Developmental research	Research in which observations are made over time to document the natural history of the phenomenon of interest
Epidemiological research	Research that documents the incidence of a disease or injury, determines causes for the disease or injury, or develops mechanisms to control the disease or injury
Evaluation research	Research conducted to determine the effectiveness of a program or policy
Historical research	Research in which past events are documented because they are of inherent interest or because they provide a perspective that can guide decision making in the present
Meta-analysis	Research process by which the results of several studies are synthesized in a quantitative way
Methodological research	Research conducted to determine the reliability and validity of clinical and research measurements
Normative research	Research that uses large, representative samples to generate norms on measures of interest
Policy research	Research conducted to inform policy making and implementation
Qualitative research	Research conducted to develop a deep understanding of the particular, usually using interview and observation
Secondary analysis	Research that reanalyzes data collected for the sole purpose of answering new research questions
Survey research	Research in which the data are collected by having participants complete questionnaires or respond to interview questions

including cases in the study was that participants have "moderate to severe" traumatic brain injury. The operational definition they used for brain injury was "an insult to the brain, not of a degenerative or congenital nature, but caused by an external physical force that may produce a diminished or altered state of consciousness, which results in impairment of cognitive abilities or physical functioning."[4(p513)] Decision rules would be established to enable the researchers to determine which of the charts they reviewed fit all of the parts of this definition. Because it is difficult to anticipate every possible variation within the medical records, the operational definitions are usually established with the help of a pilot data extraction project. Based on the pilot study, definitive decision rules and operational definitions are made before the study itself is begun.[5]

Medical record data are not the only type of retrospective work that may be of interest to the profession of rehabilitation. For example, Chevan and Chevan used U.S. Bureau of the Census data to generate a statistical profile of physical therapists in 1980 and 1990.[6] Because they were doing a *secondary analysis* of data collected for another purpose, they had to do a considerable amount of data filtering to maximize the accuracy and usefulness of the data. For example, the census data did not distinguish between physical therapists (PTs) and physical therapist assistants (PTAs). Therefore, they used educational level as a "proxy" to distinguish between PTs and PTAs. Only those identified as PTs *and* as having at least 4 years of college were selected for the sample. Although this procedure likely rejected a few retirement-aged PTs who obtained licenses before a 4-year degree was required and included a few PTAs who had 4-year degrees in addition to the 2-year degree needed to practice as a PTA, it nevertheless appeared to be the best way to filter the data to obtain a high proportion of PTs and a low proportion of PTAs.

Evaluation research is another type of descriptive nonexperimental research that is typically conducted retrospectively. Sometimes evaluation research looks at the outcomes of a program at a single facility, as was the case with Bohannon and Cooper's evaluation of rehabilitation after total knee arthroplasty at a single hospital.[7] Other times, evaluation research looks at the processes involved in delivering a service to large groups of patients across many facilities. This was the case with Jette and associates' study of the quality of home health care services.[8]

Another possible retrospective approach is *epidemiological research*. Epidemiology is the study of disease, injury, and health in a population, and epidemiological research encompasses a broad range of methods (not all of them retrospective) that are used to study population-based health issues. Lu-Yao and coworkers used retrospective methods to study the treatment of elderly Americans with hip fractures.[9] In this study, a sample of the Medicare claims database was used to determine the characteristics of patients with hip fracture, the surgical procedure used to repair the fracture, and the survival rate up to 3 years after the fracture. The very large sample size—26,434 cases—which is likely to be representative of the larger population of elderly Americans with hip fractures, is one thing that differentiates epidemiological research from smaller studies that use samples of convenience from one or just a few hospitals. See Chapter 14 for additional information on epidemiological research.

Another research approach that uses retrospective descriptive methods is *historical research*. The purpose of historical research is to document past events because they are of inherent interest or because they provide a perspective that can guide decision making in the present. One type of historical research documents the accomplishments of prominent individuals within a profession, as in a report based on information found in unpublished archival documents of Professor Nicholas Taptas's development of the artificial larynx.[10] Another form of historical research documents trends in clinical care across time, as in Richardson and colleagues' retrospective review of almost 2000 patients treated in cardiac rehabilitation programs across a 10-year period.[11] Still another form is *policy research,* which analyzes the history or impact of public policy, as in Reed's review of the history of federal legislation in the United States for persons with disabilities.[12]

Another form of research that often rests on retrospective description is the *case report* or *case study*. Although the terms are sometimes used interchangeably, they are often differentiated. When they are, the case report is described as the less controlled, less systematic of the two forms of inquiry.[13] One example of a retrospective case report is Moyers and Stoffel's report of their work with an individual whose course of occupational therapy after hand surgery was complicated by alcohol dependence.[14] The purpose of their case was to show how occupational therapists practicing in other than mental health settings, can, nevertheless, implement a holistic approach to intervention for substance use disorders. Case reports and case studies are discussed in more detail in Chapters 12 and 13.

Prospective Descriptive Research

Prospective descriptive research enables the researcher to control the data that are collected for the purpose of describing a phenomenon. The prospective nature of data collection often makes the results of such research more believable than the results of purely retrospective studies. There are four basic methods of data collection in prospective descriptive research: observation, examination, interview, and questionnaire.

OBSERVATION

An example of the observational method is a study by Geerdink and colleagues, who studied the development of kicking movements in preterm and full-term infants by videotaping them and analyzing kicking frequency and angular motion.[15] They collected data at three different periods of time: when the infants were 6, 12, and 18 weeks of age. Another term for this type of research is *developmental,* meaning that the infants were described at more than one point in time to document the effects of the passage of time. This study, then, included descriptive components (to describe movement patterns at the different times for each group) as well as analytical components (comparing the movement patterns across times and groups).

EXAMINATION

An example of prospective descriptive research that includes examination of patients is Plancher and coworkers' study of reconstruction of the anterior cruciate ligament (ACL) in patients who were at least 40 years old.[16] In this study, 40- to 60-year-olds who had an ACL reconstruction were examined at an average of 55 months after surgery. The examination included, among other things, Lachman testing, knee laxity measurements, range-of-motion measures, and tests for crepitation. The participants in this study were identified through review of medical records, but the data for the study were collected prospectively to answer the question about the status of the knees at follow-up.

Another variation on prospective descriptive research is seen in the *methodological study* of Rosa and associates,[17] who examined the ability of therapeutic touch practitioners to detect the human energy fields they claim to be able to detect and manipulate. The goals of methodological research are to document and improve the reliability and validity of clinical and research measures. This study, published in the *Journal of the American Medical Association (JAMA)*, was received with a great deal of interest because a portion of the article reported on the fourth-grade science project of one of the authors. To determine the ability of the practitioners to detect a human energy field, each practitioner placed his or her hands palm-up through a screen that kept the practitioner from seeing the experimenter. The experimenter then conducted 10 trials with each practitioner in which the experimenter hovered one of her hands over one of the hands of the practitioner. The practitioner was asked to indicate which of his or her hands was closest to the examiner's hands for each trial. Most practitioners were not able to reliably detect the correct hand. More detail about methodological research is presented in Chapters 17 and 18.

INTERVIEW

The interview method of data collection was used by Mack and colleagues to study the perceived risks to independent living of older, community-dwelling adults.[18] Data were collected by interviewing more than 100 community-dwelling elders about the importance of remaining within their homes, the factors enabling them to remain independent, the situations that might jeopardize their independence, and the resources that would help them remain independent. The interview method was ideal for this study because older adults may have visual problems that would make reading a questionnaire difficult, and some elders may have had little education, resulting in difficulties in both reading questionnaires and writing answers. In addition, the researchers were interested in these individuals' perceptions about risks to their independence; answers to a questionnaire item about such a complex notion as "risks to independence" would likely lack the depth and breadth of answers obtained in an interview. The interview method is not without hazards, however. Without the anonymity of a mailed questionnaire, participants may give what they believe to be socially acceptable answers. In this study, they might have exaggerated the importance of remaining independent if they believed that the interviewers themselves placed a great deal of importance on independence. This style of open-ended questioning, which is analyzed later for content themes, fits some definitions of qualitative research and is discussed in more detail in Chapter 13.

QUESTIONNAIRE

The questionnaire method was used by Jahnsen and associates to study fatigue in adults with cerebral palsy.[19] Because survey research typically depends on responses of participants to written questionnaires, they had to limit their sample to adults with cerebral palsy who also had no reported intellectual disabilities. In a specific variant of survey research, Ingram used the *Delphi technique* to determine the opinions of physical therapy education program directors on essential functions of physical therapist students.[20] The Delphi technique uses a series of questionnaires to elicit a consensus from a group of experts. Each round of questionnaires builds on information collected in the previous round and generally asks participants to indicate their levels of agreement or disagreement with group opinions from the previous round. The respondents were entry-level physical therapy program directors, by definition a well-educated group

whose reading and writing skills should be sufficient to respond to a questionnaire. In addition, the national sample that was desired made mailing the questionnaire far more efficient and less expensive than conducting interviews with participants. Another advantage of a mailed questionnaire is that it can maintain the anonymity of the respondent. Chapter 16 provides guidelines for survey research.

■ ANALYSIS OF RELATIONSHIPS

The second major group of nonexperimental research consists of the designs in which the primary purpose is the analysis of relationships among variables. The general format for this research is that a single group of participants is tested on several different variables and the mathematical interrelationships among the variables are studied. This type of research is sometimes called *correlational research*. The term *correlation* also refers to a specific statistical technique. Therefore, there is a temptation to consider as correlational research only those studies in which the statistical correlation technique is used. As is seen in the examples, however, analysis of relationships entails more than just statistical correlation techniques. For example, epidemiological researchers often use a variety of ratios to express the association between subject characteristics and the presence or absence of disease. Therefore, in this text, the term *correlation* is reserved for the specific statistical analysis, and the longer, but more accurate, *analysis of relationships* is used to describe a general type of research.

There are several reasons why one would want to identify relationships among variables. The first is that establishing relationships among variables without researcher manipulation may suggest fruitful areas for future experimental study. Research of this type is said to have *heuristic* value, meaning that the purpose of the study is to discover or reveal relationships that may lead to further enlightenment. The value of such heuristic research is not necessarily in its immediate results, but in the direction in which it moves the researcher.

The second specific purpose for the analysis of relationships among variables is that it allows scores on one variable to be predicted based on scores on another variable. In clinical practice, a strong relationship between certain admission and discharge characteristics in a group of patients who recently completed their course of treatment might allow better prediction of discharge status for future patients.

The third specific purpose of the analysis of relationships is to determine the reliability of measurement tools. Reliability is the extent to which measurements are repeatable. In clinical practice, we plan intervention based on certain measurements or observations. If, for example, a prosthetist cannot reliably determine whether the pelvis is level when a patient with an amputation is fitted with a new prosthesis, she might elect to shorten the prosthesis on Monday, lengthen the prosthesis on Tuesday, and leave it alone on Wednesday! The statistical determination of the reliability of measurements provides an indication of the amount of confidence that should be placed in such measures.

A fourth reason to analyze relationships among variables is to determine the validity of a measure. By comparing scores on a new test with those on a well-established, or criterion, test, the extent to which the tests are in agreement can be established. Reliability and validity of measurements are discussed in detail in Chapters 17 and 18.

Retrospective Analysis of Relationships

Relationships can be analyzed retrospectively through use of medical records or through secondary analysis of data collected for other purposes. Guccione and colleagues[21] used data from the Framingham Study to determine the effects of specific medical conditions on the functional limitations of elders. The Framingham Study collected a variety of health status measures on residents of this Massachusetts town every 2 years beginning in 1948. The data used in this study were collected on 1826 individuals during the 18th biennial examination from 1983 to 1985. Among other things, the researchers calculated an odds ratio to show the "odds of functional dependence in performing a functional task among subjects with a specific medical condition divided by the odds of dependence in that task among all subjects."[21(p353)] Compared with the total sample, those with stroke were 2.82 times as likely to be dependent in stair climbing and those with knee osteoarthritis were 1.98 times as likely to be dependent in stair climbing.

Prospective Analysis of Relationships

Analysis of relationships is often accomplished prospectively, with concomitant control over selection of subjects and administration of the measuring tools. A typical example of research in which relationships are analyzed prospectively is Powers and associates' study of the relationship between muscle force and temporal-spatial gait characteristics for patients with transtibial amputation.[22] Some of the findings were that hip extensor strength on the amputated side was correlated to gait speed, that hip abduction strength on the sound side was correlated with cadence, and that knee extensor strength on both sides was correlated with stride length. Although determining the extent of the relationship among these factors is of interest to clinicians who treat patients after transtibial amputation, identifying the relationships does not imply that manipulation of one variable will influence the others. From these results we may be tempted to conclude that an exercise program that improves hip extensor, hip abductor, and knee extensor strength will cause an increase in gait speed, cadence, and stride length. However, because the variables in this study were not subjected to controlled manipulation, such causal inferences are not justified.

Prospective analysis of relationships was also used to establish the validity of physical examination for the diagnosis of sprained ankles. To test the value of delayed physical examination versus arthrography in detecting ruptured lateral ankle ligaments, van Dijk and associates[23] performed delayed physical examinations and ankle arthrography on 160 consecutive patients who presented to the emergency department with a history of an acute injury to the lateral ankle. The arthrography was considered to be the criterion measure, or "gold standard," against which the physical examination was compared. van Dijk and associates evaluated the relationship between the physical examination result and the arthrography with the traditional epidemiological concepts of sensitivity, specificity, positive predictive value, and negative predictive value. They concluded that "physical examination gives information of diagnostic quality which is equal to that of arthrography, and causes little discomfort to the patient."[23(p958)] These epidemiological concepts are presented in more detail in Chapter 14.

Normative research is another form of descriptive research. In normative studies, large, representative groups are examined to determine typical values on the variables of interest. Andrews and associates[24] characterized their descriptive work on muscle force measurements with handheld dynamometers as "normative." They studied 156 individuals in all, with at least 50 people in each of three age groups and with at least 25 men and 25 women within each age group. Twenty-five people in each subgroup seems small for a normative study, but given the paucity of data, this information is probably as "normative" as is available at this time.

■ ANALYSIS OF DIFFERENCES

The general purpose of research in which differences are analyzed is to focus on whether groups or treatments are different in some reliable way. Although analysis of differences is often accomplished experimentally, there are many ways to analyze differences nonexperimentally. Nonexperimental analysis of differences among groups or treatments is called *ex post facto* (after the fact) or *causal-comparative* research. The independent variables in such studies are not manipulated but are the presumed cause of differences in the dependent variable. The *ex post facto* designation refers to the fact that assignment to groups is not under the control of the investigator, but rather is determined by existing characteristics of the individuals within the study. Note that ex post facto does not mean questions are developed after data collection; ex post facto designs may use either retrospective or prospective data collection.

Retrospective Analysis of Differences

Medical records provide a vast source of information about patient treatment and outcomes. When groups of patients can be identified from the medical records as having undergone certain courses of treatments or sharing certain characteristics, it is possible to study the relationship of treatment or characteristic to outcome in a retrospective manner. Four articles illustrate four different ways of developing groups in the retrospective ex post facto designs.

The first, by Timm, is a large retrospective study of postsurgical knee rehabilitation.[25] The medical charts of more than 5000 patients who had undergone surgery in one calendar year were reviewed. Four groups of patients who had completed knee rehabilitation were identified by the type of program they had completed, as documented in the medical chart: no exercise, home exercise, isotonic exercise, or isokinetic exercise. Thus the groups constituted patients treated in the same time frame but with different rehabilitation protocols. This large-group retrospective study focusing on global outcomes of treatment could be described with the contemporary term *outcomes research*.

More detail about outcomes research is presented in Chapter 15.

One disadvantage of retrospective designs such as this is that nonrandom placement into groups makes it impossible to determine why a particular patient was placed in a particular rehabilitation group. For example, did those who wanted to return to athletic competition get placed in the isokinetic group, thereby giving it a bias toward motivated patients? Unless the medical records contain information about patient goals and motivation, there is no way to determine whether or not this bias occurred.

In a second retrospective ex post facto study, successive cohorts were studied to determine whether a change in policy on the use of physical restraints for institutionalized older adults had an impact on number of falls and severity of injuries associated with falls. To do so, Dunn studied incident reports in one long-term care facility before and after a restraint-free policy was adopted, finding that the number of falls remained the same but the severity of injury decreased under the restraint-free policy.[26] The difference in patient selection between this study and Timm's study of postoperative knee rehabilitation is that answering this study question required sampling of patients from two different points in time; Timm's rehabilitation study is strengthened by its use of patients treated in a single time frame.

A third example of subject grouping within the retrospective ex post facto designs follows what is called the *case-control* design. In this design, a group of patients with the desired effect is identified, and then a group without the effect is identified. Presumed causes for the effects are then sought, and the proportions of patients with the causes in the two groups are compared. One example of a case-control design is Harding and colleagues' work on chest physiotherapy and brain damage in extremely premature infants.[27] In this study, very low birth weight infants who developed encephaloclastic porencephaly (the cases) were compared with gestation- and birth-weight–matched patients who did not develop this form of brain damage (the controls). The researchers then looked backward in time to document the number of chest physiotherapy sessions each child had undergone during the first month of life. They found that the case infants with the brain damage had received two to three times as much chest physiotherapy as the control infants without the brain damage. The confidence that can be placed in case-control research depends in large part on the criteria used to define the case and control groups.[28,29]

A fourth example of subject grouping within the retrospective ex post facto designs follows what is called the *cohort* design. Sometimes viewed as the "opposite" of a case-control study, cohort studies follow a group across time, starting with "presumed causes" and looking for "effects." This is in contrast to the case-control study in which an "effect" is identified and presumed causes are explored. In a retrospective cohort study, all of the data have already been collected at the time the research question is developed: the researcher extracts the appropriate data, groups participants based on the variable or variables of interest, and looks for differences in a variety of predictor variables. This approach was used by Cushman and associates in their study of readmissions to inpatient pediatric rehabilitation.[30] Their retrospective review of records identified children who had required oxygen or ventilator support during an inpatient pulmonary rehabilitation admission and then grouped the children according to whether they had subsequent readmissions. The children with readmissions were found to need more ventilator support, nursing care, and acute-care transfers than children without readmissions.

A final example of retrospective analysis of differences among groups is a specialized research technique called *meta-analysis*. This technique is one of three general approaches to synthesizing research results across several different studies: narrative reviews, systematic reviews, and meta-analysis.[31-33] Narrative reviews of the literature are subject to the biases of the author, as noted rather humorously, but perhaps truthfully, by Glass:

> A common method of integrating several studies with inconsistent findings is to carp on the design or analysis deficiencies of all but a few studies—those remaining frequently being one's own work or that of one's students and friends—and then advance the one or two "acceptable" studies as the truth of the matter.[34(p7)]

Systematic reviews, which require documented search strategies and explicit inclusion and exclusion criteria for studies used in the review, reduce the sorts of biases noted in the quote above. See Chapter 26 for more information on conducting and critiquing systematic reviews.

The final type of synthesis, meta-analysis, provides a quantitative way of synthesizing the results of different research studies on the same topic. Two independent research groups recently used meta-analysis to synthesize the evidence about the effectiveness of occupational therapy and physical therapy for treating persons with Parkinson's disease.[35,36] Nineteen articles on occupational therapy for Parkinson's disease were reviewed and positive effects were identified for outcomes related to capacities and abilities as well as function during activities and tasks.[35] Twelve articles on physical therapy for Parkinson's disease were reviewed and positive effects were identified for activities of daily living, walking speed, and stride length.[36] In speech-language pathology, a meta-analysis of 55 articles on treatment of aphasia supported the effectiveness of aphasia interventions.[37] The basic concept behind meta-analysis is that the size of the differences between treatment groups (the effect size) is mathematically standardized so that it can be compared between studies with different, but conceptually related, dependent variables.

Prospective Analysis of Differences

Prospective analysis of differences is the final cell of the six-cell matrix of research types. It is the only cell that is shared between the experimental and nonexperimental designs. By definition, the experimental designs must be prospective, and their purpose is to determine the effects of some intervention on a dependent variable by analyzing the differences in groups that were and were not exposed to a manipulation or the differences within a single group exposed to more than one experimental treatment. Differences between groups or within a group can also be analyzed in the absence of controlled manipulation.

An example of a nonexperimental study in which the independent variable could have been manipulated but was not is Jansen and Minerbo's comparison of early dynamic mobilization with immobilization after flexor tendon repair in the hand.[38] To make this comparison, the researchers selected subjects retrospectively by reviewing their medical records to determine who had been immobilized postoperatively and who had received early dynamic splinting. Even though the division into treatment groups was accomplished before question development, the researchers collected data themselves at $4^{1}/_{2}$ months after surgery. As was the case with our other comparisons between retrospective and prospective studies, we can place more confidence in this study because prospective data analysis allowed the researchers to standardize the measures used in the study. If the study had been completely retrospective, with group assignment and dependent measures drawn from the medical chart, the uniformity of the measures would be questioned. If the study had been completely prospective, with random group assignment, treatment, and then measurement, it no longer would have been a nonexperimental study because the manipulation would have been under the control of the investigators.

There are many examples of nonexperimental analyses of differences in which the independent variable is inherently nonmanipulable. For example, some research questions focus on differences between groups of people with different attributes, as in Page's comparison of the competitive orientation of paralympic track and field athletes with congenital disabilities to that of paralympic athletes with acquired disabilities.[39] Other common attributes used to group participants nonexperimentally are sex, age, and presence or absence of a disease or condition.

Prospective comparisons of individuals with and without a particular condition may be referred to as a cross-sectional case-control design.[40] This design is similar to the classic case-control design described earlier in that researchers must identify cases and then search for controls that are matched on important characteristics such as age. It differs from the classic case-control design in that there is no backward search for presumed causes. Rather, researchers collect prospective cross-sectional data to determine whether those with and without the condition differ on other variables. A cross-sectional cohort design was used by Wiley and Damiano to compare lower-extremity strength profiles between children with spastic cerebral palsy and their age-matched peers without cerebral palsy.[41]

Likewise, the retrospective cohort design described earlier has a prospective counterpart. Taylor and colleagues used a prospective cohort design to study patient-oriented outcomes from low back surgery.[42] Surgeons enrolled patients before surgery and researchers documented sociodemographic characteristics, preoperative signs and symptoms, diagnoses, and operative procedures. They then collected outcome data 1 year postoperatively, identifying function, quality of life, and overall treatment satisfaction. The analysis differentiated between those with better and worse outcomes, finding that older age, previous back surgery, workers' compensation, and consultation with an attorney were associated with worse outcomes. The prospective nature of this cohort study means that the collection of both predictor and outcome data was under the careful control of the investigators.

■ SUMMARY

Unlike experimental research, nonexperimental research does not require controlled manipulation of variables. Because of this permissive definition, there is a great variety of nonexperimental research designs. Descriptive studies use retrospective or prospective data collection to characterize a phenomenon of interest. In studies that involve the analysis of relationships, researchers use prospective or retrospective data collection to measure variables, which they then analyze to make predictions, establish odds, or determine reliability or validity of the measures. Nonexperimental analysis of differences can take many forms, including case control and cohort designs.

REFERENCES

1. Kerlinger FN. *Foundations of Behavioral Research*. 3rd ed. Fort Worth, Tex: Holt, Rinehart & Winston; 1986.
2. Law M, Stewart D, Pollock N, Letts L, Bosch J, Westmorland M. *Guidelines for critical review form—quantitative studies*. Available at: *http://www.fhs.mcmaster.ca/rehab/ebp*. Accessed October 24, 2003.
3. Shaughnessy JJ, Zechmeister EB. *Research Methods in Psychology*. 2nd ed. New York, NY: McGraw-Hill; 1990:217.
4. Schatz P, Hillary F, Moelter S, Chute D. Retrospective assessment of rehabilitation outcome after traumatic brain injury: development and utility of the functional independence level. *J Head Trauma Rehabil*. 2002;17:510-525.
5. Findley TW, Daum MC. Research in physical medicine and rehabilitation. III. The chart review, or how to use clinical data for exploratory retrospective studies. *Am J Phys Med Rehabil*. 1989;68:150-157.
6. Chevan J, Chevan A. A statistical profile of physical therapists, 1980 and 1990. *Phys Ther*. 1998;78:301-312.
7. Bohannon RW, Cooper J. Total knee arthroplasty: evaluation of an acute care rehabilitation program. *Arch Phys Med Rehabil*. 1993;74:1091-1094.
8. Jette AM, Smith KW, McDermott SM. Quality of Medicare-reimbursed home health care. *Gerontologist*. 1996;36:492-501.
9. Lu-Yao GL, Baron JA, Barrett JA, Fisher ES. Treatment and survival among elderly Americans with hip fractures: a population-based study. *Am J Public Health*. 1994;84:1287-1291.
10. Lascaratos JG, Trompoukis C, Segas JV, Assimakopoulos DA. Professor Nicolas Taptas (1871-1955): a pioneer of post-laryngectomy voice rehabilitation. *Laryngoscope*. 2003;113:702-705.
11. Richardson LA, Buckenmeyer PJ, Bauman BD, Rosneck JS, Newman I, Josephson RA. Contemporary cardiac rehabilitation: patient characteristics and temporal trends over the past decade. *J Cardiopulm Rehabil*. 2000;20:57-64.
12. Reed KL. History of federal legislation for persons with disabilities. *Am J Occup Ther*. 1992;46:397-408.

13. McEwen I. *Writing Case Reports: A How-To Manual for Clinicians*. 2nd ed. Alexandria, Va: American Physical Therapy Association; 2000.

14. Moyers PA, Stoffel VC. Alcohol dependence in a client with a work-related injury. *Am J Occup Ther*. 1999;53:640-645.

15. Geerdink JJ, Hopkins B, Beek WJ, Heriza CB. The organization of leg movements in preterm and full-term infants after term age. *Dev Psychobiol*. 1996;29:335-351.

16. Plancher KD, Steadman JR, Briggs KK, Hutton KS. Reconstruction of the anterior cruciate ligament in patients who are at least forty years old: a long-term follow-up and outcome study. *J Bone Joint Surg Am*. 1998;80:184-197.

17. Rosa L, Rosa E, Sarner L, Barrett S. A close look at therapeutic touch. *JAMA*. 1998;279:1005-1010.

18. Mack R, Salmoni A, Viverais-Dressler ZG, Porter E, Garg R. Perceived risks to independent living: the views of older, community-dwelling adults. *Gerontologist*. 1997; 37:729-736.

19. Jahnsen R, Villien L, Stanghelle JK, Holm I. Fatigue in adults with cerebral palsy in Norway compared with the general population. *Dev Med Child Neurol*. 2003;45: 296-303.

20. Ingram D. Opinions of physical therapy education program directors on essential functions. *Phys Ther*. 1997; 77:37-45.

21. Guccione AA, Felson DT, Anderson JJ, et al. The effects of specific medical conditions on the functional limitations of elders in the Framingham Study. *Am J Public Health*. 1994;84:351-358.

22. Powers CM, Boyd LA, Fontaine CA, Perry J. The influence of lower-extremity muscle force on gait characteristics in individuals with below-knee amputations secondary to vascular disease. *Phys Ther*. 1996;76:369-377.

23. van Dijk CN, Lim LSL, Marti RK, Bossuyt PM, Marti RK. Physical examination is sufficient for the diagnosis of sprained ankles. *J Bone Joint Surg Br*. 1996;78: 958-962.

24. Andrews AW, Thomas MW, Bohannon RW. Normative values for isometric muscle force measurements obtained with hand-held dynamometers. *Phys Ther*. 1996; 76:248-259.

25. Timm KE. Postsurgical knee rehabilitation: a five year study of four methods and 5,381 patients. *Am J Sports Med*. 1988;16:463-468.

26. Dunn KS. The effect of physical restraints on fall rates in older adults who are institutionalized. *J Gerontol Nurs*. 2001;27:40-48.

27. Harding JE, Miles FK, Becroft DM, Allen BC, Knight DB. Chest physiotherapy may be associated with brain damage in extremely premature infants. *J Pediatr*. 1998; 132:440-444.

28. Hayden GF, Kramer MS, Horwitz RI. The case-control study: a practical review for the clinician. *JAMA*. 1982; 247:326-331.

29. Newman TB, Browner WS, Cummings SR, Hulley SB. Designing an observational study: cross-sectional and case-control studies. In: Hulley SB, Cummings SR, Browner WS, Grady D, Hearst N, Newman TB, eds. *Designing Clinical Research*. 2nd ed. Philadelphia, Pa: Lippincott Williams & Wilkins; 2001.

30. Cushman DG, Dumas HM, Haley SM, O'Brien JE, Kharasch VS. Re-admissions to inpatient paediatric pulmonary rehabilitation. *Pediatr Rehabil*. 2002;5: 133-139.

31. Victor N. "The challenge of meta-analysis": discussion. Indications and contraindications for meta-analysis. *J Clin Epidemiol*. 1995;48:5-8.

32. Finney DJ. A statistician looks at meta-analysis. *J Clin Epidemiol*. 1995;48:87-103.

33. Pogue J, Yusurf S. Overcoming the limitations of current meta-analysis of randomised controlled trials. *Lancet*. 1998;351:47-52.

34. Glass GV. Primary, secondary and meta-analysis of research. *Educ Res*. 1976;5:3-9.

35. Murphy S, Tickle-Degnen L. The effectiveness of occupational therapy-related treatments for persons with Parkinson's disease: a meta-analytic review. *Am J Occup Ther*. 2000;55:385-392.

36. de Goede CJT, Keus SHJ, Kwakkel G, Wagenaar RC. The effects of physical therapy in Parkinson's disease: a research synthesis. *Arch Phys Med Rehabil*. 2001;82: 509-515.

37. Robey RR. A meta-analysis of clinical outcomes in the treatment of aphasia. *J Speech Lang Hear Res*. 1998; 41:172-187.

38. Jansen CWS, Minerbo G. A comparison between early dynamically controlled mobilization and immobilization after flexor tendon repair in zone 2 of the hand: preliminary results. *J Hand Ther*. 1990;3:20-25.

39. Page SJ. Exploring competitive orientation in a group of athletes participating in the 1996 paralympic trials. *Percept Mot Skills*. 2000;91:491-502.

40. Kazdin AE. Observational research: case-control and cohort designs. In: Kazdin AE, ed. *Research Design in Clinical Psychology*. 4th ed. Boston, Mass: Allyn & Bacon; 2003.

41. Wiley ME, Damiano DL. Lower-extremity strength profiles in spastic cerebral palsy. *Dev Med Child Neurol*. 1998;40:100-107.

42. Taylor VM, Deyo RA, Ciol M, et al. Patient-oriented outcomes from low back surgery: a community-based study. *Spine*. 2000;25:2445-2452.

12

Clinical Case Reports

Contributions of Case Reports to Theory and Practice

Purposes of Case Reports

Sharing Clinical Experiences

Illustrating Evidence-Based Practice

Developing Hypotheses for Research

Building Problem-Solving Skills

Testing Theory

Persuading and Motivating

Helping to Develop Practice Guidelines and Pathways

Format of Case Reports

Summary

Clinical case reports are the means by which clinicians explore their practice through thoughtful description and analysis of clinical information from one or more cases. Sometimes dismissed as "not research," several authors consider clinical case reports to be important forms of inquiry in the health sciences. In 1993, Rothstein, in an editor's note in the journal *Physical Therapy,* noted that case reports are "too rare in this journal and in the rehabilitation literature in general."[1(p492)] He believes that case reports are useful because they "clarify clinical terminology, concepts, and approaches to problem solving"[1(p493)] through the careful documentation of practice.

Sometimes the terms *case report* and *case study* are used interchangeably as labels for systematic descriptions of practice. However, the term *case study* is also used, particularly by qualitative researchers, to describe a more complex analysis of "the particularity and complexity of a single case"[2(pxi)] within its organizational, social, or environmental context. For the purpose of this text, the term *case report* refers to descriptions of clinical practice (described in this chapter) and *case study* refers to the more complete descriptions typical of research in the qualitative tradition (see Chapter 13). Case reports, which are nonexperimental descriptions of practice, should also be clearly differentiated from single-system experimental designs, which are discussed in detail in Chapter 10.

Case reports can be developed either retrospectively or prospectively. *Retrospective* case reports are developed when a practitioner realizes that there are valuable lessons to be shared from a case in which the rehabilitation episode has been completed. *Prospective* case reports are developed when a practitioner, on initial contact with a patient or sometime early in the course of treatment, recognizes that the case is likely to produce interesting findings that should be shared. When a case report is developed prospectively, there is the potential for excellent control of measurement techniques and complete

159

description of the treatments and responses as they unfold. Unfortunately, the prospective case report suffers from the possibility that the case was managed differently from usual because of the desire to publish the results in the future.

The remainder of this chapter examines the ways in which case reports can contribute to theory and practice, cites examples of case reports that fulfill different purposes within the literature, and briefly outlines the format of case reports. Although this chapter focuses on clinical case reports, readers should recognize that case reports can also be used to document educational or administrative practices.

■ CONTRIBUTIONS OF CASE REPORTS TO THEORY AND PRACTICE

The potential value of case reports is illustrated by reviewing the relationships between theory, research, and practice presented in Chapter 2. Figure 12–1, a modification of Figure 2–1 to include case reports, shows these relationships visually. Reflection upon experience and logical speculation, which contribute to the development of theory, can be documented or developed in clinical case reports. Theories are put into action in practice, and careful documentation of this practice within case reports can help test the theories. The information presented in case reports may be used directly to change practice, to revise theories, and to suggest areas for future research. This figure suggests, then, that case reports can contribute to the development of knowledge in rehabilitation by contributing to theory development, by testing theory, by leading to the revision of theory, and by suggesting areas for further research. This figure also suggests that the information gleaned from case reports can contribute directly or indirectly to changes in practice. This suggestion, however, is not supported by everyone.

Haynes,[3] a physician and epidemiologist, identified several purposes of various forms of scholarly communications and presented a

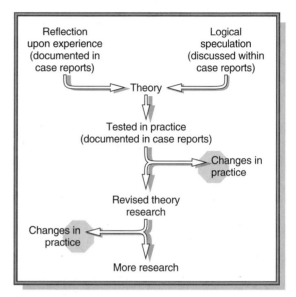

FIGURE 12–1. Modified version of Figure 2–1 showing the contribution of case reporting to the relationship between theory, practice, and research.

thoughtful analysis of the usefulness of clinical case reports. His analysis is shown in the matrix in Figure 12–2. Research reports of basic science research (sometimes called "bench research") and preliminary reports of clinical research ("field studies") are viewed as communications between scientists because their results are not yet applicable enough or rigorous enough to be applied in routine practice. Research reports of rigorous clinical trials are viewed as communications from scientists to practitioners because the findings within these definitive clinical studies are ready for application to practice. Articles that synthesize the findings of others are seen as communications between practitioners, because they can help clinicians identify and rectify gaps in their knowledge base. Finally, case reports are viewed as communications from practitioners to scientists. This view, which differs from the common perception of case reports as valuable contributions to practice, is supported as follows:

> Clinicians who use case reports and case series as guidance for management of their own patients

Authors	
Scientists	Practitioners

(Matrix — rows labeled by Audience: Scientists, Practitioners)

	Scientists	Practitioners
Scientists	Basic science "bench studies" and preliminary "field trials"	Case reports and case series
Practitioners	Rigorous clinical trials	Review articles

FIGURE 12–2. Matrix showing the purposes of various scholarly communications, delineated by the author and the audience for the communication.
Generated from information presented in Haynes RB. Loose connections between peer-reviewed clinical journals and clinical practice. *Ann Intern Med.* 1990;113: 724-728.

are at risk for deceiving themselves and hurting their patients....Some case reports eventually prove to be important; most do not. Unfortunately, their methods do not permit discrimination of the valid from the interesting but erroneous, and they cannot provide a sound basis for clinical action. Case reports are, however, a fertile source of hypotheses that could lead to systematic observation.[3(pp725-726)]

Thus, Haynes believes that the primary value of case reports is in their contributions to theory and research, rather than their direct contributions to practice. This view of case reports is not presented to discourage practitioners from reading and learning from case reports. Rather, this alternate view is presented to remind practitioners that they need to thoughtfully critique the findings of case reports, just as they would assess the validity of more traditional research reports. In addition, because case reports are presented in the familiar language of practice, rather than the sometimes foreign language of research, clinicians may find that their reading habits

gravitate toward case reports. Haynes's matrix of scholarly communications reminds us to broaden our reading habits to include review articles and the reports of rigorous clinical trials.

■ PURPOSES OF CASE REPORTS

Although the general purpose of case reports is to carefully describe practice, the case reports that are presented in the literature show that there are many ways in which this general purpose can be fulfilled. McEwen,[4] in her manual on writing case reports, identifies seven functions of case reports: (1) sharing clinical experiences, (2) illustrating evidence-based practice, (3) developing hypotheses for research, (4) building problem-solving skills, (5) testing theory, (6) persuading and motivating, and (7) helping to develop practice guidelines and pathways. Recent examples of case reports that fulfill these seven functions are presented.

Sharing Clinical Experiences

One clinical experience that is commonly shared through a case report is that of the diagnostic enigma. For example, Leerar reported on a case in which a difficult diagnosis of tarsal coalition was made[5] and Ferraro-Herrera and colleagues[6] reported on a patient for whom autonomic dysfunction was the presenting feature of Guillain-Barré syndrome.

Another common clinical experience that is shared through case reports is the presentation of unusual patients. Manktelow and colleagues[7] presented the case of a patient who experienced a late lateral femoral condyle fracture 2 years after anterior cruciate ligament reconstruction and Fiala and associates documented the treatment of a traumatic hemarthrosis of a collegiate athlete.[8]

The clinical experiences documented in case reports do not, however, need to focus on the odd or the unusual in clinical practice. Careful documentation and discussion of commonplace cases can also be instructive. For example, Page and colleagues combined constraint-induced therapy and botulinum toxin A to treat an individual with residual upper limb spasticity following a stroke[9] and Bruce and colleagues reported on the use of a voice recognition system as a writing aid for a man with aphasia.[10] In both cases, neither the diagnosis nor the treatments were particularly unusual. However, in both cases, unique combinations or applications of treatments were documented with the common diagnosis.

Illustrating Evidence-Based Practice

Some case reports may be used to illustrate how a practitioner used evidence-based practice principles to manage the case. Parker did just this in a report showing the literature-based decision-making process used to determine medical and surgical management for an older woman with a fractured femur.[11] Likewise, Whitman and associates reviewed the literature related to nonsurgical management of lumbar spinal stenosis and documented a case series using techniques supported in the literature.[12]

Developing Hypotheses for Research

Although most case reports have the potential to help develop hypotheses for research, some authors include an explicit discussion of the research applications of their work. For example, Barlow and Gierut describe the application of a linguistic approach with word pairs for a child with a phonological delay.[13] This approach included development of a series of treatment options with different levels of hypothesized effectiveness. This pattern of hypothesized effectiveness can form the basis for further research.

Another case with an explicit connection to future research is the report by Fritz and colleagues of the results of a nonsurgical treatment approach for patients with lumbar spinal stenosis (LSS).[14] They provided readers with a clear indication of the line of research that needs to flow from the case report:

> In our view, experimental studies can be performed only after an approach to evaluation, treatment, and outcome assessment has been defined for the population being studied. This case report of two patients with short-term follow-up needs to be followed by reports describing larger series of patients with LSS treated with this approach with longer follow-up periods. If the treatment approach we are recommending produces favorable long-term outcomes in larger series of patients, then a randomized clinical trial would be warranted to compare this approach with the present "standard of care," which consists of the use of medications and nonspecific exercises. Only a randomized clinical trial could produce experimental evidence for the efficacy of the treatment approach we suggest.[14(p971)]

Note that the sequence of events they described corresponds closely to the types of research described in the matrix of communication presented earlier in this chapter. The first research approach that is recommended—a larger descriptive series—is a limited "field trial." If the field trial is promising, then a formal randomized clinical trial is recommended to compare this new treatment with existing ones.

Building Problem-Solving Skills

Some clinical case reports contribute to practice by presenting frameworks for problem solving by clinicians. Zimny[15] accomplished this purpose in her case report of the clinical reasoning involved in the evaluation and management of undiagnosed chronic hip pain in a 21-year-old woman. Before describing the case, she reviewed various protocols for examination of the hip and presented several organizational models for reasoning about musculoskeletal pain. The description of the case then showed how these protocols and models could be applied in practice. The results were divided into an "examination" section, in which the results of clinical testing were reported, and an "evaluation" section, in which the author's judgments about the meaning of the clinical test results were articulated. This section gave the reader an insider's view of the clinical reasoning that was applied to this case.

Problem-solving skills in relation to teaching children who are congenitally deaf-blind was the topic of Bruce's case report on the impact of an inservice training program on the teaching practices of teachers without formal preparation for working with these children.[16] This case report used qualitative methods to document the process by which the teachers learned to implement the principles presented in the inservice program.

Testing Theory

Case reports can provide preliminary tests of various theories about patient management. For example, Moyers and Stoffel[17] presented a case report of a client with a work-related injury and alcohol dependence. A theoretical model of behavior change was presented and this theory was applied to the client described in the report. Likewise, Ross[18] described the evaluation and treatment of a patient with foot dysfunction using a tissue stress model.

Thai and colleagues[19] presented a case in which basic research findings related to the use of ultraviolet light C to kill methicillin-resistant *Staphylococcus aureus* (MRSA) were applied to treatment of three people with chronic wounds infected with MRSA.

Persuading and Motivating

Although some are uncomfortable with the idea of immediate application of the results of case reports, others find it appealing that "case reports can help practitioners deal with change, influence administrators, and persuade physicians and insurers of the value of services for particular patients."[4(p11)] One example of a case report with persuasion potential is Schindler and colleagues' report on the functional effect of bilateral tendon transfers on a person with quadriplegia.[20] Rather than reporting on a new technique, this case report extended the findings of almost 20 years of experience with tendon transfers for persons with quadriplegia. The authors of this case indicated that, although previous reports had documented improvements in hand function tests and some activities of daily living after tendon transfer, none had examined the impact of the surgeries on the amount of assistance needed with various tasks or the amount of equipment needed to accomplish the tasks. For individuals with quadriplegia who are considering tendon transfer surgery, it is exceedingly important to answer the question of whether the well-documented improvements in hand function lead to any meaningful changes in independence. Although this single case report does not provide a definitive answer to that question, the data in the case report, coupled with the well-documented experiences of the past 20 years, may assist with the decision-making process.

Other examples of the role of case reports in persuading and motivating include Wills' report on the role of physical therapists in skin cancer screening[21] and Frost's report on the role of physical, occupational, and speech therapy in hospice.[22] In both of these reports the authors used particular cases to illustrate what the authors believe are important roles for rehabilitation professionals.

Helping to Develop Practice Guidelines and Pathways

McEwen's final purpose for presenting case reports is that they may help develop practice guidelines and pathways.[4] An excellent example of a case report that accomplishes this purpose is Fritz's report of the application of a classification approach to the treatment of three patients with low back syndrome.[23] This approach to care of patients with low back pain classifies patients according to clusters of signs and symptoms and then provides treatment that "matches" the classification. If adequate testing demonstrates the validity of the classification and the effectiveness of the matched treatments, then classification approaches can be the basis for developing practice guidelines or preferred clinical pathways.

Fritz[23] contributed to these efforts by describing three patients who appeared to have similar pathology, but fell into three different classifications and were successfully treated three different ways with treatments that matched their classifications. This case-based evidence is not sufficient to conclude that this classification approach is valid, but, combined with the positive results of a similar field trial,[24] suggests that this approach may be appropriate to study with rigorous randomized clinical trials.

In a variation that applies guidelines rather than develops them, Kayser-Jones described and analyzed ethical issues surrounding end-of-life decisions made in the case of a 101-year-old resident of a nursing home.[25]

■ FORMAT OF CASE REPORTS

Case reports that appear in peer-reviewed journals typically follow the format—or a modified format—of more traditional research reports. First there is an introduction, critical review of the literature, and purpose statement to place the case into the context of what is already known about the phenomenon. Next, the equivalent of the methods section describes the subject, analyzes the presenting problem, presents examination data, outlines the conclusions drawn from the examination data, and describes the intervention. The equivalent of the results section presents the outcomes of care. As is the case with a traditional research report, the results are then placed into context in a discussion and conclusion section in which the authors discuss the meaning and application of the case. Detailed instructions for writing case reports can be found in McEwen's "how-to" manual.[4]

■ SUMMARY

Case reports are systematic descriptions of practice. It is clear that the information in case reports can be used to contribute to the development of theory and the design of research. There are differing opinions about the extent to which the information in case reports should be used directly to change practice. The written format of case reports is analogous to traditional research reports, with introduction, methods, results, and discussion sections.

REFERENCES

1. Rothstein JM. The case for case reports [Editor's Note]. *Phys Ther.* 1993;73:492-493.
2. Stake RE. *The Art of Case Study Research.* Thousand Oaks, Calif: Sage Publications; 1995.
3. Haynes RB. Loose connections between peer-reviewed clinical journals and clinical practice. *Ann Intern Med.* 1990;113:724-728.
4. McEwen I. *Writing Case Reports: A How-To Manual for Clinicians.* 2nd ed. Alexandria, Va: American Physical Therapy Association; 2001.
5. Leerar PJ. Differential diagnosis of tarsal coalition versus cuboid syndrome in an adolescent athlete. *J Orthop Sports Phys Ther.* 2001;31:702-707.
6. Ferraro-Herrera AS, Kern HB, Nagler W. Autonomic dysfunction as the presenting feature of Guillain-Barré syndrome. *Arch Phys Med Rehabil.* 1997;78:777-779.
7. Manktelow AR, Haddad FS, Goddard NJ. Late lateral femoral condyle fracture after anterior cruciate ligament reconstruction: a case report. *Am J Sports Med.* 1998; 26:587-590.
8. Fiala KA, Hoffmann SJ, Ritenour DM. Traumatic hemarthrosis of the knee secondary to hemophilia A in a collegiate soccer player: a case report. *J Athl Train.* 2002;37:315-319.
9. Page SJ, Elovic E, Levine P, Sisto SA. Modified constraint-induced therapy and botulinum toxin A: a promising combination. *Am J Phys Med Rehabil.* 2003;82:76-80.
10. Bruce C, Edmundson A, Coleman M. Writing with voice: an investigation of the use of voice recognition system as a writing aid for a man with aphasia. *Int J Lang Commun Disord.* 2003;38:131-148.
11. Parker MJ. Evidence-based case report: managing an elderly patient with a fractured femur. *BMJ.* 2000;320: 102-103.
12. Whitman JM, Flynn TW, Fritz JM. Nonsurgical management of patients with lumbar spinal stenosis: a literature review and case series of three patients managed with physical therapy. *Phys Med Rehabil Clin N Am.* 2003; 14:77-101, vi-vii.

13. Barlow JA, Gierut JA. Minimal pair approaches to phonological remediation. *Semin Speech Lang.* 2002; 23:57-68.

14. Fritz JM, Erhard RE, Vignovic M. A nonsurgical treatment approach for patients with lumbar spinal stenosis. *Phys Ther.* 1997;77:962-973.

15. Zimny NJ. Clinical reasoning in the evaluation and management of undiagnosed chronic hip pain in a young adult. *Phys Ther.* 1998;78:62-73.

16. Bruce SM. Impact of a communication intervention model on teachers' practice with children who are congenitally deaf-blind. *J Visual Impairment Blindness.* 2002; 96:154-168.

17. Moyers PA, Stoffel VC. Alcohol dependence in a client with a work-related injury. *Am J Occup Ther.* 1999;53:640-645.

18. Ross M. Use of the tissue stress model as a paradigm for developing an examination and management plan for a patient with plantar fasciitis. *J Am Podiatr Med Assoc.* 2002;92:499-506.

19. Thai TP, Houghton PE, Campbell KE, Woodbury MG. Ultraviolet light C in the treatment of chronic wounds with MRSA: a case study. *Ostomy Wound Manage.* 2002; 48:52-60.

20. Schindler L, Robbins G, Hamlin C. Functional effect of bilateral tendon transfers on a person with C-5 quadriplegia. *Am J Occup Ther.* 1994;48:750-757.

21. Wills M. Skin cancer screening. *Phys Ther.* 2002;82: 1232-1237.

22. Frost M. The role of physical, occupational, and speech therapy in hospice: patient empowerment. *Am J Hosp Palliat Care.* 2001;18:397-402.

23. Fritz JM. Use of a classification approach to the treatment of 3 patients with low back syndrome. *Phys Ther.* 1998; 78:766-777.

24. Delitto A, Cibulka MT, Erhard RE, Bowling RW, Tenhula JA. Evidence for use of an extension-mobilization category in acute low back syndrome: a prescriptive validation pilot study. *Phys Ther.* 1993;73:216-222.

25. Kayser-Jones J. A case study of the death of an older woman in a nursing home: are nursing care practices in compliance with ethical guidelines. *J Gerontol Nurs.* 2000; 26:48-54.

13

Qualitative Research

Assumptions of the Qualitative Paradigm	Data Collection
Qualitative Designs	*Interview*
Case Study	*Observation*
Ethnography	*Artifacts*
Phenomenology	**Data Analysis**
Grounded Theory	*Data Management*
Qualitative Methods	*Generating Meaning*
Sampling	*Verification*
	Summary

Research conducted in the tradition of the qualitative paradigm is of growing importance to rehabilitation literature. As health care practitioners begin to conceptualize what they do according to biopsychosocial models of care, rather than focusing solely on disease-based biomedical models of care, so too must health care researchers embrace research methods that capture the complexity of these new models of care. The qualitative research paradigm and the methods that flow from that paradigm provide a means by which researchers can match their research methods to the complex phenomena they wish to study. This chapter reviews the assumptions of the qualitative research paradigm (originally presented in Chapter 5), introduces the various research designs associated with the qualitative tradition, and discusses a variety of methods and issues related to qualitative research.

■ ASSUMPTIONS OF THE QUALITATIVE PARADIGM

Five central assumptions of the qualitative paradigm are introduced in Chapter 5 and are reviewed here. The first assumption is that the world consists of multiple constructed realities. There are always several versions of reality and the meaning that participants construct from events is an inseparable component of the events themselves. The second assumption is that the investigator and the subject are interdependent and the process of inquiry itself changes both the investigator and the subject. The third assumption is that knowledge is time and context dependent. As a consequence, qualitative research is *idiographic,* meaning that it pertains to a particular case in a particular time and context. The fourth assumption is that it is impossible to distinguish causes from effects. Researchers who adopt the qualitative paradigm believe it is more useful to describe and interpret events than to attempt to control them to establish oversimplified causes and effects. The fifth assumption is that inquiry is value bound. This value-ladenness is exemplified in the type of questions qualitative researchers ask, the way they define and measure constructs, and the way they interpret the results of their research.

QUALITATIVE DESIGNS

The qualitative research paradigm encompasses a wide range of designs that flow from the five basic assumptions previously outlined. In fact, the boundaries between different types of qualitative research are far less clear than the boundaries between different quantitative designs. Denzin and Lincoln,[1] in the preface to the second edition of their *Handbook of Qualitative Research,* articulate this as they describe the process of developing the volume:

> It did not take us long to discover that the "field" of qualitative research had undergone quantum leaps since the spring of 1991, when we began to plan the first edition. We once again learned that the field of qualitative research is defined primarily by a series of essential tensions, contradictions, and hesitations. These tensions—many of them emerging after 1991—work back and forth among competing definitions and conceptions of the field.[1(pxi)]

Whereas there is relatively well-standardized terminology for the different classifications of quantitative designs, the terminology for the different types of qualitative research is far less universally accepted. Four sometimes overlapping design strategies are discussed in this section of the chapter. Although it is useful to categorize the design strategies into a manageable number of approaches, readers should recognize that there is disagreement about what defines each approach and that there is considerable overlap among the methods used in the approaches.

To illustrate the similarities and differences between the methods, a single hypothetical research problem is developed in different ways using the four design strategies. Table 13–1 introduces this problem, which focuses on shifts in how the rehabilitation team is conceptualized and implemented in the United States.

Case Study

Case study, rather than being a complete design strategy, is one way of structuring a qualitative research project; it is "not a methodological choice, but a choice of what is to be studied."[2(p435)] By nature, a case has boundaries that define the limits of the inquiry.[3,4] In the context of the hypothetical problem defined in Table 13–1, the case is identified as the rehabilitation team at one inpatient rehabilitation facility. The purpose of such a study would be to gain an in-depth perspective on the evolution of rehabilitation team roles in the contemporary health care environment. Having identified the case, the qualitative researcher still has a choice of studying the case through any single or combination of the remaining designs, which are discussed in subsequent sections of this chapter. The researcher who studies a case chooses to emphasize the idiographic nature of qualitative research and recognizes that the results of the study will be particularly time and context dependent. Another researcher might choose to study the same problem, also guided by the qualitative paradigm, by studying rehabilitation teams at several different inpatient rehabilitation centers. The purpose of this research would be to understand the phenomenon of rehabilitation teams, rather than gaining an in-depth view of the evolution of a single rehabilitation team.

The previous paragraph identifies what is and is not a case study by contrasting the study of a single rehabilitation team with the study of several rehabilitation teams at different centers. This example leaves open the possibility of two ways of identifying what is and what is not a case: the number of elements and the relationship among the elements. The relationship among the elements

TABLE 13-1	**Hypothetical Research Problems That Match Different Qualitative Design Strategies**
Given:	During the 1980s and 1990s comprehensive rehabilitation teams were used routinely to plan, implement, and manage the care of individuals being treated in inpatient rehabilitation centers. All of the members of the team routinely evaluated each new admission, made management recommendations, and participated in regular team meetings about each patient.
However:	As widespread health care cost containment efforts have became the norm in the late 1990s and early 2000s, the routine, comprehensive rehabilitation team approach has come under scrutiny from health care insurers and facility administrators. Rehabilitation professions are being asked to reduce the number of different professionals involved in each case, to eliminate services perceived to be duplications of effort, and to reduce the amount of time spent in team meetings. The simultaneous demand to provide quality, comprehensive care while reducing costs has required rehabilitation teams to redefine themselves and the roles of the individual professionals who constitute the team.
Therefore:	(Case Study) We did an in-depth case study of the evolution of rehabilitation team roles at one inpatient rehabilitation facility.
Therefore:	(Ethnography) We used participant-observation to develop an understanding of the functioning of a contemporary rehabilitation team at an inpatient rehabilitation center.
Therefore:	(Phenomenology) The purpose of our study was to describe the experience of being a member of a contemporary rehabilitation team in an inpatient rehabilitation center.
Therefore:	(Grounded Theory) The purpose of our study was to develop a preliminary theory to explain how members of contemporary rehabilitation teams work to provide high-quality, cost-effective care.

is the key. If several different rehabilitation teams at one facility were studied, the "case study" would be of the evolution of rehabilitation teams at that particular facility. The researchers would seek information about each team's story, but would also find out about how facility-wide change was accomplished. Because of the facility boundary, different things would be learned from this case than would be learned in a qualitative study of several rehabilitation teams at different, unaffiliated facilities.

There are several good examples of qualitative case studies in rehabilitation. In a study of a single individual, an occupational therapist with chronic pain, Neville-Jan documented her own experiences with chronic pain.[5] In a multiple case study with very clear boundaries—both in identifying the activity of interest and the people to study— Taylor and colleagues examined the meaning of sea kayaking for three individuals with incomplete quadriplegia.[6] In another example, with

boundaries determined by membership in a single community-based stroke club, Sabari and colleagues collected qualitative information about personal experiences with stroke rehabilitation.[7] Finally, Jensen and colleagues studied dimensions that distinguished master from novice clinicians working in orthopedic settings.[8] In this example, the six cases were selected to represent two ends of a continuum of experience. In addition to studying each case, the researchers examined commonalities among the three master clinicians and among the three novice clinicians, as well as between the master and novice clinicians. These four articles, then, illustrate four different ways of defining the "case" or "cases" of interest.

Ethnography

The purpose of ethnography is to describe a culture. Broadly, *culture* can be defined as the knowledge, beliefs, and behaviors that define a group. The group can be a societal group such as "Americans," "French-Canadians," or "Southeast Asian immigrants." The group can also be a small, specialized unit such as "burn therapists," "members of a wheelchair basketball team," or "physical medicine and rehabilitation faculty members at a particular institution."

The ethnographic approach requires that the researcher, usually an outsider to the culture, describe the culture from the perspective of an insider. Spradley indicated that "rather than *studying people,* ethnography means *learning from people.*"[9(p3)] The way that one learns from people is often described as *participant-observation.* Participant-observers immerse themselves in a new culture so that they can participate in and experience, in part, what it means to be within this culture. Rather than being complete insiders, however, participant-observers maintain a level of detachment that enables them to analyze, reflect on, and place the happenings within the observed culture into a broader framework. The concept of the researcher as both observer and participant illustrates clearly the qualitative research assumption that the investigator and subject are interdependent. Table 13–1 includes a purpose statement for an ethnographic study consistent with the background information on evolution of rehabilitation team roles. Whereas the purpose statement for the case study identifies only who is to be studied, the purpose statement for the ethnographic study also includes information about the methods to be used as well as the interest in the broader culture surrounding the person being studied.

Clinicians who undertake ethnographic research are required to shift their "gaze" from being the expert professional observer to being a different kind of observer. Lawlor has described this shift as involving vulnerability (entering into someone else's unfamiliar world rather than controlling the familiar clinical environment), being present (watching attentively rather than doing), human sociality and social graces (establishing social connections rather than maintaining professional distance), and self-consciousness and reflexivity (focusing on the role of self as researcher rather than on the client).[10]

The nature of ethnography can be illustrated by contrasting quantitative and ethnographic approaches to studying the rehabilitation team. A quantitative approach to studying these teams might focus on the cost of services provided by each member of the team, the average number of different professionals involved in the care of patients with different diagnoses, the amount of time spent in team meetings by each professional, and scores on a written questionnaire seeking patient and family opinions about the effectiveness of the team. The ethnographic approach would require observation and documentation of some of the same activities explored by the quantitative approach but would also focus on the emotions, feelings, and perceptions of team members and the patients and families with whom they interact. To do so, the ethnographer needs to request this information from the participants in the culture being studied. To become a participant-observer, the ethnographer would spend a great deal of time with the team members being studied, participating in the team for a period of time. For example, the researcher might participate by eating lunch with team members who dine together regularly, by attending a softball game in the recreational league that staff members participate in, and by accompanying team members to professional meetings where the researcher could observe interactions of team members with other members of their own profession.

As an observer the researcher might privately note how much spontaneous conversation is focused on defining team roles, on how the heroes and villains of a team are depicted in conversations in which all members are not present, or how much conversation focuses on past team functions versus contemporary realities. As a participant, the researcher would ask direct questions about what had been observed: "One member of the team seems to dominate during team meetings and nobody challenges her—why is that?" "Today you saw your physician, three therapists, and a social worker—how well do you think they are working together to help you meet your goal of returning home?" "I noticed today that you and the occupational" therapist came to a quick resolution about which one of you would focus on treating Mrs. Henry's shoulder—what factors go into making decisions about the division of labor when more than one professional is qualified to implement certain interventions?" In addition to asking questions of the team members being studied, the ethnographic researcher would likely question other important members of the "culture": patients and their families, facility administrators, outside vendors, colleagues outside of the facility. As a participant, the researcher would recognize that his or her presence changed things in some way—people would say things for the researcher's benefit or would fail to do or say things they might have otherwise done or said if the researcher were not present. In addition, reflecting on and articulating feelings and concerns might change the way that the participants deal with those concerns.

A health-related example of an ethnographic study is Shidler's perspective on life-prolonging treatment decision making in two long-term care centers in Quebec.[11] Methods of study included more than 100 hours of interviews with informants who held many different roles within the long-term care setting, 400 hours of participant-observation, and examination of various documents. The informants included the older adults living in the long-term care centers, their family members, and personnel including physicians, registered and practical nurses, psychosocial workers, clinical administrators, nurse aides, and housekeeping staff. The extensive time spent within each facility and the wide range of informants who were interviewed and observed meant that the researcher was able to generate a complex description of the culture in which life-prolonging treatment decisions were made.

Another example of an ethnographic approach is Camp's study of the use of service dogs as an adaptive strategy for individuals with disabilities.[12] Before beginning the study, Camp volunteered with a service dog organization, attended its national conference, and spent a great deal of time talking with service dog owners, health care professionals, and dog trainers. With this background information, she felt prepared to enter the world of service dogs and their owners, interviewing and observing five different owner–dog pairs in their homes and in the community.

Phenomenology

The purpose of the phenomenological approach to qualitative inquiry is to focus on the "ways in which ordinary members of society attend to their everyday lives."[13(pp488-489)] The distinction between the phenomenological and ethnographic approaches, as defined here, can be seen if the ethnographic study of the culture of rehabilitation teams is recast as a phenomenological study. The purpose of the ethnography was to develop an understanding of the functioning of a contemporary rehabilitation team, and the methods included participant-observation of team members in work and leisure settings as well as interviews with patients and families. As observers as well as participants, ethnographers interpret the many sources of data to provide a unique combination of insider and outsider insights into the situation. Phenomenological research "gives voice" to the person being studied and requires that the researcher present the subject's view of his or her world. In a phenomenological study of rehabilitation teams, the only informants would be members of the team. For example, what patients think of the level of teamwork among the rehabilitation professionals would not be relevant to a phenomenological study. However, team member perceptions of how patients are affected by teamwork would be of great importance in describing the experience of being a member of a rehabilitation team. Table 13–1 lists a sample purpose statement that would be consistent with a phenomenological approach.

The case study described earlier, about the meaning of sea kayaking for individuals with quadriplegia,[6] used a phenomenological approach. The only informants were the individuals with quadriplegia, and the questioning started with an open-ended invitation to relate their views: "Tell me about sea kayaking." In other examples, Crichton-Smith studied the communicative experiences of adults who stammer,[14] Pitney and colleagues studied the professional socialization of certified athletic trainers working in U.S. National Collegiate Athletic Association Division I universities,[15] and Dudgeon and associates studied the experience of chronic pain for nine individuals with disabilities.[16] Thus, it can be seen that the scope of the "life world" described within a phenomenological study can vary greatly—from a narrow slice of life about a recreational activity to an all-encompassing view of life with a chronic condition.

Grounded Theory

The grounded-theory approach was developed by Glaser in the 1960s.[17] Grounded theory methods "consist of systematic inductive guidelines for collecting and analyzing data to build middle-range theoretical frameworks that explain the collected data. Throughout the research process, grounded theorists develop analytic interpretations of their data to focus further data collection, which they use in turn to inform and refine their developing theoretical analyses."[18(p509)] Because of this interplay between data collection and analysis, grounded theory is often referred to as a constant comparative method. Although initially viewed as a means of generating new theory, contemporary writers also allow that grounded-theory approaches may be used to elaborate and modify existing theories.[19,20] Although the grounded-theory approach shares interview and observational methods with other qualitative approaches, the goal of the research is different. Ethnography and phenomenology

are distinguished from grounded-theory research in that the goals of the former are to describe the phenomenon of interest and the goal of the latter is to explain the phenomenon through the analysis of the relationships among concepts. In the hypothetical example of the changing role of rehabilitation teams, a purpose consistent with a grounded-theory approach would focus on the development of a theory to explain how members of rehabilitation teams work together to balance high-quality care with cost effectiveness (see Table 13–1).

Jensen and associates' study of novice and experienced clinicians, discussed earlier as a general example of a case study, could be classified as grounded-theory research because one of its purposes was to "develop an initial conceptual framework"[8(p712)] about the work of physical therapists. In this instance, the study was used to elaborate on a previous set of themes distinguishing between novice and experienced physical therapy clinicians.

Other rehabilitation researchers have followed the more classic approach to grounded theory—going in without a theoretical framework and seeing what emerges. For example, Dubouloz and colleagues studied occupational therapists' perceptions of evidence-based practice[21] and Graham studied conceptual learning processes of physical therapy students.[22]

As noted previously, the boundaries between the qualitative approaches are not clear. Some studies may not fit any of the categories; others may fit more than one of the categories. Labels such as "case study," "grounded theory," "ethnography," and "phenomenology" are important because they provide a way to organize what we know about qualitative research. However, arguments about which definition is the "one true definition" tend to be counterproductive in that they violate one of the basic tenets of qualitative research—the acceptance of multiple realities. Thus, readers should use this classification of qualitative research as one way to organize information and recognize that others may use equally useful alternate classification systems.

■ QUALITATIVE METHODS

The methods of qualitative research are consistent with the assumptions presented earlier in the chapter and often cross the lines between the various research designs associated with qualitative research. This section of the chapter introduces sampling, data collection, and data analysis procedures commonly used by qualitative researchers. More detail about these procedures can be found in several excellent textbooks devoted to qualitative research.[23-25]

Sampling

Qualitative researchers use nonprobability sampling methods, originally described in Chapter 8, to identify the individuals who participate within their studies. These individuals are typically referred to as *informants* rather than subjects, reflecting the emphasis on gaining access to their point of view rather than on manipulating them in some way as would be typical in quantitative experimental studies.

In the broadest sense, the sampling method is one of convenience because researchers often study informants they know who meet their study criteria, or facilities or organizations with whom they have connections. Beyond the initial convenient selection of sites or subjects, qualitative researchers often use a combination of purposive sampling and snowball sampling techniques. Recall that purposive sampling involves selecting individuals not for representativeness, but for diversity of views. Researchers studying the evolution of rehabilitation teams in inpatient rehabilitation centers might believe that it is important to include both male and female physiatrists, therapists with extensive clinical experience as well as new graduates, and professionals who have worked in other settings in the past. They might also believe that they should have the perspectives of professionals working with patients of differing socioeconomic status and of teams that appear to work well together as well as those who do not.

Because there is no established sampling frame of rehabilitation teams, researchers would likely use snowball sampling techniques to assemble the purposive sample. To do so, they might ask a few key colleagues to identify rehabilitation teams that appear to have made a particularly good or a particularly poor response to new pressures to work together differently. If these key colleagues happen to identify two urban teams that work with individuals with spinal cord injuries, the researcher might then seek out additional teams that serve rural communities or that work with individuals with brain injuries and stroke. In qualitative research, the sampling design may change as the study progresses. In the first few interviews with teams, informants may indicate that working with patients who do not speak English is a special challenge for the team and that an effective translator is critical to maintaining a patient-focused effort. If the researchers had not anticipated this as an important dimension of the study, they might now change their purposive sampling procedure to identify some teams that include translators.

If a researcher plans an ethnographic study, then the informants would include individuals other than the members of the rehabilitation team. At the beginning of the study, the researcher would likely anticipate some groups of informants that would be important to the study—patients, families, facility administrators. However, the researcher would not have enough knowledge of the phenomenon of rehabilitation teams to anticipate all of the relevant informants. During contact with initial informants, then, a common question should therefore be, "Who else could provide me with information about xxx?" At a given facility, for example, the evening shift housekeeper may be someone who always seems to know everything about everybody. At the outset, she might not be identified as a potential informant, but some of the initial informants would likely say "Talk to Bea, she knows everything!" This variation on snowball sampling helps identify additional informants who meet criteria the researcher had anticipated as well as additional classes of informants that had not been anticipated.

Several reports of qualitative research illustrate these sampling principles. Pitney and colleagues, in their study of professional socialization of certified athletic trainers, used snowball sampling to expand their informants from an original six participants to the final 16.[15] A variation on snowball sampling was used by Jensen and associates to identify their "master" clinicians.[8] The researchers asked academic clinical education coordinators in three different regions to identify, or nominate, several therapists who would be considered master clinicians in orthopedic physical therapy. Potential informants who were identified as master clinicians by more than one clinical coordinator were then contacted by one of the researchers to determine their willingness to participate.

Data Collection

Although there are many different design strategies for qualitative research, their implementation rests on a common core of methods. These methods include interviewing, observation, and examination of artifacts.

INTERVIEW

"Asking questions and getting answers is a much harder task than it may seem at first. The spoken or written word has always a residue of ambiguity, no matter how carefully we word the questions and how carefully we report or code the answers."[26(p645)] Interviewing, with all of its ambiguity, is one of the primary ways in which qualitative researchers collect data. Interviews can be classified by the extent of structure, the number of interviewees, and the proximity of the interviewer and interviewee.

With respect to structure, interviews can generally be classified as structured, semistructured, and unstructured. A *structured interview* is essentially an oral administration of a written questionnaire. When a surveyor stops you in the shopping mall to determine whether you have purchased a certain brand of facial tissue within the past 6 weeks, he or she is using a structured interview. The surveyor asks the same questions of everyone and does not deviate from the wording in the question. Structured interviews are most appropriate when relatively factual information is sought. In qualitative research, structured interviews might be used to collect a core of basic information from informants. However, structured interviews are rarely the choice for capturing the depth and breadth of response that is desired in qualitative research.

Semistructured interviews are based on predeveloped questions, but the format permits the interviewer to clarify questions to help the participant provide more information for the study. Semistructured interviews are appropriate when information of a somewhat abstract nature is sought. Qualitative researchers who are testing theory (rather than developing it) or verifying information (rather than collecting it for the first time) may use semistructured interviews for these components of their data collection efforts. Pizzari and colleagues used semistructured interviews to study adherence to anterior cruciate ligament rehabilitation.[27] Although they were guided by a schedule of questions, the unstructured format left them free to elaborate on questions as requested by the informants or to follow up on information volunteered by the informants.

Unstructured interviewing is the general method used by qualitative researchers to come to an understanding of the opinions and beliefs of informants. In an unstructured interview, researchers have a general idea of the topics that they hope to cover during the interview. However, the order and way in which the topics are covered are left to the interviewer as he or she interacts with subjects. The interviewer is free to follow up on unexpected responses that lead in a direction that was unanticipated by the researcher. In addition, unstructured interviews can change from interviewee to interviewee as the researcher gains more insight into the situation being studied. Suppose that Informant A volunteers his belief that the changes in rehabilitation team roles are specifically directed at decreasing or eliminating a particular service from the facility. The researcher, who may not have anticipated a need to determine beliefs about the motives behind the evolution of team roles, might follow this thread in subsequent interviews to determine whether others share Informant A's belief. Graham used unstructured interviewing to collect data from the students in her study of conceptual learning processes of physical therapy students.[22] Because she went into the study without a preconceived theory about conceptual learning processes of physical therapy students, it was appropriate that she go into the interviews in a consistent manner—without a preconceived set of questions.

With respect to the number of interviewees, researchers must determine whether they wish to interview informants singly or in groups. Individual interviews may elicit more confidential information about the informant or more frank information about other individuals within the setting. Group interviews may make the interviewer seem less intimidating and the responses of some group members may prompt other members to remember or share additional information. In any given study, it may be appropriate to conduct individual interviews, group interviews, or both.

With respect to the proximity of the interviewer and interviewee, the options are expanding because of the availability of new communication technologies. In-person interviews allow for the best opportunity to establish rapport and observe nonverbal cues of the interviewee. Telephone interviews do not permit observation of nonverbal behaviors, but may give the interviewer access to informants who are unavailable in person. Interactive two-way video hookups provide an opportunity to see the informants being interviewed at a distance. Electronic mail provides an opportunity to communicate with others in an informal conversational way, and various forms of electronic conferencing offer an electronic equivalent of the group interview situation.

Whichever style of interviewing is used, the researcher must consider several common concerns. First, the interviewer's vocabulary must match that of the individuals being interviewed, including the use of lay versus health care terminology when appropriate. Second, interviewers must be sensitive to the meaning of specific words that they use. For example, when interviewing individuals who are members of racial or ethnic groups, the interviewers should determine informants' preferences for identifying terms such as *black* versus *African American, American Indian* versus *Native American,* and *Latino* versus *Hispanic.*

Third, interviewers must do what they can to establish rapport and make the interviewee comfortable. Friendly chit-chat and social conventions such as talking about the weather, taking coats, offering coffee or soft drinks, and the like can all be used to place the participant at ease in the research situation. The interviewees' comfort may be enhanced if the interview takes place on their "turf"—their office, their home, or a public place of their choosing.

Fourth, interviewers must ensure that subjects give their informed consent to participate in the interview. The interviewer should specify the purposes of the study, emphasize the provisions for confidentiality of responses, and make it clear that the participant can terminate the interview at any time. If the researcher is going to audiotape or videotape the interview, the participant needs additional assurances about the provisions for confidentiality of the recorded information. In research conducted using interviews, the primary risk to the participant is often the breach of confidentiality. Therefore, informed consent sometimes may be accomplished verbally rather than in writing so there is no written record of the names of those who participated in the study.

OBSERVATION

Qualitative researchers frequently use observation as an adjunct to interviews. The observational role has been described as a continuum between complete observation and complete participation. Along this continuum, four points have been defined: complete participant, participant-as-observer, observer-as-participant, and complete observer. These terms, originated by Gold in the 1950s, have been reconceptualized by contemporary qualitative researchers.[28]

When the researcher is a complete participant, this means that he or she is a full, legitimate member of the setting being studied. This may involve "opportunistic research" wherein a researcher recognizes a good research opportunity within an organization to which he or she already belongs or "participatory" or "action" research in which the researcher and informants become genuine partners in generating new knowledge that is expected to lead to changes within an organization or system.[29] An interesting variation on the researcher as complete participant can be found in Neville-Jan's autoethnography describing her experiences with chronic pain.[5]

In the participant-as-observer model the researcher assumes limited membership roles within a community for the purpose of conducting the research. This role has generated controversy in past research, mostly in sociological studies of illegal or socially unacceptable behavior, when researchers inserted themselves into a community without disclosing their role as a researcher. In today's electronic world, this issue has arisen anew in conjunction with the use of Internet communities, such as mailing lists and chat rooms, for qualitative research.[30] This model of observation can, however, be accomplished with the knowledge and consent of the members of the community. If, for example, a speech-language pathologist researcher wished to gain an insider perspective to the work of rehabilitation teams, he or she might work as a clinician within the facility for several hours a day and assume a visible role as researcher for the rest of each day.

In the observer-as-participant model, the researcher does not assume membership roles within the community. Rather, the researcher is available for relatively brief periods during which interviews and observations take place. Despite the relatively brief contact, the researcher recognizes that the very process of implementing the study changes the environment. The concept of the participant-observer, discussed earlier in the chapter, is generally broad enough to include both the observer-as-participant and participant-as-observer levels along this continuum.

In the complete observer model, the researcher assumes the role of the "objective observer" who does not change the situation being observed. Qualitative researchers generally believe that this end of the continuum is not possible to achieve, because the mere presence of the investigator changes the dynamics of the situation.

The kinds of observations that one makes are dependent on the purpose of the research. In general, observations relate to the nonverbal behaviors of individual informants, interpersonal exchanges among informants, and the physical setting associated with the problem. In the study of the evolution of rehabilitation teams, the researcher might note posture, hand gestures, and the tone of voice of individual informants; might note that Informants A, E, and G not only share similar views of the situation but also tend to sit together at team meetings; and might observe that an old schedule of team meetings is posted on one ward with two scrawled notes in different handwriting reading "the good old days" and "the bad old days." Some of these observations may confirm information gained in the interviews and other observations may require follow-up in interviews. For example, a researcher might ask the following: "I notice that an old schedule of team meetings, with graffiti added, is still posted on the ward—what are your views on the impact of fewer routine team meetings?"

There are several ethical issues involved with observation in qualitative research. When one interviews informants, there is a formal opportunity to discuss the study and gain the informed consent of the informant. Observation, however, may result in the inclusion of information about the behavior of members of the community who did not specifically agree to participate in the research. Even if observation occurs in public places, people who are observed may feel that their privacy has been violated. If descriptions of observations are sufficiently detailed, readers of the research results may be able to identify the participants, even if an attempt has been made to disguise the identity of the setting or of the particular informants. As discussed earlier, researchers who assume increasingly legitimate membership roles within the communities they study will likely interact with many people who are unaware of their research role—even if key members of the community have given informed consent to the project.

ARTIFACTS

Artifacts are sometimes known as the "material traces" associated with the research, or as the "material culture" of the setting.[31] Artifacts include any physical evidence that contributes to the understanding of the problem at hand. Some artifacts are readily available and observable to the researcher; others require that the researcher inquire about their existence or look in archives or public document depositories to locate them. Artifacts can be broadly divided into written documents, written records, objects, and the environment.

Although the terms "documents" and "records" are often used interchangeably, Hodder believes that it is useful to distinguish between them.[31] He defines *written documents* as unofficial or personal writings. For our hypothetical study of the evolving role of rehabilitation teams, one set of relevant documents might include informal correspondence on the job—perhaps a trail of electronic mail messages between members of a team or working papers of a reorganization committee. Personal writings might include a journal that a therapist keeps, or a letter to the team from a former coworker who moved out of state.

Records are then defined as official documents. In our hypothetical study, records that are relevant might include licenses of the practitioners involved, annual performance reviews, and transcribed notes documenting team meetings. Some records, such as birth, death, marriage, and professional licensure, are public and can be obtained by the researcher—or anyone else. Other records, including medical records, are private and require the cooperation and permission of those who have access to the private records.

Objects can send powerful qualitative messages. Think about the gift that might be given by coworkers to a team member moving to another job. A carefully wrapped memory book of photos and letters from coworkers says one thing; a gift basket with cheeses and jams says another; and an unwrapped gift that everyone recognizes as coming from the facility gift shop says another! Clearly, the researcher would not conclude that the relationship between team members was close, distant, or dysfunctional based on the gift alone—but the gift would be a part of the pattern of evidence that would describe team relationships. Other common objects to be studied include photographs and personal effects in the offices or homes of informants.

The environment offers other artifactual evidence that may be important to the research. For example, in my own back yard, the pattern of beaten down grass provides clear evidence of the movement patterns of the dogs during the day and the pattern of brown foliage on the lower branches of isolated shrubs indicates their status as "watering" points! In a more relevant example, the retention of memos on the bulletin board, described earlier as an observation, might also be considered an artifact. Whether one considers them to be artifacts or observations, they can provide evidence that supplements the data gathered directly from informants.

Artifacts, then, provide material evidence that contributes to the breadth and depth of information collected by the qualitative researcher. Unlike archaeologists or criminal forensic investigators, qualitative researchers rarely base their conclusions on the analysis of artifacts alone. Rather, they use artifacts to supplement the data they collect through interview and observation.

Data Analysis

Data analysis in qualitative research is a process that differs greatly from data analysis in quantitative research. Whereas quantitative researchers typically describe their conclusions in statistical, probabilistic terms, qualitative researchers typically describe their conclusions in interpretive narratives that provide "thick description" of the phenomenon being studied. Generating this narrative rests on three general steps in the data analysis process—data management, generating meaning, and verification.

DATA MANAGEMENT

Data management relates to the collection, storage, and retrieval of information collected within the study. One of the consequences of seeking depth and breadth of information from multiple sources is that the amount of data becomes voluminous. A 30-minute interview with one informant might yield 20 pages of verbatim transcript based on an audiotape of the interview, 12 marginal notes on the transcript to remind the researcher of things to follow up on with future informants, and two pages of handwritten observations. If one does three interviews with each of 10 informants, this could easily result in more than 600 pages of data! Clearly, the qualitative researcher needs to develop a system for organizing and storing the information collected throughout the study.

One of the keys to the organization of data is the identification of the source of the data. Researchers come up with an identification code that enables them to determine where a piece of data came from originally. For example, a code of JP/I/02/07 might refer to the seventh page of the transcript of the second interview conducted with an informant with the code initials JP. A code of MM/R/12/02 might refer to the second page of the twelfth record that was authored by an informant with the code initials MM.

A second key to the organization and reduction of data is a code-and-retrieve system. The coding system is the means by which the researcher labels the themes that emerge as the data are amassed. Box 13–1 shows a coded portion of Stikeleather's study of injured workers' perceptions of the workers' compensation process.[32] The nine text fragments included in Box 13–1 are only a small proportion of the hundreds of fragments that were coded for this participant. Although this code-and-retrieve process is, in part, a data management project, deciding how to code the data becomes a highly analytical process. This process involves several levels of coding as basic concepts are consolidated into larger groupings of ideas. Thus, the process of managing and analyzing the data generally occurs simultaneously.

From a technical standpoint, qualitative researchers used to (and some still do) generate hundreds, sometimes thousands, of index cards in the course of a study. Each card would include a coded snippet of interview, observation, or reflection, cross-referenced to the original source of the data. The researchers would sort and resort the cards, seeking to understand the relationships among the various themes that emerged. Today, many qualitative researchers use word processing or relational database programs with search and sort properties to manage this process. In addition, several commercial software products have been designed to help qualitative researchers with the code-and-retrieve process, as well as the process of identifying relationships among concepts.[25(p316)]

GENERATING MEANING

After the data are coded, the researcher's job is to generate meaning from the data by noting themes, patterns, and clusters within the data, as well as identifying relationships among the themes and clusters. This is a reflective process that requires that the researcher "try on" ideas based on a portion of the data, test them against other portions of the data, and modify them as needed. In Stikeleather's study of the workers' compensation process, she began to group codes together under larger themes.[32] For example, the codes "health over work," "report

BOX 13-1

Excerpt of Coded Data

Jill Stikeleather, a physical therapist interested in work-related injury, conducted an exploratory qualitative study of injured workers' perspectives of the workers' compensation process.[32] Stikeleather used HyperRESEARCH, a coding and theory building program,[25(p316)] to assist in managing the coding process. The excerpt reported here has been sorted by codes and is not the continuous narrative of the interview. Each piece of text is linked to this particular interview by the letter-and-number identifier generated by the researcher, by the conceptual code words she assigned to the text, and by whether the statements are by the participant (P) or the interviewer (I).

DMV00339, financial security
P: Be able to stay around to retire. That is my biggest concern. You know, I look at it this way...I've worked too long at this job not to get nothing out of it.

DMV00339, health over work
P: I'm going back with a whole different attitude. I am taking a lunch hour every day. I am taking one hour. I am not running any longer, because all that does is get you hurt. I'm gonna do the job by the book.

DMV00339, learned to protect against injury
P: I've learned an awful lot being in therapy. How to keep yourself from getting hurt, you know. And I'm learning finally after all these years to slow down and think about what I'm doing before I try to do it.

DMV00339, learned to protect against injury
P: Well, I'm getting so that any injury on the job, I report, regardless of how small it is. Because now I know it can escalate into something worse.
I: So you sort of learned your lesson with the knee?
P: Yes. And the best thing I ever did was report my shoulder the day it happened, too.

DMV00339, learned to protect against injury
P: So you know, if you do it the wrong way, and that's why when I'm out on the job, or even at home, but I don't lift heavy things at home, if I can get out of it.

DMV00339, legitimacy questioned
P: I mean, I was shocked, because any doctor that the clinic has ever referred me to has either told me that "my backache was due to my period," "my ankle was all right even though I didn't look at the x-rays," or "you have arthritis." You know, it was like, "Go on, out of here, goodbye."

DMV00339, legitimacy questioned
P: The first time they put it in a cast for 6 weeks. Then the second time, "Well, there's nothing wrong with you, go back to work." That's basically what it was.

DMV00339, legitimacy questioned
P: But on like ankle and sometimes back, they tend to talk among themselves and say "Oh, she's faking." But now they've got a younger girl to pick on, so...and she is faking half the time!

DMV00339, pushing self/no choice
P: And it's like, I retire in 3.5 years, you know, and it's like I'm just going to have to grin and bear it. I can't quit my job.

injury quickly," "learned to protect against injury," and "educate" were all grouped into an "educate/protect self" theme. Other codes were grouped to generate the themes of "continued health problems," "physician caring," "work environment," and so forth. Finally, the relationships among the various themes were examined. For each of the participants in her qualitative study, Stikeleather generated a diagram showing the relationships among the themes for that participant. The diagram and a narrative story line expounding on the meaning of each theme and the relationship among the themes constituted the "within-case" portion of her study. In addition, when there is more than one case, researchers typically do a "cross-case" comparison to search for similarities and differences among the cases. Stikeleather, for example, noted that one of her participants found the workers' compensation system to be more supportive than the other participants and explored reasons why the one worker's experience was so different from the rest.

Generating meaning from qualitative data, then, involves an interpretive process in which data are reduced into small components (coding), reorganized into larger components (themes), and then displayed in ways that illustrate the relationships among components. This process is an iterative one, meaning that the researcher goes back and forth among the steps several times, making modifications along the way until the final analysis of relationships among themes fits with the data. Graham's description of data analysis in her study of conceptual learning processes of physical therapist students illustrates these iterative steps:

> As I transcribed the first set of interviews, I made notes about potential categories and trends. After the transcriptions were complete, I read each transcribed interview several times. I then coded the data to identify emerging categories and trends. The second set of interviews focused on the trends that emerged from the first set of interviews. The process continued through the final set of interviews. The previously collected data were compared with the newly collected data to identify emerging or changing trends. In this way, existing trends were discarded as new trends developed.[22(pp857-858)]

This sequence of steps is illustrated nicely in a diagram of the determinants of adherence to anterior cruciate ligament rehabilitation, from the research of Pizzari and colleagues.[27] Reproduced here as Figure 13–1, the ovals represent the codes, the boxes represent the themes, and the placement of arrows connecting the many codes to the three themes that feed into the core concept of adherence indicate the relationships between concepts. Several texts provide detailed guidance on the process of generating meaning from qualitative data.[23,25,33]

VERIFICATION

A final step in data analysis is the process of verifying the conclusions that have been drawn.[25] Without some verification process, qualitative research results remain open to the criticism that the researcher found what he or she was hoping to find. One form of verification is the triangulation of results. This is done by comparing multiple sources of information to determine whether they all point to similar conclusions.

A second form of verification is the use of multiple researchers to code data independently. Typically, two or more researchers independently code a small amount of data at the beginning of the study, compare their results, discuss discrepancies, and code another small set of data until they are satisfied that they have a common understanding of what the codes mean. If they then divide the data so that each researcher codes just a portion of the data, they may complete periodic reliability checks to ensure that they remain consistent throughout the course of the study.

A third form of verification is called *member checking*. In this process, informants review the interpretive "story" that the researcher has generated and have the opportunity to correct technical errors or take issue with ways in which the researcher has interpreted their situation. The researcher uses this information to revise the story, or at least to indicate points of departure

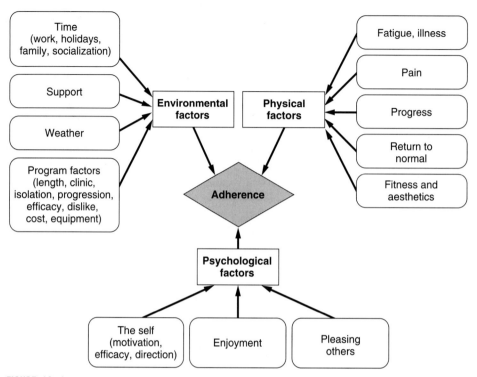

FIGURE 13–1. Flowchart representing factors influencing adherence to anterior cruciate ligament rehabilitation. The ovals correspond to codes, the boxes to themes, and the arrangement of arrows to the relationship among codes, themes, and the core concept of adherence.
From Pizzari T, McBurney H, Taylor NF, Feller JA. Adherence to anterior cruciate ligament rehabilitation: a qualitative analysis. *J Sport Rehabil.* 2002;11:90-102.

between his or her views and the views of the informants.

A fourth way of verifying the data analysis process is to have an outside researcher audit the analysis. Through this process, the outsider does a detailed "walk through" of the data analysis to determine whether the steps the researcher took and the conclusions that were drawn at each step make logical sense and appear to fit the data. Comments from the auditor are carefully considered and, as is the case with member checks, used to either revise the results or indicate points of departure between the researcher and the auditor.

A final way of enhancing the quality of qualitative research is to present reflexive accounts of ways in which the subjectivity of the researcher

had an impact on all phases of the study, from the conceptualization of the research problem to the analysis of data. In a reflexive account researchers reflect on the ways in which they affected and were affected by the qualitative research process. In a recent article, Primeau both describes reflexive analysis and presents a reflexive account of her role in a qualitative study of work and play in families.[34]

The various pieces of qualitative research that have been cited throughout this chapter illustrate, in the aggregate, all of the first four classes of verification techniques. Graham,[22] Pitney and associates,[15] and Jensen and colleagues[8] used multiple sources of data to triangulate results. Pizzari and colleagues[27] and

Dudgeon and associates[16] used two researchers to independently code data. Graham,[22] Pitney and colleagues,[15] Dudgeon and associates,[16] and Taylor and colleagues[6] used member checks to solicit feedback from their participants. Finally, Graham[22] and Pitney and associates[15] asked colleagues to audit their data analysis process. By implementing these verification steps, qualitative researchers help to establish the credibility of qualitative findings by subjecting themselves to external review and demonstrating to skeptics that "qualitative" is not synonymous with "arbitrary."

For final thoughts on data analysis in qualitative research, the words of Dickie, an occupational therapist and anthropologist, say it well:

> Qualitative research data analysis should not be easy. Ultimately it takes an enormous amount of intellectual "sweat" by the humans who are trying to make sense out of a situation, a setting, or a culture they thought was interesting enough to study…. Different research traditions and methodologies require different sorts of data analysis activities and call them by different names even when they are essentially the same…. Coding of some sort lays the foundation for most analytical processes, … but the nature of the coding process is specific to the researcher(s). The development and explication of the categories that are defined through reading and coding the data can become the "secret world" of the researcher, where magic does indeed take place but is never shared. But it shouldn't be that way. We need to learn what the labels and the jargon mean, then throw out the terms and describe what we do. We need to tell the research story, including the challenges of data analysis and how we resolved them, to support our interpretations. Researchers must be present in the stories they tell.[35(pp50-51)]

■ SUMMARY

Qualitative research includes a broad group of designs that generally follow five assumptions: that reality is constructed by participants, that researchers and subjects are interdependent, that research results are time and context dependent, that differentiating between causes and effects is not generally possible, and that research is a value-laden process. Although many different terms are used to describe qualitative design strategies, major approaches include case studies, ethnography, phenomenology, and grounded theory. Sampling in qualitative research generally includes convenience sampling, often selecting informants purposively through snowball sampling procedures. Common data collection methods include interviews, observation, and collection and review of artifacts. The data analysis process includes methods for managing large volumes of data from different sources; ways of generating meaning from codes, themes, and relationships among themes; and techniques to verify the conclusions.

REFERENCES

1. Denzin NK, Lincoln YS. Preface. In: Denzin NK, Lincoln YS, eds. *Handbook of Qualitative Research.* 2nd eds. Thousand Oaks, Calif: Sage Publications; 2000.
2. Stake RE. Case studies. In: Denzin NK, Lincoln YS, eds. *Handbook of Qualitative Research.* 2nd ed. Thousand Oaks, Calif: Sage Publications; 2000.
3. Stake RE. *The Art of Case Study Research.* Thousand Oaks, Calif: Sage Publications; 1995.
4. Yin RK. *Applications of Case Study Research.* 2nd ed. Thousand Oaks, Calif: Sage Publications; 2002.
5. Neville-Jan A. Encounters in a world of pain: an autoethnography. *Am J Occup Ther.* 2003;57:88-98.
6. Taylor LPS, McGruder JE. The meaning of sea kayaking for persons with spinal cord injuries. *Am J Occup Ther.* 1996;50:39-46.
7. Sabari JS, Meisler J, Silver E. Reflections upon rehabilitation by members of a community based stroke club. *Disabil Rehabil.* 2000;22:330-336.
8. Jensen GM, Shepard KF, Gwyer J, Hack LM. Attribute dimensions that distinguish master and novice physical therapy clinicians in orthopedic settings. *Phys Ther.* 1992;72:711-722.
9. Spradley JP. *The Ethnographic Interview.* Fort Worth, Tex: Holt, Rinehart & Winston; 1979.
10. Lawlor MC. Gazing anew: the shift from a clinical gaze to an ethnographic lens. *Am J Occup Ther.* 2003;57:29-39.
11. Shidler S. A systemic perspective of life-prolonging treatment decision making. *Qual Health Res.* 1998;8:254-269.
12. Camp MM. The use of service dogs as an adaptive strategy: a qualitative study. *Am J Occup Ther.* 2001;55:509-517.
13. Gubrium JF, Holstein JA. Analyzing interpretive practice. In: Denzin NK, Lincoln YS, eds. *Handbook of Qualitative*

Research. 2nd ed. Thousand Oaks, Calif: Sage Publications; 2000.

14. Crichton-Smith I. Communicating in the real world: accounts from people who stammer. *J Fluency Disord.* 2002;27:333-351.

15. Pitney WA, Ilsey P, Rintala J. The professional socialization of Certified Athletic Trainers in the National Collegiate Athletic Associate Division I context. *J Athl Train.* 2002;37:63-70.

16. Dudgeon BJ, Gerrard BC, Jensen MP, Rhodes LA, Tyler EJ. Physical disability and the experience of chronic pain. *Arch Phys Med Rehabil.* 2002;83:229-235.

17. Glaser BG, Strauss AL. *The Discovery of Grounded Theory: Strategies for Qualitative Research*. Chicago, Ill: Aldine Publishing; 1967.

18. Charmaz K. Grounded theory: objectivist and constructivist methods. In: Denzin NK, Lincoln YS, eds. *Handbook of Qualitative Research*. 2nd ed. Thousand Oaks, Calif: Sage Publications; 2000.

19. Strauss A. *Qualitative Analysis for Social Scientists*. Cambridge, England: Cambridge University Press; 1987.

20. Vaughan D. Theory elaboration: the heuristics of case analysis. In: Becker H, Ragin C, eds. *What is a Case?* Cambridge, England: Cambridge University Press; 1992.

21. Dubouloz C-J, Egan M, Vallerand J, von Zweck C. Occupational therapists' perceptions of evidence-based practice. *Am J Occup Ther.* 1999;53:445-453.

22. Graham CL. Conceptual learning processes in physical therapy students. *Phys Ther.* 1996;76:856-865.

23. Denzin NK, Lincoln YS, eds. *Handbook of Qualitative Research*. 2nd ed. Thousand Oaks, Calif: Sage Publications; 2000.

24. Morse JM, Field PA. *Qualitative Research Methods for Health Professionals*. 2nd ed. Thousand Oaks, Calif: Sage Publications; 1995.

25. Miles MB, Huberman AM. *Qualitative Data Analysis: An Expanded Sourcebook*. 2nd ed. Thousand Oaks, Calif: Sage Publications; 1994.

26. Fontana A, Frey JH. The interview: from structured questions to negotiated text. In: Denzin NK, Lincoln YS, eds. *Handbook of Qualitative Research*. 2nd ed. Thousand Oaks, Calif: Sage Publications; 2000.

27. Pizzari T, McBurney H, Taylor NF, Feller JA. Adherence to anterior cruciate ligament rehabilitation: a qualitative analysis. *J Sport Rehabil.* 2002;11:90-102.

28. Angrosino MV, Mays de Pérez KA. Rethinking observation: from method to context. In: Denzin NK, Lincoln YS, eds. *Handbook of Qualitative Research*. 2nd ed. Thousand Oaks, Calif: Sage Publications; 2000.

29. Letts L. Occupational therapy and participatory research: partnership worth pursuing. *Am J Occup Ther.* 2003;57:77-87.

30. Eysenbach G, Till JE. Ethical issues in qualitative research on Internet communities. *BMJ.* 2001;323:1103-1105.

31. Hodder I. The interpretation of documents and material culture. In: Denzin NK, Lincoln YS, eds. *Handbook of Qualitative Research*. 2nd ed. Thousand Oaks, Calif: Sage Publications; 2000.

32. Stikeleather S. *Injured Workers' Perspective on Claiming Compensation for Work-Related Injuries. PhD dissertation*. West Lafayette, Ind: Purdue University; 1998.

33. Coffey A, Atkinson P. *Making Sense of Qualitative Data: Complementary Research Strategies*. Thousand Oaks, Calif: Sage Publications; 1996.

34. Primeau LA. Reflections on self in qualitative research: stories of family. *Am J Occup Ther.* 2003;57:9-16.

35. Dickie VA. Data analysis in qualitative research: a plea for sharing the magic and the effort. *MJ Occup Ther.* 2003;57:49-56.

Epidemiology

Epidemiology has been defined as the "study of the distribution and determinants of states of health and illness in human populations."[1(p4)] This definition articulates a descriptive role for epidemiological research (studying distributions of health and illness), as well as an analytical role (studying determinants of health and illness). There is an implied element of diagnosis and screening in this definition, in that both are necessary for distinguishing between those who are healthy and those who are ill. The other critical component of this definition is the emphasis on populations—epidemiological research tends to focus on large groups of people. As such, it has important applications in public and community health. This public health function is illustrated in Box 14–1, which relates a classic story of an early epidemiological project that helped establish the transmission of cholera via contaminated water.

With its emphasis on the study of large groups, epidemiological research tends to focus on describing the characteristics of existing groups of people or analyzing the relationships among various health and demographic factors as they unfold within certain subgroups or across time. Both of these foci are nonexperimental in nature because they document existing health and illness states rather than attempting to change these states by introducing a controlled treatment. Despite this predominantly nonexperimental focus, some epidemiological research may be experimental in nature and follows the principles outlined in Chapter 9.

This chapter is organized around three major sections. The first section examines the use of

---

BOX 14–1

Dumping in and Pumping from the Thames: An Epidemiological Study of Cholera in Nineteenth-Century London

Routine collection of population data allowed British physician John Snow to investigate the epidemic of cholera that took place from 1848 to 1854. He noticed that deaths from cholera were particularly high in those areas of London that were supplied by two water companies, the Lambeth Company and the Southwark and Vauxhall Company. The two companies served about two thirds of London's residents, and their water mains were often interwoven in such a manner that houses on the same street or even next door to each other were receiving water from different sources. Both companies obtained water from an area of the Thames River heavily polluted with sewage. However, at some time between 1849 and 1854, the Lambeth Company changed its source of water to a part of the Thames River that was less contaminated. The rates of cholera declined in those areas that were supplied by the Lambeth Company, but rates of cholera remained the same in those areas supplied by the Southwark and Vauxhall Company. Snow recognized the opportunity to test his hypothesis that contaminated water was related to cholera by making use of the natural experiment that existed. He actually walked house to house in the area served by the two water companies and was able to determine the source of water for every dwelling. He noted that no experiment could have been devised that would test the relationship between cholera and the water supply more thoroughly. More than 300,000 people of each sex and every age, occupation, and socioeconomic group were divided into two groups without their choice and, often, without their knowledge. One group received water contaminated with the sewage of London, and the other group did not. The results in 1853-1854 were dramatic:

Water Company	Number of Houses	Deaths from Cholera	Deaths per 10,000 Houses
Southwark and Vauxhall	40,046	1263	315
Lambeth	26,107	98	37
Rest of London	256,423	1422	59

However, Snow also was aware that many other factors could account for the differences in cholera rates, and he investigated variations in the data as possible clues to further understanding of the epidemic. Snow's achievements were remarkable for the times. As one of the first epidemiologists, he outlined the frequency and distribution of cholera and found evidence of a cause or determinant of the outbreak. Snow logically organized data, and recognized and analyzed a natural experiment, and he did so before the era of bacteriology.

Excerpted from Harkness GA. *Epidemiology in Nursing Practice.* St Louis, Mo: Mosby–Year Book; 1995:6-9. Used with permission. The data within the excerpt are originally from Snow J. *On the Mode of Communication of Cholera.* 2nd ed. London: Churchill; 1855.

---

ratios, proportions, and rates to describe various health and illness phenomena. The second section presents a variety of concepts that are important to the understanding of screening and diagnostic processes. The third section presents nonexperimental epidemiological designs that compare health and illness in different naturally occurring groups.

■ RATIOS, PROPORTIONS, AND RATES

Researchers and practitioners are often interested in documenting "how many" cases of particular diseases or injuries occur in different groups, regions, or time frames. However, raw frequency counts of cases are rarely valuable because they

TABLE 14-1	Hypothetical Data on Ankle Sprains, University A, 2004-2005
Number at risk during the year	12,237
Athletes	1216
Nonathletes	11021
Number surveyed at beginning of year	9857
Number of ankle sprains at beginning of year	61
Total new ankle sprains during year	436
Distribution by type of sprains	
Inversion sprains	401
Eversion sprains	35
Distribution by activity level of individual	
Athletes	170
Nonathletes	266

are not directly comparable across groups of different sizes or across varied time frames. In Box 14–1, for example, the number of deaths from cholera in households supplied by the different water companies was not meaningful until it was expressed as the number of deaths per 10,000 houses supplied by each company. Changing frequencies into meaningful epidemiological data depends on the calculation of various ratios, proportions, and rates. The discussion of these concepts is accompanied by a hypothetical example related to ankle sprains on a college campus (Table 14–1).

Ratios

A *ratio* expresses the relationship between two numbers by dividing the numerator by the denominator. The numerator of a ratio is not necessarily a subset of the denominator. The simple formula for a ratio is therefore:

$$\text{Ratio} = a/b \qquad \text{(Formula 14–1)}$$

An example is the ratio of inversion to eversion ankle sprains. The hypothetical data shown

in Table 14–1 show that, of a total of 436 new ankle sprains documented during the 2004-2005 academic year, 401 were inversion sprains (*a* in Formula 14–1) and 35 were eversion sprains (*b* in Formula 14–1). This divides out to a ratio of 11.46 to 1 (401 ÷ 35 = 11.46). The notation for ratios is that a colon (:) is used for the "to" so that the ratio of inversion to eversion ankle sprains would be expressed as 11.46:1. The interpretation of this ratio is that there were almost 11½ inversion ankle sprains for every eversion ankle sprain reported on the campus of University A during the 2004-2005 academic year.

Proportions

A *proportion* is a fraction in which the numerator is a subset of the denominator. The formula for a proportion is:

$$\text{Proportion} = a/a + b \qquad \text{(Formula 14–2)}$$

If we wish to know what proportion of ankle sprains are inversion sprains, then we must divide the number of inversion sprains (*a*) by the total number of ankle sprains, or the sum of the inversion sprains (*a*) and the eversion sprains (*b*). Thus, the proportion of inversion sprains is $401/(401 + 35) = .9197$. Proportions are often converted to percentages by multiplying by 100. Thus, we find that 91.97% of ankle sprains at University A are inversion sprains. Sometimes very small proportions are multiplied by constants larger than 100 in order to express them as whole numbers rather than decimals.

Rates

A *rate* is a proportion expressed over a particular unit of time. In epidemiology, rates are used to express the change in a health variable in the population at risk over a period of time. Because rates often describe fairly rare events in large populations, the number that is calculated is often a decimal beginning with one or more zeros.

At University A, the rates of new inversion and eversion ankle sprains in a year are as follows:

Rate of new inversion sprains per year =
$$401/12{,}237 = .03277$$

Rate of new eversion sprains per year =
$$35/12{,}237 = .00286$$

Because it is difficult to conceptualize these small decimal values, rates are multiplied by a constant to obtain values that are whole numbers. To use the same constant to express both inversion and eversion ankle sprain rates as whole numbers, multiply each rate by 1000, as follows:

Rate of new inversion sprains = [401/12,237]
$$\times\ 1000 = 32.77 \text{ per 1000 people per year}$$

Rate of new eversion sprains = [35/12,237]
$$\times\ 1000 = 2.86 \text{ per 1000 people per year}$$

When rates are multiplied by a constant, it is important to include the constant when listing the rate so that readers know whether the rate is, for example, for 1000 people or 1 million people.

Epidemiologists use ratios, percentages, and rates to express many important concepts. Two of the most common are *prevalence* and *incidence*. Each of these can be expressed in crude, specific, and adjusted forms.

Prevalence

Prevalence expresses the proportion of a population that exhibits a certain condition at a given point in time.

Prevalence = Existing cases/Population
examined at a given point in time
(Formula 14–3)

Because the proportion is often small, it is usually multiplied by an appropriate constant. Because prevalence is a value at a given time, rather than a value calculated over a given period of time, it is a proportion rather than a rate.

To determine prevalence, one must consider which individuals to count in the numerator and denominator of Formula 14–3.

The numerator contains all of the cases of the desired condition at the time of measurement. Consider the example of multiple sclerosis. Because the symptoms of multiple sclerosis come and go and may resemble other disorders, at any one point in time, there are many individuals who have the disease but have not been diagnosed. Once diagnosed, however, the condition is presumed to exist for a lifetime. Therefore, the difficulty in defining cases of multiple sclerosis is in knowing when the disease begins, not when it ends.

Contrast this with the case of acute conditions that have more distinct beginnings, but less clear endpoints. An ankle sprain might be defined as posttraumatic pain, swelling, bruising, or instability that results in an inability to participate fully in desired activities. With this definition, one would count all of the following as cases: an individual who sprained her ankle 2 days ago and is still walking gingerly, an intercollegiate athlete who sprained his ankle 3 weeks ago and is now practicing with the team but is not yet back on the game roster, and a recreational athlete who sprained her ankle 3 years ago and gave up racquetball because of chronic instability. One would not count an individual who "twisted" his ankle but did not experience swelling, bruising, or functional difficulties, nor would one count an individual who sustained a sprain in the past but has no residual swelling or instability and has returned to full function.

The denominator contains all of the people "examined" to determine whether they have the condition. Sometimes this number represents an actual examination of the individuals in the population; other times the number is determined from responses to a survey or numbers of cases within a large health care system or health insurer database.

To determine the prevalence of ankle sprains at University A, researchers need to pick a reporting date and a mechanism to obtain the information. Knowing that all members of the community need to renew parking permits during the first week of September, the researchers might set up shop at the parking permit window and administer a brief survey to all members of the campus who are willing to participate. If they administered 9857 questionnaires and identified 61 cases of ankle sprain, then prevalence would be calculated as follows:

$$\text{Prevalence of ankle sprains at the beginning of the academic year} = [61/9857] \times 1000 = 6.19$$

When reporting the prevalence it is important to include the constant and the point in time that the data were collected. In a report about ankle sprains at University A, the researchers might, after presenting their definition of what constituted an ankle sprain, write that "the prevalence of ankle sprains in the academic community at the beginning of the academic year was 6.19 sprains per 1000 people."

The "point in time" used to define prevalence can vary, yielding "point prevalence" and "period prevalence." When determining the point prevalence, the point in time is literally the time of measurement, for example, if a researcher asks study participants "Do you currently have low back pain?" When determining period prevalence, the point in time is a longer time frame defined by the researcher. For example, the 1-year period prevalence could be calculated if a researcher asks study participants "Have you had low back pain any time in the past 12 months?"

Because of the complexities in defining the numerator and denominator to determine prevalence, it is not always feasible to provide definitive estimates of prevalence for any number of common conditions seen by rehabilitation professionals. For example, Loney and Stratford reviewed the literature and found 13 different studies on the prevalence of low back pain in adults.[2] The point prevalence estimates in the studies they reviewed ranged from 4.4% to 33.0% and the 1-year prevalence rates were from 3.9% to 63.0%.

Incidence

Incidence is the rate of new cases of a condition that develop during a specified period of time. The numerator represents the number of new cases and the denominator represents the number in the population at risk:

$$\text{Incidence} = \text{New cases during time period} / \text{Population at risk during time period}$$
(Formula 14–4)

As with other values, the incidence is often multiplied by a constant so that it can be expressed as a whole number rather than as a decimal.

To determine the incidence of ankle sprains at University A, researchers would need to set up a monitoring system to ensure good reporting of ankle sprains among members of the university community. In this example, the following (unrealistic) assumptions are made: (1) all members of the community will seek care for sprained ankles, (2) all will seek care at the campus health center or the athletic training center, and (3) all the professionals providing the care will use the same operational definition of ankle sprain and will report the number of new cases accurately. In the real world, determining incidence is complicated because people do not always seek medical care for new conditions, the care they receive occurs in many different places, and the providers they see define conditions differently and report them inconsistently. In our ideal world, we have already established the number of new cases of ankle sprain at University A to be 436 during the 2004-2005 academic year (see Table 14–1). Thus, 436 is the numerator of the incidence formula.

The denominator for incidence is the population at risk during the time period being measured. Determining this number is harder than it seems. First, one must determine the number in the "population." However, the number of individuals in a population usually varies over the course of the time period being studied. One common way to handle this is to use the number in the population at the midpoint of the period of study. For this ankle sprain example, the 2004-2005 academic year could be defined as September 1, 2004, to August 31, 2005, with a midpoint at March 1, 2005. This is probably a good date in the academic calendar because it avoids the peak enrollment time of early September as well as the valley of summer enrollments. Incidence studies frequently use the calendar year as the reporting period with July 1 as the midpoint for determining the denominator.

The second difficulty in determining the denominator for an incidence calculation is in determining who is "at risk." If some conditions affect only one sex, or are virtually unheard of in certain age groups, then the population at risk should include only those of the appropriate sex or age. If having the condition means that one is no longer at risk of developing a new case of the disease (e.g., multiple sclerosis), then individuals with the condition at the start of the reporting period should be excluded from the denominator. In contrast, if the condition of interest can occur multiple times in the same individuals, then even those with the condition at the start of the reporting period remain at risk for new events. In the example of ankle sprains, the 61 people with ankle sprains during the first week of September 2004 remain at risk for a new ankle sprain during the academic year and are not excluded from the denominator. Therefore, the incidence of ankle sprains at University A would be calculated as follows:

$$\text{Incidence of ankle sprains during 2004-2005} = [436/12,237] \times 1000 = 35.63$$

Note that the constant of 1000 is used, even though we could have multiplied by a constant of 100 to get a value that was a whole number. Because incidence and prevalence are often reported together, it is helpful to express them in terms of the same multiple of the population. Because the constant of 1000 was used to express the prevalence, it was also used to express the incidence. When reporting incidence rates, it is important to include the time

period studied and the population multiplier. In a report about ankle sprains at University A, researchers would indicate that the "incidence of ankle sprains during the 2004-2005 academic year was 35.63 per 1000 people in the academic community."

Like prevalence, incidence estimates for a particular condition can vary greatly based on differences in how the numerator and denominator are defined. For example, Krotenberg and colleagues reviewed the literature on the incidence of dislocation in the acute care setting following total hip replacement surgery and found estimates from 0% to almost 7%, with an incidence across studies of 1.27%.[3] They then conducted their own study of the incidence of dislocation in the rehabilitation setting following total hip arthroplasty, finding an incidence of 2.15%.

Relationship Between Incidence and Prevalence

The relationship between incidence and prevalence depends on the nature of the condition being examined. For diseases or injuries that are of short duration (either rapidly resolving or quickly fatal), the incidence is often greater than the prevalence. Consider the common cold—during the course of a year, most people get a new cold at some point (high incidence), but far fewer have colds at the same time (lower prevalence). This general statement is complicated by the seasonal nature of colds—it sometimes seems like everyone has them at once. The hypothetical ankle sprain example in this chapter exhibits this relationship between incidence and prevalence: the incidence is high (35.63 per 1000 people during the 2004-2005 academic year) compared with the prevalence (6.19 sprains per 1000 people at the beginning of September 2004).

For conditions that are of long duration, incidence is often lower than prevalence. Consider Parkinson's disease. Reports of crude prevalence range from approximately 65 to 187 cases per

100,000 population, depending on geographical region.[4] The annual incidence is much lower, ranging from approximately 4 to 20 new cases per 100,000 population across the same regions.[4] Similar patterns can be expected with conditions such as multiple sclerosis, spinal cord injury, cerebral palsy, and diabetes.

Even though "incidence" and "prevalence" have the specific meanings outlined here, sometimes the terms are used inaccurately as general measures of frequency. The following mnemonic device, based on the first three letters of each word, helps readers remember which is which:

Incidence = **N**ew **C**ases (**INC**idence)

PRevalence = **E**xisting cases (**PRE**valence)

Crude, Specific, and Adjusted Rates

Although rates are sometimes calculated for purely descriptive purposes, researchers often wish to compare the rates with one another. They may wish to compare their sample with established population norms, they may wish to determine whether the rate within their population has changed over time, or they may wish to see whether their rates are approaching some desirable target rate. Making valid comparisons, however, depends on comparing the rates for similar populations. To generate the data appropriate for these "apple-to-apple" comparisons, researchers often modify their rates in several different ways.

Crude rates are rates calculated using the entire population at risk. Generating a crude rate is usually the starting point for the researcher's calculations. The incidence rate of 35.63 ankle sprains per 1000 people during the 2004-2005 academic year is a crude rate. In certain circumstances, crude rates are systematically modified to become specific and adjusted rates.

Specific rates are rates for specified subgroups of the population. In the ankle sprain example, we might wonder whether athletes and nonathletes had different rates of ankle sprains. To determine this, we would first need an operational definition of athlete (perhaps someone who participates in recreational or intercollegiate team sports or individual physical activities an average of two times per week). Next, we would need to determine the number of athletes and nonathletes for the denominators of our specific rates. Finally, we would need to know how many of our 436 new cases occurred in athletes versus nonathletes. Figure 14–1, which presents a 2 × 2 matrix containing this hypothetical information, shows that the specific incidence for athletes appears to be much higher (139.80 per 1000 athletes) than it is for the nonathletes (24.14 per 1000 nonathletes).

If we wished, we could get even more specific. Among athletes, we might generate sport-specific incidence rates to determine whether there is a higher incidence among basketball, volleyball, and soccer players than among

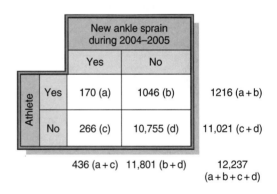

FIGURE 14–1. Crude and specific incidence rates of ankle sprain at University A during the 2004-2005 academic year.

Crude incidence rate: [(a + c)/(a + b + c + d)] × constant = [436/12,237] × 1000 = 35.63 per 1000 people

Specific incidence rate for athletes: [a/(a + b)] × constant = [170/1216] × 1000 = 139.80 per 1000 athletes

Specific incidence rate for nonathletes: [c/(c + d)] × constant = [266/11,021] × 1000 = 24.14 per 1000 nonathletes

swimmers, golfers, and baseball/softball players. We also might determine competition-specific rates to look at incidence in recreational versus intercollegiate athletes. In addition, we might suspect that there are age or gender differences in ankle sprain incidence and calculate age- and sex-specific rates as well.

Adjusted rates are used when one wishes to compare rates across populations with different proportions of various subgroups. Let's assume that the injury statistics for University B report that their ankle sprain incidence for the year was only 100.8 sprains per 1000 athletes. Initially concerned because University A's incidence for athletes seems so much higher, you realize that the rates must be adjusted before you can make a valid comparison. Table 14–2 shows the

specific, unadjusted rates for each university. A much higher proportion of athletes are soccer players at University A than at University B. Furthermore, soccer players at both universities have a high incidence of ankle sprains. To compare "apples to apples," you need to mathematically adjust the proportion of athletes in each sport at one university so that it matches the proportion at the other university, and then adjust the presumed number of injuries and the incidence rates in light of the new proportions. Table 14–3 shows how this is done, by adjusting the University A data to match the proportions at University B. For example, at University B, only 1.6% of the athletes are soccer players. If University A, with 1216 athletes overall, had only 1.6% soccer players, then they would have

TABLE 14–2 Hypothetical Sport-Specific Incidence Rates at Universities A and B

Category	University A			University B		
	No. of Sprains	*No. (%) in Group*	*Incidence of Sprains (per 1000)*	*No. of Sprains*	*No. (%) in Group*	*Incidence of Sprains (per 1000)*
Recreational	109	968 (79.6)	112.6	81	821 (84.5)	98.7
Intercollegiate						
Soccer	49	92 (7.6)	532.6	9	16 (1.6)	562.5
Baseball/Softball	8	74 (6.1)	108.1	5	68 (7.0)	73.5
Swimming	4	82 (6.7)	48.7	3	67 (6.9)	44.8
Total	170	1216 (100.0)	139.8	98	972 (100.0)	100.82

TABLE 14–3 Adjusted Hypothetical Sport-Specific Incidence Rates at University A

Category	University A			University A—Adjusted		
	No. of Sprains	*No. (%) in Group*	*Incidence of Sprains (per 1000)*	*No. of Sprains*	*No. (%) in Group*	*Incidence of Sprains (per 1000)*
Recreational	109	968 (79.6)	112.6	115.70	1027.52 (84.5)	112.6
Intercollegiate						
Soccer	49	92 (7.6)	532.6	10.36	19.46 (1.6)	532.6
Baseball/Softball	8	74 (6.1)	108.1	9.20	85.12 (7.0)	108.1
Swimming	4	82 (6.7)	48.7	4.09	83.90 (6.9)	48.7
Total	170	1216 (100.0)	139.8	139.35	1216 (100.0)	114.60

19 soccer players (1216 × .016 = 19.456). If these 19.46 players sustained ankle injuries at the same rate that the original 92 players did (532.6 per 1000 players), you would expect them to have sustained roughly 10.36 injuries during the year (19.46 × 0.5326 = 10.36). First, the University B subgroup proportions are used to adjust the proportions in the University A population. Then, the University A incidence rates are applied to the new proportions to calculate the adjusted injury numbers.

This adjustment is done for each subgroup within the population, as shown in Table 14–3. If University A had the same distribution of athletes as University B, then you would expect University A to have 139.35 ankle sprains among its 1216 athletes for an adjusted incidence of 114.60 sprains per 1000 athletes. This process shows that the adjusted incidence rates are more similar to University B (114.60 compared with 100.82) than the original unadjusted rates (139.80 compared with 100.82).

Relative Risk: Risk Ratios and Odds Ratios

Epidemiologists often wish to move beyond describing groups to compare the probability that different groups with different characteristics will be affected by disease or injury in some way. That is, they seek to determine the relative risk of disease or injury of two different groups. There are two important ways in which relative risk is calculated—using risk ratios and using odds ratios. The distinction between the two is important and warrants careful consideration of the examples that follow.

The risk ratio is calculated by creating a ratio of the incidence rate for one subgroup and the incidence rate for another subgroup. In the example of ankle sprain, athletes sustained ankle sprains at a rate of 139.8 per 1000 people and nonathletes sustained ankle sprains at a rate of 24.14 per 1000 people (see Figure 14–1). If we create a ratio out of these two numbers (139.8/ 24.14), we find that the athletes are 5.79 times as

likely to sustain ankle sprains as nonathletes. Earlier, a 2 × 2 matrix was used to organize the data. The formula for determining the risk ratio is often given with a standard form of this table in mind (Figure 14–2). The risk ratio is defined as:

$$\text{Risk ratio} = [a/(a + b)]/[c/(c + d)]$$

$$\text{(Formula 14–5)}$$

Note that this is calculated by "working" the table horizontally—determining the incidence of ankle sprains for the row that represents athletes and then determining the incidence for the row that represents nonathletes. We can compute relative risks this way because we have measured the entire population of interest, and the totals for each row [(a + b) and (c + d)] give us meaningful information about the number of athletes and nonathletes in the population.

Emery and Meeuwisse determined the relative risks of groin injuries in different subgroups of professional hockey players.[5] The researchers had access to the entire population of interest through the electronic injury surveillance system required by teams participating in the North American National Hockey League. They found that players who participated in fewer than 18 sport-specific training sessions in the off season were 3.38 times more likely to sustain a groin injury than those players who participated in 18 or more off-season, sport-specific training sessions.

Many epidemiological researchers, however, do not have access to an entire population of

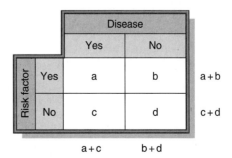

FIGURE 14–2. Standard table for determining relative risk.

interest. Instead of measuring the entire population of interest, the researcher identifies a number of individuals who have the condition or risk factor of interest. The researchers then seek out matched controls without the condition or risk factor in order to create a comparison group. Figure 14–3 shows two new sets of hypothetical data used to determine the relative risk of ankle sprains in athletes and nonathletes. In Figure 14–3, *A,* the researchers identified one control for each case; in Figure 14–3, *B,* they identified three controls for each case. In both parts of Figure 14–3, the numbers for those with ankle sprains remains constant. In addition, the distribution of athletes and nonathletes without ankle sprains remains the same even though the absolute numbers change from Part A to Part B. Watch what happens mathematically if we apply the risk ratio formula to these tables. Figure 14–3 shows that the risk ratio is different for the two parts of the figure. This is because the totals in the margin change as the number of control subjects changes. Because the totals in the margins reflect the sampling design and not the actual totals in the population, it is not valid to use the risk ratio in this situation.

When computing risk ratios is not valid, then a value known as the odds ratio is used to estimate relative risk. To understand the difference between these two ratios, the difference between proportions and odds must be clarified. To use a common example,[6(p91)] consider a baseball player who has one hit (and three misses) in four times at bat in a game. A hit is represented by *a* and a miss is represented by *b*. The formula for a proportion is a/(a + b), which in this case means that the proportion of hits is 1/4, or 0.25. The proportion divides the "part" by the "whole." In contrast, odds are determined by creating a ratio between hit and misses, or a/b. The odds divides one "part" by the other "part." In this baseball example, the odds of getting a hit is 1:3 or 0.333.

Returning to the ankle sprain example, the totals in the margins of the rows in Figure 14–3 are not meaningful because they do not represent the "whole" population of interest; instead

they reflect the sampling design of the researchers. When this is the case, researchers use an odds ratio, rather than a risk ratio based on proportions, to estimate relative risk among subgroups.

The odds ratio uses only the numbers found within the table (not those in the margin) and works the table "vertically." In Figure 14–3, *A,* the odds of a person with an ankle sprain being an athlete is 18/32, or 0.5625. The odds of a person without an ankle sprain being an athlete is 6/44, or 0.1364. The odds ratio is simply the ratio of these two odds. The conceptual formula for the odds ratio is given below, along with a common algebraic simplification:

$$\text{Odds ratio} = (a/c)/(b/d) = ad/bc$$

$$(\text{Formula } 14\text{–}6)$$

In contrast to the changing value of the risk ratio between Figures 14–3, *A,* and 14–3, *B,* the odds ratio remains the same whether the researcher selects one or three controls for each case.

Epidemiologists use measures such as incidence, prevalence, risk ratios, and odds ratios to describe the distribution of disease and injury within populations and population subgroups. Epidemiological studies frequently report these measures or variations on these measures. Readers who encounter a rate, proportion, or ratio with which they are unfamiliar should be able to apply the general principles in this section to gain a general understanding of the unfamiliar measure.

■ SCREENING AND DIAGNOSIS

A common function of epidemiological research is to evaluate the usefulness of various screening and diagnostic tests. Four key proportions are used to compare the usefulness of the test being evaluated to a criterion test that is considered the "gold standard." These four proportions are the sensitivity, specificity, positive predictive value, and negative predictive value. They are generally

A

	Ankle sprains September 1998		
	Yes	**No**	
Athlete **Yes**	18 (a)	6 (b)	24 (a+b)
Athlete **No**	32 (c)	44 (d)	76 (c+d)

50 (a+c)   50 (b+d)

B

	Ankle sprains September 1998		
	Yes	**No**	
Athlete **Yes**	18 (a)	18 (b)	36 (a+b)
Athlete **No**	32 (c)	132 (d)	164 (c+d)

50 (a+c)   150 (b+d)

FIGURE 14–3. Relative risk of sustaining an ankle sprain for athletes and nonathletes. The two parts of the figure demonstrate the problem of calculating risk ratios when the total population of interest has not been studied. Because the totals in the row margins reflect the sampling design rather than the proportion of injury in the population, the risk ratio changes from A to B. The odds ratio, which does not depend on the totals in the margins, remains the same.

A, Hypothetical study in which one control subject is identified for each case.

Proportion of athletes with ankle sprains = a/(a + b) = 18/24 = 0.75

Proportion of nonathletes with ankle sprains = c/(c + d) = 32/76 = 0.42

Risk ratio = [a/(a + b)]/[c/(c + d)] = 0.75/0.42 = 1.79

Odds of someone with an ankle sprain being an athlete = a/c = 18/32 = 0.5625

Odds of someone without an ankle sprain being an athlete = b/d = 6/44 = 0.1364

Odds ratio = (a/c)/(b/d) = 0.5625/0.1364 = 4.124

B, Hypothetical study in which three controls are identified for each case.

Proportion of athletes with ankle sprains = a/(a + b) = 18/36 = 0.500

Proportion of nonathletes with ankle sprains = c/(c + d) = 32/164 = 0.195

Risk ratio = [a/(a + b)]/[c/(c + d)] = 0.500/0.195 = 2.56

Odds of someone with an ankle sprain being an athlete = a/c = 18/32 = 0.5625

Odds of someone without an ankle sprain being an athlete = b/d = 18/132 = 0.1364

Odds ratio = (a/c)/(b/d) = 0.5625/0.1364 = 4.124

		Condition according to gold standard		
		Present	Absent	
Condition according to test being evaluated	Present	a	b	(a+b)
	Absent	c	d	(c+d)
		(a+c)	(b+d)	

FIGURE 14–4. Illustration of traditional epidemiological concepts.

Sensitivity = a/(a + c)

Specificity = d/(b + d)

Positive predictive value = a/(a + b)

Negative predictive value = d/(c + d)

represented by a standard 2 × 2 table, as shown in Figure 14–4.

Sensitivity and Specificity

Sensitivity and specificity compare the conclusions of the new test with the results on the criterion test. They are determined by "working" the 2 × 2 table vertically. The *sensitivity* of a test is the proportion or percentage of individuals with a particular diagnosis who are correctly identified as positive by the test. The *specificity* is the proportion or percentage of individuals without a particular diagnosis who are correctly identified as negative by the test.

Sensitivity = a/(a + c)   (Formula 14–7)

Specificity = d/(b + d)   (Formula 14–8)

Continuing with the ankle injury examples already presented, these two epidemiological concepts are illustrated in Figure 14–5, which uses data from Clark and associates' study of ankle joint effusion and occult ankle fractures.[7]

		Fracture found with computed tomography		
		Yes	No	
Ankle effusion found on plain radiograph	≥15 mm	10 (a)	2 (b)	12
	< 15 mm	2 (c)	12 (d)	14
		12	14	

FIGURE 14–5. Calculation of sensitivity, specificity, positive predictive value, and negative predictive value.
From data in Clark TWI, Janzen DL, Logan PM, Connell DG. Improving the detection of radiographically occult ankle fractures: positive predictive value of an ankle joint effusion. *Clin Radiol.* 1996;51:632-636.

Sensitivity = a/(a + c) = 10/12 = 0.833 = 83.3%

Specificity = d/(b + d) = 12/14 = 0.857 = 85.7%

Positive predictive value = a/(a + b) = 10/12 = 0.833 = 83.3%

Negative predictive value = d/(c + d) = 12/14 = 0.857 = 85.7%

In this example, the sensitivity and the positive predictive value are the same, and the specificity and negative predictive value are the same. This is because the number of false-positive results and the number of false-negative results are the same in this example. In most examples, this is not the case and all four of the proportions take different values.

A series of patients with severe ankle sprains, but without apparent fractures on plain radiographs, was studied with plain radiographs and computed tomography (CT). The gold standard for identifying ankle fractures was CT of the ankle. The new test involved measuring the extent of ankle joint effusion on the plain radiographs. The researchers found that an ankle effusion of 15 mm or more on plain radiography had a sensitivity of 83.3% for detecting occult ankle fractures. This means that 83.3% of patients with fractures also had an effusion of

15 mm or more. When testing patients without occult fractures, they found that an effusion of less than 15 mm had a specificity of 85.7%. This means that 85.7% of the patients without occult fractures had effusions of less than 15 mm.

When test results can take more than two values, as in this study, then the researchers need to determine the "cutoff" score for differentiating between positive and negative results. Figure 14–6

shows an approximate reconstruction of the results of the two tests for all 26 patients in the series. If the criterion for a positive result is set at 12 mm or more of effusion, then the sensitivity of the test would be 100%, because all 12 patients with fractures visualized by CT had an effusion of 12 mm or more. However, the specificity would be only 64.3%, because this permissive criterion would result in many false-positive results. If the criterion for a positive result is set at 18 mm or more of effusion, then the specificity of the test would be 100%, because all 14 patients without fractures had effusions of less than 18 mm. However, the sensitivity would be only 58.3% because this stringent criterion would result in many false-negative results. Test developers work to determine an intermediate cutoff score that results in a desirable balance between the sensitivity and specificity of the test.

	Computed tomography results	
	Fracture	No fracture
21		
19,19,19		
18,18,18		
		17,17
16,16		
15		
14		14,14
12		12
		11,11,11,11
		10
		9,9
		6
		5

Size of effusion (mm) (vertical axis label)

FIGURE 14–6. Illustration of how changing the cutoff score influences sensitivity and specificity. If the cutoff is between 11 and 12 mm, sensitivity is maximized. If the cutoff is between 17 and 18 mm, specificity is maximized.

Sensitivity if cutoff is set at 12 mm or more:
$(12/12) \times 100 = 100.0\%$

Specificity if cutoff is set at 12 mm or more:
$(9/14) \times 100 = 64.3\%$

Sensitivity if cutoff is set at 18 mm or more:
$(7/12) \times 100 = 58.3\%$

Specificity if cutoff is set at 18 mm or more:
$(14/14) \times 100 = 100.0\%$

Data from Clark TWI, Janzen DL, Logan PM, Connell DG. Improving the detection of radiographically occult ankle fractures: positive predictive value of an ankle joint effusion. *Clin Radiol.* 1996;51:632-636.

RECEIVER-OPERATOR CURVES

One way that this process is visualized is through development of a receiver-operator curve (ROC). Clark and colleagues created such a curve with their data, as shown in Figure 14–7.[7] The heavy line with the triangles for points represents a test

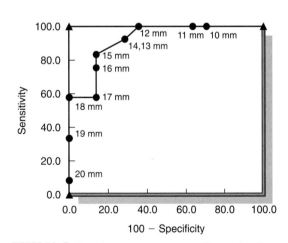

FIGURE 14–7. Receiver-operator curve illustrating how changing the cutoff score influences the sensitivity and specificity of a test. In general, the ideal cutoff score is the one closest to the upper left-hand corner of the graph.

with an ideal cutoff point—at 100% sensitivity and 100% specificity (the upper left-hand corner of the graph). In practice, tests generally deviate from this ideal, as is the case with the use of the extent of ankle effusion to predict occult ankle fractures (the circular points on the graph). These points demonstrate visually that cutoff scores of 20, 19, and 18 mm result in perfect specificity but low sensitivity; and the cutoff scores of 12, 11, and 10 mm result in perfect sensitivity but low specificity. The cutoff score of 15 mm results in the best balance between sensitivity and specificity—it is the point closest to the ideal point in the upper left-hand corner. When two points are approximately equidistant from this ideal point, then researchers consider the impact of false-positive results (needlessly worrying the healthy) or false-negative results (falsely reassuring the ill) in determining which cutoff score to select. If the disease being screened for is serious but treatable in early stages, then the researchers would probably choose the cutoff score with somewhat lower specificity and higher sensitivity so that the probability of false-negative results would be lower. If the disease being screened for is less serious and can be effectively treated even at later stages of the disease, then the researchers would probably choose a cutoff score with lower sensitivity and higher specificity so that the probability of false-positive results would be lower.

LIKELIHOOD RATIOS

The following is an important way that sensitivity and specificity are used in the calculation of likelihood ratios:

Likelihood ratio of a positive test =
  Sensitivity%/(100 − Specificity%)
  (Formula 14–9)

Likelihood ratio of a negative test =
  (100 − Sensitivity%)/Specificity%
  (Formula 14–10)

A likelihood ratio of a positive test of 1.0 does not help to rule in disease because the false-positive results (100 − specificity) are as likely as true positive results (sensitivity). The higher the likelihood ratio of a positive test, the more information the test gives for ruling in a disease or injury.

A likelihood ratio of a negative test of 1.0 does not help to rule out disease because the false-negative results (100 − sensitivity) are as likely as the true negative results (specificity). The lower the likelihood of a negative test, the more information the test gives for ruling out a disease or injury.[8(pp178-179)] Likelihood ratios are also a good way to determine the information provided by tests that have multiple levels of cutoff points.[6(p92)]

One important characteristic of sensitivity and specificity is that they are unaffected by the proportion of individuals with the disease or injury of interest. Because they are each calculated from one column of the 2 × 2 table, the number of individuals in the other column does not affect their value. Thus, ankle effusion measurement should yield similar sensitivity and specificity whether it is applied to a group with minor ankle sprains with few fractures or to a group with severe sprains and many fractures.

Predictive Value

Although sensitivity and specificity are useful concepts, they only tell half the story about diagnostic and screening tests. The other half of the story is told by the positive and negative predictive values. The *positive predictive value* is the percentage of individuals identified by the test as positive who actually have the diagnosis. The *negative predictive value* is the percentage of those identified by the test as negative who actually do not have the diagnosis. These values are found by "working" the table horizontally:

Positive predictive value = a/(a + b)
  (Formula 14–11)

Negative predictive value = d/(c + d)
  (Formula 14–12)

Because the table is worked horizontally, the predictive values vary greatly depending on the proportion of individuals with and without the disease or injury. This is illustrated in Figure 14–8, which maintains the sensitivity and specificity values of the original study. What is varied, though, is the proportion of total cases with and without an ankle fracture. In the original study, 46% of the cases had an ankle fracture identified through CT. In Figure 14–8, A, only 4% of the cases have an ankle fracture; in Figure 14–8, B, 94% of cases have an ankle fracture. When dealing with a population with only a 4% probability of having a fracture, the predictive value of a positive test is only 20%—this means that 80% of positive test results would be false-positive. Although this sounds bad, the upside is that the predictive value of a negative test is 99%—there would be very few false-negative results. Conversely, when dealing with a population with a 94% probability of having a fracture, the predictive value of a positive test is 99%, and the predictive value of a negative test is only 23%. Because the positive and negative predictive values are dependent on the proportion of diseased or injured individuals within the population studied, this proportion should always be specified when the predictive values are reported.

This characteristic of the predictive values has a great deal of impact for clinicians who are performing diagnostic or screening tests. To know how to interpret the predictive value of a test, the clinician should estimate the "pretest" probability of the patient having the condition. If an asymptomatic individual is being screened, then the probability of having the condition is low. In this instance, the predictive value of a positive test is likely to be low, but the predictive value of a negative test is likely to be high. If an individual with a history and physical examination that is highly suggestive of the condition is tested, then the predictive value of a positive test is likely to be high and the predictive value of a negative test is likely to be low. Applying this information to the example of ankle effusion, a clinician who notes a 15-mm ankle effusion on the plain radiograph of a

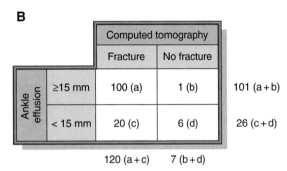

FIGURE 14–8. Changing the prevalence of fractures influences the predictive values, but not the sensitivity and specificity.

A, Illustration with prevalence of 4%.

Sensitivity = a/(a + c) = 5/6 = 83%

Specificity = d/(b + d) = 120/140 = 86%

Positive predictive value = a/(a + b) = 5/25 = 20%

Negative predictive value = d/(c + d) = 120/121 = 99%

B, Illustration with prevalence of 94%

Sensitivity = a/(a + c) = 100/120 = 83%

Specificity = d/(b + d) = 6/7 = 86%

Positive predictive value = a/(a + b) = 100/101 = 99%

Negative predictive value = d/(c + d) = 6/26 = 23%

patient experiencing an uncomplicated recovery from ankle sprain would likely not order a CT to look for an occult fracture. The assumption would be that the patient belongs to a population similar to the one in Figure 14–8, *A,* and the positive ankle effusion has a high probability of being a false-positive finding. In contrast, if a clinician notes a 15-mm ankle effusion on the radiograph of a patient with a great deal of swelling and discoloration, malleolar tenderness, and inability to bear weight 72 hours after injury, a follow-up CT would likely be ordered to look for an occult fracture. The assumption would be that the patient belongs to a population similar to the one in Figure 14–8, *B,* and the positive ankle effusion has a high probability of being a true indication of an occult fracture.

This section of the chapter has only introduced the complex interrelationships among sensitivity, specificity, likelihood ratios, prevalence, and predictive values. Several excellent texts and articles present a fuller description of these topics.[8-12] A number of contemporary articles in the rehabilitation literature use these concepts to examine screening and diagnostic tests of importance to rehabilitation professionals. Smith and colleagues[13] and Peruzzi and associates[14] studied the sensitivity and specificity of two different methods of bedside assessment of swallowing function in individuals with stroke and tracheostomy, respectively. In both cases the bedside measures were compared against the gold standard of videofluoroscopy. Law and colleagues conducted a systematic review of the literature to identify the feasibility of universal screening of children for speech and language delay.[15] McFarland and colleagues assessed the usefulness of three common clinical tests for diagnosing superior labral anterior-posterior lesions of the shoulder.[16] Kuhlman and Hennessy evaluated the sensitivity and specificity of a number of signs of compression of the median nerve within the carpal tunnel.[17] Flegel and Kolobe studied usefulness of the Test of Infant Motor Performance for predicting motor performance in the early school years.[18] In addition to their use in evaluating diagnostic and screening

tests, these concepts can be used to identify factors that are predictive of other events, such as discharge location, development of postoperative complications, or response to treatment, as in Wagner and colleagues' use of trauma scores to predict discharge after traumatic brain injury,[19] Hulzebos and associates' identification of preoperative risk factors for pulmonary complications in patients with coronary artery bypass surgery,[20] and Flynn and colleagues' use of clinical examination items to predict which patients with low back pain would respond to spinal manipulation.[21]

■ NONEXPERIMENTAL EPIDEMIOLOGICAL DESIGNS

Three common nonexperimental designs are used to implement epidemiological research: cross-sectional, case-control, and cohort designs. Figure 14–9 shows how each design is related to the timing of various elements of the design. Cross-sectional studies are used to document the status of a group at a particular point in time. With case-control studies, researchers identify individuals with the condition of interest (the cases) and individuals without the condition of interest (the controls). They then look into the

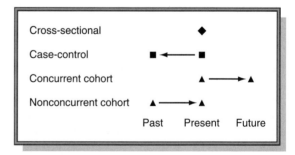

FIGURE 14–9. The epidemiological designs can be characterized by the timing of measurements, as well as the direction in which the logic of the design proceeds. Data are collected at one point in time for cross-sectional studies, researchers work from effects to causes in case-control designs, and they work from causes to effects in two variations on cohort designs.

past for the presence or absence of risk factors that might explain the presence or absence of the condition. In effect, in case-control studies, the researchers start with an effect and go looking for a cause. With cohort studies (also termed *concurrent cohort studies*), researchers identify individuals with various risk factors and look into the future to see if the condition of interest develops. In a variation on cohort studies, sometimes termed *historical cohort studies* or *nonconcurrent cohort studies*, the researchers identify a group of interest, identify risk factors from the past, and then determine whether a condition of interest is present or absent. In both variations of cohort studies, the researchers start with the cause and look for the effect.

In the research design overview presented in Chapter 6, the terms *prospective* and *retrospective* are defined in terms of the timing of data collection in relation to the development of the research problem. It is also noted that alternate definitions of these two terms are sometimes used to describe the "direction" in which the research proceeds. According to these alternate definitions, a *prospective study* proceeds from cause to effect, as do the cohort designs. A *retrospective study* proceeds from effect to cause, as do the case-control designs. In this text, the terms refer to the timing of data collection, as recommended by Friedman.[11] When referring to the direction in which the research proceeds, the terms cohort and case-control are used.

Cross-Sectional Studies

Cross-sectional studies are used to document health status at a single point in time for each participant within the study. In some instances, the point in time may be a range of calendar dates (e.g., a study in which fitness levels of top executives in a particular company are collected between January and March of 1 year); in other instances, the point in time may be a particular event (e.g., a study of fitness levels of top executives as they turn 60 years old). In studies that document health status, the point in time is

often the point of entry into a health system. This was the case for Fallat and associates' study of sprained ankle syndrome.[22] During a 33-month period, they conducted a standardized examination of all patients presenting to a hospital emergency department with acute "twisted" ankles. Even though the study was conducted over an almost 3-year period, each of the more than 600 patients within the study was assessed only once. The "point in time" that makes this a cross-sectional study was the "event" of presenting to an emergency department with a complaint of a twisted ankle.

Many reports of case-control and cohort research include a cross-sectional component that describes the patient groups at a single point in time. For example, Prencipe and colleagues[23] conducted a study of stroke, disability, and dementia among elders in rural Italy. Although their main purpose was to document the relationship between stroke and dementia (done through a nonconcurrent cohort design, to be described later), their results also included age- and sex-specific prevalence rates for stroke in the population they surveyed.

Case-Control Studies

The defining characteristic of a case-control study is that the researchers start with "effects" and look for "causes." First, the researchers identify individuals with the effect of interest (the cases). Second, they identify appropriately matched individuals without the effect of interest (the controls). Third, they evaluate all the participants (cases and controls alike) to determine the presence or absence of various factors hypothesized to cause the effect of interest. This evaluation may involve review of records to determine previous health status, may involve collection of new information that asks subjects to recall past behaviors or events, or may involve observation of characteristics that were presumed to have existed before the effect of interest occurred. Finally, they conduct statistical analyses to determine whether individuals with the presumed causes have a higher relative risk of being a case than a control.

Morris and colleagues used case-control methods to determine the effect of preexisting conditions on mortality in trauma patients.[24] A computerized database with information on all discharges from California acute care hospitals assured a large, representative sample. The effect of interest was death from trauma and the cases were 3074 of almost 200,000 trauma patients in the database who died from their injuries. The researchers matched each case with up to four trauma survivors discharged from the same hospital, within the same age grouping, and with a similar severity of injury. They then collected information about 11 preexisting health conditions. Finally, they determined the relative risk of dying (the risk of having the "effect" of interest) for patients with the various preexisting conditions (the presumed "causes"). Using odds ratios, they determined that individuals with cirrhosis were 4.7 times more likely to die of trauma than individuals without cirrhosis, and that individuals with chronic obstructive pulmonary disease were 1.8 times more likely to die of trauma than those without the disease.

Harding and colleagues used case-control methods to determine the impact of early chest physiotherapy on the development of brain damage in extremely premature infants.[25] An initial review of the medical records of more than 400 low birth weight infants from one New Zealand hospital was undertaken. The effect of interest was development of a specific type of brain damage (encephaloclastic porencephaly), and 13 infants with this form of brain damage were identified in 1993 and 1994 as the "cases." The researchers matched each case with two controls who did not have brain damage and who were admitted close to the time of the case, had similar gestation times and birth weights, and survived their first week. They then reviewed the medical records to identify 51 factors they believed could be related to the development of the brain damage. Of these 51 factors, only breech presentation, hypotension in the first week of life, and number of

chest physiotherapy treatments during the first month of life were different between the cases and controls. Based on this work, the hospital discontinued the use of chest physiotherapy for very low birth weight infants during the first month of life and, at the time the study was published, had not seen any further cases of encephaloclastic porencephaly in this group of infants.

However, the authors published a follow-up study that examined injury and physiotherapy data on babies in their hospital from 1985 (9 years before the cluster of cases occurred) to 1998 (4 years after chest physiotherapy was discontinued).[26] They found that the number of chest physiotherapy treatments delivered to babies with these gestational ages and birth weights had been considerably higher in the mid-1980s than during 1993-1994 when the cases emerged. However, no cases of encephaloclastic porencephaly were documented outside of the original cluster in 1993-1994. Based on this follow-up study, the authors concluded that the association between injury and number of chest physiotherapy treatments during 1993-1994 cannot be a complete explanation for the emergence of the cases. This pair of studies reminds us of two things: (1), that case-control designs do not provide direct evidence of cause and effect, and (2), that research results from isolated studies are not definitive, requiring clinicians to continually update their knowledge of research literature in their areas of practice.

Another case-control study is Clemson and associates' study of hazards in the home and risk of falls and hip fractures.[27] Their method of identifying cases and controls yielded, in effect, two studies within a single report. For one study, the cases were 43 patients with recurrent falls (two or more falls in the past year) and the controls were 157 nonfallers; for the other study, the cases were 52 patients with hip fractures compared with 195 patients without hip fractures. Thus, the effects of interest were falls and fractures. The presumed causes were hazards in the home, as assessed by occupational therapists. Using odds ratios, the researchers found, among other things, that individuals in homes with hazardous toilet railings had more than 11 times the risk of falls or hip fractures as those with safe railings.

These three studies illustrate some of the positive and negative features of case-control methods. In the study of the association between preexisting conditions and death from trauma, the case-control methods enabled the researchers to study a large number of trauma cases cost effectively. If the researchers had tried to implement this study with a cohort design, they would have had to enroll tens of thousands of patients and follow them for years until enough of the subjects sustained trauma for which they were hospitalized—and until they had a large enough subgroup of patients who died of the trauma. This illustrates one of the chief advantages of the case-control design over other designs—the ability to study a reasonable number of individuals with relatively rare conditions without needing to observe the entire population at risk for long periods. This issue of feasibility also came into play in the study of factors associated with brain damage in very low birth weight infants. In this study, reviews of 3 years of medical records were needed to identify 13 cases. It would have been very expensive to initiate and maintain a cohort study of all incoming low birth weight infants for the 3 years needed to identify this modest number of cases.

A second advantage of the case-control design is that it enables researchers to study things that might not otherwise be ethical to study. In the study of home hazards, one would clearly not be able to study this experimentally by randomly placing patients into hazardous and nonhazardous home environments. One would not even be able to study this ethically with a nonexperimental cohort design. To do so would involve identifying a group of older persons to study, evaluating their homes for hazards, and then doing nothing about those hazards until you saw who did and who did not fall or fracture their hips. Ethical practice would demand that subjects at least be given advice about how to remedy the hazards that were identified—and, if enough patients took that advice, the level of

hazards across the homes would become much more uniform, and one of the variables of interest would be nearly eliminated. Therefore, the case-control method, in which hazards that were presumed to exist before the fall or fracture are identified after the return home, provides an ethical way to study this potential relationship.

One of the chief concerns about case-control designs is the manner in which the presumed causes are documented or identified. In the study of brain damage of very low birth weight infants, 51 different factors were extracted from the medical records. Because of the emergent nature of care for extremely premature infants, not all of the factors may have been well documented for all the cases and controls.

In the study of hazards in the home, the hazards were evaluated after the fall or fracture and after the patient had returned home. The assumption was made that the home environment was similar at discharge to what it was before the fall. If a sufficient number of concerned children or neighbors have taken up throw rugs, installed toilet safety rails, replaced burned out light bulbs, and tightened rickety stair railings during the hospitalization of the person who fell or fractured the hip, then this assumption would not be valid. In addition, if this effort to reduce hazards is done more often for those who fall or fracture a hip and less often for those who have not fallen, then this selective reduction in hazards for certain groups of subjects would be of particular concern to the validity of the project.

Cohort Studies

Cohort designs are characterized by their progression from cause to effect. In a cohort study, individuals are selected because they do not have the disease or injury of interest, and they can be classified as to their status on a risk factor or factors of interest. The "healthy" individuals (at least with respect to the disease or injury of interest) in the different risk categories are followed for a period of time to compare their relative risks of developing the disease or injury of interest.

There are several variants of the cohort design. In the first, the subjects are identified in the present and followed into the future to see who does and does not develop the outcome of interest. This variant is either known simply as a cohort design or as a *prospective* or *concurrent cohort design.* In the second variant, the subjects are placed into risk factor groupings based on data collected in the past. Then, they are measured in the present or future to determine who develops the outcome of interest. This variant is either known as a *historical cohort design* or a *nonconcurrent cohort design.* In the third variant, the *retrospective cohort design,* all of the data have already been collected at the time the research question is developed; the researchers extract the appropriate data, group participants based on a variable or variables of interest, and look for differences in a variety of predictor variables. In all of the variants, the researcher establishes the presence or absence of the risk factor first and then determines the presence or absence of the outcome of interest. This is the reverse of the case-control design, in which the outcome is established before the risk factors are identified.

A concurrent cohort design was used by Rothweiler and colleagues to study the effect of age at the time of injury on psychosocial outcomes in traumatic brain injury.[28] More than 400 patients with brain injury were studied at 1 month and 1 year after injury to determine their psychosocial functioning. The independent variable was age, with five levels: 18 to 29 years, 30 to 39 years, 40 to 49 years, 50 to 59 years, and 60 years and older. The dependent variable was psychosocial functioning as measured by the Glasgow Outcome Scale, postinjury living situation, and postinjury employment status. They found that, in general, older individuals who sustain traumatic brain injury experience more psychosocial dysfunction than younger individuals.

Likewise, Taylor and colleagues used a prospective cohort design to study outcomes after low back surgery.[29] They collected baseline and 12-month follow-up information on individuals undergoing low back surgery. Using the 12-month follow-up information, they divided the group into those who responded well to the surgery and those who did not respond well. Then, they looked back at the baseline information to identify factors that were different between the two outcome groups. They found that older age, previous low back surgery, workers' compensation coverage, and consultation with an attorney before surgery were related to worse outcomes.

The study of stroke, disability, and dementia, mentioned earlier when describing cross-sectional studies, used a nonconcurrent cohort design to answer the main question of interest of whether patients with stroke have a higher risk of dementia than individuals without stroke.[23] The grouping of patients into stroke and stroke-free categories was based on a door-to-door survey done by a lay researcher. The strokes that were identified had to have occurred before the "prevalence day" established by the researchers. This ensured that the "direction" of the study was from possible cause (a stroke, in the past) to effect (dementia, in the present). Odds ratios, adjusted for age and sex differences between the stroke and stroke-free groups, showed that the individuals with stroke had 5.8 times the risk of dementia than those without stroke.

Finally, a retrospective cohort design was used by Cushman and associates in their study of readmissions to inpatient pediatric pulmonary rehabilitation.[30] Their retrospective review of records identified children who had required oxygen or ventilator support during an inpatient pulmonary rehabilitation admission, and then grouped the children according to whether they had subsequent readmissions. The children with readmission were found to need more ventilator support, more nursing care, and more acute-care transfers than children without readmissions.

■ SUMMARY

Epidemiology is the study of the distribution and determinants of disease and injury in populations.

Common measures used in epidemiology include ratios, proportions, and rates. Prevalence is the proportion of existing cases of a disease or injury in a population at a particular point of time. Incidence is the rate of development of new cases of a disease or injury in a population at risk. Relative risk of disease or injury in different groups is expressed with risk ratios and odds ratios. Screening and diagnostic tests are evaluated by measures of sensitivity (the proportion of patients with the condition who test positive), specificity (the proportion of patients without the condition who test negative), and the likelihood ratios (usefulness for ruling in and ruling out diagnoses). In addition, predictive values for positive and negative tests can be calculated for populations with different proportions of individuals with disease or injury. Common epidemiological research designs include cross-sectional studies (subjects measured at one point in time), case-control studies (researchers work backward from effect to cause), and cohort studies (researchers work forward from cause to effect).

REFERENCES

1. Harkness GA. *Epidemiology in Nursing Practice*. St. Louis, Mo: Mosby–Year Book; 1995.
2. Loney PL, Stratford PW. The prevalence of low back pain in adults: a methodological review of the literature. *Phys Ther*. 1999;79:384-396.
3. Krotenberg R, Stitik T, Johnston M. Incidence of dislocation following hip arthroplasty for patients in the rehabilitation setting. *Am J Phys Med Rehabil*. 1995;74:444-447.
4. Tanner CM, Goldman SM. Epidemiology of Parkinson's disease. *Neurol Clin*. 1996;14:317-335.
5. Emery CA, Meeuwisse WH. Risk factors for groin injuries in hockey. *Med Sci Sports Exerc*. 2001;33:1423-1433.
6. Jekel JF, Elmore JG, Katz DL. *Epidemiology, Biostatistics, and Preventive Medicine*. 2nd ed. Philadelphia, Pa: WB Saunders; 2001.
7. Clark TW, Janzen DL, Logan PM, Ho K, Connell DG. Improving the detection of radiographically occult ankle fractures: positive predictive value of an ankle joint effusion. *Clin Radiol*. 1996;51:632-636.
8. Riegelman RK, Hirsch RP. *Studying a Study and Testing a Test: How to Read the Health Science Literature*. 4th ed. Boston, Mass: Little, Brown & Co; 1999.
9. Sackett DL, Haynes RB, Guyatt GH, Tugwell P. *Clinical Epidemiology: A Basic Science for Clinical Medicine*. 2nd ed. Philadelphia, Pa: Lippincott-Raven Publishers; 1991.
10. Gerstman BB. *Epidemiology Kept Simple: An Introduction to Classic and Modern Epidemiology*. 2nd ed. New York, NY: Wiley-Liss; 2003.
11. Friedman GD. *Primer of Epidemiology*. 5th ed. New York, NY: McGraw-Hill; 2003.
12. Fritz JM, Wainner RS. Examining diagnostic tests: an evidence-based perspective. *Phys Ther*. 2001;81:1546-1564.
13. Smith HA, Lee SH, O'Neill PA, Connolly MJ. The combination of bedside swallowing assessment and oxygen saturation monitoring of swallowing in acute stroke: a safe and humane screening tool. *Age Aging*. 2000;29:495-499.
14. Peruzzi WT, Logemann JA, Currie D, Moen SG. Assessment of aspiration in patients with tracheostomies: comparison of the bedside colored dye assessment with videofluoroscopic examination. *Respir Care*. 2001; 46:243-247.
15. Law J, Boyle J, Harris F, Harkness A, Nye C. The feasibility of universal screening for primary speech and language delay: findings from a systematic review of the literature. *Dev Med Child Neurol*. 2000;42:190-200.
16. McFarland EG, Kim TK, Savino RM. Clinical assessment of three common tests for superior labral anterior-posterior lesions. *Am J Sports Med*. 2002;30:810-815.
17. Kuhlman KA, Hennessey WJ. Sensitivity and specificity of carpal tunnel syndrome signs. *Am J Phys Med Rehabil*. 1997;76:451-457.
18. Flegel J, Kolobe TH. Predictive validity of the Test of Infant Motor Performance as measured by the Bruininks-Oseretsky Test of Motor Proficiency at school age. *Phys Ther*. 2002;82:762-771.
19. Wagner AK, Hammond FM, Grigsby JH, Norton HJ. The value of trauma scores: predicting discharge after traumatic brain injury. *Am J Phys Med Rehabil*. 2000;79:235-242.
20. Hulzebos EH, Van Meeteren NL, DeBie RA, Dagnelie PC, Helders PJ. Prediction of postoperative pulmonary complications on the basis of preoperative risk factors in patient who had undergone coronary artery bypass graft surgery. *Phys Ther*. 2003;83:8-16.
21. Flynn T, Fritz J, Whitman J, et al. A clinical prediction rule for classifying patients with low back pain who demonstrate short-term improvement with spinal manipulation. *Spine*. 2002;24:2835-2843.
22. Fallat L, Grimm DJ, Saracco JA. Sprained ankle syndrome: prevalence and analysis of 639 acute injuries. *J Foot Ankle Surg*. 1998;37:280-285.
23. Prencipe M, Ferretti C, Casini AR, Santini M, Giubilei F, Culasso F. Stroke, disability, and dementia: results of a population survey. *Stroke*. 1997;28:531-536.

24. Morris JA, Mackenzie EJ, Edelstein SL. The effect of preexisting conditions on mortality in trauma patients. *JAMA*. 1990;263:1942-1946.

25. Harding JE, Miles FK, Becroft DM, Allen BC, Knight DB. Chest physiotherapy may be associated with brain damage in extremely premature infants. *J Pediatr*. 1998;132:440-444.

26. Knight DB, Bevan CJ, Harding JE, et al. Chest physiotherapy and porencephalic brain lesions in very preterm infants. *J Paediatr Child Health*. 2001;37:554-558.

27. Clemson L, Cumming RG, Roland MA. Case-control study of hazards in the home and risk of falls and hip fractures. *Age Aging*. 1996;25:97-101.

28. Rothweiler B, Temkin NR, Dikmen SS. Aging effect on psychosocial outcome in traumatic brain injury. *Arch Phys Med Rehabil*. 1998;79:881-887.

29. Taylor VM, Deyo RA, Ciol M, et al. Patient-oriented outcomes from low back surgery: a community-based study. *Spine*. 2000;25:2445-2452.

30. Cushman DG, Dumas HM, Haley SM, O'Brien JE, Kharasch VS. Re-admissions to inpatient paediatric pulmonary rehabilitation. *Pediatr Rehabil*. 2002;5: 133-139.

Outcomes Research

The outcomes movement in health care policy, practice, and research has received widespread recognition during the 1990s and 2000s. Most writers attribute the emergence of the outcomes movement to (1) the need for cost containment in the health care sector,[1-3] (2) the need to examine outcomes other than mortality when dealing with the increasingly prevalent chronic diseases of an aging society,[2,4] and (3) the need to determine "best practices" and thereby reduce the great variations in health care that occur for reasons apparently unrelated to the characteristics of the group receiving the care.[1-5] Contemporary authors[4-6] credit the conceptual basis for outcomes assessment to Donabedian, whose "structure, process, outcomes" framework influenced the design of the *Medical Outcomes Study* (MOS), an important outcomes project initiated in the late 1980s.[7]

As with many developing movements, there is neither widespread agreement about the definitions of various components related to health care outcomes nor agreement as to the boundaries of the outcomes movement. Consequently, the terms "outcomes" and "outcomes research" are used in different ways by the many participants in and observers of the health care system. One area of commonality, however, is the shift in emphasis from looking for narrow biological effects of treatments delivered under highly controlled conditions to assessing the broad biopsychosocial impact of treatments implemented in typical clinical settings.[1,2,4,8] This shift, from what is termed "efficacy" to what is characterized as "effectiveness" has profound implications for the conduct of outcomes research. These implications extend from the nature of the overall research design to the selection of the dependent measures of interest. A general text that addresses many of these issues is Kane's *Understanding Health Care Outcomes Research*.[9]

The purpose of this chapter is to present an overview of the outcomes movement in rehabilitation research. First, the purpose of outcomes research is explored by contrasting the concepts of efficacy and effectiveness. Second, broad frameworks for outcomes research are presented. Third, a variety of measurement tools consistent with these frameworks are described. Finally, design and implementation issues related to outcomes research are addressed.

■ PURPOSE OF OUTCOMES RESEARCH

One thing that has consistently been used to characterize the outcomes movement is the differentiation between "efficacy" and "effectiveness." Although he does not use these words, Kane[10] identified the tension between these two concepts and between the research models that support each concept:

> If the practice of medicine (including rehabilitation) is to become more empiric, it will have to rely on epidemiological methods. Although some may urge the primacy of randomized clinical trials as the only path to true enlightenment, such a position is untenable for several reasons. First, the

exclusivity of most trials is so great that the results are difficult to extrapolate to practice. Such trials may be the source of clinically important truths, but these findings will have to be bent and shaped to fit most clinical situations. Second, researchers do not have the time or resources to conduct enough trials to guide all practice. Instead, we need a more balanced strategy that combines targeted trials with well-organized analysis of carefully recorded clinical practice.[10(pJS22)]

This observation emphasizes the importance of studying health care under ideal conditions through highly controlled experimental studies (randomized clinical trials) as well as through well-organized analysis of clinical practice as it actually occurs (outcomes research). These contrasting approaches are often thought of as assessing "efficacy" versus "effectiveness."

Efficacy

Efficacy is usually defined as the biological effect of treatment delivered under carefully controlled conditions. The research method that is best suited to determining efficacy is the randomized controlled trial, in which researchers control for a variety of factors that would interfere with an understanding of the impact of the treatment of interest. Thus, participants are selected to be relatively homogeneous, treatments are implemented in uniform ways, and dependent variables are selected because they are objective and relate directly to the expected biological effect of the treatment. Research to determine efficacy focuses on the "does it work?" and "is it safe?" questions, and does not often examine issues of cost, feasibility, and acceptability to practitioners and patients.

Effectiveness

In contrast, effectiveness is defined as the usefulness of a particular treatment to the individuals receiving it under typical clinical conditions. Nonexperimental research methods are often used to determine effectiveness. Rather than manipulating the treatment patients receive, as well as the conditions under which they receive it, researchers implementing nonexperimental designs examine the effectiveness of actual treatment that has already occurred or observe actual treatment as it is delivered. This is a messy process that usually results in heterogeneous groups of subjects, treatments that are implemented in various ways by different clinicians and patients, and dependent variables that focus on broader outcomes of interest to patients, payers, and practitioners.

■ FRAMEWORKS FOR OUTCOMES RESEARCH

The shift from looking at narrow efficacy to broader effectiveness has required that practitioners develop broad-based frameworks to guide the way that they think about disease and injury, as well as the consequences of disease and injury. Three frameworks that have received widespread discussion within the rehabilitation literature include the Nagi model,[11] the World Health Organization's (WHO's) original *International Classification of Impairments, Disabilities and Handicaps* (ICIDH)[12] and the revised WHO *International Classification of Functioning, Disability, and Health* (ICF).[13] Each of the three frameworks is presented here, followed by a summary of issues and refinements that have been articulated by others.

Nagi Model

Saad Nagi, a sociologist, first presented his model in 1965.[14] He revisited this original model as an appendix to a report of the Committee on a National Agenda for the Prevention of Disabilities,[11] a group appointed jointly by the Centers for Disease Control and Prevention and the National Council on Disabilities. His scheme describes active pathology, impairment, functional limitation, and disability, as shown in the top row of Figure 15–1. For example, a man with osteoarthritis experiences inflammation (the active pathology, manifested at the cellular level), which contributes to muscle weakness and valgus deformity at the knees (the impairments, at the tissue, organ, or system level). He has difficulty walking long distances or climbing stairs (the functional impairment, at the level of the person) and he gives up his position as a field-based police officer because it involves more walking and stair climbing than is tolerable (the disability, at the level of social functioning).

International Classification of Impairments, Disabilities, and Handicaps

The WHO published its initial ICIDH in 1980.[12] This classification, a supplement to the *International Classification of Diseases, Ninth Revision* (ICD-9), was needed because of the inadequacies of the ICD-9 in addressing the long-term impact of chronic diseases. The ICIDH, as can be inferred from its name and as shown in the middle row of Figure 15–1, conceptualized the long-term sequelae of disease as impairments, disabilities, and handicaps. For example, a man with osteoarthritis experiences inflammation (the disease, manifested at the cellular level) that leads to muscle weakness and valgus deformity at the knees (the impairments, at the tissue, organ, or system level). The person has difficulty walking long distances or climbing stairs (the disability, at the level of the person) and he changes from a field position as a police officer to a desk job because the demands of and architectural barriers in the field involve more walking and stair climbing than is tolerable (the handicap, at the level of society and the environment). Although the ICIDH has been replaced by the newer ICF described in the following section, it remains an important framework for rehabilitation professionals because much of the rehabilitation literature from the 1980s and 1990s uses ICIDH concepts and terminology.

Nagi			
Active Pathology	*Impairment*	*Functional Limitation*	*Disability*
Interruption or interference with normal processes and efforts of the organism to regain normal state	Anatomical, physiological, mental, or emotional abnormalities or loss	Limitation in performance at the level of the whole organism or person	Limitation in performance of socially defined roles and tasks within a sociocultural and physical environment

ICIDH			
Disease	*Impairment*	*Disability*	*Handicap*
Intrinsic pathology or disorder	Loss or abnormality of psychological, physiological, or anatomical structure or function at organ level	Restriction or lack of ability to perform an activity in a normal manner	Disadvantage resulting from impairment or disability that limits or prevents fulfillment of a normal role (depends on age, sex, sociocultural factors for the person)

ICF		
Body Functions and Structures	*Activities*	*Participation*
Changes in body functions (physiological) or structures (anatomical). When these changes are positive, they result in functional and structural integrity; when these changes are negative, they result in impairment	Functioning at an individual level	Functioning at a societal level
	Both activities and participation can be viewed in terms of capacity (ability to execute a task in a standard environment) and performance (executing tasks in the current environment)	
	Disability occurs when activities are limited or participation in societal roles is restricted. Disability is modified by the environmental and personal context in which the individual functions	

FIGURE 15–1. Frameworks for Outcomes Research: Nagi Model; the International Classification of Impairments, Disabilities, and Handicaps (ICIDH); and the International Classification of Functioning, Disability, and Health (ICF).

The verbal descriptions of the Nagi and ICIDH models are from Jette AM. Physical disablement concepts for physical therapy research and practice. *Phys Ther.* 1994;74:380-386. Their presentation has been modified to show how the categories are related across the models.

Used with permission of the American Physical Therapy Association. ICF descriptions are from World Health Organization. *International Classification of Functioning, Disability, and Health.* Available at: *www.who.int/classification/icf.* Accessed October 27, 2003.

International Classification of Functioning, Disability, and Health

A major reformulation of the ICIDH occurred with the endorsement of the *International Classification of Functioning, Disability and Health* (ICF) by the WHO Assembly in 2001.[13] Seen by some as a synthesis of the Nagi and ICIDH frameworks,[15] the ICF uses a different set of terms for key concepts (see bottom row of

Figure 15–1). The concept of impairment is known in the ICF by "changes in body functions or structures." The terms "functional limitation" (Nagi), "disability" (Nagi and ICIDH), and "handicap" (ICIDH) are either not used or are used differently. The new terms are "activities," "participation," and "disability." Activities refer to functioning at an individual level and participation to functioning at a societal level. Disability is seen as the consequence of either activity limitations or participation restrictions. Both activities and participation can be viewed in terms of "capacity" (the ability to execute a task in a standard environment) and performance (executing tasks in the current environment). Disability is seen as modifiable by the environment and personal context in which the individual functions. In ICF language, the same man with osteoarthritis of the knees would have impairments related to inflammation (a change in body function) and joint space narrowing (a change in body structure). Although he can walk more than a mile and climb stairs if the terrain is level and there is only one flight of stairs (he retains walking and stair climbing capacity in standard environmental contexts), he rarely performs these tasks in his daily life (his performance is indicative of an activity limitation, which is a disability at the individual level). He changes from a field position as a police officer to a desk job because the demands of and architectural barriers in the field involve more walking, running, and stair climbing than is tolerable (this restriction in a societal job role is also a disability). His work disability is modified by environmental and personal contexts. For example, the field environment cannot change to accommodate his activity limitations, but an alternate administrative environment that meets his activity needs is available. This particular police officer has the personal attributes and abilities—organizational and computer skills, for example—to make the transition from field to desk work possible; others would not have these skills and the disability would be much greater because the personal context would be a barrier to changing job roles.

The ICF appears to have addressed many of the concerns that individuals and groups had identified with either or both of the other frameworks. For example, Jette was critical of the ICIDH scheme because it mingled both attribute (individual level) and relational (societal level) concepts within the "disability" category and because the "handicap" category did not clearly differentiate among individual characteristics and the social and environmental circumstances that place an individual with a disability at a disadvantage.[16] The ICF clearly separates attribute (activities) and relational (participation) concepts, redefines disability to reflect limitations or restrictions at either level, and adds the modifying concepts of personal and environmental factors.

Another criticism of the earlier frameworks was the lack of differentiation between capacity and performance. For example, in a 1994 article, Verbrugge and Jette discussed the importance of distinguishing between intrinsic disability (difficulty experienced when external assistance, either equipment or personnel, is not available) and actual disability (difficulty experienced when external assistance is available).[17] Similarly, in 1997, Liang identified three domains that enter into function: capacity (the level of impairment), will (psychological factors such as motivation and self-confidence), and need (the social and environmental context).[18] The ICF tries to capture the complex interplay between these factors by differentiating between capacity (the ability to execute a task in a standard environment) and performance (executing tasks in the current environment).

Despite the differences between the frameworks, the complexity of the disablement process, and the difficulties with measurement within any of the models, these frameworks convey a central message that has shaped outcomes research in rehabilitation. The message is that simply measuring changes in body structures and functions is insufficient for the study of person-level concepts such as activity, participation, and disability. Rehabilitation professionals have received this message and have changed the ways in which they measure outcomes in both clinical and research settings. The next section of this chapter highlights measures that reflect the person-level categories within the disablement models.

MEASUREMENT TOOLS FOR OUTCOMES RESEARCH

Clinicians and researchers have long used measures of pathology (e.g., laboratory values and imaging techniques) and measures of changes in body functions and structures (e.g., range of motion, muscle performance) to guide their practice and to serve as dependent measures in research studies. Outcomes research, or an outcomes focus to practice, generally means that researchers and practitioners supplement these measures of pathology and bodily changes with person-level measures of activity, participation, or disability. This section of the chapter is designed to provide an overview of these person-level measures.

Quality of Life

Quality of life is a global concept that can include elements as diverse as perceptions of health, satisfaction with the work environment, quality of family and social relationships, satisfaction with schools and neighborhoods, productive use of leisure time, connections with one's spiritual nature, and financial well-being. Although problems in many of these areas can lead to health-related problems associated with stress, poor eating habits, sedentary lifestyles, and tobacco, alcohol, and drug use, global measures of quality of life are so broad as to have limited use in health care research and practice settings.

Health-Related Quality of Life

Because quality of life, as a global concept, is limited in its usefulness in health care research, a variety of measures of health-related quality of

life (HRQL) have been developed. These measures have also been termed "health status" and "outcomes" measures. They may also be referred to as "generic" tools because they are designed for use with individuals with health conditions of all types, although their suitability for use with some populations has been questioned. For example, in a study of the performance of five HRQL instruments with a population of individuals with spinal cord injury, Andresen and colleagues found that some of the longer instruments were difficult for more impaired individuals to complete and that some language in the instruments (e.g., references to walking) was offensive to individuals with spinal cord injuries.[19] There is general agreement that measures of HRQL should include elements related to physical, psychological, and social functioning. Because many of these measures have been well described by others,[20-22] only a few are described here.

SF-36

The Medical Outcomes Study (MOS), begun in the late 1980s, was designed to develop patient outcome tools and to monitor variations in outcome based on differences in health care systems, clinician styles, and clinician specialties.[7] One of the major tools to come out of this study is the Short Form-36, commonly known as the SF-36. The self-report includes 36 items covering eight domains of functioning: role limitation due to physical problems, role limitation due to emotional problems, social functioning, mental health, pain, energy, fatigue, and general health perceptions. The SF-36 is scored to produce a profile of the eight domains, each with scores ranging from 0 to 100, with higher scores representing better health. The eight scores are used to derive two summary scales, the physical component summary (PCS) and the mental component summary (MCS). Although this tool takes only about 10 minutes to complete, the desire for an even briefer tool has led to its modification into a shorter tool known as the SF-12. This 12-item tool includes one or two items from each of the eight components of the SF-36.[23]

The SF-36 has been used as one of the major health status measures in any number of rehabilitation research studies—including randomized controlled trials, outcomes research as defined in this chapter, and many descriptive and relationship analysis studies. For example, McAllister and colleagues used the SF-36 to determine the impact of injury severity and training time on the HRQL of collegiate athletes,[24] Smith and colleagues used it in a study of the relationship between self-reported HRQL and a performance measure of walking in individuals with peripheral neuropathy,[25] Jones and associates used it as a measure of global function in a study that determined preoperative predictors of function after total knee arthroplasty,[26] Clark and colleagues used it as a dependent measure in their randomized controlled trial of occupational therapy for independent living adults,[27] Wilson and coworkers used it to describe the quality of life of individuals with dysphonia compared with age-matched healthy controls,[28] and Alexander and colleagues used it to correlate the amount of different rehabilitation services received by patients with their health outcomes.[29]

SICKNESS IMPACT PROFILE

The Sickness Impact Profile (SIP) is a 136-item self-report that takes about 30 minutes to complete.[30] It also exists in a shorter 68-item version.[31] It is used to evaluate the physical dimensions of ambulation, mobility, and body care; the psychosocial dimensions of social interaction, communication, alertness, and emotional behavior; and other dimensions related to sleep/rest, eating, work, home management, and recreational pastimes. The instrument is scored on a percentage basis, with higher scores representing greater levels of disability. Mueller and colleagues used the SIP to document the health status of patients with transmetatarsal amputation and diabetes, compared with age- and sex-matched individuals without either condition,[32] Kwakkel and colleagues used it to determine the long-term effects of upper and lower extremity training after stroke,[33] Schoppen and associates used it as

a measure of functional outcome in a study of predictors of function for individuals with unilateral lower-limb amputations,[34] and DePalma and coworkers used it to study the quality of life of severely injured trauma survivors 6 months after discharge from the hospital.[35]

FUNCTIONAL STATUS QUESTIONNAIRE

The Functional Status Questionnaire (FSQ) is a 34-item self-report that, like the SF-36, takes about 10 minutes to complete.[20,22] It measures physical function (basic and instrumental activities of daily living), emotional function (anxiety and depression and quality of social interaction), social performance (occupational function and social activities), and a group of other functions (sexual function, global disability, global health satisfaction, and social contacts). Boström and colleagues used the FSQ to study predictors of disability in patients with rheumatoid arthritis,[36] Binder and associates used it as a dependent measure in their randomized controlled trial of the effects of intensive exercise training on frailty of older adults,[37] and Brach and associates used it to study the relationship between performance-based and self-reported measures of function in older women.[38]

Condition-Specific Tools

In addition to generic health status instruments, a variety of condition-specific tools have been developed. Two book references provide additional insight into condition-specific tools: Atherly provides an overview of differences between condition-specific and generic measures[39] and Pynsent and associates provide information about a variety of condition-specific or region-specific outcome tools in orthopedics.[40] Hundreds of condition-specific tools exist, ranging from well-tested tools that have been translated into many languages and used widely in research to little-tested tools that are never used by researchers other than the instrument developer. Table 15–1 presents a sampler of different

TABLE 15-1 A Sampler of Condition-Specific Tools for Rehabilitation

Tool	Characteristics	Research About the Tool	Research Using the Tool
Stroke-Adapted Sickness Impact Profile	30-item, 8-scale, version of the Sickness Impact Profile, adapted for individuals with stroke.	van Straten, 1997[41] Buck, 2000[43]	van Straten, 2000[42]
Quadriplegic Index of Function	Assesses 10 domains of function: transfers, grooming, bathing, feeding, dressing, wheelchair mobility, bed activities, bowel and bladder programs, and understanding personal care.	Gresham, 1986[44] Meyers, 2000[45]	Rothwell, 2003[46]
Oswestry Disability Index	Measures 10 areas of perceived disability related to low back pain: pain intensity, changing pain status, personal hygiene, lifting, walking, sitting, standing, sleeping, social activity, and traveling. Scoring is converted to percentage, with a higher score representing a higher percentage of disability.	Fairbank, 2000[47]	Flynn, 2003[48]
Western Ontario and McMaster University Osteoarthritis Index (WOMAC)	24-item tool with 3 subscales: joint pain, physical joint function, and joint stiffness. Available in 60 alternative language forms.	Bellamy, 2002[49] Angst, 2001[50]	Jones, 2003[26]
Lysholm Knee Rating Scale	Assesses 8 areas of knee dysfunction: limp, support, locking, instability, pain, swelling, ability to squat, ability to negotiate stairs. Scored from 0 to 100 with higher scores representing better function.	Johnson, 2001[51]	McAllister, 2003[52]
Disabilities of the Arm, Shoulder, and Hand (DASH)	30-item scale measuring self-reported upper-extremity disability and symptoms. Scores on individual items are summed and converted to a scale with a range from 0 to 100 with higher scores representing greater disability.	Gummesson, 2003[53] Beaton, 2001[54]	Murphy, 2003[55]
Fatigue Questionnaire	11 items assessing physical and mental fatigue and duration and extent of fatigue. Maximum score of 33, with physical and mental fatigue subscores.	Chalder, 1993[56]	Jahnsen, 2003[57]
Brief Symptom Inventory for Depression	53 items focus on how much an individual has been bothered by depressive symptoms over the past 7 days. Each item scored from 1 (not at all) to 5 (extremely distressed); 9 symptom dimensions and 3 global indices can be calculated. Scores are standardized, with higher scores indicating greater distress.	Vahle, 2000[58] Morlan, 1998[59]	Wiegner, 2000[60]

condition-specific tools that are relevant to rehabilitation research, providing basic information about the tools, one or more references about the measurement characteristics of the tool, and one or more references to research using the tool as an outcome measure.[26,41-60] Note that the "conditions" to which the tools are "specific" range from specific primary diagnoses (e.g., stroke, spinal cord injury), to general primary diagnoses (e.g., low back pain and osteoarthritis), to secondary conditions seen in rehabilitation (e.g., fatigue and depression), and to body regions (e.g., the knee or the arm, shoulder, and hand).

Patient-Specific Instruments

Although the use of generic and condition-specific outcomes measures for research with groups of individuals has ballooned over the past two decades, many of the tools are not very responsive to individual changes in functional status, thereby limiting their clinical utility. The patient-specific class of outcome measures is a group of tools designed to identify individualized goals and detect individual changes in status related to those goals.[61]

Generic patient-specific instruments can be used with patients or clients with any type of problem. One scale with a long history of use in psychotherapy and more recent use in rehabilitation is Goal Attainment Scaling (GAS).[61] With GAS, individualized problems are identified and a continuum of five possible outcomes related to each problem is developed. Scoring is standardized, with the most unfavorable outcome scored as −2, less than the expected outcome as −1, the expected outcome as 0, a greater than expected outcome as +1, and the most favorable outcome likely as +2.[62] The same highly individualized approach, but with a different scoring system, is found in the Canadian Occupational Performance Measure (COPM) and the Patient Specific Functional Scale (PSFS).[61] The GAS approach has been used for measuring outcomes in geriatric rehabilitation.[63] Both GAS scores and the COPM were used by Trombly and colleagues to document achievement of self-identified goals by adults with traumatic brain injury.[64] Chatman and colleagues studied the measurement characteristics of the PSFS in individuals with knee dysfunction.[65]

In a variation of generic patient-specific instruments, providers and clients choose from a menu of goal statements rather than generating highly individualized problems and goals.[66,67] For example, in Beurskens and colleagues' study of a patient-specific approach to measuring functional status in individuals with low back pain, they presented patients with a list of 36 activities that are often limited by low back pain.[67] Patients could, however, identify problematic activities not on the list.

Patient-specific tools that are also disorder-specific are available. The McMaster Toronto Arthritis (MACTAR) scale includes a list of activities expected to be affected by arthritis. Five priority items are selected and changes in status are scored on the 3-point scale of worse, no change, and improved.[61] The American Speech-Language-Hearing Association (ASHA) uses a disorder-specific, patient-specific tool as the outcome measure in its National Outcomes Measurement System.[68] A large set of Functional Communication Measures, with subsets specific to different communication disorders, has been developed by the ASHA, with each measure scored on a 7-point scale appropriate to the item and disorder.

Satisfaction

Satisfaction is seen as an important outcome of treatment, as well as an indicator of the effectiveness of various structures and processes within the health care system. The health status measures described in the previous section may demonstrate changes in status over the course of treatment yet still fail to indicate whether the extent of change met the expectation of the patient. Measurements of patient satisfaction provide this important perspective. In addition to satisfaction with the outcomes of care, patients' opinions may be sought on other structural and process dimensions of the health care system: accessibility and convenience of care, availability of resources, continuity of care, efficacy/outcomes of care, finances, humaneness, information gathering, information giving, pleasantness of surroundings, and quality of caregivers. Input into the structure and process of health care is seen as important because it can help health care entities organize themselves more effectively. For example, in a quality improvement program for patients with acute hip fracture implemented in Sweden in the late 1990s, the success of the program, which was designed to improve pain management, decrease surgery waiting times, and reduce development of pressure ulcers, was reported in a 2003 research article.[69] In this approach to satisfaction, the authors did not ask patients about their satisfaction with care; rather, they studied factors generally accepted to be important to patients.

Satisfaction is also important because it may be indirectly related to clinical outcomes if it affects appointment-keeping and adherence to treatment recommendations. In a review article about satisfaction research, Di Palo discussed several national efforts to collect satisfaction data.[70] As is the case with health status tools, both global and condition-specific satisfaction tools have been developed. In addition, many tools are developed by individual facilities for their own use each year. In contrast to the health status tools, a few of which enjoy widespread popularity for clinical and research use, there seems to be, as yet, no clear "winners" in the satisfaction instrument sweepstakes. Maciejewski and associates provide an overview of many of the issues related to measurement of satisfaction in health care settings.[71]

■ DESIGN ISSUES FOR OUTCOMES RESEARCH

Although research of any type can have person-level outcomes as dependent measures, outcomes research, as defined by the focus on effectiveness, is about much more than simply broadening the measurement tools used in research. It also involves a commitment to studying care as it actually occurs, rather than under the ideal, controlled conditions of experimental research. Therefore, for the purpose of this chapter, outcomes research is also assumed to imply a set of methods related to the assessment of care as it occurs in the real world. The design elements that characterize outcomes research, as they are presented here, include nonexperimental design and the analysis of information contained in various health care databases.

Database Research

The databases used in outcomes research can be medical records themselves, computerized abstracts of medical records, health care insurance claims databases, databases generated within one's own facility or within a network of facilities associated with a large health care conglomerate, or participation in national databases that combine data from clinical entities from many regions. In the United States and the United Kingdom, recent changes to health care privacy regulations have presented outcomes researchers with new challenges related to gaining access to these databases, as noted in Chapters 3 and 28.[72,73]

REVIEW OF EXISTING MEDICAL RECORDS

Medical records themselves may be used as sources of data in outcomes projects. The biggest advantage to using medical records is that they contain a great deal of information that can be evaluated in context. However, this advantage is balanced by at least two disadvantages. First, reviewing records is a time-consuming process that requires the personnel extracting the data to make judgment calls about which of the many pieces of information is relevant to the questions at hand. Second, the information in medical records is often inconsistent and incomplete. Both of these disadvantages have the impact of reducing the available sample size that can be generated for a given project.

ABSTRACTS OF MEDICAL RECORDS

The various reporting mechanisms required for billing, reporting, and accreditation processes mean that records of hospitalization are routinely abstracted, summarized on a "facesheet," and computerized at discharge. Use of this computerized information is time efficient for the researcher and generally ensures that there is a common data set on all patients of interest. One problem with the abstracted information is that there may be errors in coding the information, including diagnoses, comorbidities, and complications. A study that compared facesheet information with information in the medical chart of patients with hip fracture found that there was an error rate of 12% related to diagnoses, 17% related to complications, and 16% related to surgical procedures.[74]

In addition to this concern about the accuracy of the data, the information in the abstract is often less specific than desired by the researcher, so "proxy" measures are used instead of the real measures of interest. For example, researchers who wish to eliminate chronically depressed patients from their sample might screen out patients taking antidepressant medication. If antidepressant medications are used for conditions other than chronic depression, or if many patients receive antidepressants for a short period of time after an acute health care event, then many relevant patients may be excluded from the study. Conversely, if depression is prevalent but often untreated, then many depressed patients may not be screened from the analysis.

INSURANCE CLAIMS DATABASES

Insurance claims databases, which often share a great deal of information with administrative facesheets, are frequently used for outcomes studies. Examples relevant to rehabilitation include research on hip fracture outcomes using Medicare claims data,[75] and use of Blue Cross–Blue Shield claims to assess the number of visits and costs of care when patients were seen for physical therapy with and without physician referrals.[76]

In a review of the use of claims databases for outcomes research, Motheral and Fairman[77] identified several challenges to the effective use of this data source. One central advantage to claims databases is that, because of their link to reimbursement for services, they tend to be complete. In addition, they offer access to large numbers of patients at relatively low cost, without ethical concerns related to how treatment is delivered. However, claims databases suffer from limitations on the number of diagnoses, comorbidities, and procedures that are listed, making it difficult to adjust for differences in severity of illness among groups of patients that the researcher hopes to compare. Another potential disadvantage is that when reimbursement policies change, concomitant changes in coding strategies may reflect the policy change rather than a change in practice. In addition, person-level outcomes, such as HRQL, which are so important to determining effectiveness, are generally not available through insurance claims databases. Outcomes such as mortality, discharge location, or readmission dates may provide the only insights into the impact of the treatment episodes for the people being treated. Finally, insurance claims data are only available on individuals who are insured, making it difficult to generalize results to groups that are uninsured. Chan and colleagues have summarized specific issues involved in using the U.S. Medicare database for outcomes research.[78]

IN-HOUSE DATABASES

To solve many of the problems with the use of medical records, abstracts of medical records, and insurance claims databases, facilities may choose to develop and manage their own outcomes databases. Experience in developing such databases was described by Shields and colleagues[79] and Weinstein and associates.[80]

Developing one's own database is a time-consuming, expensive venture. For example, in the project described by Shields and colleagues,[79] staff at the University of Iowa Hospitals and Clinics began the development process in 1986, began collecting data in 1991, and began retrieving data in 1993. This long-term commitment was feasible for a teaching hospital with a research mission and access to university resources in instrument development, computer systems, and research design and analysis. Hospitals in large systems, extended care and rehabilitation facilities that are part of a nationwide system, or outpatient clinics that are affiliated with a national corporation may also have the resources to pursue this type of a database and may find competitive business reasons to collect this information even if they do not have primary research missions.

Despite the time and money involved in creating an in-house database, there are many benefits to doing so. In-house outcomes systems may have high levels of utilization by staff members who participate in the development process, have local control of the training process for staff members who contribute information to the database, and have staff who are able to design data collection tools to answer specific questions of interest within the setting.

NATIONAL OUTCOMES DATABASES

Clinical leaders who wish to involve their facilities in outcomes research may not believe that developing an in-house database is the best solution. They may not have the resources to develop and maintain a system, and they may wish to be able to compare the care at their facilities with that delivered in other centers. Participating in a national outcomes database gives clinics access to the needed resources and allows them to "benchmark" their practices against other similar clinics in the database. In addition, in comparison to in-house databases, the pooling of data from many clinics may increase sample size, enhance statistical power, and improve the generalizability of research results generated from the database.

National databases in the United States exist as government, professional, and commercial enterprises. For example, the National Institute on Disability and Rehabilitation Research (NIDRR) sponsors three model systems in burn, spinal cord injury (SCI), and traumatic brain injury care. One component of each model system is an outcomes database.[81-83] By 1998, the National Spinal Cord Injuries Collaborative Database (established in 1973) associated with the Spinal Cord Injury Model Systems contained data on more than 25,000 individuals with SCI.[45] Despite the promise of such a database, it is estimated that only 15% of individuals in the United States with SCIs are included in the database, the longitudinal data are spotty because treatment centers have moved in and out of the model system, HRQL data have only been collected for the last few years, and there are large gaps in the economic data within the database.[45] Despite these limitations, the SCI model system database has been used for outcomes research about individuals with SCI, as in Krause and associates' study of employment after SCI.[84]

The Uniform Data System for Medical Rehabilitation (UDSMR), with relationships with more than 1400 facilities worldwide, sponsors outcomes databases that currently house more than 2,500,000 patient records that include scores on its well-known Functional Independence Measure (FIM) and WeeFIM (the FIM instrument adapted for children and adolescents) instruments. The UDSMR was established in the 1980s with government funding from the NIDRR and cosponsorship from the American Congress of Rehabilitation Medicine, the American Academy of Physical Medicine and Rehabilitation, and several other national professional organizations.

The National Outcomes Measurement System (NOMS) of the National Center for Treatment Effectiveness in Communication Disorders of the American Speech-Language-Hearing Association is an example of an association-sponsored national outcomes database.[68] As noted earlier in this chapter, the outcomes measures used in this database are a set of ASHA-developed Functional Communication Measures (FCMs) selected for each patient according to their individual presentation and their communication disorder. Health care facilities and schools can participate in NOMS and individual speech-language pathologists and audiologists can contribute data once they are trained and registered in the use of the FCMs. Data collection for the adult health care subset of the database began in 1998. By July 2003, more than 50,000 cases had been contributed to the adult component of NOMS (Tobi Frymark, personal communication).

Focus on Therapeutic Outcomes, Inc., (FOTO) is a widely used commercial outcomes database for rehabilitation.[85] Developed in 1993 through a grant from several national rehabilitation companies, it is now privately owned. Subscribers collect a number of standard outcome measures (such as the SF-36 and the Oswestry and Lysholm scales) on their patients and submit to FOTO for inclusion in the database. FOTO provides benchmarking reports to subscribers that enable them to compare their outcomes against national norms.

Although participation in national outcomes databases, such as those outlined in the previous paragraphs, has the advantages of access to resources and benchmarking information, there may be considerable reluctance on the part of rehabilitation professionals to participate in the process. For example, several national outcomes projects in prosthetics and orthotics did not garner the necessary participation from prosthetists and orthotists in the field,[86] and Russek and colleagues were disappointed by the level of therapist participation in data collection for a database for a multisite corporation with 71 clinics nationwide.[87] Conversely, the ASHA National Outcomes Measurement System has collected more than 50,000 cases from 1998 to 2003 in its adult component alone and the National Athletic Trainers' Association completed its high school athletics injury surveillance project with a database of 23,566 injuries documented by athletic trainers at more than 250 different schools nationwide.[88]

Russek and colleagues[87] explored these participation issues by surveying therapists who should have been able to participate in their data collection effort. Five major factors concerning attitudes about standardized data collection were identified: inconvenience of the data collection tool, acceptance of the operational definitions used for the data collection effort, lack of automation of the process, the paperwork load within the clinic in general, and training issues. They also found that clinics with a staff member responsible for the organization and management of the data collection effort tended to have higher levels of participation. Together, these factors seem to indicate that administrators who wish for their facilities to participate in national outcomes databases should attend to the convenience of doing so for individual staff members, and should also work to enhance "buy-in" by providing local support to the effort and improving the training of staff for the data collection effort.

Analysis Issues

The design of outcomes research studies has a major impact on the way in which the data are analyzed. Because the foundation needed to understand statistical analysis issues has not yet been laid (see Section 6, Chapters 19 through 23), these statistical issues are introduced briefly here and followed up in more detail in Section 6.

CASE MIX ADJUSTMENTS

Because outcomes research studies tend to be nonexperimental in nature, the researcher has little or no control over which patients are placed into which groups within the study. Thus, there are often important differences among study groups, some of which occur because there are systematic biases in the way that clinical decisions are made. For example, older adults with more active lifestyles may seek total knee replacement as a treatment for osteoarthritis, whereas less active patients may choose more conservative care. Differences in outcomes between these two groups, then, might be the result of preoperative lifestyles rather than the treatment of interest. In addition, if the outcomes reported are to be compared with outcomes in other facilities or regions, then researchers need to assure that they are "benchmarking" themselves against comparable groups.[89,90]

There are two general ways to deal with case mix problems in outcomes research. The first is to stratify the groups and compare only those subgroups that have, for example, similar ages, comorbidities, or disease severity. The second way of managing case mix problems is to mathematically adjust the data so that two groups with, for example, different average ages are equalized in some way. Sometimes this is done by "weighting" subgroups within the analysis, much as epidemiological rates are adjusted for valid comparisons between groups (see Chapter 14). Smith,[91] Nitz,[92] and Derose[93] provide guidance about risk adjustment for severity, comorbidity, and demographic and psychosocial factors, respectively.

TECHNIQUES FOR DEALING WITH MISSING DATA

Because the databases used for outcomes research are often developed for other purposes, missing data is a frequent problem. One solution is to simply delete variables or patients for which there is incomplete data. The other general solution is to use a variety of statistical methods to estimate, or "impute" what the missing score might have been. If the researcher has good ways of imputing missing data, this is often preferred to deleting cases, because it maintains larger sample sizes.

SURVIVAL ANALYSIS

Because the data in existing databases often include events such as death, readmission, and discharge, outcomes research reports often use a technique called *survival analysis* to analyze the timing of these events. In general, survival analysis involves creating a graph that indicates the cumulative proportion of individuals for whom an event has or has not occurred (y axis) against time (x axis). There are several different ways of creating survival analysis graphs, some of which result in smooth curves and some of which result in stair-step graphs (Kaplan-Meier method).[94(pp154-158)] Survival analysis can be used to show the pattern of achievement of the milestone for a single group, or it can be used to compare patterns across groups. Figure 15–2 shows the survival curves generated in Hoenig and colleagues' study of the timing of surgery and rehabilitation care after hip fracture.[95] In this study, most of the surviving patients regained ambulation ability after hip fracture. Therefore, the outcome of "ambulation," per se, was not a good indicator of differences between treatment regimens. However, the time it took until ambulation occurred turned out to be a useful measure. The survival curves, for example, show that those receiving high-frequency physical therapy (PT), occupational therapy (OT), or both (more than five visits per week) ambulated earlier than those who received low-frequency PT or OT, regardless of whether the surgical repair was done early (within 2 days of hospitalization) or late.

COMPARISONS ACROSS SCALES

Outcome studies often involve several different dependent variables, and some of these dependent variables contain multiple subscales. Often, the different tools are scored differently and have different scales of measurement. In addition, the groups being studied may show more or less variability on the different measures, which also influences the interpretation of changes in scores. If a researcher wishes to know which of the many different variables changed the most, then the changes need to be expressed on a common scale that captures both the size of the change as well as the variability within the group. The usual scale that is used is a measure of *effect size,* which expresses the difference between two means in terms of the amount of variability within the data. An effect size of 1.0 indicates that the difference between the means

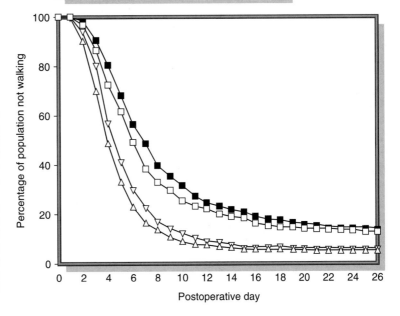

		Median number of days to ambulation
△	Early surgical repair and high-frequency PT/OT	3.9
▽	Late surgical repair and high-frequency PT/OT	4.4
□	Early surgical repair and low-frequency PT/OT	5.9
■	Late surgical repair and low-frequency PT/OT	6.7

FIGURE 15–2. Illustration of the use of survival curves. The curves show the probability and timing of ambulation according to timing of surgical repair and the frequency of physical and occupational therapy (PT/OT).
From Hoenig H, Rubenstein LV, Sloane R, et al. What is the role of timing in the surgical and rehabilitative care of community-dwelling older persons with acute hip fracture? *Arch Intern Med.* 1997;157:513-520. Used with permission of the American Medical Association.

of two groups is the same size as the standard deviation, a measure of variability within each group. Effect sizes less than 1.0 mean that the difference between the means is smaller than the standard deviation, and effect sizes larger than 1.0 mean that the difference is greater than the standard deviation. The conceptual basis for effect size becomes clearer after a review of the statistics chapters, which lay the statistical foundation needed for a full understanding of effect sizes. For now, it is enough to know that the use of effect sizes enables the researcher to compare the magnitude of change across many different variables. Jette and Jette used effect sizes to evaluate changes in SF-36 scores and Lysholm Knee Rating Scale scores over an episode of physical

therapy for patients with knee impairments.[96] Figure 15–3 shows a radar graph of their results. In a radar graph, each dependent variable is displayed as a "spoke" coming from a common center. The scale on each spoke is the same, and in this example represents effect size, marked in one-tenth of a standard deviation increments. It is readily apparent from this graph that the biggest changes were seen in Lysholm scores and in the bodily pain and physical function subscales of the SF-36.

MULTIVARIATE STATISTICS

The final analysis issue covered here also stems from the multiple dependent variables that are

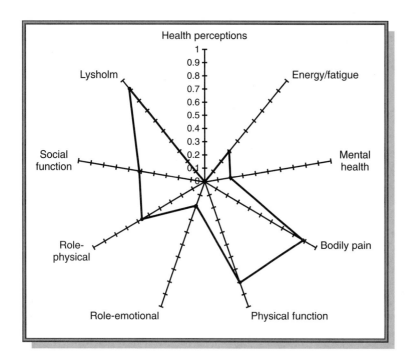

FIGURE 15–3. Use of effect sizes in a radar graph format to display changes in SF-36 and Lysholm scores over a physical therapy episode for patients with knee impairments. Changes are presented as effect sizes for each outcome and are represented by a point on an arm of the radar graph. The center of the graph is no change. Each hatch mark represents a change of one-tenth of a standard deviation.
From Jette DU, Jette AM. Physical therapy and health outcomes in patients with knee impairments. *Phys Ther.* 1996;76:1178-1187. Used with permission of the American Physical Therapy Association.

often measured in outcomes studies. Because of these many variables, researchers often use statistical tools that enable them to analyze many dependent variables simultaneously. The general term for these types of statistical tools is *multivariate*. Although the descriptions of multivariate results often appear intimidating, they rest on many of the same statistical foundations as do the simpler univariate statistics that handle one dependent variable at a time.

■ SUMMARY

Outcomes research refers to a broad group of research designs that evaluate the overall effectiveness of clinical care as it is delivered in actual practice, rather than the physiological efficacy of treatments given under tightly controlled circumstances to narrowly defined groups of subjects. Evaluations of effectiveness in rehabilitation are often guided by one of three widely used frameworks: the Nagi model, the WHO's original *International Classification of Impairments, Disabilities, and Handicaps* (ICIDH), or its newer *International Classification of Functioning, Disability, and Health* (ICF). These frameworks add the concepts of activity, participation, and disability to traditional measures of changes in bodily functions or structures. Elements of this broader conceptualization of health status can be measured by a number of generic, condition-specific, person-specific, or satisfaction tools. Outcomes research studies generally rely on databases that are generated by review of medical records, computerized abstracts of medical records, insurance claims data, in-house data collection efforts, or national databases that provide standardized data collection forms and analysis services. Statistical analysis of outcomes research is often complex and must address issues of case mix, missing data, survival analysis, comparisons across different scales, and analysis of many dependent variables simultaneously.

REFERENCES

1. Keller RB, Rudicel SAZ, Liang MH. Outcomes research in orthopaedics. *J Bone Joint Surg Am.* 1993;75:1562-1574.

2. Nyiendo J, Haas M, Hondras MA. Outcomes research in chiropractics: the state of the art and recommendations for the chiropractic research agenda. *J Manipulative Physiol Ther.* 1997;20:185-200.

3. Ellenberg DB. Outcomes research: the history, debate, and implications for the field of occupational therapy. *Am J Occup Ther.* 1996;50:435-441.

4. Bradham DD. Outcomes research in orthopedics: history, perspectives, concepts, and future. *Arthroscopy.* 1994;10: 493-501.

5. Birkmeyer JD. Outcomes research and surgeons. *Surgery.* 1998;124:477-483.

6. Jette AM. Outcomes research: shifting the dominant research paradigm in physical therapy. *Phys Ther.* 1995; 75:965-970.

7. Tarlov AR, Ware JE, Greenfield S, Nelson EC, Perrin E, Zubkoff M. The Medical Outcomes Study: an application of methods for monitoring the results of medical care. JAMA. 1989;262:925-930.

8. Faust HB, Mirowski GW, Chuang T-Y, et al. Outcomes research: an overview. *J Am Acad Dermatol.* 1997;36: 999-1006.

9. Kane RL. *Understanding Health Care Outcomes Research.* Gaithersburg, Md: Aspen Publishers; 1997.

10. Kane RL. Improving outcomes in rehabilitation: a call to arms (and legs). *Med Care.* 1997;35(suppl):JS21-JS27.

11. Nagi SA. Disability concepts revisited: implications for prevention. In: Pope AM, Tarlov AR, ed. *Disability in America: Toward a National Agenda for Prevention.* Washington, DC: National Academy Press; 1991.

12. *International Classification of Impairments, Disabilities, and Handicaps.* Geneva, Switzerland: World Health Organization; 1980.

13. World Health Organization. *International Classification of Functioning, Disability, and Health.* Available at: *www.who.int/classification/icf.* Accessed October 27, 2003.

14. Nagi S. Some conceptual issues in disability and rehabilitation. In: Sussman M, ed. *Sociology and Rehabilitation.* Washington, DC: American Sociological Association; 1965:100-113.

15. Stucki G, Ewert T, Cieza A. Value and application of the ICF in rehabilitation medicine. *Disabil Rehab.* 2002;24: 932-938.

16. Jette AM. Disablement outcomes in geriatric rehabilitation. *Med Care.* 1997;35(suppl):JS28-JS37.

17. Verbrugge LM, Jette AM. The disablement process. *Soc Sci Med.* 1994;38:1-14.

18. Liang MH. Comments on: Jette AM. Disablement outcomes in geriatric rehabilitation. *Med Care.* 1997; 35(suppl): JS28-JS37.

19. Andresen EM, Fouts BS, Romeis JC, Brownson CA. Performance of health-related quality-of-life instruments in a spinal cord injured population. *Arch Phys Med Rehabil.* 1999;80:877-884.

20. McHorney CA, Tarlov AR. Individual-patient monitoring in clinical practice: are available health status surveys adequate? *Qual Life Res.* 1995;4:293-307.

21. Maciejewski M. Generic measures. In: Kane RL, ed. *Understanding Health Care Outcomes Research.* Gaithersburg, Md: Aspen Publishers; 1997:19-52.

22. Jette AM. Using health-related quality of life measures in physical therapy outcomes research. *Phys Ther.* 1993;73:528-537.

23. Ware JE, Kosinski M, Keller SD. A 12-item short-form health survey: construction of scales and preliminary tests of reliability and validity. *Med Care.* 1996;34:220-223.

24. McAllister DR, Motamedi AR, Hame SL, Shapiro MS, Dorey FJ. Quality of life assessment in elite collegiate athletes. *Am J Sports Med.* 2001;29:806-810.

25. Smith DG, Domholdt E, del Aguila M, Coleman K, Boone D. Ambulatory activity in men with diabetes: relationship between self-reported and real-world performance-based measures. *J Rehabil Res Dev.* 2004;41:(in press).

26. Jones CA, Voaklander DC, Suarez-Alma ME. Determinants of function after total knee arthroplasty. *Phys Ther.* 2003;83:696-706.

27. Clark F, Azen SP, Zemke R, et al. Occupational therapy for independent-living older adults: a randomized controlled trial. *JAMA.* 1997;278:1321-1326.

28. Wilson JA, Deary IJ, Millar A, Mackenzie K. The quality of life impact of dysphonia. *Clin Otolaryngol.* 2002;27: 179-182.

29. Alexander H, Bugge C, Hagen S. What is the association between the different components of stroke rehabilitation and health outcomes? *Clin Rehabil.* 2001;15:207-215.

30. Bergner M, Bobbitt RA, Carter WB, Gilson BS. The Sickness Impact Profile: development and final revision of a health status measure. *Med Care.* 1981;19:787-805.

31. de Bruin AF, Diederiks JP, de Witte LP, Stevens FC, Philipsen H. The development of a short generic version of the Sickness Impact Profile. *J Clin Epidemiol.* 1994;47: 407-418.

32. Mueller MJ, Salsich GB, Strube MJ. Functional limitations in patients with diabetes and transmetatarsal amputations. *Phys Ther.* 1997;77:937-943.

33. Kwakkel G, Kollen BJ, Wagenaar RC. Long term effects of intensity of upper and lower limb training after stroke: a randomised trial. *Neurol Neurosurg Psychiatry.* 2003;72:473-479.

34. Schoppen T, Boonstra A, Groothoff JW, de Vries J, Goeken LN, Eisma WH. Physical, mental, and social predictors of functional outcome in unilateral lower-limb amputees. *Arch Phys Med Rehabil.* 2003;84:803-811.

35. DePalma JA, Fedorka P, Simko LC. Quality of life experienced by severely injured trauma survivors. *AACN Clin Issues.* 2003;14:54-63.

36. Boström C, Harms-Ringdahl K, Nordemar R. Shoulder, elbow and wrist movement impairment-predictors of

disability in female patients with rheumatoid arthritis. *Scand J Rehabil Med.* 1997;29:223-232.

37. Binder EF, Schechtman KB, Ehsani AA, et al. Effects of exercise training on frailty in community-dwelling older adults: results of a randomized, controlled trial. *J Am Geriatr Soc.* 2002;50:1921-1928.

38. Brach JS, VanSwearingen JM, Newman AB, Kriska AM. Identifying early decline of physical function in community-dwelling older women: performance-based and self-report measures. *Phys Ther.* 2002;82:320-328.

39. Atherly A. Condition-specific measures. In: Kane RL, ed. *Understanding Health Care Outcomes Research.* Gaithersburg, Md: Aspen Publishers; 1997:53-66.

40. Pynsent P, Fairbank J, Carr A. *Outcome Measures in Orthopaedics.* Oxford, England: Butterworth-Heinemann; 1993.

41. van Straten A, de Haan RJ, Limburg M, Schuling M, Bossuyt PM, van den Bos GA. A stroke-adapted 30-item version of the Sickness Impact Profile to assess quality of life (SA-SIP30). *Stroke.* 1997;28:2155-2161.

42. van Straten A, de Haan RJ, Limburg M, van den Bos GA. Clinical meaning of the Stroke-Adapted Sickness Impact Profile-30 and the Sickness Impact Profile-136. *Stroke.* 2000;31:2610-2615.

43. Buck D, Jacoby A, Massey A, Ford G. Evaluation of measures used to assess quality of life after stroke. *Stroke.* 2000;31:2004-2010.

44. Gresham GE, Labi ML, Dittmar SS, Hicks JT, Joyce SZ, Stehlik MA. The Quadriplegia Index of Function (QIF): sensitivity and reliability in a study of thirty quadriplegic patients. *Paraplegia.* 1986;24:38-44.

45. Meyers AR, Andresen EM, Hagglund KJ. A model of outcomes research: spinal cord injury. *Arch Phys Med Rehabil.* 2000;81(12 suppl 2):S81-S90.

46. Rothwell AG, Sinnott KA, Mohammed KD, Dunn JA, Sinclair SA. Upper limb surgery for tetraplegia: a 10-year re-review of hand function. *J Hand Surg [Am].* 2003;28: 489-497.

47. Fairbank JC, Pynsent PB. The Oswestry Disability Index. *Spine.* 2000;25:2940-2952.

48. Flynn TW, Fritz JM, Wainner RS, Whitman JM. The audible pop is not necessary for successful spinal high-velocity thrust manipulation in individuals with low back pain. *Arch Phys Med Rehabil.* 2003;84:1057-1060.

49. Bellamy N. WOMAC: a 20-year experiential review of a patient-centered self-reported health status questionnaire. *J Rheumatol.* 2002;29:2473-2476.

50. Angst F, Aeschlimann A, Steiner W, Stucki G. Responsiveness of the WOMAC osteoarthritis index as compared with the SF-36 in patients with osteoarthritis of the legs undergoing a comprehensive rehabilitation intervention. *Ann Rheum Dis.* 2001;60:834-840.

51. Johnson DS, Smith RB. Outcome measurement in the ACL deficient knee–what's the score? *Knee.* 2001;8: 51-57.

52. McAllister DR, Tsai AM, Dragoo JL, et al. Knee function after anterior cruciate ligament injury in elite collegiate athletes. *Am J Sports Med.* 2003;31:560-563.

53. Gummesson C, Atroshi I, Ekdahl C. The disabilities of the arm, shoulder and hand (DASH) outcome questionnaire: longitudinal construct validity and measuring self-rated health change after surgery. *BMC Musculoskelet Disord.* 2003;4:11.

54. Beaton DE, Katz JN, Fossel AH, Wright JG, Tarasuk V, Bombardier C. Measuring the whole or the parts? Validity, reliability, and responsiveness of the Disabilities of the Arm, Shoulder, and Hand outcome measure in different regions of the upper extremity. *J Hand Ther.* 2001;14:128-146.

55. Murphy DM, Khoury JG, Imbriglia JR, Adams BD. Comparison of arthroplasty and arthrodesis for the rheumatoid wrist. *J Hand Surg [Am].* 2003;28: 570-576.

56. Chalder T, Berelowitz G, Pawlikowska T, et al. Development of a fatigue scale. *J Psychosom Res.* 1993; 37:147-153.

57. Jahnsen R, Villien L, Stanghelle JK, Holm I. Fatigue in adults with cerebral palsy in Norway compared with the general population. *Dev Med Child Neurol.* 2003;45: 296-303.

58. Vahle V, Andresen EM, Hagglund KJ. Depression measures in outcomes research. *Arch Phys Med Rehabil.* 2000;81(suppl 2):S53-S62.

59. Morlan KK, Tan SY. Comparison of the Brief Psychiatric Rating Scale and the Brief Symptom Inventory. *J Clin Psychol.* 1998;54:885-894.

60. Wiegner S, Donders J. Predictors of parental distress after congenital disabilities. *J Dev Behav Pediatr.* 2000; 21:271-277.

61. Donnelly C, Carswell A. Individualized outcome measures: a review of the literature. *Can J Occup Ther.* 2002; 69:84-94.

62. Ottenbacher KJ, Cusick A. Goal attainment scaling as a method of clinical service evaluation. *Am J Occup Ther.* 1990;44:519-525.

63. Stolee P, Stadnyk K, Myers AM, Rockwood K. An individualized approach to outcome measurement in geriatric rehabilitation. *J Gerontol A Biol Sci Med Sci.* 1999; 54:M641-M647.

64. Trombly CA, Radomski JV, Davis ES. Achievement of self-identified goals by adults with traumatic brain injury: phase I. *Am J Occup Ther.* 1998;52:810-818.

65. Chatman A, Hyams S, Neel J, et al. The Patient-Specific Functional Scale: measurement properties in patients with knee dysfunction. *Phys Ther.* 1997;77:820-829.

66. Smith A, Cardillo JE, Smith SC, Amezaga A. Improvement scaling (rehabilitation version): a new approach to measuring progress of patients in achieving their individual rehabilitation goals. *Med Care.* 1998;36: 333-347.

67. Beurskens AJ, de Vet HC, Koke AJ, et al. A patient-specific approach for measuring functional status in low back pain. *J Manipulative Physiol Ther*. 1999;22: 144-148.

68. American Speech-Language-Hearing Association. *National Outcomes Measurement System: gaining the support of your staff and administration: health care*. Available at: *http://professional.asha.org/resources/ noms/health.cfm*. Accessed October 24, 2003.

69. Hommel A, Ulander K, Thorngren K-G. Improvements in pain relief, handling time and pressure ulcers through internal audits of hip fracture patients. *Scand J Caring Sci*. 2003;17:78-83.

70. Di Palo MT. Rating satisfaction research: is it poor, fair, good, very good, or excellent? *Arthritis Care Res*. 1997;10:422-430.

71. Maciejewski M, Kawiecki J, Rockwood T. Satisfaction. In: Kane RL, ed. *Understanding Health Care Outcomes Research*. Gaithersburg, Md: Aspen Publishers; 1997: 67-89.

72. Durham ML. How research will adapt to HIPAA: a view from within the healthcare delivery system. *Am J Law Med*. 2002;28:491-502.

73. Cassell J, Young A. Why we should not seek individual informed consent for participation in health services research. *J Med Ethics*. 2002;28:313-317.

74. Fox KM, Reuland M, Hawkes WG, et al. Accuracy of medical records in hip fracture. *J Am Geriatr Soc*. 1998; 46:745-750.

75. Lu-Yao GL, Baron JA, Barrett JA, Fisher ES. Treatment and survival among elderly Americans with hip fractures: a population-based study. *Am J Public Health*. 1994; 84:1287-1291.

76. Mitchell JM, de Lissovoy G. A comparison on resource use and cost in direct access versus physician referral episodes of physical therapy. *Phys Ther*. 1997;77:10-18.

77. Motheral BR, Fairman KA. The use of claims databases for outcomes research: rationale, challenges, and strategies. *Clin Ther*. 1997;19:346-366.

78. Chan L, Houck P, Prela CM, MacLehose RF. Using Medicare databases for outcomes research in rehabilitation medicine. *Am J Phys Med Rehabil*. 2001;80:474-480.

79. Shields RK, Leo KC, Miller B, Dostal WF, Barr R. An acute care physical therapy clinical practice database for outcomes research. *Phys Ther*. 1994;74:463-470.

80. Weinstein JN, Brown PW, Hanscom B, Walsh T, Nelson EC. Designing and ambulatory clinical practice for outcomes improvement: from vision to reality—The Spine Center at Dartmouth-Hitchcock, year one. *Qual Manage Health Care*. 2000;8:1-20.

81. *COMBI: The Center for Outcome Measurement in Brain Injury*. Available at: *http://www.tbims.org/combi*. Accessed August 2, 2003.

82. *UCHSC Burn Model System Data Coordination Center (BMS/DCC)*. Available at: *http://mama.uchsc.edu/pub/ nidrr/*. Accessed August 2, 2003.

83. *The 16 Model Spinal Cord Injury Systems*. Available at: *http://www.ncddr.org/rpp/hf/hfdw/mscis/map.html*. Accessed August 2, 2003.

84. Krause JS, Kewman D, DeVivo MJ, et al. Employment after spinal cord injury: an analysis of cases from the Model Spinal Cord Injury System. *Arch Phys Med Rehabil*. 1999;80:1492-1500.

85. *FOTO Inc*. Available at: *http://www.fotoinc.com*. Accessed August 2, 2003.

86. Jerrell ML. Revisiting outcomes research in O & P. *O & P Business News*. 2003;12:18-19,21-22,24.

87. Russek L, Wooden M, Ekedahl S, Bush A. Attitudes toward standardized data collection. *Phys Ther*. 1997;77: 714-729.

88. Powell JW, Barber-Foss KD. Injury patterns in selected high school sports: a review of the 1995-1997 seasons. *J Ath Train*. 1999;34:277-284.

89. Pryor DB, Lee KL. Methods for the analysis and assessment of clinical databases: the clinician's perspective. *Stat Med*. 1991;10:617-628.

90. LaValley MP, Anderson JJ. Statistical and study design issues in assessing the quality and outcomes of care in rheumatic diseases. *Arthritis Care Res*. 1997;10:431-440.

91. Smith M. Severity. In: Kane RL, ed. *Understanding Health Care Outcomes Research*. Gaithersburg, Md: Aspen Publishers; 1997:129-152.

92. Nitz NM. Comorbidity. In: Kane RL, ed. *Understanding Health Care Outcomes Research*. Gaithersburg, Md: Aspen Publishers; 1997:153-174.

93. Derose S. Demographic and psychosocial factors. In: Kane RL, ed. *Understanding Health Care Outcomes Research*. Gaithersburg, Md: Aspen Publishers; 1997: 175-209.

94. Jekel JF, Elmore JG, Katz DL. *Epidemiology, Biostatistics, and Preventive Medicine*. 2nd ed. Philadelphia, Pa: WB Saunders; 2001.

95. Hoenig H, Rubenstein LV, Sloane R, Horner R, Kahn K. What is the role of timing in the surgical and rehabilitative care of community-dwelling older persons with acute hip fracture? *Arch Intern Med*. 1997;157:513-520.

96. Jette AM, Jette DU. Physical therapy and health outcomes in patients with knee impairments. *Phys Ther*. 1996;76: 1178-1187.

Survey Research

Survey research is a form of inquiry that rests on the assumption that meaningful information can be obtained by asking the parties of interest what they know, what they believe, and how they behave. This chapter defines the scope of survey research, identifies the type of information that can be gleaned from survey research, presents a variety of types of items that are used within questionnaires, and addresses a variety of implementation details for mailed surveys, Internet surveys, and in-person or telephone interviews.

■ SCOPE OF SURVEY RESEARCH

A survey has been defined as a "system for collecting information from or about people to describe, compare, or explain their knowledge, attitudes, and behavior."[1(p1)] More specifically, survey research relies on self-reported information from participants, rather than on observations or measurements taken by the researcher. For example, consider ways of studying the extent to which patients adhere to a prescribed regimen. One way to study this topic would be to ask patients how often they are taking their medications or performing a home therapy regimen or to ask questions to determine their recall of important details about the regimen. This self-report information could be collected with survey methods in a face-to-face interview, by administering a questionnaire over the telephone, or with a mailed or Internet questionnaire. An assumption of the survey approach is that patients would provide accurate information about their activities.

In contrast, this topic could also be studied by having researchers score patients in some way as they observe them demonstrating the prescribed regimen. An assumption of the observational approach is that patients who were adherent to the regimen would, for example, set up a week's worth of medications correctly without prompting and those who were not adherent would set up the medications incorrectly or would require prompting from the researcher. Neither the survey approach nor the observational approach is inherently superior for studying this topic. Each rests on assumptions that will not be met in all cases—some patients would exaggerate their adherence if surveyed and some patients who faithfully take their medications may become flustered in front of the researcher and require prompting to demonstrate the regimen. Researchers need to consider which of the potential problems to avoid when they make decisions among the approaches that could be taken with a given topic.

To place survey research into the context of other forms of research, recall the six-celled matrix of research types presented earlier in Chapter 6 (see Figure 6–4) and repeated in Chapter 11 (see Figure 11–1). One dimension of the matrix is the purpose of the research. Survey techniques can be used for all three purposes: describing phenomena, analyzing relationships among variables, and analyzing differences among groups or across time.

The second dimension of the matrix is the timing of data collection. Clearly, surveys can be prospective, with self-reported information collected to answer specific research questions developed by the researchers. It is equally clear that self-reported information may be used retrospectively—that is, data collected for one purpose might be extracted and reanalyzed to meet another research need. For example, Chevan and Chevan used U.S. Bureau of the Census data to develop a profile of physical therapists.[2] However, most would not label this study "survey research." Instead, they would refer to it as a secondary analysis. The term *survey research* is generally used to describe original, prospective collection of self-reported data.

The third dimension of the matrix is whether the research is experimental or nonexperimental in nature. Clearly, survey research can be nonexperimental, with no controlled manipulation of independent variables. It is equally clear that self-reported information can be used in experimental research—as was the case when Balogun and associates studied the impact of educational programs on physical therapist and occupational therapist student attitudes toward working with individuals with acquired immunodeficiency syndrome.[3] This project was experimental in that there was controlled manipulation of the type of education received. Researchers surveyed participants to determine self-reported attitudes across time (preeducation, mideducation, and posteducation). However, most would not label this study as "survey" research; they might label it as an experimental, educational research project. Thus, although survey research can be experimental in nature, the term is often reserved for nonexperimental studies using self-reported information.

In summary, survey research can be used to meet the purposes of description, analysis of relationships, or analysis of differences. The term "survey research" is generally reserved for nonexperimental research with prospective collection of self-reported data. It is important to recognize that although all survey research projects use self-reported information, not all research projects that use self-reported information are considered survey research. Studies that use self-reported information retrospectively or in the context of experimental research are often referred to by more specific names.

TYPES OF INFORMATION

The scope of information that can be obtained through self-report instruments is vast. Concrete facts, knowledge, and behavior can be documented, as can abstract opinions and personal characteristics. The rehabilitation literature contains many examples of each of the five types of survey information just mentioned; one example of each follows. Hagberg and Brånemark[4] collected factual information about prosthetic use from individuals with transfemoral amputation and Nadler and associates[5] collected factual information from athletic trainers about complications encountered when delivering therapeutic modalities. Wagner and associates did preprogram and post-program surveys of college students enrolled in a physical medicine and rehabilitation internship to determine whether their knowledge of physical medicine and rehabilitation increased after completing the internship.[6] Tepe and associates[7] and Tharpe and colleagues[8] used survey methods to determine behaviors—the vocal habits and hygiene of young choir singers and the hearing aid fitting practices of audiologists for children with multiple impairments, respectively. Rubery and Bradford explored the opinions of spinal surgeons about athletic activity after spine surgery in children and adolescents.[9] As a part of a study of career success factors, Rozier and colleagues used self-reported information to determine a personal characteristic of respondents—their self-esteem as measured by the Rosenberg Self-Esteem Scale.[10]

TYPES OF ITEMS

Although the format of interview and questionnaire items is limited only by the creativity of the researcher, several standard item formats exist. The broadest distinction among item types is

open- versus closed-format items. The closed-format items presented in this chapter are divided further into multiple-choice, Likert-type, semantic differential, and Q-sort items.

Open-Format Items

Open-format items permit a flexible response. Interviews frequently include open-format items, and it is these open-format items that allow for the greater breadth of response that is a major advantage of using the interview in survey research. Suppose that a researcher is interested in identifying the sources of job satisfaction and dissatisfaction for rehabilitation professionals. An open-format interview question might be "What about your job is satisfying to you?" Respondents would be free to structure their responses as desired. Some might emphasize aspects of patient care, others might focus on working with a respected leader, others might discuss the quality of interactions among coworkers, and others might list several different satisfying aspects of their work.

Questionnaires may also include open-format items, although the depth of response depends on the respondents' ability to communicate in writing and their willingness to provide an in-depth answer in the absence of an interviewer who can prompt them and provide encouragement during the course of their response.

The major difficulty with open-format items is their analysis. The researcher must sift and categorize the responses into a relatively small number of manageable categories. The literature on the qualitative research paradigm provides guidelines for the classification of responses from open-format items, as discussed in Chapter 13. The categorization of responses from open-format items is sometimes used to generate the fixed alternatives needed for closed-format items.

Closed-Format Items

Closed-format items restrict the range of possible responses. Mailed questionnaires often include a high proportion of closed-format responses. In addition, highly structured interviews may use closed-format responses. In such a case, the interview becomes nothing more than an orally administered questionnaire and the breadth of response characteristic of most interview formats is lost. Four types of closed-format items are discussed below: multiple-choice, Likert-type, semantic differential, and Q-sort items.

MULTIPLE-CHOICE

Multiple-choice items can be used to measure knowledge, behavior, opinions, or personal characteristics. Some researchers design closed-format items that allow some flexibility of response by including "other" as a possible response category and permitting respondents to write in a response of their choice.

In a variation of the multiple-choice item, a vignette may be used as the stem of the item. A vignette is a short story or scenario that sets a scene. Colón-Emeric and associates used a vignette about a man with an osteoporotic hip fracture to elicit patient management recommendations from physicians[11] and Hasenbein and associates used vignettes to elicit physician opinions about optimal rehabilitation settings and outcomes for individuals with traumatic brain injury.[12] Vignettes permit researchers to evaluate responses to a complex circumstance that may better approximate clinical settings than traditional multiple-choice items.

LIKERT-TYPE

Likert-type items, named for their originator, are used to assess the strength of response to a declarative statement. The most typical set of responses includes "strongly agree," "agree," "undecided," "disagree," and "strongly disagree." Many others are available, a few of which are "very important" to "very unimportant," "strongly encourage" to "strongly discourage," and "definitely yes" to "definitely no."[13] Likert-type items (with ratings from "negative effect" to "positive effect") were used by Rozier and colleagues to

determine the perceived impact of various factors (i.e., age, family responsibilities) on the career success of physical therapists.[10]

SEMANTIC DIFFERENTIAL

Semantic differential items are based on the work of Osgood and colleagues in the 1950s.[14] Semantic differential items consist of adjective pairs that represent different ends of a continuum. The respondent indicates the place on the continuum that best represents the item or person being described. If semantic differential items were used to study rehabilitation professionals' opinions about their department, word pairs such as "cohesive–fragmented," "invigorating–dull," and "organized–disorganized" might be used to elicit their opinions. Semantic differential items were used by Streed and Stoecker to assess the levels of stereotyping in physical therapy and occupational therapy students.[15]

Q-SORT

A Q-sort is a method of forced-choice ranking of many alternatives.[16] It could be used to study job satisfaction of rehabilitation professionals. To do so, the researcher would generate a set of, say, 50 items about the job that might be important to rehabilitation professionals. Example items might be "chance to rotate among services," "collegial team relationships," and "availability of support staff." Each item would be written on a single card. Each clinician in the study would be asked to sort the cards into categories based on a preset distribution. For example, for our 50-card sort there might be five categories with the following forced distribution: exceedingly important (four cards), very important (10 cards), moderately important (22 cards), minimally important (10 cards), and of negligible importance (four cards). This distribution would force clinicians to differentiate among a set of job satisfaction items by identifying the very few that are most important as well as the very few that are least important.

Responses could be quantified by assigning numerals to each category (exceedingly important = 5; of negligible importance = 1) and adding the scores for each item across therapists. Items with the highest scores would be those that were consistently placed in the more important categories. Kovach and Krejci used Q-sort methodology to determine the factors that staff members in long-term care facilities perceived were most important in improving care for residents with dementia.[17]

■ IMPLEMENTATION OVERVIEW

There are three classic methods of collecting survey data: personal interviews, telephone interviews, and written questionnaires. An emerging method is to collect survey data through the Internet. Each of these four methods has its advantages and disadvantages, as indicated in Table 16–1.

TABLE 16–1 **Advantages and Disadvantages of Interviews and Questionnaires**

	Method			
Characteristics	Personal Interviews	Telephone Interviews	Mailed Questionnaires	Internet Questionnaires
Time	Very time consuming	Time consuming	Time efficient	Time efficient
Cost	Personnel to conduct interviews, clerical or data entry personnel, travel	Personnel to conduct interviews, clerical or data entry personnel, long-distance telephone	Clerical or data entry personnel, printing and mailing	Internet and e-mail access, survey software
Geographic distribution	Greatly limited unless very well funded	Somewhat limited by long-distance telephone costs	Broad geographic distribution feasible because mailings can reach long distances at low cost	Very broad geographic distribution feasible because of quick world-wide Internet availability
Depth of response	Can be extensive	Somewhat limited	Limited	Limited
Anonymity	Difficult to achieve	Difficult to achieve	Easily achieved	Easily achieved
Literacy of respondents	Can sample those unable to read/write	Can sample those unable to read/write	Respondents must be able to read/write	Respondents must be able to read/write
Ability to clarify questions	Possible	Possible	Difficult, depends on respondent initiative	Difficult, depends on respondent initiative
Scheduling	Must coordinate researchers' and respondents' schedules	Must coordinate researchers' and respondents' schedules	Completed at respondents' convenience	Completed at respondents' convenience
Data entry	By researcher or assistant	By researcher or assistant	By researcher or assistant	By respondents as they complete the questionnaire

Need for Rigor

Survey research is sometimes viewed as an "easy" approach to research—write a few questions, interview participants or mail out questionnaires, and wait for the information to come pouring in. Unfortunately, this view sometimes leads to surveys that are conducted casually and lead to a superficial or distorted understanding of a topic based on the responses of a few. In contrast, well-designed and well-implemented survey research involves meticulous attention to the details of sampling, interview, or questionnaire design; interview implementation or questionnaire distribution; and follow-up. Dillman's classic text on the "total design method" of implementing surveys,[18] Fink and Kosecoff's overview text on conducting surveys,[19] and the *Survey Kit*[20] (a set of 10 slim volumes covering different aspects of survey research) provide prospective researchers with the information needed to implement survey research in rigorous ways to produce valid and reliable information. In addition, survey researchers, just like researchers who study health care interventions,[21] need to attend to the ethical implications of their research, including issues of informed consent, anonymity of responses, and psychological impact of answering sensitive questions. Procedural guidelines for conducting mailed surveys, Internet surveys, and interviews are discussed in the next three main sections of this chapter.

Sample Size and Sampling

One task common to all surveys is the sampling process. First, the population of interest is defined, for example, pediatric physical therapists. Second, the sampling frame is created, for example, physical therapists who belong to the Pediatric Section of the American Physical Therapy Association (APTA) or physical therapists who are board-certified pediatric clinical specialists. Either one of these sampling frames is limited because it will not contain all physical therapists who work with children. In addition, the two sampling frames differ and researchers need to consider which sampling frame best meets their needs—one is larger and includes therapists with an interest in pediatrics, but who may not have much experience or expertise in the area; the other is smaller and includes only those who have undergone a certification process in pediatric physical therapy. In some instances, the population and the sampling frame are the same, and the researcher wishes to study the entire population of interest—in these cases the sampling process is complete after just two steps. This was the case with Sneed and colleagues' study of pediatric physiatrists and training programs,[22] with Domholdt and colleagues' study of physical therapist program directors,[23] and with Sim and Adams' study of therapeutic approaches of occupational therapists and physical therapists in the United Kingdom for individuals with fibromyalgia syndrome.[24] In most instances, though, the sampling frame is much larger than is needed or than is practical, and the researcher must determine how to sample from among the many elements within the sampling frame.

The third step, then, is determining how many responses to the survey are desired. To do so for questionnaires that will result in proportions (e.g., what proportion of pediatric physical therapists work in school systems), the researchers need to determine the level of confidence they wish to have in their results (typically 95%, which corresponds to a Z score of approximately 2), the proportion they expect to answer "yes" to the questions of interest (often simplified to $p = .50$, which maximizes the sample size estimate), and the amount of error they are willing to tolerate in their results.[25] The formula for determining sample size with these factors is:

$$n = \frac{Z^2(p)(1 - p)}{error^2} \qquad \text{(Formula 16–1)}$$

Inserting "2" for the Z and ".05" for the p yields a simplified formula of:

$$n = \frac{1}{error^2} \qquad \text{(Formula 16–2)}$$

A researcher, then, who wishes to estimate a proportion with a 5% error in either direction, would require a sample size of 400:

$$n = \frac{1}{.05^2} = 400 \qquad \text{(Formula 16–3)}$$

A researcher who wants considerably more precision, within 2% in either direction, would require a much larger sample of 2500:

$$n = \frac{1}{.02^2} = 2500 \qquad \text{(Formula 16–4)}$$

When the sample size exceeds 5% to 10% of the size of the population, the sample size can be reduced from these estimates. More detail on sample size determination for surveys can be found in other texts.[25,26]

The fourth step is determining the number of surveys to distribute. Once the desired number of respondents is determined, the researchers must estimate what proportion of individuals will respond to the survey to determine how many surveys must be distributed. If, for example, 400 responses from pediatric physical therapists are desired and a 50% response rate is expected, then 800 surveys must be distributed. The expected response rate is affected by the length of the questionnaire, the connection between researchers and respondents, and the level of interest respondents are expected to have in the topic. A survey on a "hot" topic, studied with a brief questionnaire, by researchers who are known to the respondents, with incentives for respondents, may yield a response rate of 90%. A lengthy, unsolicited survey on an obscure topic from researchers not known to respondents may yield a response rate of 10%.

The final step is determining how to select the prospective respondents from the larger sampling frame. If, for example, there are 4000 pediatric physical therapists in the Pediatric Section of the APTA and we wish to send surveys to 800 of them, then we need to determine how to select the 800 from the 4000. The various probability and nonprobability sampling methods described in Chapter 8 are all possible methods of selecting the sample. When working with organizations that sell mailing labels to researchers, it is often possible to request a random or systematic sample of labels so the researchers do not have to undertake the sampling process themselves. For example, the researcher for our hypothetical study of pediatric physical therapists could purchase a systematic sample of 800 mailing labels for members of the Pediatric Section of the APTA. Clearly, researchers will tailor these general sample size and sampling guidelines to fit the needs of their particular survey.

■ MAILED SURVEYS

Compared with interviews, mailed surveys cost less and permit a broader sampling frame and larger numbers of participants. Despite these advantages, mailed surveys may also have the disadvantages of unavailability of appropriate mailing lists of participants, low response rates, inability to gain information from individuals who cannot read, and lack of control over who actually responds to the questionnaire. Borque and Fielder present the details of conducting mailed surveys in one volume of the *Survey Kit*.[27] This section presents an overview of details related to the following: access to a sampling frame, deciding between researcher-developed and existing self-report instruments, questionnaire development, motivating prospects to respond, and implementation details.

Access to a Sampling Frame

When survey data are collected through a mailed questionnaire, potential participants can often be identified from the mailing lists of various groups. Mailing labels or directories of member addresses are available from sources such as professional associations. For example, when Deen and associates conducted their study of the practice characteristics of occupational therapists working in occupational health settings, they used the membership lists of several state or territorial Occupational Therapy Associations in Australia.[28] A researcher interested in surveying rehabilitation directors at acute care hospitals across the United States might purchase American Hospital Association labels as a route to the appropriate people. When labels are ordered, the researcher can often specify several inclusion and exclusion criteria, as well as ask for a random sampling of labels meeting those criteria. In one step, then, the researcher can define the population, sample from that population, and obtain the labels needed to do the mailing. More details about sampling procedures are provided in Chapter 8.

Researcher-Developed Versus Existing Instruments

Researchers who wish to collect data through survey methods are faced with the question of whether to develop their own questionnaire or use an existing self-report instrument. A literature review should be done to determine what instruments have been used in related studies. Existing instruments that are commercially available and frequently cited in the literature can be identified from references such as the *Mental Measurements Yearbook*[29] and *Tests in Print*.[30] The text *Instruments for Clinical Health Care Research* includes descriptions of existing measures for constructs such as quality of life, coping, hope, self-care, and body image.[31] An instrument that was developed for a single study can often be obtained by writing the researcher. Even if an instrument has been used only once before, there is a base of information about the tool on which subsequent research can build. Researchers are encouraged to use or adapt

existing self-report tools that meet their needs before they develop their own.

Questionnaire Development

When researchers determine that they require unique information for their study, they must develop their own questionnaire. There are five basic steps to questionnaire development: drafting, expert review, first revision, pilot test, and final revision.

DRAFTING

The first step in developing a questionnaire is to draft items for consideration for inclusion in the questionnaire. In some cases, researchers may conduct focus groups or other interview studies to assist with this first step, as was the case in a report of the use of a small focus group to help identify needs of individuals with multiple sclerosis.[32] These needs, along with information found in the literature, were then used as the basis for the development of a written needs assessment questionnaire. Before writing any items, the researcher needs to reexamine the purposes of the study and outline the major sections the questionnaire needs to include to answer the questions under study. Researchers seem to have an almost irresistible urge to ask questions because they seem interesting, without knowing how the answers will be used. This lengthens the questionnaire and may decrease the number of participants who respond. Several authors have provided specific suggestions for questionnaire design and format.[13,18,33]

Even for the first draft, the researcher must begin to consider issues of format and comprehensibility. The items in a questionnaire are often divided into topical groups to break the questionnaire into more easily digestible parts. In addition, because different topics may require items with different formats, the section headings provide for a transition between different types of items. Some recommend that easier items be placed first on the questionnaire, with more difficult items presented later. The thought behind this is that the easy initial questions will get respondents interested in the questionnaire so that they will follow through with the more difficult questions that come later. For similar reasons, some recommend that demographic questions come last. It is thought that completing the demographic questions first will either bore respondents or offend them with questions about sensitive areas such as salary.

The readability of the type used in the questionnaire is important. The smallest readable type is generally considered to be 10-point type. Twelve-point type is more readable and is probably preferable for most questionnaires. If the population is expected to have difficulty with vision or if reading skills are likely to be low, 14-point type may be useful.

The type font is also important; researchers should not use atypical fonts that may be difficult to read. With the widespread availability of personal computers and low-cost desktop publishing services, any researcher should be able to produce an attractive, inviting questionnaire at a reasonable cost.

A second aspect of readability is the reading level required to understand the questionnaire. College-educated researchers are so accustomed to reading and writing that they forget that their writing is likely to be at an academic level that many will not be able to comprehend. To increase readability, researchers should write clearly and avoid jargon.

The instructions on how to complete the survey also must be clear and specific (e.g., "Check one box," "Circle as many items as apply," and "Write in your age in years at your last birthday"). If the same format of questions is used throughout a questionnaire, the instructions need to be given only once. If the format of questions changes from item to item, instructions should be provided for each item.

Researchers designing questionnaires must decide whether to include space for data coding on the questionnaire itself. Data coding is used to turn answers to questions into numbers suitable

for statistical analysis. Figure 16–1 shows an example of a questionnaire page with a data coding column completed, based on a survey conducted by Bashi and Domholdt.[34] Some researchers do not like to include a data-coding column on questionnaires because they believe it is distracting to the respondent and takes up unnecessary space.

The researcher must also consider format and printing decisions such as the color of paper, the size and arrangement of pages, and the amount of white space on the questionnaire. The color of paper should be fairly light to ensure good readability. Good quality paper should be used because it is the first means by which the potential respondent determines whether the questionnaire is worth responding to. One format that has been recommended is a booklet.[18] A four-page questionnaire could be made by printing on both sides of a single sheet of 11- × 17-inch paper and folding it in half to make an 8½- × 11-inch booklet. In such a booklet, because multiple sheets of paper are not needed, none are inadvertently separated from one another. Another benefit is that the familiar booklet form should lead to fewer skipped questions; if single pages are printed front and back and stapled together, the reverse side of one sheet may be omitted by some respondents. The booklet may also have the appearance of being more professional, thereby increasing the return rate for the study.

EXPERT REVIEW

Once the draft is written, the researcher needs to undertake the second step in questionnaire development: subjecting the questionnaire to review by a colleague or colleagues knowledgeable about the topic under study. This is essentially a check for content validity. Did the colleagues think that all the important elements of the constructs under study were addressed? Were questions understandable? Were terms defined satisfactorily? In addition to providing feedback on the content of the questionnaire, colleagues can also assess the format of the questionnaire.

27. At some point during my professional career, utilization of support personnel for patient treatment has presented me with ethical dilemmas. (Circle appropriate letter)

    a.   Strongly agree
    b.   Agree
    c.   Disagree
    (d.) Strongly disagree
    e.   Unable to decide

28. I am comfortable with support personnel involvement in patient treatment at my current job. (Circle appropriate letter)

    a.   Strongly agree
    (b.) Agree
    c.   Disagree
    d.   Strongly disagree
    e.   Unable to decide

29. I am satisfied with professional association guidelines regarding utilization of support personnel in patient treatment. (Circle appropriate letter)

    a.   Strongly agree
    b.   Agree
    c.   Disagree
    d.   Strongly disagree
    (e.) Unable to decide

This column for researcher use only

1. _4_

2. _2_

3. _5_

FIGURE 16–1. Questionnaire excerpt, with coding column. The circled letters are converted to numbers before data entry.
Items modified from a survey described in Bashi HL, Domholdt E. Use of support personnel for physical therapy treatment. *Phys Ther.* 1993;73:421-436.

FIRST REVISION

After the expert review, the researcher makes revisions in the questionnaire based on the feedback. If the selected colleagues make no recommendations for change, the researcher probably needs to identify other colleagues who are willing to be more critical.

PILOT TEST

The next step is to pilot test the instrument on the types of participants who will complete the questionnaire. When pilot testing, it is useful to have participants indicate the time it took them to complete the questionnaire. The final item on

the pilot questionnaire should be a request for the participants to review the questionnaire and write any comments they might have about the nature and format of the items.

When the pilot surveys are returned, the researcher should determine the return rate of the questionnaires and look for troublesome response patterns. For example, if only 40% of the pilot participants return questionnaires, then the researcher should not expect a better return rate from actual participants. The researcher should attempt to determine the reasons for nonresponse to the pilot survey so that corrective measures can be taken on the final questionnaire.

Patterns to be sought among responses to the pilot testing are missing responses, lack of range in responses, many responses in the "other" category, and extraneous comments. For example, if one used several Likert-scale items and all the respondents answered "strongly agree," this may mean the item was worded so positively that no reasonable person would ever disagree with the statement. Rewording should create an item that is more likely to elicit a range of responses. Assume that the purpose of a survey is to determine clinicians' attitudes toward long-term care of the elderly. An item worded "Quality long-term care for the elderly is an important component of the health care system in the United States" would be difficult to disagree with. Rewording the item to read "Funding for long-term care of the elderly should take priority over funding for public education" requires the respondent to make choices between funding priorities and would likely elicit a greater range of responses.

An item repeatedly left unanswered may indicate that placement of the item on the page is a problem, the item is so sensitive that people do not wish to answer it, or the item is so complicated that it takes too much energy to answer it. A multiple-choice item frequently answered with the response category of "other" may indicate that the choices given were too limited.

FINAL REVISION

Rewording of items, elimination of items, addition of items, or revision of the questionnaire format may all be indicated by the results of the pilot study. If a great many problems were identified in the pilot study, the researcher may wish to retest the questionnaire with a new group of pilot participants before investing the money and time in the final questionnaire.

Motivating Prospects to Respond

Once the individuals to whom a questionnaire will be sent are identified, it is the researcher's job to sell them on the idea of completing the questionnaire. The cover letter that accompanies the survey is the major sales tool. It must be attractive, be brief but complete, and provide potential respondents with a good reason to complete the study. Figures 16–2 and 16–3 provide two examples of cover letters annotated with comments on their good and bad points. Other methods of motivating participants are the inclusion of incentives in the initial mailing (e.g., inexpensive, lightweight items like a packet of instant cocoa or a dollar bill), entry into a random drawing for a more valuable incentive when the completed questionnaire is returned, or offering the results of the study when the analysis is complete.

Implementation Details

There are a number of implementation details that need to be planned when conducting a mailed survey: addressing options, envelopes, postage, and follow-up. If the researcher has a choice between printing the address directly on the outer envelope versus using mailing labels, the former has the advantage of appearing to be more individualized. If the questionnaire packet that goes to prospective participants fits in a business-sized envelope, the researcher can choose between enclosing a folded business-sized return envelope or using a slightly smaller return envelope designed to fit flat within a business envelope. The latter option provides for a flatter packet and a more professional look. The budget may dictate whether bulk or first class mailing rates are used to send the questionnaires. Whenever possible, first class mailing should be done, because bulk mail receives lower priority and is often not delivered in a timely fashion. The researcher needs to decide whether to use first class or business-reply postage for return envelopes. First class postage must be affixed to each return envelope with the knowledge that a proportion of the investment in return postage will be lost to nonrespondents. Business-reply postage costs more per envelope than first class postage, but this higher cost is charged only on the returned envelopes.

October 8, 2004

(A)   Dear Program Director:

(B)   We are students in the master's degree program in occupational

      therapy at the University of Anytown. For our research

      project we are studying the content of occupational therapy

(C)   curriculums in geriatrics to determine whether enough

      attention is paid to geriatrics education for occupational

      therapists. Please complete this survey and return it to us

(D)   at the following address by October 15, 2004:

      University of Anytown

(E)   1256 Holt Road

      Anytown, IN   46234

(F)   Thank you for your participation. If you would like a

      summary of the results, please write your name and address

      on the last page of the survey.

      Sincerely,

(G)

(H)   Jodi Beeker   Jonathon Mills

      Occupational Therapy Student   Occupational Therapy Student

FIGURE 16–2. Example of a poor cover letter for a questionnaire. (A) There is no personalization of greeting to potential respondents. (B) When the first sentence indicates that the researchers are students, potential respondents may assume that the research is being done only because it is required. (C) The second sentence indicates a bias on the part of the researchers. (D) Because of the early return date, the potential respondents might not receive the questionnaire until 1 or 2 days before the deadline. (E) The researchers have obviously not included a self-addressed, stamped return envelope and are asking potential respondents to bear part of the cost of the study. (F) The mechanism for respondents to indicate their interest in the study results destroys the anonymity of the questionnaire. (G) Lack of signatures (or photocopied signatures) indicates an impersonal approach to potential respondents. (H) There is no way, other than through the mail, to contact the student researchers if the potential respondent has questions about the study.

(A)   ***University of Anytown***
      1256 Holt Road   *Anytown, Indiana 46234*
      Department of Occupational Therapy   *(317) 555-4300*

October 8, 2004

Elizabeth Wagner, OTR, EdD
Director, Department of Occupational Therapy
University of the Southwest
1400 SW Main Street
College Town, AZ 88735

(B)   Dear Dr. Wagner:

(C)   We are requesting your participation in a survey of occupational therapy programs in the
      United States to determine the characteristics of geriatric education within occupational
      therapy curriculums. We know that directors of occupational therapy education programs are
      faced with dilemmas about the breadth and depth of content that should be included in
      today's overcrowded occupational therapy curriculums. We believe that a compilation
      of information about geriatrics curriculum content will be helpful to occupational therapy
(D)   educators as they determine the amount of emphasis they wish to place on geriatric
      education within their own curriculums.

(E)   In pilot testing, the enclosed questionnaire took an average of less than 10 minutes to
      complete. We would greatly appreciate your time in completing the questionnaire and
(F)   returning it in the enclosed envelope by **November 8, 2004**. If you would like a copy of
      the results, please complete the enclosed postcard and return it separately from the
(G)   questionnaire.

      Thank you in advance for your consideration. If you have any questions or concerns
      about the study, please feel free to contact any of us at the address or telephone
      numbers listed.

      Sincerely,

(H)   *Jodi Beeker*   *Jon Mills*   *Jan Woolery*
      Jodi Beeker   Jon Mills   Jan Woolery, OTR, PhD
      OT Student   OT Student   Associate Professor
(I)   (317) 555-4321   (317) 555-6789   (317) 555-4378

FIGURE 16–3. Example of a good cover letter for a questionnaire. (A) Letterhead paper
is used to indicate affiliation of the researchers. (B) The greeting is personalized.
(C) Introductory paragraph is neutral on the subject matter. (D) The last sentence of the
introductory paragraph indicates the usefulness of findings; this provides a reason for
completing the questionnaire. (E) The time required of respondents is indicated.
(F) The return date gives respondents a few weeks to reply. (G) The mechanism for
obtaining survey results does not violate the anonymity of responses. (H) Signing each
cover letter individually provides a personal touch. (I) Telephone numbers for students
and the name and telephone number of a responsible faculty member provide a mechanism by which potential respondents can contact them about the survey.

The researcher needs to compare costs between these postage options, assuming various return rates, to make a good decision about which option will be more cost effective.

Plans for follow-up mailings, if needed to achieve the desired return rate, need to be made in advance of the first mailing. To provide for the possibility of following up nonrespondents, the researcher numbers the master list of participants and in the envelope going to each participant places a return envelope or postcard with that participant's number on it. If the numbering is done on the return envelope, the corresponding participant is crossed off when their numbered envelope is returned, then the questionnaire and envelope are separated from one another, and the envelope with the identifying information is discarded and never associated with the corresponding questionnaire. This maintains the confidentiality of participant responses, but depends on researcher integrity to do so.

A postcard system for follow-up maintains even greater anonymity. A numbered postcard is included with the questionnaire packet, and the participant is instructed to mail the postcard and questionnaire back separately so that the questionnaire and participant number will never be directly linked as they are if the return envelope is coded. However, a postcard system increases mailing and printing costs and participants may forget to mail the postcard.

If the return rate is lower than desired by a week to 10 days after the first responses were due, a second mailing to nonrespondents should be done. This follow-up packet should contain a new cover letter and a duplicate copy of the questionnaire. It is often appropriate to differentiate between first and second returns so that one can check to see whether there is a difference of opinions between those who initially responded and those who required a second prodding. This can be done by using a different-colored questionnaire for the follow-up mailing or by making an inconspicuous mark on all the questionnaires sent with the second mailing. If the first respondents were positive and the second respondents somewhat more negative

on the issues studied, this is an indication that overall opinion may not be as positive as that of the initial respondents.

One specialized questionnaire approach, the *Delphi technique,* assumes that several mailings will go to all participants. This technique uses several rounds of questionnaires that compensate for some of the limitations of administration of a single questionnaire. The Delphi technique was designed as a consensus-generating technique that eliminates the interpersonal factors that influence group decisions made in traditional meetings. These factors include the undue influence of a dominant personality and the willingness of less vocal members to acquiesce for the sake of achieving consensus.[35]

In a Delphi study, respondents complete and return a first-round questionnaire. A group of experts evaluates the first-round responses and compiles results; the results are returned to the respondents for review and comment (the second round). The experts review the second-round responses and compile results; again, the results are sent back to the respondents for a third round. This iterative sequence is repeated until the responses from a round are consistent with the responses of the previous round. Ingram used a Delphi approach to determine physical therapist educational program directors' opinions about essential functions for physical therapy students.[36]

■ INTERNET SURVEYS

The widespread availability of the Internet has given rise to the phenomenon of Internet-administered surveys. Internet surveys become feasible when a high proportion of the population of interest is likely to have Internet access and known e-mail addresses. For example, Domholdt and colleagues conducted an Internet-based Spring 2003 follow-up[37] to their mailed Spring 2000 survey of physical therapist program directors.[23] Because all of the physical therapist program directors have known e-mail addresses, the Internet format did not exclude any potential respondents.

Once researchers determine that an Internet-based survey is appropriate, they need to give the same careful consideration to questionnaire design, distribution, and follow-up that would be given to a mailed survey.[38] The most basic way to conduct an Internet-based survey is to send an e-mail to a group of respondents, with the questionnaire embedded within the e-mail. Respondents hit the reply button, fill out their answers within the return e-mail, and send back to the researcher. This process is fraught with difficulties, the most notable being that item formats do not translate well from researcher to respondent and anonymity of responses cannot be maintained.

Survey software products solve most of these problems. Typically, they consist of a questionnaire generation tool, mass e-mailing and follow-up capabilities, and database creation. Using the questionnaire generation tool, the researcher creates an attractive questionnaire from a menu of different types of items. The mailing features permit the researcher to send a cover e-mail to the survey sample, with an embedded link that takes the prospective respondent to the Internet site where the survey is available for completion. When a response is submitted, the researcher does not know the e-mail address from which it came, preserving anonymity for respondents. The more sophisticated products maintain a separate list of respondents, not linked to their responses, so that follow-up of nonrespondents can occur. The survey responses are placed in a database, which the researcher can typically download into a spreadsheet or statistical analysis program, eliminating the data entry task typically associated with a survey. A variety of products for constructing and administering Internet-based surveys are available—they range from inexpensive products with little support[39] to more expensive products with a great deal of support for researchers.[40,41]

Commonly cited advantages to Internet surveys are that they are useful with specific populations who have nearly universal access to the Internet, they require less time for responses and follow-up communication, they eliminate the need for manual data entry, they are convenient for the respondent, they have wide geographic coverage, and they can maintain anonymity of the survey.[42] Limitations of Internet surveys are that selection is biased to those with Internet access, there may be no e-mail address directory for some populations, there may be technological difficulties, and the survey may be seen as intrusive by some Internet users.[42] Researchers considering an Internet survey need to weigh these advantages and limitations in the context of their particular study—just as they have always weighed the advantages and limitations of conducting surveys through personal interviews, telephone interviews, or mailed surveys.

■ INTERVIEW SURVEYS

Compared with mailed and Internet surveys, interviews can achieve greater depth of response, maintain control over who actually responds, determine the opinions of those who cannot read, and may have higher response rates. Even so, interviews may also have the disadvantages of difficulty coordinating researcher and participant schedules; lack of anonymity of responses; and high personnel, travel, or telephone costs. The details of implementing telephone[43] and in-person interview[44] surveys are presented in two volumes of the *Survey Kit*. The following sections of this chapter present an overview of details related to access to prospective participants, development of the interview schedule, motivating prospects to participate, and implementation.

Access to Prospective Participants

Because of the high cost of interviews, their use is often confined to studies that require fewer participants in well-defined groups. Examples include studies of patient satisfaction with care delivered at a single location, and opinions and attitudes of students who have participated in a particular education program. Because of the focused nature of many interview studies, the need to purchase extensive lists of names, addresses, and telephone numbers is not needed, because the researcher already has access to the prospective participants. When polling of the general population is done by telephone, a variety of techniques for random digit dialing is used. As was the case with mailed questionnaires, it may be appropriate to sample from a larger population of eligible participants, according to the various procedures outlined earlier in Chapter 8.

Development of Interview Schedules

Many researchers who use interviews to collect data ask questions that they have developed themselves. The researcher must decide whether structured, semistructured, or unstructured interviews are appropriate based on the nature of information desired. Details about interview styles are discussed in Chapter 13.

When conducting a survey with interviews, the "interview schedule" is the corollary to the mailed questionnaire in mail surveys. The basic steps of drafting, reviewing, revising, and pilot testing are completed as they would be when developing a mailed questionnaire. The interview schedule needs to be formatted so that the sequence of items, along with instructions and explanatory text, is clear. If the interviews are highly structured, the instructions are usually expanded into scripts with a conversational tone. If the data are to be collected through telephone interviews, each question must be relatively simple so that respondents can comprehend all their response choices without a visual cue. In-person interviews can include more complex questions if visual aids are provided for respondents. Limperopoulos and Majnemer conducted a structured telephone survey of rehabilitation specialists (occupational therapists, physical therapists, and speech-language pathologists) at all Canadian hospitals with tertiary care neonatal

intensive care units (NICUs) to determine their roles in the NICU.[45] The 13-item interview consisting of mostly fixed response items yielded a response rate of 100%.

Motivating Prospects to Participate

When implementing mailed or Internet surveys, the cover letter or cover e-mail to the survey serves as the main tool for motivating participants to participate. In interview surveys, this same function can be served by advance letters, precalls, or introductory scripts. An advance letter outlines the purposes of the study and the requirements for participation, and notifies prospective participants how they will be contacted to determine their willingness to participate. The same general guidelines for effective cover letters for mailed surveys apply to advance letters for interview surveys. Sometimes a precall (either by telephone or in person) is used instead of a letter. This allows the interviewer to answer any questions the prospective participant may have, to secure the participant's consent, and to schedule a time for the interview. In large-scale telephone surveys, the first few sentences uttered by the interviewer may be the only "advance" notice that participants have of the study. Because many people routinely refuse to interact with telephone solicitors, researchers must develop an introductory script that clearly and quickly differentiates the study call from the many sales calls received by prospective participants.

Once a participant has agreed to participate in the study, the interviewer's role becomes one of keeping participants at ease to maximize their responses to questions and to motivate and engage them to provide thoughtful, accurate responses.

Implementation Details

Implementation details of concern to researchers conducting interview surveys include securing a location for calling or interviewing in person, providing for the comfort of in-person participants, maintaining appropriate supplies, training interviewers, and tracking contacts with prospective participants.

The location for telephone interviews needs to include a quiet environment so that the interviewer can hear participants and give them their full attention. If many interviewers are being used, a centralized calling area that enables the researcher to monitor the quality of the calls and answer questions as they arise is helpful. If in-person interviews take place on the participant's "turf," then the interviewer needs to be prompt. If the interviews are being conducted at, for example, the interviewer's office, then a receptionist should be available to greet arriving participants or take calls from participants who will be late or unable to keep their appointment. The comfort of participants should be taken into account by providing a comfortable seating area, an appropriate arrangement of interviewer and participant, and making water or soft drinks available during the interview.

The interviewer needs to be prepared with an adequate supply of paper and working pens or pencils. If the interviews are to be recorded, the interviewer needs to be familiar with the recording equipment and ensure that the supply of tapes and batteries is adequate to meet the needs of the day.

When several interviewers are used within a study, the primary researcher needs to provide for their training. An interviewer manual should be developed and ought to include information on interviewing techniques and guidelines, the responsibilities of the interviewers, the rationale for interview questions, and a complete set of forms and procedures. The training process should include demonstration of good interview techniques, practice interviews, and observation and feedback to new interviewers.

■ SUMMARY

Surveys are systems for collecting self-reported information from participants. In general, the term "survey research" is applied to nonexperimental research with prospective data collection. Self-report instruments can be used to collect facts, determine knowledge, describe behavior, determine opinion, or document personal characteristics. Self-report instruments can include open- and closed-format items. Closed-format items include multiple-choice items, Likert-type scales, semantic differentials, and Q-sorts. Sound survey design requires meticulous attention to the details of sampling, interview, or questionnaire design; interview implementation or questionnaire distribution; and follow-up. The advantages and disadvantages of personal interviews, telephone interviews, mailed questionnaires, or Internet questionnaires must be considered when determining the method of data collection.

REFERENCES

1. Fink A. *The Survey Handbook, The Survey Kit, Volume 1.* 2nd ed. Thousand Oaks, Calif: Sage Publications; 2003.
2. Chevan J, Chevan A. A statistical profile of physical therapists, 1980 and 1990. *Phys Ther.* 1998;78:301-312.
3. Balogun JA, Kaplan MT, Miller TM. The effect of professional education on the knowledge and attitudes of physical therapist and occupational therapist students about acquired immunodeficiency syndrome. *Phys Ther.* 1998;78:1073-1082.
4. Hagberg K, Brånemark R. Consequences of non-vascular trans-femoral amputation: a survey of quality of life, prosthetic use and problems. *Prosthet Orthot Int.* 2001;25:186-194.
5. Nadler SF, Prybicien M, Malanga GA, Sicher D. Complications from therapeutic modalities: results of a national survey of athletic trainers. *Arch Phys Med Rehabil.* 2003;84:849-853.
6. Wagner AK, Stewart PJB. An internship for college students in physical medicine and rehabilitation: effects on awareness, career choice, and disability perceptions. *Am J Phys Med Rehabil.* 2001;80:459-465.
7. Tepe ES, Deutsch ES, Sampson Q, Lawless S, Reilly JS, Sataloff RT. A pilot survey of vocal health in young singers. *J Voice.* 2002;16:244-250.
8. Tharpe AM, Fino-Szumski MS, Bess FJ. Survey of hearing aid fitting practices for children with multiple impairments. *Am J Audiol.* 2001;10:32-40.
9. Rubery PT, Bradford DS. Athletic activity after spine surgery in children and adolescents. *Spine.* 2002;27:423-427.
10. Rozier CK, Raymond MJ, Goldstein MS, Hamilton BL. Gender and physical therapy career success factors. *Phys Ther.* 1998;78:690-704.

11. Colón-Emeric C, Yballe L, Sloane R, Pieper CF, Lyles KW. Expert physician recommendations and current practice patterns for evaluating and treating men with osteoporotic hip fracture. *J Am Geriatr Soc.* 2000;48:1261-1263.

12. Hasenbein U, Kuss O, Baumer M, Schert C, Schneider H, Wallesch CW. Physicians' preferences and expectations in traumatic brain injury rehabilitation—results of a case-based questionnaire survey. *Disabil Rehab.* 2003;25: 136-142.

13. Fink A. *How to Ask Survey Questions, The Survey Kit, Volume 2.* 2nd ed. Thousand Oaks, Calif: Sage Publications; 2003.

14. Osgood CE, Suci GJ, Tannenbaum PH. *The Measurement of Meaning.* Urbana, Ill: University of Illinois Press; 1957.

15. Streed CP, Stoecker JL. Stereotyping between physical therapy students and occupational therapy students. *Phys Ther.* 1991;71:16-24.

16. Stephenson W. *The Study of Behavior: Q Technique and Its Methodology.* Chicago, Ill: University of Chicago Press; 1975.

17. Kovach CR, Krejci JW. Facilitating change in dementia care: staff perceptions. *J Nurs Adm.* 1998;28:17-27.

18. Dillman DA. *Mail and Telephone Surveys: The Total Design Method.* New York, NY: John Wiley & Sons; 1978.

19. Fink A, Kosecoff J. *How To Conduct Surveys: A Step-By-Step Guide.* Thousand Oaks, Calif: Sage Publications; 1998.

20. Fink A, ed. *The Survey Kit.* 2nd ed. Thousand Oaks, Calif: Sage Publications; 2003.

21. Evans M, Robling M, Maggs Rapport F, Houston H, Kinnersley P, Wilkinson C. It doesn't cost anything to ask, does it? The ethics of questionnaire-based research. *J Med Ethics.* 2002;28:41-44.

22. Sneed RC, May WL, Stencel C, Paul SM. Pediatric physiatry in 2000: a survey of practitioners and training programs. *Arch Phys Med Rehabil.* 2002;83:416-422.

23. Domholdt E, Stewart JC, Barr JO, Melzer BA. Entry-level doctoral degrees in physical therapy: status as of Spring 2000. *J Phys Ther Educ.* 2002;16:60-68.

24. Sim J, Adams N. Therapeutic approaches to fibromyalgia syndrome in the United Kingdom: a survey of occupational therapists and physical therapists. *Eur J Pain.* 2002;7:173-180.

25. *Survey Research Using SPSS.* Chicago, Ill: SPSS, Inc; 1998.

26. Fink A. *How to Sample in Surveys, The Survey Kit, Volume 7.* 2nd ed. Thousand Oaks, Calif: Sage Publications; 2003.

27. Borque LB, Fielder EP. *How to Conduct Self-Administered and Mail Surveys, The Survey Kit, Volume 3.* 2nd ed. Thousand Oaks, Calif: Sage Publications; 2003.

28. Deen M, Gibson L, Strong J. A survey of occupational therapy in Australian work practice. *Work.* 2002;19: 219-230.

29. Plake BS, Impara JC, Spies RA, Pale BS, eds. *The Fifteenth Mental Measurements Yearbook.* Lincoln, Neb.: Buros Institute of Mental Measurements of the University of Nebraska-Lincoln; 2003.

30. Murphy LL, Plake BS, Impara JC, Spies RA, eds. *Tests in Print VI.* Lincoln, Neb: Buros Institute of Mental Measurements of the University of Nebraska-Lincoln; 2002.

31. Frank-Stromborg M, Olsen SJ. *Instruments for Clinical Health Care Research.* 2nd ed. Sudbury, Mass: Jones & Bartlett Publishers; 1997.

32. Koopman W. Needs assessment of persons with multiple sclerosis and significant others: using the literature review and focus groups for preliminary survey questionnaire development. *Axon.* 2003;24:10-15.

33. Peterson RA. *Constructing Effective Questionnaires.* Thousand Oaks, Calif: Sage Publications; 2000.

34. Bashi HL, Domholdt E. Use of support personnel for physical therapy treatment. *Phys Ther.* 1993;73:421-436.

35. Goodman CM. The Delphi technique: a critique. *J Adv Nurs.* 1987;12:729-734.

36. Ingram D. Opinions of physical therapy education program directors on essential functions. *Phys Ther.* 1997;77:37-45.

37. Domholdt E, Kerr LR, Mount KA. Entry-level doctoral degrees in physical therapy: status as of Spring 2003. In preparation.

38. Dillman D. *Mail and Internet Surveys: A Tailored Design Method.* New York, NY: Wiley; 2000.

39. *Survey Suite.* Available at: *http://intercom.virginia.edu/ cgibin/cgiwrap/intercom/SurveySuite/ss_wizard.pl.* Accessed August 10, 2003.

40. *Survey Share.* Available at: *http://www.surveyshare.com.* Accessed August 10, 2003.

41. *Survey Solutions.* Available at: *http://www.perseusdevelopment.com.* Accessed August 10, 2003.

42. Klein J. Issues surrounding the use of the Internet for data collection. *Am J Occup Ther.* 2002;56:340-343.

43. Borque LB, Fielder EP. *How to Conduct Telephone Surveys, The Survey Kit, Volume 4.* Thousand Oaks, Calif: Sage Publications; 2003.

44. Oishi SM. *How to Conduct In-Person Interviews for Surveys, The Survey Kit, Volume 5.* Thousand Oaks, Calif: Sage Publications; 2003.

45. Limperopoulos C, Majnemer A. The role of rehabilitation specialists in Canadian NICUs: a national survey. *Phys Occup Ther Pediatr.* 2002;22:57-72.

Measurement

Measurement Theory

Rehabilitation professionals use measurements to help them decide what is wrong with patients or clients, how to intervene, and when to discontinue treatment. Health care insurers rely on these measurements when they make decisions about whether to reimburse for rehabilitation services. Researchers use measurements to quantify the characteristics they study. In fact, some investigators focus the majority of their research on the evaluation of rehabilitation measures. However, knowledge about the usefulness of measurements is not reserved for these research specialists—clinicians also need to understand the meaning and usefulness of the measures they use.

This chapter presents a framework for understanding and evaluating the measurements used by rehabilitation professionals. It does this by presenting several definitions of measurement, discussing scales of measurement and types of variables, introducing the statistical concepts required to understand measurement theory, and discussing measurement reliability, validity, and responsiveness to change. Chapter 18 builds on this framework by presenting strategies for conducting research about measurements.

■ DEFINITIONS OF MEASUREMENT

The broadest definition of measurement is that it is "the process by which things are differentiated."[1] A narrower definition is that measurement "consists of rules for assigning numbers to objects in such a way as to represent quantities of attributes."[2] According to the first definition, classification of patients into diagnostic groups is a form of measurement; according to the second definition, it is not. This text uses the broader definition of measurement, with the addition of one qualification: measurement is the *systematic* process by which things are differentiated. Thus, this definition emphasizes that measurement is not a random process, but one that proceeds according to rules and guidelines.

Differentiation can be accomplished with names, numerals, or numbers. For example, classifying people as underweight, normal weight, or overweight involves the assignment of names to differentiate people according to the characteristic of ideal body composition. If these groups are relabeled as Groups 1, 2, and 3 or Groups I, II, and III, then each person is assigned a numeral to represent body composition. A *numeral* is a symbol that does not necessarily have quantitative meaning[3(p392)]; it is a form of naming. Describing people not by groups but by their specific percentage of body fat (e.g., 10% or 14%) would involve the assignment of a number to represent the quantity of body fat. A *number,* then, is a numeral that has been assigned quantitative meaning.

■ SCALES OF MEASUREMENT

Four classic scales, or levels, of measurement are presented in the literature. These scales are based on the extent to which a measure has the properties of a real-number system. A real-number system is characterized by order, distance, and origin.[4(p12)] *Order* means that higher numbers represent greater amounts of the characteristic being measured. *Distance* means that the magnitude of the differences between successive numbers is equal. *Origin* means that the number zero represents an absence of the measured quality.

Nominal Scales

Nominal scales have none of the properties of a real-number system. A nominal scale provides classification without placing any value on the categories within the classification. Because there is no order, distance, or origin to the classification, the classification can be identified by name or numeral. However, it is often better to give classifications names instead of numerals so that no quantitative difference between categories is implied. Classification of patients with cerebral palsy into quadriplegic, diplegic, and hemiplegic categories is an example of a nominal measurement. The classification itself does not rank, for example, the functional impairment of the individual—that depends on level of spasticity, intellectual functioning, and a host of other factors not implied by the classification itself.

Ordinal Scales

Ordinal scales have only one of the three properties of a real-number system: order. Thus, an ordinal scale can be used to indicate whether a person or object has more or less of a certain quality. Ordinal scales do not ensure that there are equal intervals between categories or ranks. Because the intervals on an ordinal scale are either not known or are unequal, mathematical manipulations such as addition, subtraction, multiplication, or division of ordinal numbers are not meaningful.

Many functional scales are ordinal. The amount of assistance a patient needs to ambulate is often rated as maximal, moderate, minimal, standby, or independent. Is the interval between maximal and moderate assistance the same as the interval between minimal and standby assistance? Probably not. Sometimes numerals are assigned to points on an ordinal scale, but the validity of this procedure has been questioned because the numerals are often treated as if they were quantitative numbers.[5]

Figure 17–1 illustrates the phenomenon of nonequal intervals between points on an ordinal scale of gait independence. Assume that the underlying quantity represented by the assistance categories is the proportion of the total work of ambulation that is exerted by the patient. If the patient and clinician are expending equal energy to get the patient walking, then the patient is exerting 50% of the total work of ambulation. If the patient is independent and the clinician does not need to expend any energy, then the patient is exerting 100% of the total work of ambulation. The top line of Figure 17–1 shows the assistance categories. The middle two lines show numerals that could be assigned to the assistance categories. Either set of numerals would meet the order criterion—higher numerals indicate higher levels of independence. The magnitude of the two sets of numerals varies greatly and shows the danger of thinking

of ordinal numbers as real quantities. The bottom scale shows how the assistance categories might fall along a continuum of total work percentage. The categories "minimal," "standby," and "independent," as used by most clinicians, probably fall in the top 20% of the scale. The categories "maximal" and "moderate" probably fall in the bottom 80% of the scale. Thus, the gait independence classification used by clinicians is clearly an ordinal scale: the classification has order but does not represent equal intervals of the underlying construct that is being measured.

A second type of ordinal scale is a ranking. During 2003, sisters Serena Williams and Venus Williams were the first- and second-ranked women tennis players in the world, respectively. Although the interval between these two players was slight, the difference between the second-ranked and third-ranked players was much greater. The intervals between ranks are usually unknown and cannot be assumed to be equal.

Interval Scales

Interval scales have the real-number system properties of order and distance, but they lack a meaningful origin. A meaningful zero point

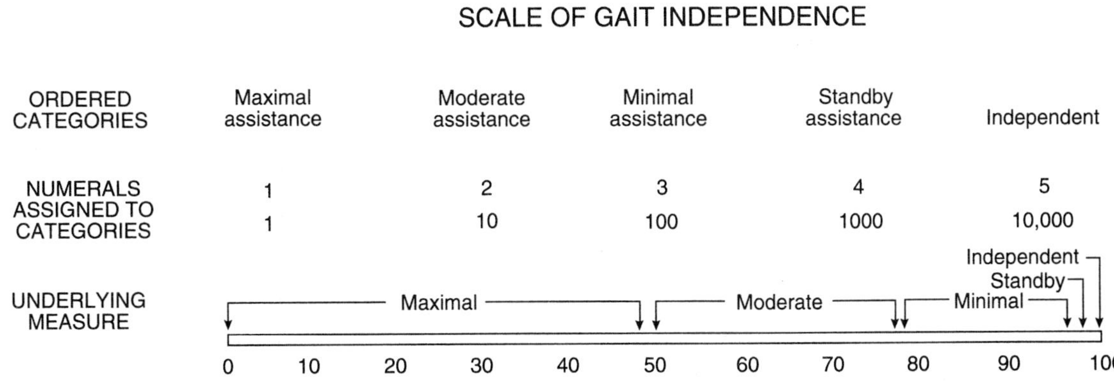

SCALE OF GAIT INDEPENDENCE

ORDERED CATEGORIES	Maximal assistance	Moderate assistance	Minimal assistance	Standby assistance	Independent
NUMERALS ASSIGNED TO CATEGORIES	1	2	3	4	5
	1	10	100	1000	10,000

UNDERLYING MEASURE

```
              |———— Maximal ————|  |—— Moderate ——|  |— Minimal
0   10   20   30   40   50   60   70   80   90   100
```

Independent ⌐
Standby ⌐
Minimal ⌐

FIGURE 17–1. Level of assistance in gait as an ordinal measurement. The top row shows the assistance categories as used by many clinicians. The bottom row shows a theoretical underlying distribution of the categories based on what percentage of effort is being exerted by the patient. The middle two rows show two vastly different numbering schemes; in both schemes the numbers get larger as the amount of effort exerted by the patient increases.

represents the absence of the measured quantity. The Celsius and Fahrenheit temperature scales are examples of interval scales. The zero points on the two temperature scales are arbitrary: On the Fahrenheit scale it is the temperature at which salt water freezes, and on the Celsius scale it is the temperature at which fresh water freezes. Neither implies the absence of the basic property of heat—the temperature can go lower than zero on both scales. Both scales, however, have regular (but different) intervals. Because of the equal intervals, addition and subtraction are meaningful with interval scales. A 10° increase in temperature means the same thing whether the increase is from 0° to 10° or from 100° to 110°. However, multiplication and division of Fahrenheit or Celsius temperature readings are not useful because these operations assume knowledge of zero quantities. A Fahrenheit temperature of 100° is not twice as hot as a temperature of 50°; it is merely 50° hotter.

Ratio Scales

Ratio scales exhibit all three components of a real-number system: order, distance, and origin. All the arithmetic functions of addition, subtraction, multiplication, and division can be applied to ratio scales. Length, time, and weight are generally considered ratio scales because their absence is scored as zero, and the intervals between numbers are known to be equal. The Kelvin temperature scale is an example of a ratio scale because the intervals between degrees are equal and the zero point represents the absence of heat.

Determining the Scale of a Measurement

To determine the scale of a measure, the researcher must ascertain whether there is a true zero (origin), whether intervals between numbers are equal (distance), and whether there is an order to the numbers or names that constitute the measure (order). Although this

sounds simple enough, a number of twists come into play when determining the scale of a measurement.

For example, does the classification of patients as underweight, normal weight, and overweight represent a nominal or ordinal scale? The numbers are placed into classes, but these classes also have an order. As another example, do scores on the Sickness Impact Profile (SIP), represent ordinal or interval data? Summed scales, that is, those scored by summing the values of responses on many questions, are often treated as interval scales even though it can be argued that the underlying construct being measured is too abstract to permit the assumption that intervals between scores are equal. When ordinal scales can take many values (e.g., with a summed score that can range from 0 to 100 as opposed to a gait assistance scale with only five values), data may have the mathematical characteristics of an interval scale. Because the scale of measurement determines which mathematical manipulations are meaningful, controversy about measurement scales soon becomes controversy about which statistical tests are appropriate for which types of measures. These statistical controversies are discussed in Chapter 20.

■ TYPES OF VARIABLES

With respect to measurement, variables can be classified as continuous or discrete. A *discrete* variable is one that can assume only distinct values. Nominal scale variables are, by definition, discrete: The individuals being classified must fit into a distinct category; they cannot be placed between the categories. Discrete variables that can assume only two values are called *dichotomous* variables. Examples of dichotomous variables are sex (male vs. female) or disease state (present vs. absent). Variables that are counts of behaviors or persons are discrete variables because fractional people or behaviors are not possible. If the measure of interest is the number of times a child names an object correctly in 10 trials, it is not possible to get a score of 7.5 on a single trial. Note, however, that it is possible to have an *average* score of 7.5 if the 10-trial sequence is repeated on 4 subsequent days with scores of 8, 6, 9, and 7 (8 + 6 + 9 + 7 = 30; 30/4 = 7.5). If discrete variables can assume a fairly large range of values, have the properties of a real-number system, or are averaged across trials, then they become similar to continuous variables.

A *continuous* variable is one that theoretically can be measured to a finer and finer degree.[4(p15)] Clinicians interested in hand function might record the time it takes for someone to transfer 25 objects from one tray to another. Depending on the sophistication of the measurement tools, the clinician might measure time to the nearest second or to the nearest one-thousandth of a second. If the smallest increment on a clinician's watch is the second, then measurements cannot be recorded in smaller increments even though the clinician knows that the true time required for completion of a task is not limited to whole seconds. Thus, the limits of technology dictate that continuous variables will always be measured discretely.

■ STATISTICAL FOUNDATIONS OF MEASUREMENT THEORY

Seven basic concepts underlie most of measurement theory: frequency distribution, mean, variance, standard deviation, normal curve, correlation coefficient, and standard error of measurement (SEM). These concepts are introduced here and are expanded upon in Chapters 19 and 22.

Frequency Distribution

A *frequency distribution* is nothing more than the number of times each score is represented in the data set. If a therapist measures a patient's knee flexion 10 times during 1 day, the following scores might be obtained: 100, 100, 90, 95, 110, 110, 95, 105, 95, 100. Table 17–1 and Figure 17–2 show two ways of presenting the frequency distribution for these 10 scores.

TABLE 17–1	Frequency Distribution of 10 Knee Flexion Measurements
Score	**Frequency**
90	1
95	3
100	3
105	1
110	2

Mean

The arithmetic *mean* of a data set is the sum of the observations divided by the number of observations. Mathematical notation for the mean is:

$$\overline{X} = \frac{\Sigma X}{N}$$ (Formula 17–1)

$\overline{X}$ is the symbol for the sample mean and is sometimes called "X-bar." Σ is the uppercase Greek letter sigma and means "the sum of." X is the symbol for each observation. N is the symbol for the number of observations. In words, the mean equals the sum of all the observations divided by the number of observations. The mean of the data set presented earlier is calculated as follows:

$$\overline{X} = (90 + 95 + 95 + 95 + 100 + 100$$
$$+ 100 + 105 + 110 + 110)/10 = 100$$

The population mean, μ, is calculated the same way, but is rarely used in practice because researchers do not have access to the entire population.

Variance

The *variance* is a measure of the variability around the mean within a data set. To calculate

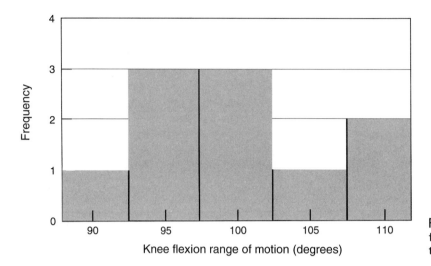

FIGURE 17–2. Histogram of the frequency distribution of hypothetical knee flexion data.

the variance, a researcher converts each of the raw scores in a data set to a deviation score by subtracting the mean of the data set from each raw score. In mathematical notation,

$$x = X - \overline{X} \qquad \text{(Formula 17–2)}$$

The lowercase italic x is the symbol for a deviation score. The *deviation score* indicates how high or low a raw score is compared with the mean. The first two columns of Table 17–2 present the raw and deviation scores for the knee flexion data set, followed by their sums and means. Note that both the sum and the mean of the deviation scores are zero. In order to generate a nonzero index of the variability within a data set, the deviation scores must be squared. The variance is then calculated by determining the mean of the squared deviations. In mathematical notation,

$$\sigma^2 = \frac{\Sigma x^2}{N} \qquad \text{(Formula 17–3)}$$

σ is the lowercase Greek sigma and when squared is the notation for the population variance. The third column in Table 17–2 shows the squared deviations from the group mean, the sum of the squared deviations, and the mean of

	X	**x**	**x²**	**z score**
	90	−10	100	−1.59
	95	−5	25	−.79
	95	−5	25	−.79
	95	−5	25	−.79
	100	0	0	0
	100	0	0	0
	100	0	0	0
	105	+5	25	+.79
	110	+10	100	+1.59
	110	+10	100	+1.59
Σ	1000	0	400	
μ	100	0	40.0 = σ², variance	

TABLE 17–2 Computation of the Variance in the 10 Knee Flexion Measurements

the squared deviations. The variance is the mean of the squared deviation scores. In practice there are different symbols and slightly different formulas for the variance, depending on whether the observations represent the entire population of interest or just a sample of the population. This distinction is addressed in Chapter 19.

Although the variance is useful in many statistical procedures, it does not have a great deal of intuitive meaning because it is calculated from squared deviation scores. A measure that does have intuitive meaning is the standard deviation.

Standard Deviation

The *standard deviation* is the square root of the variance and is expressed in the units of the original measure:

$$\sigma = \sqrt{\sigma^2} = \sqrt{\frac{\Sigma x^2}{N}} \qquad \text{(Formula 17–4)}$$

The mathematical notations for the standard deviation and the variance make their relationship clear: The notation for the variance (σ^2) is simply the square of the notation for standard deviation (σ). The standard deviation of the knee flexion data presented in Table 17–2 is the square root of 40, or 6.3°.

Normal Curve

Groups of measurements frequently approximate a bell-shaped distribution known as the normal curve. The *normal curve* is a symmetric frequency distribution that can be defined in terms of the mean and standard deviation of a set of data. Any raw score within the distribution can be converted into a *z score,* which indicates how many standard deviations the raw score is above or below the mean. A z score is calculated by subtracting the mean from the raw score, creating a deviation score, and then dividing the deviation score by the standard deviation:

$$z = \frac{x}{\sigma} \qquad \text{(Formula 17–5)}$$

The fourth column of Table 17–2 shows each raw score as a z score. Raw scores were transformed into z scores by dividing each of the deviation scores (x) by the standard deviation

of 6.3°. The z score tells us, for example, that a measurement of 90° is 1.59 standard deviations below the mean.

In a normal distribution, 68.27% of the scores fall within 1 standard deviation above or below the mean, 95.44% of the scores fall within 2 standard deviations above or below the mean, and 99.74% of the scores fall within 3 standard deviations above or below the mean. Figure 17–3 shows a diagram of the normal curve, with the percentages of scores that are found within each standard deviation. Figure 17–4, *A,* shows the normal curve that corresponds to the knee flexion data set. The mean is 100°, and the standard deviation is 6.3°. Figure 17–4, B, shows that if the knee flexion scores are normally distributed, we could expect about 98% of our measurements to exceed the score of 87.4° (the shaded area in the figure). Figure 17–4, C, shows that we could expect about 68% of our measures to fall between 93.7° and 106.3°. Predicting the probability of obtaining certain ranges of scores is one of the most basic of statistical functions.

Correlation Coefficient

A *correlation coefficient* is a statistical summary of the degree of relationship that exists between two or more measures. The relationship can be between either different variables (such as bone density and age) or repeated measures of the same variables (such as blood pressures of the same individual taken by three different clinicians). There are many different types of correlation coefficients (Table 17–3); the computational distinctions between them are discussed in Chapter 22. A group of correlations known as intraclass correlation coefficients are commonly used to document reliability.

A correlation coefficient of 0.0 means that there is no relationship between the variables; a correlation coefficient of 1.0 indicates that there is a perfect relationship between the variables. Values in between these two extremes indicate intermediate levels of relationship. Some correlation coefficients can also have values from

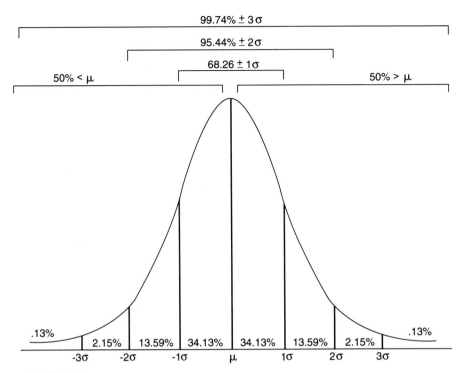

FIGURE 17–3. Probabilities of the normal curve. μ = mean; σ = standard deviation.

0.0 to −1.0. A negative correlation indicates an inverse relationship between variables (i.e., as the values for one variable become larger, the values for the other become smaller). In this text, r is used as a general symbol for a correlation coefficient. The specific notation for each type of coefficient is introduced when needed.

Standard Error of Measurement

In addition to knowing the relationship between repeated measurements, the researcher may wish to know how a given score is related to a "true" score for the person, as well as how much a score might vary with repeated measurements of the same individual. To determine the amount of measurement error, a researcher can take many repeated measures of the same participant and calculate the standard deviation of the scores; this standard deviation is known as the *standard error of measurement* (SEM). In practice, it is difficult to determine the SEM directly. Consider the effect of measuring wrist flexion up to 100 times in someone with limited wrist motion to determine the SEM. The individual's wrist flexion

FIGURE 17–4. Probabilities of the normal curve applied to hypothetical range-of-motion data with a mean of 100 and a standard deviation of 6.3. **A,** The range-of-motion values that correspond to 1, 2, and 3 standard deviations above the mean. **B,** The probability of obtaining a score greater than 87.4° (the shaded area) is 97.72%. **C,** The probability of obtaining a score between 93.7° and 106.3° (the shaded area) is 68.26%. μ = mean; σ = standard deviation.

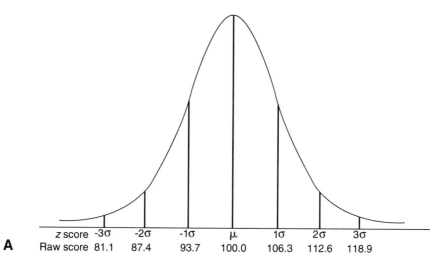

A

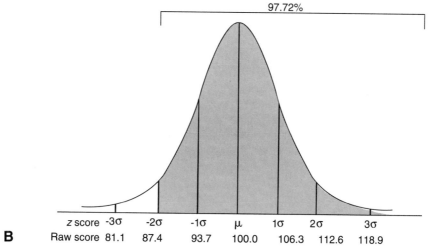

B

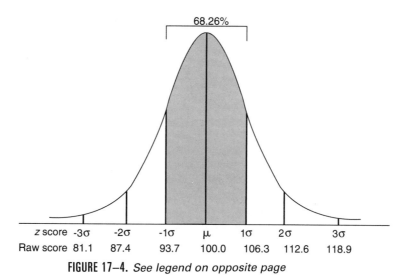

C

FIGURE 17–4. *See legend on opposite page*

	Type of	
	Data	No. of Repeated
Name of Coefficient	Required	Measures Compared
Pearson product moment correlation	Continuous	Two
Intraclass correlation	Continuous	Two or more
Spearman rank order correlation	Ranked	Two
Kendall's tau	Ranked	Two
Cohen's kappa	Nominal	Usually two; can be modified to accommadate more than two

TABLE 17-3 Correlation Coefficients

might improve during the course of testing by virtue of the exercise associated with taking so many measurements. Conversely, the individual's wrist flexion might be reduced as the joint became progressively more painful. In any event, taking so many repeated measurements would likely result in a confounding of measurement error with actual treatment effects.

Because of the difficulty in directly determining the SEM, it is often estimated as follows[6,7(p119)]:

$$SEM = \sigma\sqrt{1 - r} \qquad \text{(Formula 17–6)}$$

Assume that a researcher takes two wrist flexion measurements on each of 10 patients. If the standard deviation of the measures is 5° and the intraclass correlation coefficient between the two measures is .80, then the estimated SEM is 2.2°.

$$\begin{aligned} SEM &= 5\sqrt{1 - .80} \\ &= 5\sqrt{.20} \qquad \text{(Formula 17–7)} \\ &= 5(.44) = 2.2 \end{aligned}$$

The SEM is a standard deviation of measurement errors, and measurement errors are assumed to be normally distributed. Thus, by combining our knowledge of the probabilities of the normal curve with this value for the SEM, we can conclude there is a 68% probability that person's true wrist flexion would be within 1 SEM or ±2.2°

of the original measurement. Approximately 96% of the time, true wrist flexion would be within 2 standard errors of measurement or ±4.4° of the original measurement.

To determine how much a measure would be expected to vary with repeated measurement, the SEM is multiplied by the square root of the number of measurements and added and subtracted from the original measurement, as above.[6,7(p120)]

$$\begin{aligned} SEM_{repeated} &= \sqrt{2}\left(5\sqrt{1 - .80}\right) \\ &= 1.414\left(5\sqrt{.20}\right) \\ &= (1.414)(2.2) \qquad \text{(Formula 17–8)} \\ &= 3.1 \end{aligned}$$

There is a 68% probability that a repeated measure of wrist flexion would be within ±3.1° of the original measurement. Approximately 96% of the time, a repeated measure of wrist flexion would be within ±6.2° of the original measurement.

■ MEASUREMENT FRAMEWORKS

There are two basic frameworks in which measurement is conducted and evaluated: norm referenced and criterion referenced. *Norm-referenced* measures are those used to judge individual performance in relation to group norms. The statistical concepts of the mean and standard deviation are integral to norm-referenced measures. Measurements that use norm-referenced frameworks may use raw scores that are compared with tables of raw-score norms. More commonly, raw scores are standardized in some way to present them in relationship to the mean and standard deviation of the sample on which the norms were established. These standardized scores may be z scores (based on a mean of 0 and a standard deviation of 1), T scores (based on a mean of 50 and a standard deviation of 10, thereby eliminating negative scores), percentile ranks (converting the z scores to a percentile ranking based on the normal distribution), or a measure-specific system such as the Scholastic Achievement Test (SAT) based on a mean of 500 and a standard deviation of 100.[8]

Many clinical measurements are norm referenced. Blood pressure and pulse rates are evaluated against a range of normal values, muscle performance can be compared with average performance for age- and sex-matched groups, a patient's function after a stroke may be compared with that of patients with comparable lesions, and developmental status may be compared against norms established with typically developing children. Clinicians who often work with norm-referenced measures may wish to consult a more detailed measurement text to develop a stronger knowledge base in the use of norm-referenced tests.[8]

A *criterion-referenced* measure is one in which each individual's performance is evaluated with respect to some absolute level of achievement. When a teacher establishes 75% as the minimum passing score in a course, this is a criterion-referenced measurement. If all students exceed the 75% criterion, all pass. If only 25% exceed the criterion, only 25% pass. Clinicians use a criterion-referenced framework when they set specific performance criteria that patients have to meet in order to resume athletic competition, be released from an inpatient setting, or take an assistive device home.

■ MEASUREMENT RELIABILITY

Reliability is the "degree to which test scores are free from errors of measurement."[9(p19)] Other terms that are similar to reliability are *accuracy, stability,* and *consistency.* Despite its conceptual simplicity, one pair of writers notes that "it is devilishly difficult to achieve a real understanding of…reliability."[7(p104)] Despite this difficulty, this section of the chapter forges ahead and introduces reliability theories, components, and measures.

Two Theories of Reliability

Two basic measurement theories—classical measurement theory and generalizability theory—provide somewhat different views of reliability. *Classical measurement theory* rests on the assumption that every measurement, or obtained score, consists of a true component and an error component. In addition, each person has a single true score on the measurement of interest. Because we can never know the true score for any measure, the relationship between repeated measurements is used to estimate measurement errors. A measurement is said to be reliable if the error component is small, thus allowing consistent estimation of the true quantity of interest. With classical measurement theory, all variability within a person's score is viewed as measurement error.[10]

Classical theories of reliability have been extended into what is known as generalizability theory. *Generalizability theory* recognizes that there are different sources of variability for any measure. Measurements are studied in ways that permit the researcher to divide the measurement error into sources of variability, or *facets,* of interest to the researcher.

To understand the differences between these two approaches, consider the measurement of forward head position with a device that provides a measurement in centimeters. Classical measurement theory assumes that every person has a true value for forward head position and that variations in a person's scores are measurement errors about the true score. In contrast, generalizability theory recognizes that differences in scores may be related to any number of different facets. Facets of interest to a given researcher for this example might be the subject's level of relaxation, his or her level of comfort with the particular examiner taking the measurement, the skill of the examiner, and the accuracy of the device used to measure forward head position. The generalizability approach seems to have a great deal of promise for the study of measurements in rehabilitation because it acknowledges and provides a way to quantify the many sources of variability that rehabilitation professionals see in their patients or clients from day to day.

Components of Reliability

Several components of reliability are examined frequently: instrument, intrarater, interrater, and intrasubject reliability. Although it is often difficult to completely separate these components from one another, readers of the literature need to be able to conceptualize the different components so that they can determine which components or combinations of components are being studied.

INSTRUMENT RELIABILITY

The reliability of the instrument itself may be assessed. There are three broad categories of rehabilitation measurements: biophysiological, self-report, and observational. Different instruments are used to take the different types of measurements, and the appropriate approach for determining an instrument's reliability depends on the type of instrument.

Biophysiological measurements are obtained through the use of mechanical or electrical tools such as the dynamometer, goniometer, spirometer, scale, and electromyograph. The reliability of these instruments is assessed by taking repeated measurements across the range of

values expected to be found in actual use of the device. Assessment of scores on two or more administrations of a test is often called *test-retest reliability*. For example, Stratford and colleagues determined the test-retest reliability of a hand-held dynamometer by repeated application of known loads from 10 to 60 kg.[11] If the output of a device is in analog format (i.e., the tester determines the value by examining a scale on the device), then it is impossible to separate the reliability of the device from the examiner's ability to read the scale accurately. If the device output is in digital format, separation of device reliability from examiner reliability is easier because the digital reading leaves little room for examiner interpretation.

Self-report measurements are obtained through the use of instruments that require participants to give their own account of the phenomenon under study. Written surveys, standardized tests, pain scales, and interviews are examples of self-report measures. Forms of reliability for self-report tests include test-retest reliability, in which subjects take the same test on two or more occasions; parallel-form reliability, in which similar forms of a test are each administered once; split-half reliability, in which portions of a test are compared with each other; and internal consistency, in which responses to individual items are evaluated. The reader is referred to standard texts on health, educational, or psychological measurement for a fuller description of assessment of the reliability of written tests.[12(pp37-42),13,14]

Observational measurements require only a human instrument with systematic knowledge of what to observe. The examiner may be an unobtrusive observer or may play a more active role by requesting that the participant execute a series of actions. The knowledge may be in the examiners' head, as is often the case when a clinician observes gait patterns or other movement strategies, or examiners may use formal checklists to organize their observations.

Manual muscle testing, placement of patients into gait or transfer independence categories, determining developmental status, and documenting the accessibility of home or work environments are additional examples of rehabilitation measures that require only a human instrument with the knowledge of what to observe. The reliability of observational scales with multiple items can be examined for internal consistency in much the same manner as are written tests. Because the tester is the instrument, determining the reliability of observational measures is linked to determining intrarater and interrater reliability, described next.

INTRARATER RELIABILITY

A strict definition of *intrarater reliability* is "the consistency with which one rater assigns scores to a single set of responses on two occasions."[15(p141)] If a researcher is using a video clip to analyze speech patterns, he or she can watch and listen on two different dates. Because the behavior being assessed both times is identical, any variability in scores is, in fact, related to measurement errors of the researcher. For most of the measurements we take in rehabilitation, however, we do not have the ability to exactly reproduce the movement of interest, as a videotape would. If a clinician wishes to assess intrarater reliability of knee extension performance as measured by a handheld dynamometer, the patient will have to perform the movement two or more times. In doing so, any variability in the force measurements can be attributed to either the examiner's measurement error or the subject's inconsistent performance. It is often difficult to separate the two.

INTERRATER RELIABILITY

A strict definition of *interrater reliability* holds that it is the "consistency of performance among different raters or judges in assigning scores to the same objects or responses.... [It] is determined when two or more raters judge the performance of one group of subjects at the same point in time."[15(p140)] If two clinicians simultaneously observe and rate an infant's spontaneous movements as part of a developmental assessment, the comparison between their scores would be a pure measure of interrater reliability because they observed the exact same episode of movement. If they observed the child at two different times, however, it would be impossible to separate the variability attributable to differences in the examiners from the variability attributable to actual differences in the child's behavior from time to time.

A variation of intertester reliability, triangulation, is used to document the consistency of the results of qualitative research. *Triangulation* consists of comparing responses across several different sources,[16] which in effect become different raters of the phenomenon of interest. The literature of qualitative research provides additional detail about reliability issues in qualitative research.[16,17]

INTRASUBJECT RELIABILITY

The final component of reliability is associated with actual changes in subject performance from time to time. Some measurements in rehabilitation may appear to be unreliable simply because the phenomenon being measured is inherently variable. It may be unreasonable to think, for example, that single measurements of spasticity could be reproducible because spasticity is such a changing phenomenon. Unless one has a perfectly reliable instrument and a perfectly reliable examiner, it is impossible to derive a pure measure of subject variability. Thus, most test-retest reliability calculations reflect some combination of instrument errors, tester errors, and true subject variability. Chapter 18 presents research designs for evaluating the different reliability components or combinations of components.

Quantification of Reliability

Reliability is quantified in two ways, as either relative or absolute reliability. *Relative reliability* examines the relationship between two or more sets of repeated measures; *absolute reliability* examines the variability of the scores from measurement to measurement.[10]

RELATIVE RELIABILITY

Relative reliability is based on the idea that if a measurement is reliable, individual measurements within a group will maintain their position within the group on repeated measurement. For example, people who score near the top of a distribution on a first measure would be expected to stay near the top of the distribution even if their actual scores changed from time to time. Relative reliability is measured with some form of a correlation coefficient, which, as mentioned earlier in this chapter, indicates the degree of association between repeated measurements of the variable of interest. Different correlation coefficients are used with different types of data, as shown in Table 17–3.[18-20] The mathematical basis of correlation coefficients and the rationale for choosing a particular coefficient are discussed in greater detail in Chapter 22.

We know that a correlation coefficient of 1.0 indicates a perfect association between repeated measures. How much less than 1.0 can a correlation be if it is to be considered reliable? This question is not easily answered. Currier cites two different sources in which adjectives were used to describe ranges of reliability coefficients (e.g., 0.80 to 1.00 was described as "very reliable" and 0.69 and below was said to constitute "poor reliability").[21(p167)] Streiner and Norman cite two different authors who recommend minimum reliability coefficients of 0.94 and 0.85—but then imply that such arbitrary judgments are foolish.[7(p121)] There are several problems with using adjectives to describe ranges of correlation coefficients or setting minimum acceptable reliability coefficients. First, there are many different formulas for correlation coefficients, and these different formulas may result in vastly different coefficients for the same data.[22] Second, there is not universal agreement about the appropriateness of the different formulas.[23,24] Third, acceptable levels of reliability may differ depending on whether one is using the measurement to make judgments about individual change (as in clinical practice) or group change (as in traditional group research designs), with judgments about individual change requiring higher levels of reliability.[7(p121), 12(p41)]

Fourth, the value of a correlation coefficient is greatly affected by the range of scores used to calculate the coefficient. Correlation coefficients evaluate the consistency of an individual's position within a group; if the group as a whole shows little variability on the measure of interest, there is little mathematical basis for determining relative positions and the correlation between the repeated measurements will be low. Thus, other things being equal, the interrater reliability correlation coefficient calculated on a group of patients with knee flexion range-of-motion values between 70° and 90° would be lower than one calculated on a group with a broader range of values, say, between 30° and 90°.

Fifth, most of the correlation coefficients are not very good at detecting systematic errors. A systematic error is one that is predictable. For example, assume that on a first measurement of limb girth a researcher used one tape measure and on a second measurement used a different tape measure that was missing the first centimeter. There would be a systematic measurement error of 1 cm on the second measure. However, if each subject's position within the group were maintained, the correlation coefficients would remain high despite the absolute difference.

Because of these five issues, a rigid criterion for acceptable reliability is inappropriate. In addition, the component of reliability being studied affects the interpretation of the correlation coefficient. For example, one would ordinarily expect there to be less variability in scores recorded on a single day than in scores recorded over a longer time period. Similarly, intrarater reliability coefficients are generally higher than interrater reliability coefficients. Finally, if a researcher is deciding which of two measurement tools to use and has found that one has an intrarater reliability of .99 and the other an intrarater reliability of .80, then .80 seems unacceptable. On the other hand, if a highly abstract concept is being measured and a researcher is deciding between two instruments with intertester reliability coefficients of .45 and .60, then .60 may become acceptable. Because of the limitations of determining relative reliability with correlation coefficients, researchers should often supplement relative information with absolute information.

ABSOLUTE RELIABILITY

Absolute reliability indicates the extent to which a score varies on repeated measurement. The statistic used to measure absolute reliability is the SEM, described earlier in the chapter. For a clinician or researcher to make meaningful statements about whether a patient's or participant's condition has changed, he or she must know how much variability in the scores could be expected solely because of measurement errors. This is illustrated in Mawdsley and associates' study of the reliability of the figure-of-eight method of measuring ankle edema.[25] The intrarater reliability coefficient (an intraclass correlation coefficient) for repeated girth measurements was 0.99. The SEM of the measurement was calculated to be 0.45 cm. This indicates that approximately 96% of the time, the true value for ankle girth would be expected to fall within ±0.90 cm of the observed measurement (observed score ±2 SEMs), and a repeated measurement would be expected to fall within ±1.27 cm of the first measurement [first measurement ±2 $(\sqrt{2})$ (SEM)].

Thus, the correlation coefficient and the SEM provide different types of information about a measure. From the very high correlation coefficient we learned that the relative reliability of the measure was very high: participants in the group must have maintained their relative positions almost perfectly on repeated measurements. From the SEM we learned how much error, expressed in the units of the measure, we might expect with this measurement. Knowing the SEM of a measurement—and a little bit about the normal curve—enables rehabilitation professionals to evaluate clinical changes in patients in comparison to changes that might be expected solely from measurement error.

■ MEASUREMENT VALIDITY

Measurement validity is the "appropriateness, meaningfulness, and usefulness of the specific inferences made from test scores."[9(p9)] Reliability is a necessary, but not sufficient, condition for validity. An unreliable measure is also an invalid measurement, because measurements with a great deal of error have little meaning or utility. A reliable measure is valid only if, in addition to being repeatable, it provides meaningful information.

Earlier we defined *research validity* as the extent to which the conclusions of research are believable and useful (see Chapter 7). Note that although the two types of validity relate to different areas—measurement and research design, respectively—they are similar in that they both relate to the *utility* of findings and not to the findings themselves. Thus, measurement validity is not a quality associated with a particular instrument or test, but rather is a quality associated with the way in which test results are applied.

For example, the size of a child's spoken vocabulary may provide a valid gross indication of cognitive function in children without communication disorders. The same measure of spoken vocabulary may not be a valid indicator of cognitive function in children who have difficulty producing certain sounds and who may therefore elect to limit the words they choose to speak. Measurement validity is often subdivided into several categories: construct, content, and criterion validity.

Construct Validity

Construct validity is the validity of the abstract constructs that underlie measures. For example, strength is a construct that is poorly delineated in the rehabilitation literature. When rehabilitation professionals speak of strength, they may mean many different things. Strength may be conceptualized as the ability to move a body part against gravity, the ability to generate speed-specific torque, the ability to lift a certain weight a certain number of times in a certain time period, or the ability to accomplish some functional task. Manual muscle tests, isokinetic tests, work performance tests, and functional tests may all be valid measures of a particular conceptualization of strength or muscle performance.

To maximize construct validity, rehabilitation researchers must first be very clear about the constructs they wish to measure. If strength is an important construct within a study, is it best conceptualized as functional strength, static strength, eccentric strength, or some other aspect of this extremely broad construct? Once the underlying construct of interest is clarified, it must be operationalized to make it measurable. An *operational definition* is a specific description of the way in which a construct is presented or measured within a study. For example, Mathiowetz studied fatigue in persons with multiple sclerosis.[26] He chose his measurement tool based on an operational definition of fatigue found in a clinical practice guideline for multiple sclerosis: "a subjective lack of physical and/or mental energy that is perceived by the individual or caregiver to interfere with usual and desired activities."[27(p2)] The Fatigue Impact Scale used within the study appears to be consistent with the construct, in that it includes subscales related to physical, cognitive, and social impact of fatigue. Although developing operational definitions is necessary for construct validity, it does not *guarantee* construct validity. One might, for example, argue that Mathiowetz did not determine the perceptions of both individuals with multiple sclerosis and their caregivers (for those who were not independent in all activities), thereby failing to include all elements of the operational definition within the measurement design of his study. Supplying readers with the operational definitions used in a study allows them to form their own opinion of the validity of the measurements.

In addition to the intellectual task of determining the match between constructs and their measurement, another way to determine construct validity is to use "known-group" comparisons. In this approach, groups of individuals who are expected to perform differently on a measurement are compared to determine whether the hypothesized differences materialize. For example, in a validation study of the Hong Kong Chinese Version of the Lawton Instrumental Activities of Daily Living (IADL) scale, the authors administered the test to older adults living in a hostel and to those in a care-and-attention home.[28] The construct validity of the scale was demonstrated when the scale successfully differentiated between individuals in the different living situations.

Content Validity

Content validity is the extent to which a measure is a complete representation of the concept of interest. Content validity is more often a concern with self-report or observational tools than with biophysiological ones. When students come away from a test saying "Can you believe how many questions there were on…?," they are talking about the content validity of the test, because they are questioning whether the emphasis on the examination was an accurate representation of the course content.

Murney and Campbell tested a form of content validity of the Test of Infant Motor Performance when they tested what they referred to as the "ecological relevance" of the test items.[29] They found that 98% of the items in the test corresponded to environmental demands placed on the infant during normal daily activities. In a more traditional way of testing content validity, the test developers also asked a panel of experts to review the items in the test to ensure that a wide range of possible environmental demands was included within the test. When a researcher is designing a questionnaire or a functional scale, he or she should have its content validity evaluated by knowledgeable peers or evaluated in natural settings as part of the pilot testing of the instrument. These evaluation procedures may lead to the addition of items, the deletion of irrelevant or redundant items, or reassessment of the emphasis given to particular topics.

Criterion Validity

Criterion validity is the extent to which one measure is systematically related to other measures or outcomes. Whereas relative reliability compares repeated administrations of the *same* measurement, criterion validity compares administration of *different* measures. The mathematical basis for determining the degree of association between two different measures is similar to that for determining the association between repeated administrations of the same measurement. Therefore the correlation coefficients used to determine relative reliability are often used to measure criterion validity as well. The epidemiological concepts of specificity and sensitivity, described in Chapter 14, are also useful for determining criterion validity. Criterion validity can be subdivided into concurrent and predictive validity on the basis of the timing of the different measures.

Concurrent validity is at issue when one is comparing a new tool or procedure with a measurement standard. Clark and colleagues determined the concurrent validity of a new procedure to detect occult ankle fracture (presence of a 15-mm ankle effusion on a plain radiograph) with that of the "gold standard" of computed tomography.[30] Often, however, a true gold standard against which the new measurement can be compared does not exist. For example, in the study of the measurement of fatigue in individuals with multiple sclerosis, introduced earlier in the chapter, the Fatigue Impact Scale (FIS) was validated by correlating FIS scores with those of another self-reported fatigue scale and with the various subscales of the SF-36 instrument used to document health-related quality of life.[26] None of these comparison tools can be considered gold standards in the way that computed tomography is the definitive tool for diagnosing some conditions.

Predictive validity relates to whether a test done at one point in time is predictive of future status. Flegel and Kolobe studied the predictive validity of the Test of Infant Motor Performance (TIMP) by comparing scores on the TIMP at up to 4 months of age with scores on the Bruininks-Oseretsky Test of Motor Proficiency (BOTMP) of the same children at 4 to 7 years of age.[31] More than 89% of children were correctly classified by the TIMP. That is, 89% of children were "true positives" (classified as at risk for developmental delay by the TIMP and later classified as developmentally delayed by the BOTMP) or "true negatives" (classified as not at risk for developmental delay by the TIMP and later classified as not developmentally delayed by the BOTMP). Only 11% of children were "false positives" (classified as at risk by the TIMP and not delayed by the BOTMP) or "false negatives" (classified as not at risk by the TIMP but as delayed by the BOTMP). Determining the predictive validity of a screening measure such as the TIMP is an essential but time-consuming process. The premise of many screening tests is that they allow early identification of some phenomenon that is not usually apparent until some later date. The usefulness of such measures cannot be determined unless their predictive validity is known.

■ RESPONSIVENESS TO CHANGE

A third critical issue is the responsiveness to change of a measurement. Practitioners are generally hoping to effect change in their patients or clients, so measures that can reflect such changes in individuals are desirable. Consider two individuals, both of whom have goals related to weight change. One is a man who weighs 250 pounds and wishes to reduce to 190 pounds. The other is a premature infant who weighs 2500 grams and is fighting to get to 4000 grams. For the man who is dieting, a bathroom scale with increments of 1 pound will be responsive enough to document his weight loss. For the premature infant, a bathroom scale obviously will not be responsive enough to measure the small changes in weight that are expected to occur; a more precise scale that can measure to the nearest gram is needed. Measurements, then, must be selected with an eye to how responsive to change they will be given the characteristics of the individuals being studied. Also referred to in the literature as "sensitivity to change," in this text the term "responsiveness" is used instead to eliminate any confusion with the epidemiological concept of sensitivity.

Responsiveness to change can be defined as "the extent to which practically or theoretically significant changes in the subject's 'state' are reflected in substantive changes in observed values."[6(p335)] Responsiveness of a measure is related to both the reliability and validity of the measure. If a measure is not very reliable, as indicated by a large SEM, then changes that indicate true change in the status of clinical clients or research participants must be larger still to represent more than measurement error. Conversely, if the measure is very reliable, with a small SEM, then even small changes in the measure will represent true changes in a participant's state, thereby being "responsive" to change.

A measure that is not a good conceptual fit with the construct being measured (i.e., it does not have construct validity) is unlikely to be responsive to change. For example, the Barthel Index of activities of daily living has been used as a generic outcomes tool for individuals with spinal cord injury. However, some have questioned whether its items are specific enough to document the small changes in function that might be expected for some individuals with quadriplegia. In response to these concerns Gresham and colleagues developed a Quadriplegia Index of Function (QIF) and tested its responsiveness to change compared with the Barthel Index.[32] They found that the average percent improvement from admission to discharge for individuals with quadriplegia at a rehabilitation hospital was 46% for the QIF, but only 20% for the Barthel Index, demonstrating better responsiveness to change for the QIF compared with the Barthel Index.

Responsiveness to change is also a function of the number of values that a scale can take. If a scale can take only a few values (e.g., the familiar grading scale of A, B, C, D, F), then relatively large changes in performance are needed before a change in grade is registered on the scale. Conversely, if the grading scale includes + and − grades, then relatively small changes in performance may change a grade from B− to B and then to B+.

Ceiling and floor effects also have an impact on the responsiveness of a measure. A floor effect occurs when an individual scores at the bottom of a scale and no further declines in the quantity being measured can be registered. Ceiling effects occur at the top of a scale so that no further improvement can be registered. Depending on how far "under" the floor (or "over" the ceiling) an individual's true state, substantial change may occur without registering a change on the measurement scale. In Smith and associates' study of the relationship between generic measures of health-related quality of life and ambulatory function, they documented large floor and ceiling effects on some of the SF-36 subscales for their study sample of veterans with peripheral neuropathy.[33] For example, they found that 46% of their sample was at the floor of the role limitation/physical subscale and that 30% were at the ceiling of the social function subscale. Had this been a longitudinal study of physical and social impact of peripheral neuropathy, they would have been unable to detect declines in physical role limitations or improvements in social functioning for substantial numbers of individuals within their study.

Researchers or clinicians who wish to use measures that are responsive to change should look for measures with good reliability and validity for the population they are studying or treating, that can take a number of different values, and that are unlikely to have large floor or ceiling effects for the population of interest. Like reliability and validity, responsiveness to change is not an invariant characteristic of the measure; rather, it varies based on the conditions under which it is applied and the population in which it is used.

■ SUMMARY

Measurement is a systematic process by which things are differentiated. Measurements can be identified by scale (nominal, ordinal, interval, or ratio), type (discrete or continuous), and framework (norm referenced or criterion referenced). Statistical concepts of importance to measurement theory include the frequency distribution, mean, variance, standard deviation, normal curve, correlation, and SEM. Reliability is the extent to which a measure is free from error. The components of reliability include instrument, tester, and subject variability. Relative measures of reliability are correlation coefficients; the absolute measure of reliability is the standard error of measurement. Validity is the meaningfulness and utility of an application of a measurement. The components of validity include construct, content, and criterion validity. Responsiveness to change is the extent to which a change in status is reflected in a change in the measured value. Responsiveness to change depends on both the reliability and validity of a measure and is specific to the population being measured.

REFERENCES

1. Hopkins KD, Stanley JC. *Educational and Psychological Measurement and Evaluation*. 6th ed. Englewood Cliffs, NJ: Prentice-Hall; 1981:3.

2. Nunnally JC. *Psychometric Theory*. 2nd ed. New York, NY: McGraw-Hill; 1978:3.

3. Kerlinger FN, Lee HB. *Foundations of Behavioral Research*. 4th ed. Fort Worth, Tex: Harcourt College Publishers; 2000.

4. Safrit MJ. An overview of measurement. In: Safrit MJ, Wood TM, ed. *Measurement Concepts in Physical Education and Exercise Science*. Champaign,Ill: Human Kinetics; 1989.

5. Merbitz C, Morris J, Grip JC. Ordinal scales and foundations of misinference. *Arch Phys Med Rehabil*. 1989;70:308-312.

6. Hyde ML. Reasonable psychometric standards for self-report outcomes measures in audiological rehabilitation. *Ear Hear*. 2000;21:24S-36S.

7. Streiner DL, Norman GR. *Health Measurement Scales: A Practical Guide to Their Development and Use*. 2nd ed. Oxford: Oxford University Press; 1995.

8. Anastasi A, Urbina S. Norms and the meaning of test scores. In: Anastasi A, Urbina S, ed. *Psychological Testing*. 7th ed. Upper Saddle River, NJ: Prentice Hall; 1997.

9. American Educational Research Association, American Psychological Association, National Committee on Measurement in Education. *Standards for Educational and Psychological Testing*. Washington, DC: American Psychological Association; 1999.

10. Morrow JR. Generalizability theory. In: Safrit MJ, Wood TM, ed. *Measurement Concepts in Physical Education and Exercise Science*. Champaign, Ill: Human Kinetics; 1989.

11. Stratford PW, Norman GR, McIntosh JM. Generalizability of grip strength measurements in patients with tennis elbow. *Phys Ther*. 1989;69:276-281.

12. McDowell I, Newell C. *Measuring Health: A Guide to Rating Scales and Questionnaires*. New York, NY: Oxford University Press; 1996.

13. Anastasi A, Urbina S. Reliability. *Psychological Testing*. 7th ed. Upper Saddle River, NJ: Prentice Hall; 1997.

14. Litwin MS. *How to Assess and Interpret Survey Psychometrics, The Survey Kit, Volume 5*. Thousand Oaks, Calif: Sage Publications; 2003.

15. Waltz CF, Strickland OL, Lenz ER. *Measurement in Nursing Research*. Philadelphia, Pa: FA Davis; 1984.

16. Denzin NK, Lincoln YS. *Handbook of Qualitative Research*. 2nd ed. Thousand Oaks, Calif: Sage Publications; 2000.

17. Miles MB, Huberman AM. *Qualitative Data Analysis: An Expanded Sourcebook*. 2nd ed. Thousand Oaks, Calif: Sage Publications; 1994.

18. Cohen J. A coefficient of agreement for nominal scales. *Educational and Psychological Measurement*. 1960;20: 37-46.

19. Haley SM, Osberg JS. Kappa coefficient calculation using multiple ratings per subject: a special communication. *Phys Ther*. 1989;69:970-974.

20. Bartko JJ. The intraclass correlation coefficient as a measure of reliability. *Psychol Rep*. 1966;19:3-11.

21. Currier DP. *Elements of Research in Physical Therapy*. 3rd ed. Baltimore, Md: Williams & Wilkins; 1990.

22. Shrout PE, Fleiss JL. Intraclass correlations: uses in assessing rater reliability. *Psychol Bull*. 1979;86:420-428.

23. Bartko JJ, Carpenter WT. On the methods and theory of reliability. *J Nerv Ment Dis*. 1976;163:307-317.

24. Hart DL. Invited commentary. *Phys Ther*. 1989;69: 102-103.

25. Mawdsley RH, Hoy DK, Erwin PM. Criterion-related validity of the figure-of-eight method of measuring ankle edema. *J Orthop Sports Phys Ther*. 2000;30:149-153.

26. Mathiowetz V. Test-retest reliability and convergent validity of the Fatigue Impact Scale for persons with multiple sclerosis. *Am J Occup Ther*. 2003;57:389-395.

27. Multiple Sclerosis Council for Clinical Practice Guidelines. *Fatigue and multiple sclerosis: evidence-based management strategies for fatigue in multiple sclerosis*. Washington, DC: Paralyzed Veterans of America; 1998.

28. Tong AYC, Man DWK. The validation of the Hong Kong Chinese Version of the Lawton Instrumental Activities of Daily Living scale for institutionalized elderly persons. *OTJR: Occupation Participation Health*. 2002;22: 132-142.

29. Murney ME, Campbell SK. The ecological relevance of the Test of Infant Motor Performance elicited scale items. *Phys Ther.* 1998;78:479-489.

30. Clark TWI, Janzen DL, Logan PM, Ho K, Connell DG. Improving the detection of radiographically occult ankle fractures: positive predictive value of an ankle joint effusion. *Clin Radiol.* 1996;51:632-636.

31. Flegel J, Kolobe THA. Predictive validity of the Test of Infant Motor Performance as measured by the Bruininks-Oseretsky Test of Motor Proficiency at school age. *Phys Ther.* 2002;82:762-771.

32. Gresham GE, Labi ML, Dittmar SS, Hicks JT, Joyce SZ, Stehlik MA. The Quadriplegia Index of Function (QIF): sensitivity and reliability in a study of thirty quadriplegic patients. *Paraplegia.* 1986;24:38-44.

33. Smith DG, Domholdt E, Coleman KL, del Aguila MA, Boone DA. Ambulatory activity in men with diabetes: relationship between self-reported and real-world performance-based measures. *J Rehabil Res Dev.* 2004;41: (in press).

Methodological Research

The goals of methodological research are to document and improve the reliability, validity, and responsiveness of clinical and research measurements. Because measurement is an integral part of clinical and research documentation, research that examines measurements is important to all of the rehabilitation professions. In addition to the importance of measurement as a topic in its own right, documentation of the reliability and validity of the measures used within a study is a necessary component of all research. This chapter provides a framework for the design of methodological research. Reliability designs are presented first, followed by validity designs and responsiveness designs.

■ RELIABILITY DESIGNS

The reliability of a measurement is influenced by many factors, including (1) the sources of

variability studied, (2) the participants selected, and (3) the range of scores exhibited by the sample. Each of these factors is illustrated in this chapter by a hypothetical example of measurement of joint range of motion. The hypothetical example is supplemented by relevant examples from the literature. After these three general factors are discussed, two specialized types of reliability studies are considered: reliability optimization and reliability documentation within nonmethodological research.

Sources of Variability

Differences found in repeated measurements of the same characteristic can be attributed to instrument, intrarater, interrater, and intrasubject components. Within each of these four reliability components there are many additional sources of variability. When designing reliability studies, researchers must clearly delineate which of the reliability components they wish to study and which sources of variability they wish to study within each component. To assist with this task, it is helpful to list the four reliability components and all possible sources of variation for each component. Box 18–1 shows some potential sources of variability in passive range-of-motion scores as measured with a universal goniometer.

Once the sources of variability within the measurement are delineated, the researcher must determine which of the components will be the focus of his or her methodological study. As is the case with all research design, the investigator designing methodological research must identify a problem that needs to be studied. Is there a knowledge deficit about the interinstrument reliability of goniometers of different sizes or designs? Is it important to establish the degree of variation that can be expected in a particular measurement made by a single clinician? What is the magnitude of differences that could be expected if several clinicians take measurements of the same person? Is participant or patient performance consistent across days or weeks?

Each of these questions relates to one of the four components of reliability: instrument, intrarater, interrater, and intrasubject. However, in many methodological studies, more than one of the reliability components are examined, or the reliability components are intertwined and cannot be separated clearly. For example, Nussbaum and Downes[1] examined the reliability of a pressure-pain algometer by using two measurers, with three measurements of each taken on 3 different days. Intrarater, interrater, and intrasubject reliability are examined, although they cannot necessarily be completely separated from one another. For example, the day-to-day reliability involves consistency of examiners across the 3 days as well as consistency across days of the participants' perceptions of pain in response to the pressure of the instrument.

Levels of Standardization

Once the sources of variability have been determined, it is necessary to determine the degree of standardization in the measurement protocol. The degree of standardization is the number of sources of variability within a reliability component that are controlled.

Consider three different reasons to study intertester reliability of goniometric measurements. The purpose of one study might be to determine interrater reliability of goniometric measurements

---

BOX 18–1

Sources of Variability in Passive Range-of-Motion Measurements with a Universal Goniometer

INSTRUMENT

Loose axis (slips during measurement)
Tight axis (too difficult to move precisely)
Interinstrument differences

INTRARATER

Variations in participant positioning
Inconsistent identification of landmarks
Variable end-range pressure
Inconsistent stabilization
Reading errors

INTERRATER

Variations in participant positioning
Inconsistent identification of landmarks
Variable end-range pressure
Inconsistent stabilization
Differing ability to gain participants' trust
Different end-digit preference
Reading errors

INTRASUBJECT

Varying levels of pain
Differing tolerance to end-range pressure
Mood changes
Differing activities before measurement
Biological variation

as they occur in the clinic, without any standardization of technique between clinicians. The purpose of a second study might be to determine the upper limits of interrater reliability with a highly standardized protocol. The purpose of a third study might be to determine interrater reliability with a level of standardization that would be feasible for most clinics to achieve.

The preceding three purpose statements correspond to three general approaches to reliability that are seen in the literature: nonstandardized, highly standardized, and partially standardized. The three approaches differ in the extent to which the sources of variability are controlled within each of the reliability components under study. For intertester reliability in the measurement of passive motion with a goniometer, Box 18–1 lists seven possible sources of variability: positioning, landmark identification, end-range pressure, stabilization, patient trust in the clinician, end-digit preference (some clinicians always round measurements to the nearest 5°, others round to even numbers only, and others do not round off at all), and reading errors. Let's consider how nonstandardized, highly standardized, and partially standardized studies would be applied to these sources of variability to determine intertester reliability of goniometric measurement.

NONSTANDARDIZED APPROACH

A completely nonstandardized approach would control none of these sources of variability and would establish the lower limit for the reliability component studied. The basic design of a nonstandardized study of intertester reliability would be to have each clinician take measurements privately so as not to influence the technique of the other clinicians within the study.

Watkins and associates studied the reliability of goniometric measures of knee range of motion.[2] Because they wished to study reliability under typical clinical conditions, they did not train their examiners in standardized procedures. In fact, they ensured that the second clinician never saw the first clinician taking measurements,

nor did they require standardized positioning of the patient or the goniometer.

HIGHLY STANDARDIZED APPROACH

In contrast to a nonstandardized approach, a highly standardized approach would control many of the possible sources of variability to determine the upper limits of the reliability of the component. Whereas a nonstandardized approach seeks to document the reliability of measurements as they commonly occur, a highly standardized approach seeks to document reliability in an ideal situation. A highly standardized approach to taking measurements may be a useful way of separating measurement error from participant variability.

In a highly standardized study of intertester goniometric reliability, positioning, stabilization, landmarks, end-range pressure, and end-digit preference would all be controlled. Positioning for shoulder internal rotation, for example, could be controlled by having all clinicians take the measurements with the patient supine on the same firm plinth. Stabilization could be controlled by strapping the patient's chest to prevent substitution of scapular or trunk movements. To control inconsistent identification of landmarks, landmarks could be marked on the participants and left in place while all clinicians take their measurements. End-range pressure could be standardized by having an assistant provide a predetermined force as documented by a handheld dynamometer. Finally, end-digit preference could be controlled by instructing clinicians to report the measurement to the nearest degree. The experimental protocol for such a study might be that one clinician positions each patient and three other clinicians each take a measurement in rapid succession. Such a protocol would establish the upper limits of intertester reliability and would eliminate the effects of participant variation because the participant would not be moved between measurements.

Mayerson and Milano used a highly standardized approach to study goniometric measurement reliability.[3] A healthy participant was positioned in 22 consistent extremity joint positions; two clinicians each took two measurements at each position. The protocol eliminated variability resulting from participant positioning, stabilization, end-range pressure, and changes in participant motion. Thus, the protocol provided a test of the reliability of goniometer placement and reading. They found that both intertester and intratester differences could confidently be expected to fall within 4° of each other in a highly standardized measurement protocol.

PARTIALLY STANDARDIZED APPROACH

The third approach to determining the sources of variability to be studied within an investigation of reliability is the partially standardized approach. As indicated by its name, this approach falls between the extremes of the nonstandardized and highly standardized approaches by standardizing a few sources of variability while leaving others nonstandardized. The sources of variability that are standardized often reflect the realities of the clinic. The hypothetical, highly standardized study of internal rotation range of motion described previously is probably unrealistic for routine clinical use: an assistant is not always available to position the patient, and landmarks are likely to be washed off between treatment sessions. A partially standardized measurement protocol might therefore standardize positioning and stabilization but allow landmark determination and end-range pressure to vary among clinicians. The experimental protocol for a partially standardized study requires educating the examiners in the standardized methods to be employed in the study.

Youdas and colleagues used a partially standardized approach to study the reliability of cervical range-of-motion measurements taken by visual estimation, with a universal goniometer, and with a cervical range-of-motion instrument.[4] Clinicians were trained in the use of a standardized protocol for positioning of the participants; placement of the measuring devices and a warm-up protocol for participants were also standardized.

The appropriate level of standardization for reliability studies depends on the research question and each approach can be useful for specific purposes. Nonstandardized studies describe reliability as it is; highly standardized studies present idealized reliability estimates and examine the impact of limited sources of variability on reliability; partially standardized studies describe reliability with moderate levels of standardization that could be achievable in clinical settings.

Participant Selection

As is the case with all types of research, participant selection in reliability studies influences the external validity of the study; the study results can be generalized only to the types of participants studied. Therefore, the reliability of an instrument should be determined using the individuals on whom the instrument will be used in practice. If the measure is a clinical one, it is best to determine its reliability on patients who would ordinarily require this measurement as part of their care. Watkins and associates did this in their study of the reliability of knee range-of-motion measurements.[2] They even divided their patients into diagnostic categories to determine whether the measurements were more reliable for patients with certain types of knee dysfunction. The inappropriate use of normal participants to establish the reliability of clinical measures has the potential to inflate reliability estimates because normal participants may be easier to measure than patients. Pain, obliteration of landmarks because of deformity, or difficulty following directions because of neurological impairment may make it difficult to take measurements in patients.

If a researcher ultimately wishes to determine norms for certain characteristics, it is appropriate to determine the reliability of the measurements using normal participants. If the measurement in question is part of a screening tool, such as a flexibility test that might be administered at a fitness fair, then a broad sampling of the individuals likely to be screened should be used to establish the reliability of the measurement.

Range of Scores

The reliability of a measure should be determined over the range of scores expected for that measure. There are two reasons for this. First, as discussed in Chapter 17, a restricted range of scores leads to low reliability coefficients, even in the presence of small absolute differences in repeated measurements. The use of normal participants can restrict the range of scores within a study, thereby reducing the reliability coefficients and underestimating the reliability of the measure in clinical use. In contrast, using an extremely heterogeneous group (e.g., a mixed group of patients and nonpatients) would generally overestimate the reliability of the measure for clinical use, but might be the ideal mix of individuals for establishing the reliability of the tool for screening purposes.

Second, reliability may vary at different places in the range of scores because of difficulties unique to taking measurements at particular points in the range. For example, Nussbaum and Downes[1] found that interrater reliability was greatest when testing participants with lower pain thresholds. Researchers need to carefully consider the characteristics of the individuals on whom the test or tool will be used and select a research sample that matches those characteristics.

Optimization Designs

In many instances, researchers have found less than optimal reliability for rehabilitation measures. Such research is useful because it may lead to a healthy skepticism about the measurements we use. In and of itself, however, *documenting* the reliability of a clinical measure does nothing to *improve* its reliability. Improving the reliability of rehabilitation measures requires that researchers study ways to optimize reliability. There are two basic designs for optimization research: standardization and mean designs.

STANDARDIZATION DESIGNS

Standardization designs compare the reliabilities of measurements taken under different sets of conditions. For example, suppose that the result of a nonstandardized reliability study was that the standard error of measurement (SEM) for passive internal rotation range of motion was 10°. Furthermore, suppose the result of a highly standardized, but clinically unfeasible, study was that the SEM was 1°. A standardization study might be developed with a goal of determining what level of standardization is needed to achieve an SEM of 3°. To do so, a researcher might determine reliability with standardized positioning. If, despite the positioning change, the SEM is still too large, both position and upper chest stabilization might be standardized. The level of standardization would be increased until the reliability goal was met. A reverse sequence could also be implemented by starting with a highly standardized procedure and eliminating standardization procedures that are not feasible in the clinic.

MEAN DESIGNS

Mean designs compare the reliabilities of single measurements and also compare the reliabilities of measurements averaged across several trials. This design is particularly appropriate for measures that are difficult to standardize for clinical use or for characteristics that are expected to show a great deal of natural variation.[5] Connelly and colleagues used a mean strategy to study the reliability of walking tests in a frail elderly population.[6] Two raters took three measures on each of 2 days. They then computed reliability coefficients comparing the means for each day between raters, the best score for each day between raters, and the first measure for each day between raters. They found that the reliability coefficients were highest when they used the mean of three measures, were worst when they used the first measure, and were intermediate when they used the best measure. Such information helps clinicians and researchers make knowledgeable decisions about whether to rely on single measures or whether to average the results of repeated measurements.

Reliability in Nonmethodological Studies

Useful research studies are based on reliable measurements. Measurement reliability in nonmethodological studies should often be addressed at two times during the study: during the design phase and during the implementation phase.

In the design phase, the researcher must determine which of several possible instruments to choose, which of several possible measurement protocols to follow, and which of several raters to use. Studies of interinstrument, interrater, or intrarater reliability components may be needed to make these decisions.

When conducting a pilot reliability study, the researcher needs to simulate the research conditions as closely as possible. The same types of participants, settings, time pressures, and the like should be employed. The results of a pilot reliability study conducted after clinic hours, when researchers and participants have much time and few distractions, may differ from those of the actual study if the actual study takes place during clinic hours, when time is short and distractions abound.

Reliability measures should also be taken during implementation of a study, as in some instances the reliability attained during training phases has been shown to decline during experimental phases.[7,8] Researchers can establish reliability during the course of a study by taking repeated measures of all participants, using pretest and posttest scores of a control group as the reliability indicator, or taking repeated measures of selected participants at random. Which strategy is adopted depends on factors such as the expense of the measures, the risks of

repeated measurements to participants, and the number of participants in the study.

■ VALIDITY DESIGNS

As discussed previously, the validity of a measurement is the extent to which a particular use of the measurement is meaningful. Measures are validated through argument about and research into the soundness of the interpretations made from them. To make sound interpretations, a researcher must first be confident that the measurements are reproducible, or reliable. Recall that although reliability is necessary for validity, it does not validate the meaning behind the measure. This section of the chapter presents several designs for research to determine the construct, content, and criterion validity of measurements.

Construct Validation

Constructs are artificial frameworks that are not directly observable. Strength, function, and pain are constructs used frequently in rehabilitation. Because the constructs themselves are not directly observable, there are no absolute standards against which measurements can be compared to determine whether they are valid indicators of the constructs. Consider, for example, all the different measures that rehabilitation professionals use to represent the construct of strength: manual muscle testing, the number of times that a particular weight can be lifted, handheld dynamometers, and a multitude of isokinetic tests. All are appropriate for some purposes, but none is a definitive measure of strength.

In the absence of a clear-cut standard, persuasive argument becomes one means by which the construct validity of measurements is established.[9] A researcher who wishes to assess strength gains following a particular program of exercise must be prepared to defend the appropriateness of the measurements he or she used for the type of exercise program studied. Such considerations include whether the measure should test concentric or eccentric contractions, whether the test should be isometric or should sample strength throughout the range of motion, and whether the test should be conducted in an open or closed kinetic chain position.

A second way in which construct validity is established is by making predictions about the patterns of test scores that should be seen if the measure is valid.[10(p152-157)] One method is to examine the convergence and divergence of measures thought to represent similar and different constructs, respectively. For example, one study that sought to validate the Short Form-36 (SF-36) health survey questionnaire as a measure of general health status in the British population did so by having almost 2000 patients take both the SF-36 and the Nottingham health profile.[11] If the SF-36 was valid in this population, the researchers predicted that the overall score would correlate fairly well with the overall score on the Nottingham health profile. In addition, they predicted that there would be higher correlations between the physical scales on the two tests than there would be between the physical and mental scales. For the most part, they found this to be true. For example, the strength of the correlation between the physical functioning scale on the SF-36 and the physical morbidity scale on the Nottingham health profile was 0.52; between the physical functioning scale on the SF-36 and the social isolation scale on the Nottingham health profile it was only 0.20. Construct validity is best supported when the scores on items thought to represent the same construct are highly associated (convergence) and when scores on items that are theoretically different have a low association (divergence).

Another set of predictions that is often used to establish construct validity relates to the performance of "extreme groups" or "known groups" on the test of interest. Tong and Man did this in their study of the validation of the Hong Kong Chinese version of the Lawton Instrumental Activities of Daily Living (IADL) Scale for institutionalized elderly individuals living in two different levels of institutions.[12]

They predicted that the scale would differentiate between groups living in hostel versus care-and-attention homes, and in 78% of cases they were able to predict living situation correctly based on the IADL scale. Creative researchers are able to envision the optimal performance of their tests and then set up research situations to determine how closely the tests come to meeting their predictions for optimal performance.

Content Validation

Content validation involves documenting that a test provides an adequate sampling of the behavior or knowledge that it is measuring. To determine the content validity of a measure, a researcher compares the items in the test against the actual practice of interest. There are four basic issues a researcher must consider when determining content validity: (1) the sample on whom the measure is validated, (2) the content's completeness, (3) the content's relevance, and (4) the content's emphasis. For example, consider the content validity of the Clinical Performance Instrument (CPI), an assessment tool used widely to evaluate students on clinical rotations in physical therapy.[13] The CPI consists of more than 40 clinical behaviors that should be exhibited by physical therapy students. If the CPI has content validity, then it should accurately represent the demands that clinical practice places on clinicians.

To determine content validity, a researcher needs to determine an appropriate group on whom the content can be validated. To determine the content validity of the CPI, should a random sampling of clinicians be selected for observation of their practice? Should clinicians with less than 2 years of experience constitute the sample? Should students on clinical rotations be studied? If the CPI is viewed as a tool that determines readiness for entry-level physical therapy practice, then the group of new clinicians may be the most appropriate group on whom the content should be validated. If the CPI is viewed as a tool that assesses performance on clinical rotations, then the student group may be the appropriate group on whom the tool should be validated.

Once the participant group has been identified, test content can be compared with actual practice. If the validity were perfect, all activities of the observed clinicians would be represented in the CPI, and all items in the CPI would be demonstrated in actual practice. In addition, more emphasis would be placed on items that are frequently performed in actual practice and less emphasis would be placed on infrequently performed items.

Criterion Validation

The criterion validation of a measure is determined by comparing it with an accepted standard of measurement. The major considerations in designing a criterion validation study are selecting the criterion, timing the administration of the tests, and selecting a sample for testing.

Three different criteria against which a test is compared are found in the literature. The first criterion is essentially *instrumentation accuracy*. The accuracy of the measurement provided by an instrument is determined by comparing the reading on the device with a standard measure. Examples in the literature include comparing the angular measurements of a goniometer with known angles[2] and testing a digitizer against known lengths.[14] Complex instruments have specific standardization procedures that allow the investigator to check the instrument against known standards and either make adjustments until the device readings accurately reflect the standard or develop equations that can be used to correct for inaccuracies.[15]

The second criterion is a concurrent one. A concurrent criterion is applied at the same time the test in question is validated. Irrgang and colleagues determined the *concurrent validity* of their Activities of Daily Living Scale of the Knee Outcome Survey with the Lysholm Knee Rating Scale by administering both scales multiple times for almost 400 patients with knee impairments.[16]

The third criterion is predictive. A measure has *predictive validity* if the result of its administration at one point in time is highly associated with future status. There are three difficulties in doing predictive studies: determining the criterion itself, determining the timing of administration of the criterion, and maintaining a good sample of participants measured on both occasions. Flegel and Kolobe studied the predictive validity of the Test of Infant Motor Performance (TIMP) by comparing children's scores on the test when they were less than 4 months old with an assessment of their motor proficiency between the ages of 4 and 7 years.[17]

The importance of timing is also illustrated in the TIMP validity study. By assessing motor proficiency between the ages of 4 and 7 years, Flegel and Kolobe could test a broad range of skills including fine motor skills needed for handwriting and drawing. If they had tested at only 1 to 2 years of age, they would not have been able to look at these skills. On the other hand, if they had tested children at the age of 12 years, they might have identified more subtle coordination problems as the children began to participate in sports activities.

The third difficulty with predictive validity studies is the sample available for study. Because these studies extend over time, there may be differential loss of participants. For example, in Flegel and Kolobe's study, only 65 children from the initial sample of 137 who were tested with the TIMP could be located for the later testing.[17] If, for example, a disproportionate number of children determined by the TIMP to be at high risk for developmental delay were within the 65 children available for later testing, this might lead to inflated predictive validity estimates. Flegel and Kolobe were able to guard against this possibility by stratifying the 65 children into age and risk groups and then randomly sampling children within each group for their study.

■ RESPONSIVENESS DESIGNS

Studies of the responsiveness of a measure to changes in status generally involve (1) identification of a group of patients who can be assumed to have made a true change in the underlying construct of interest, (2) use of the measure of interest at pretreatment and posttreatment to calculate various measures of responsiveness, and (3) comparison of the responsiveness of the measure of interest to other related measures to determine the relative responsiveness of the different measurement tools.

For example, Beaton and colleagues conducted a study of the validity, reliability, and responsiveness of the Disabilities of the Arm, Shoulder, and Hand (DASH) outcome measure for different regions of the upper extremity.[18] They first identified a sample of patients who were awaiting treatment for a variety of upper extremity conditions. They assumed that the group as a whole would improve following treatment and that measurements taken before treatment and 12 weeks after treatment would reflect these improvements. However, they recognized that not everyone in the sample might improve, so they created two subgroups of patients about whom the assumption of improvement was more likely to be valid: one subgroup was for those who said their upper-limb *condition* had improved with treatment, and one subgroup was for those who said their upper-limb *function* had improved with treatment. In addition, for their question about the responsiveness to change for conditions affecting different parts of the upper extremity, they further subdivided their patients into those with shoulder conditions and those with wrist and hand conditions.

The primary measure of interest was the DASH, and pretreatment and posttreatment measures of the DASH were recorded for all of the participants. The extent to which the DASH changed was represented by three different measures: a change score, an effect size, and a standardized response mean (SRM). A change score is simply the difference between the posttreatment and pretreatment scores. If a study is only examining responsiveness of a single measurement tool, then examining change scores may be sufficient to determine responsiveness. The effect size is the mean change score divided by the standard deviation of the pretreatment score, and the SRM is the mean change score divided by the standard deviation of the change scores. Effect size or SRM is used when comparing the responsiveness of different measurement tools with different measurement scales. By dividing the change score by some measure of variability (either variability at baseline for the effect size or variability of the change scores for SRM), the level of responsiveness is standardized and can be compared across tools with different measurement scales. Beaton and colleagues found that DASH scores were reduced by an average of 13.3 points for all patients and by an average of 19.7 points for the subset of patients who reported that their function was better.

Because they were not just interested in the responsiveness of the DASH by itself, but in the responsiveness of the DASH compared with some more specific tools, they also took pretreatment and posttreatment measures using the Shoulder Pain and Disability Index (SPADI) and the Brigham carpal tunnel questionnaire. To compare across these tools, they moved beyond change scores by calculating effect scores and SRM scores. For a subset of shoulder patients who rated their function as better after treatment, the DASH SRM of 1.44 showed more responsiveness to change than the SPADI SRM of 1.13. For a subset of wrist and hand patients who rated their function as better after treatment, the DASH SRM of 0.91 showed marginally more responsiveness to change than the Brigham carpal tunnel questionnaire SRM of 0.87.[18]

Similar methods have been used to compare the responsiveness of the Quadriplegia Index of Function with the Barthel Index[19] and the Western Ontario and McMaster Universities Osteoarthritis Index (WOMAC) with the SF-36[20,21] and Knee Society Clinical Rating System.[21]

■ SUMMARY

Methodological research is conducted to document and improve measuring tools by assessing their reliability, validity, and responsiveness. The major components of reliability are instrument, intrarater, interrater, and intrasubject reliability. Reliability research can be classified according to whether the measurement protocol used is nonstandardized, partially standardized, or highly standardized. Participants should be selected based on whether they would likely be assessed with the tool in clinical situations; in addition, participants who demonstrate a wide range of scores should be selected. Construct validity is determined through logical argument and assessment of the convergence of similar tests and divergence of different tests. Content validity is determined by assessing the completeness, relevancy, and emphasis of the items within a test. Criterion validity is determined by comparing one measure with an accepted standard of measurement. Responsiveness of a measure is determined by examining the change scores, effect scores, or standardized response means for the measure for a group that is assumed to have undergone a true change in the underlying construct of interest.

REFERENCES

1. Nussbaum EL, Downes L. Reliability of clinical pressure-pain algometric measurements obtained on consecutive days. *Phys Ther.* 1998;78:160-169.
2. Watkins MA, Riddle DL, Lamb RL, Personius WJ. Reliability of goniometric measurements and visual estimates of knee range of motion obtained in a clinical setting. *Phys Ther.* 1991;71:90-97.
3. Mayerson NH, Milano RA. Goniometric reliability in physical medicine. *Arch Phys Med Rehabil.* 1984;65:92-94.
4. Youdas JW, Carey JR, Garrett TR. Reliability of measurements of cervical spine range of motion-comparison of three methods. *Phys Ther.* 1991;71:98-104.
5. Stratford PW. Summarizing the results of multiple strength trials: truth or consequence. *Physiotherapy Can.* 1992;44:14-18.
6. Connelly DM, Stevenson TJ, Vandervoort AA. Between- and within-rater reliability of walking tests in a frail elderly population. *Physiother Can.* 1996;48:47-51.
7. Mitchell SK. Interobserver agreement, reliability, and generalizability of data collected in observational studies. *Psychol Bull.* 1979;86:376-390.
8. Taplin PS, Reid JB. Effects of instructional set and experiment influence on observer reliability. *Child Dev.* 1973;44:547-554.
9. Cronbach LJ. *Essentials of Psychological Testing.* New York, NY: Harper & Row; 1990:185.
10. Streiner DL, Norman GR. *Health Measurement Scales: A Practical Guide to Their Development and Use.* 2nd ed. Oxford: Oxford University Press; 1995.
11. Brazier JE, Harper R, Jones NMB, et al. Validating the SF-36 health survey questionnaire: new outcome measure for primary care. *Br Med J.* 1992;305:160-164.
12. Tong AYC, Man DWK. The validation of the Hong Kong Chinese Version of the Lawton Instrumental Activities of Daily Living scale for institutionalized elderly persons. *OTJR: Occupation Participation Health.* 2002;22:132-142.
13. *Clinical Performance Instrument.* Alexandria, Va: American Physical Therapy Association; 1998.
14. Norton BJ, Ellison JB. Reliability and concurrent validity of the Metrecom for length measurement on inanimate objects. *Phys Ther.* 1993;73:266-274.
15. Geddes LA, Baker LE. *Principles of Applied Biomedical Instrumentation.* 3rd ed. New York, NY: John Wiley & Sons; 1989:8-9.
16. Irrgang JJ, Snyder-Mackler L, Wainner RS, Fu FH, Harner CD. Development of a patient-reported measure of function of the knee. *J Bone Joint Surg Am.* 1998;80:1132-1145.
17. Flegel J, Kolobe THA. Predictive validity of the Test of Infant Motor Performance as measured by the Bruininks-Oseretsky Test of Motor Proficiency at school age. *Phys Ther.* 2002;82:762-771.
18. Beaton DE, Katz JN, Fossel AH, Wright JG, Tarasuk V, Bombardier C. Measuring the whole or the parts? Validity, reliabililty, and responsiveness of the Disabilities of the Arm, Shoulder, and Hand outcome measure in different regions of the upper extremity. *J Hand Ther.* 2001;14:128-146.
19. Gresham GE, Labi ML, Dittmar SS, Hicks JT, Joyce SZ, Stehlik MA. The Quadriplegia Index of Function (QIF): sensitivity and reliability in a study of thirty quadriplegic patients. *Paraplegia.* 1986;24:38-44.
20. Angst F, Aeschlimann A, Steiner W, Stucki G. Responsiveness of the WOMAC osteoarthritis index as compared with the SF-36 in patients with osteoarthritis of the legs undergoing a comprehensive rehabilitation intervention. *Ann Rheum Dis.* 2001;60:834-840.
21. Lingard EA, Katz JN, Wright J, Wright EA, Sledge CB, Kinemax Outcomes Group. Validity and responsiveness of the Knee Society Clinical Rating System in comparison with the SF-36 and WOMAC. *J Bone Joint Surg Am.* 2001;83:1856-1864.

Data Analysis

Statistical Reasoning

Statistics has a bad name. Consider this tongue-in-cheek sampling from the irreverent *Journal of Irreproducible Results*:

We all know that you can prove anything with statistics. So I recently proved that nobody likes statistics, except for a few professors. If you don't believe that, just ask the person on the street. I did. The first person I saw referred to the subject as "sadistics." The second person, an old gentleman along the Mississippi River, muttered something about "liars, damned liars, and statisticians."[1(p13)]

Although quips about statistics may be amusing, the discipline of statistics should not be confused with the conclusions that researchers draw from statistical analyses. Statistics is a discipline in which mathematics and probability are applied in ways that allow researchers to make sense of their data. Although there are many different statistical tests and procedures—too many to include even in textbooks devoted solely to statistics—there are remarkably few central concepts that underlie all of the tests.

In this chapter, the central concepts of statistics are introduced. Readers should be prepared to read this chapter, and Chapters 21 through 24, which cover particular statistical tests, very slowly. Careful reading, examination of the tables and figures, and independent calculation of the examples in this chapter should provide a strong basis for understanding not only the following chapters but, more importantly, the data analysis and results portions of research articles in the rehabilitation literature.

The chapter begins by presenting a data set that is used for all of the statistical examples in this and the following four chapters. Next, the concepts of frequency distribution, central tendency, variability, and normal distribution, which were introduced in Chapter 17, are reviewed and expanded. Then the new concepts of sampling distribution, significant difference, and power are explained. Finally, the concepts are integrated by a discussion of statistical conclusion validity.

■ DATA SET

Achieving a conceptual understanding of statistical reasoning is greatly enhanced by performing simple computational examples. Thus, a small hypothetical data set has been developed for use throughout this and the following four chapters. Because it would be difficult to develop a small data set relevant to the practice of all of the rehabilitation professions, the data set was developed around a set of hypothetical patients who have undergone the common surgical procedure of total knee arthroplasty. If readers do not have experience treating individuals who have had total knee replacement, surely they have relatives or acquaintances who have undergone this common procedure. Our data set consists of 30 hypothetical patients, 10 at each of three clinics, who have undergone rehabilitation for a total knee arthroplasty. Eighteen pieces of information are available for each patient:

> Case number
> Clinic attended
> Sex
> Age
> Three-week knee flexion range of motion (ROM)
> Six-week knee flexion ROM
> Six-month knee flexion ROM
> Six-month knee extensor torque
> Six-month knee flexor torque
> Six-month gait velocity
> Four 6-month activities of daily living (ADL) indexes
> Four 6-month deformity indexes

The ADL and deformity indexes were adapted for the purposes of this data set from a knee rating system used at Brigham and Women's Hospital in Boston.[2] Table 19–1 provides an outline of the data set, indicating abbreviations for each variable, the unit of measurement when appropriate, and the meaning of any numerical coding. Table 19–2 presents the actual data set.

■ FREQUENCY DISTRIBUTION

A *frequency distribution* is a tally of the number of times each score is represented in a data set. There are four ways of presenting a frequency distribution: frequency distribution with percentages, grouped frequency distribution with percentages, frequency histogram, and stem-and-leaf plot.

TABLE 19-1 Data Set Specifications for Patients Who Underwent Rehabilitation after Total Knee Arthroplasty

Variable Code	Variable Name	Variable Values
CASE	Case number	01-30
CN	Clinic number	1 = Community Hospital
		2 = Memorial Hospital
		3 = Religious Hospital
SEX	Patient sex	0 = male
		1 = female
AGE	Patient age	In years at last birthday
W3R	Three-week range of motion (ROM) at each clinic	To nearest degree
W6R	Six-week ROM	To nearest degree
M6R	Six-month ROM	To nearest degree
E	Six-month extension torque	To nearest Newton • meter(N•m)
F	Six-month flexion torque	To nearest N•m
V	Gait velocity	To nearest cm/sec
DFC	Deformity: flexion contracture	1 = >15°
		2 = 6-15°
		3 = 0-5°
DVV	Deformity: varus/valgus angulation in stance	1 = >10° valgus
		2 = >5° varus or 6-10° valgus
		3 = 5° varus to 5° valgus
DML	Deformity: mediolateral stability	1 = marked instability
		2 = moderate instability
		3 = stable
DAP	Deformity: anteroposterior stability with knee at 90° flexion	1 = marked instability
		2 = moderate instability
		3 = stable
ADW	Activities of daily living (ADL): distance walked	5 = unlimited
		4 = 4-6 blocks
		3 = 2-3 blocks
		2 = indoors only
		1 = transfers only
AAD	ADL: assistive device	5 = none
		4 = cane outside
		3 = cane full-time
		2 = two canes or crutches
		1 = walker or unable to walk
ASC	ADL: stair climbing	5 = reciprocal, no rail
		4 = reciprocal, with rail
		3 = one at a time, with or without rail
		2 = one at a time, with rail and assistive device
		1 = unable to climb stairs
ARC	ADL: rising from a chair	5 = no arm assistance
		4 = single arm assistance
		3 = difficult with two-arm assistance
		2 = needs assistance of another
		1 = unable to rise

TABLE 19–2 Data Set for Patients Who Underwent Rehabilitation After Total Knee Arthroplasty

Case	CN	Sex	Age	W3R	W6R	M6R	E	F	V	DFC	DVV	DML	DAP	ADW	AAD	ASC	ARC
01	1	1	50	95	90	100	170	100	165	2	1	2	1	5	5	5	5
02	1	0	87	32	46	85	100	60	100	2	2	1	1	3	4	4	2
03	1	0	66	67	78	100	130	70	130	1	1	2	2	4	5	5	4
04	1	0	46	92	85	105	175	95	170	2	2	1	2	5	5	5	5
05	1	0	53	87	85	105	157	86	150	1	2	2	2	5	4	5	5
06	1	0	76	58	50	95	88	52	135	2	1	2	2	4	4	4	4
07	1	1	43	92	95	110	120	75	153	1	1	1	1	5	5	5	5
08	1	1	46	88	90	100	130	90	145	2	3	3	2	4	5	5	5
09	1	1	43	84	80	95	132	92	147	1	1	1	2	5	5	5	4
10	1	1	48	81	90	105	156	98	145	2	2	3	2	5	5	4	5
11	2	0	92	34	63	90	87	53	95	3	2	2	2	3	3	3	3
12	2	0	65	56	71	90	160	95	150	2	3	2	2	4	4	5	5
13	2	0	76	45	63	78	92	60	120	1	2	1	2	4	3	3	4
14	2	0	92	27	35	65	85	49	85	3	3	3	3	2	1	1	2
15	2	1	68	76	70	95	170	102	165	2	3	2	2	4	3	5	5
16	2	1	79	49	56	98	81	37	93	2	2	2	1	3	2	3	2
17	2	1	85	47	58	84	87	46	70	3	2	2	2	2	1	2	2
18	2	1	82	50	60	80	93	63	94	1	1	2	2	3	2	2	2
19	2	0	81	40	40	83	96	58	101	2	2	2	2	3	2	1	2
20	2	1	90	67	70	95	103	63	103	1	1	3	3	2	2	2	3
21	3	0	66	32	67	105	180	105	180	1	2	1	1	5	5	5	5
22	3	0	72	50	67	105	150	85	150	2	3	3	2	5	4	4	4
23	3	0	68	60	65	95	154	89	156	2	3	3	2	4	4	4	4
24	3	0	77	84	80	105	141	83	146	2	2	2	1	3	3	4	3
25	3	0	60	81	85	100	168	93	178	3	3	3	2	4	5	5	5
26	3	1	75	81	94	110	146	84	135	2	1	3	3	5	5	5	5
27	3	1	73	84	90	100	120	74	134	2	2	2	3	4	4	4	4
28	3	1	72	81	95	103	110	68	120	2	1	2	3	4	5	3	4
29	3	1	72	82	90	104	116	74	126	3	2	3	1	4	3	4	3
30	3	1	63	91	95	106	137	86	131	2	1	3	3	4	5	5	5

Note: All variables are identified in Table 19–1.

Frequency Distribution with Percentages

Table 19–3 shows a frequency distribution with percentages for the variable 3-week ROM. The first column lists the scores that were obtained. The second column, absolute frequency, lists the number of times that each score was obtained. For example, two patients had 3-week ROM values of 67°. The third column, relative frequency, lists the percentage of patients who received each score. This is calculated by dividing the number of patients with that score by the total number of patients. From this column we find that the four patients who had scores of 81 represent 13.3% of the sample

$[(4/30) \times 100 = 13.3\%]$. The fourth column, cumulative frequency, is formed by adding the relative frequencies of the scores up to and including the score of interest. For example, a researcher might be interested in the percentage of patients who had ROM scores of less than 50° 3 weeks postoperatively. From the cumulative frequency column one finds that 26.7% of the sample had ROM values of 49° or less.

A variation of this basic display is needed if there are missing values in the sample. Suppose that Patients 3 through 5 missed their 3-week evaluation appointments. Table 19–4 presents a revised frequency distribution that accounts for these three missing pieces of data. Note that another column, adjusted frequency, has been added. The adjusted frequency is calculated by dividing the number of observations for each score by the number of valid scores for each variable, rather than by the number of participants. In this case, there are 27 valid scores. The relative frequency of a ROM score of 81° is now 14.8% $[(4/27) \times 100 = 14.8\%]$. The cumulative frequency is the sum of the adjusted frequencies. If many data points are missing, it is often misleading to present the frequencies as percentages of the total sample; use of adjusted frequencies corrects the problem.

Grouped Frequency Distribution with Percentages

The grouped frequency distribution is another way frequency information is commonly presented. When there are many individual scores in a distribution, the characteristics of the distribution may be grasped more easily if scores are placed into groups. Table 19–5 presents a grouped frequency distribution for the 3-week ROM values. From this grouped distribution it is readily apparent that the group with the highest frequency is that with scores from 80° to 89°.

A disadvantage of the grouped frequency distribution is that information is lost. Table 19–5 indicates that there are three subjects whose

TABLE 19–3	Frequency Distribution of 3-Week Range-of-Motion Values

Score (°)	Absolute Frequency	Relative Frequency (%)	Cumulative Frequency (%)
27	1	3.3	3.3
32	2	6.7	10.0
34	1	3.3	13.3
40	1	3.3	16.7
45	1	3.3	20.0
47	1	3.3	23.3
49	1	3.3	26.7
50	2	6.7	33.4
56	1	3.3	36.7
58	1	3.3	40.0
60	1	3.3	43.3
67	2	6.7	50.0
76	1	3.3	53.3
81	4	13.3	66.6
82	1	3.3	70.0
84	3	10.0	80.0
87	1	3.3	83.3
88	1	3.3	86.6
91	1	3.3	90.0
92	2	6.7	96.7
95	1	3.3	100.0
TOTAL	30	100.0	

scores range from 30° to 39°. But what does this mean? This could mean all three patients had scores of 39, three patients had scores of 30, or the three had a variety of scores within this range.

Frequency Histogram

Another way to present a grouped frequency distribution is a histogram. A histogram presents each grouped frequency as a bar on a graph. The height of each bar represents the frequency of observations in the group. Figure 19–1 shows a histogram of the 3-week ROM data. As with the grouped frequency distribution from which the histogram is generated, information is lost

because one does not know how the scores are distributed within each group.

Stem-and-Leaf Plot

A final way of presenting frequency data is the stem-and-leaf plot. This plot presents data concisely, without losing information in the grouping process. Each individual score is divided into a "stem" and a "leaf," as shown in Table 19–6. In this instance, the stem is the digit representing the multiple of 10 (20, 30, 40, and so on), and the leaf is the digit representing the multiple of 1 (1, 2, 3, 4, and so on). The row with the stem of 5 has leaves of 0, 0, 6, and 8. The stems and leaves together represent the four scores of 50,

TABLE 19–4	**Frequency Distribution of 3-Week Range-of-Motion Scores, Modified for Missing Values**			
Score (°)	Absolute Frequency	Relative Frequency (%)	Adjusted Frequency (%)	Cumulative Frequency (%)
27	1	3.3	3.7	3.7
32	2	6.7	7.4	11.1
34	1	3.3	3.7	14.8
40	1	3.3	3.7	18.5
45	1	3.3	3.7	22.2
47	1	3.3	3.7	25.9
49	1	3.3	3.7	29.6
50	2	6.7	7.4	37.0
56	1	3.3	3.7	40.7
58	1	3.3	3.7	44.4
60	1	3.3	3.7	48.1
67	1	3.3	3.7	51.8
76	1	3.3	3.7	55.5
81	4	13.3	14.8	70.3
82	1	3.3	3.7	74.3
84	3	10.0	11.1	85.1
88	1	3.3	3.7	88.8
91	1	3.3	3.7	92.5
92	1	3.3	3.7	96.2
95	1	3.3	3.7	100.0
Missing	3	10.0	Missing	
TOTAL	30	100.0	100.0	

50, 56, and 58. The stem-and-leaf plot, like the histogram, provides a good visual picture of the frequency distribution.

■ CENTRAL TENDENCY

Researchers often wish to collapse a set of data into a single score that represents the whole set, that is, the researcher is interested in the central tendency of the data. The measures of central tendency, along with the measures of variability that will follow, are known as *descriptive statistics*. The three commonly used measures of central tendency are the mean, the median, and

the mode. If a distribution is perfectly symmetric, then the mean, median, and mode are all identical. If the distribution is asymmetric, they differ.

Mean

The arithmetic *mean* of a data set is the sum of the observations divided by the number of observations. Recall from Chapter 17 that mathematical notation for the mean is as follows:

$$\overline{X} = \frac{\Sigma X}{N} \qquad \text{(Formula 19–1)}$$

In words, this equation says the mean is the sum of all the observations divided by the number of observations. The mean of the 3-week ROM scores for Clinic 1 is 77.6°– [(95 + 32 + 67 + 92 + 87 + 58 + 92 + 88 + 84 + 81)/10 = 77.6]. The mean is a versatile measure of central tendency because it uses information from all the scores in the distribution. However, extreme values can distort the mean. In this example, seven of the 10 scores are greater than 80°, but the very low score of 32° pulls the mean down to 77.6°.

Median

The *median* is the "middle" score of a distribution, or the score above which half of the distribution

Scores (°)	Frequency	Relative Frequency (%)	Cumulative Frequency (%)
20-29	1	3.3	3.3
30-39	3	10.0	13.3
40-49	4	13.3	26.7
50-59	4	13.3	40.0
60-69	3	10.0	50.0
70-79	1	3.3	53.3
80-89	10	33.3	86.7
90-99	4	13.3	100.0
TOTAL	30	100.0	

TABLE 19-5 Grouped Frequency Distribution for 3-Week Range-of-Motion Values

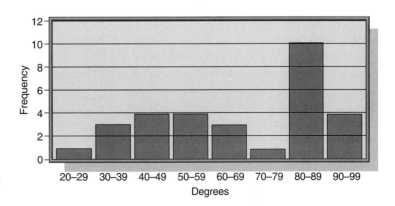

FIGURE 19–1. Histogram of 3-week range-of-motion scores.

lies. To calculate the median, a researcher must first rank the scores. When the distribution has an odd number of scores, the middle score is easy to locate: $(N + 1)/2$ = the middle-ranked score. Thus, in a sample of 987 scores, the 494th ranked score is the median. When the number of scores in a distribution is even, as in our example, the median is calculated by finding the mean of the two middle scores: $[N/2]$ and $[(N/2) + 1]$. In a sample with 988 scores, the median is the mean of the 494th and 495th ranked scores. Table 19–7 presents the frequency distribution for the ten 3-week measurements we are considering. The median, as shown, is 85.5°. The median is a useful measure of central tendency when the distribution contains a few extreme values that distort the mean. In addition, the median is often used to describe the central tendency of ordinal measurements, particularly if further statistical analysis of the measures will be done with nonparametric statistics (to be described in more detail in Chapter 20). The disadvantage of the median is that it does not include information from all of the scores in the distribution.

Mode

The *mode* is the score that occurs most frequently in a distribution. If there are two modes, the distribution is termed *bimodal*. Our example of 3-week ROM scores has a mode of 92, as shown in Table 19–7. The mode is often used to describe nominal data, which have neither the property of order nor the property of distance and therefore cannot provide a median and mean (see Chapter 17).

TABLE 19-6	Stem-and-Leaf Plot of 3-Week Range-of-Motion Frequency Distribution	
Stem	**Leaf**	**Total**
2	7	1
3	2 2 4	3
4	0 5 7 9	4
5	0 0 6 8	4
6	0 7 7	3
7	6	1
8	1 1 1 1 2 4 4 4 7 8	10
9	1 2 2 5	4
TOTAL		30

TABLE 19-7	Median and Mode Calculations for 3-Week Range-of-Motion Values for Clinic 1			
Score (°)	**Absolute Frequency**	**Cumulative (%)**	**Median***	**Mode†**
32	1	10.0		
58	1	20.0		
67	1	30.0		
81	1	40.0		
84	1	50.0		
			85.5	
87	1	60.0		
88	1	70.0		
92	2	90.0		92
95	1	100.0		

*Median is the "middle" score. When there is an even number of scores, the two middle scores are averaged. In this example, the median is (84 + 87)/2 = 85.5.
†Mode is the score that occurs most frequently.

■ VARIABILITY

The variability of a data set is the amount of spread in the data. Two different groups might have the same mean score, yet have very different characteristics. For example, a sample of female college athletes might have the same mean weight as a sample of female nonathletes at the school. However, the athletes would be expected to have a relatively narrow range of weights, whereas the nonathletes would be expected to range in weight from the very underweight to the very overweight. The three measures of variability are range, variance, and standard deviation.

Range

The *range* is the difference between the highest and lowest values in the distribution. In the group of 10 patients from Clinic 1, the range is 63° (95 − 32 = 63). Although the range is technically a single score, it is often reported by presenting both the high and low scores so that readers will understand not only the range but also the magnitude of the scores in the distribution. The range can be used as a measure of variability with any of the measures of central tendency, but is particularly appropriate for use with the median.

Variance

The *variance* is a measure of variability that, like the mean, requires that every score in the distribution be used in its calculation. Therefore, the variance, along with the closely related standard deviation, are generally reported in concert with the mean. Although the calculation of the variance is presented in Chapter 17, it is reviewed here with our 3-week ROM data from Clinic 1. To calculate the variance, we convert each of the raw scores in the data set to a *deviation score* by subtracting the mean of the data set from each raw score. In mathematical notation,

$$x = X - \overline{X} \qquad \text{(Formula 19–2)}$$

Recall from Chapter 17 that the lowercase, italic x is the symbol for a deviation score. The deviation score indicates how high or low a raw score is compared with the mean. The first two columns of Table 19–8 present the raw and deviation scores for the knee flexion data set and, below them, their sums and means. Note that both the sum and the mean of the deviation scores are zero. To generate a nonzero index of the variability within a data set, we must square the deviation scores. We can then calculate the *population variance* by determining the mean of the squared deviations. In mathematical notation,

$$\sigma^2 = \frac{\sum x^2}{N} \qquad \text{(Formula 19–3)}$$

We know from Chapter 17 that σ is the lowercase Greek sigma and when squared is the notation for the variance. The third column in Table 19–8 shows the squared deviations from the group mean and, below them, their sum and mean. The population variance is used when all of the members of a population are known. In practice this rarely occurs, so the *sample variance* is used to *estimate* the population variance. The sample variance is calculated by dividing the sum of the squared deviations by N − 1, as follows:

$$s^2 = \frac{\sum x^2}{N - 1} \qquad \text{(Formula 19–4)}$$

The symbol for the sample variance is s^2. In our example, the sample variance is calculated by dividing 3542.40 (the sum of the squared deviations) by 9 (N − 1), as shown in Table 19–8.

The rationale for dividing the sum of the squared deviations by N − 1 rests on the concept of *degrees of freedom*. Although an abstract concept, degrees of freedom can be understood in a general sense through the use of an illustration. In a sample of 10 values with a known mean, nine of the values are "free" to fluctuate, as long as the investigator has control over the final

	X	x	x^2	z score	p
TABLE 19-8					

TABLE 19-8 Computation of the Variance, z Scores, and Probabilities for 3-Week Range-of-Motion Scores at Clinic 1

	X	x	x^2	z score	p
	32	− 45.6	2,079.36	−2.30	.011
	58	− 19.6	384.16	−.99	.161
	67	− 10.6	112.36	−.53	.298
	81	3.4	11.56	.17	.433
	84	6.4	40.96	.32	.374
	87	9.4	88.36	.47	.319
	88	10.4	108.16	.52	.302
	92	14.4	207.36	.73	.233
	92	14.4	207.36	.73	.233
	95	17.4	302.76	.88	.189
$\Sigma =$	776	0	3,542.40		
$\overline{X} =$	77.6	0	354.24	= population variance (σ^2)	
			18.82	= population standard deviation (σ)	
$s^2 = \dfrac{\Sigma x^2}{N - 1}$			393.60	= sample variance (s^2)	
			19.84	= sample standard deviation (s)	

value. For our sample of 10 observations with a mean of 77.6°, the sum of those 10 observations is 776. If we wanted to generate another sample with a mean of 77.6°, we could select nine numbers randomly as long as we could manipulate the tenth value. If nine randomly selected numbers each have a value of 100, then they add to a total of 900. The sample can still have a mean value of 77.6° if the tenth value is manipulated to be −124 (900 − 124 = 776; 776/10 = 77.6). This phenomenon is termed *degrees of freedom*, or the number of items that are free to fluctuate. Thus, for the mean, there are always N − 1 degrees of freedom. Statisticians have found that using the degrees of freedom for the mean as the denominator of the sample variance formula leads to an unbiased estimation of the population variance. The degrees of freedom concept is used in the computation of many different statistical tests.

Standard Deviation

As just defined, the population variance is the mean of the squared deviations from the mean, and the sample variance is the sum of the squared deviations from the mean, divided by the degrees of freedom for the mean. Although the variance is useful in many statistical procedures, it does not have a great deal of intuitive meaning because it is calculated from squared deviation scores. A measure that has such meaning is the *standard deviation*. The standard deviation is the square root of the variance and is expressed in the units of the original measure. The population standard deviation is the square root of the population variance; the sample standard deviation is the square root of the sample variance:

$$s = \sqrt{s^2}$$

The mathematical notations for the sample standard deviation and the sample variance make their relationship clear: The notation for the variance (s^2) is simply the square of the notation for standard deviation (s). In practice, the entire population is not usually measured, so the sample standard deviation is used as an estimate of the population standard deviation. The sample standard deviation of the knee flexion data presented in Table 19–8 is the square root of 393.60, or 19.84°.

Taken together, the measures of central tendency and variability are referred to as descriptive measures. When these measures are used to describe a population, they are known as *parameters;* when they are used to describe a sample, they are known as *statistics.* Because researchers can rarely measure all the individuals within a population, they use sample statistics such as the mean and standard deviation as estimates of the corresponding population parameters.

■ NORMAL DISTRIBUTION

The normal distribution is central to many of the statistical tests that are presented in subsequent chapters. Groups of measurements frequently approximate a bell-shaped distribution known as the normal curve. The *normal curve* is a symmetric frequency distribution that can be defined in terms of the mean and standard deviation of a set of data.

z Score

Any score within a distribution can be standardized with respect to the mean and standard deviation

of the data. That is, each score can be expressed in terms of how many standard deviations it is above or below the mean. The result of such a standardization procedure is called a *z score.* A *z* score is calculated by dividing the deviation score ($x = X - \bar{X}$) by the standard deviation:

$$z = \frac{x}{s} \qquad \text{(Formula 19–5)}$$

When a normally distributed set of data is converted to *z* scores, the distribution of the *z* scores is known as the *standard normal distribution.* The standard normal distribution has a mean of zero and a standard deviation of 1.0. The fourth column of Table 19–8 shows our 10 raw 3-week ROM scores as *z* scores. This was done by dividing each of the deviation scores (x) by the standard deviation (s) of 19.84°. The magnitude and sign of the *z* score tell us, for example, that a measurement of 32° is 2.30 standard deviations below the mean.

Percentages of the Normal Distribution

In a normal distribution, the percentage of scores that fall within a certain range of scores is known. Approximately 68% of scores fall within 1 standard deviation above or below the mean. Approximately 96% of the scores fall within 2 standard deviations of the mean, and almost 100% of the scores fall within 3 standard deviations of the mean. Figure 19–2 shows a diagram of the normal curve, with the exact percentages of scores that are found within each standard deviation.

Figure 19–3, *A,* shows the normal curve that corresponds to our 3-week ROM data for Clinic 1. The sample mean is 77.6°, and the sample standard deviation is 19.84°. The x axis is labeled with both *z* scores and the raw scores that correspond to 1, 2, and 3 standard deviations above and below the mean. Figure 19–3, *B,* shows that if the knee flexion scores are normally distributed,

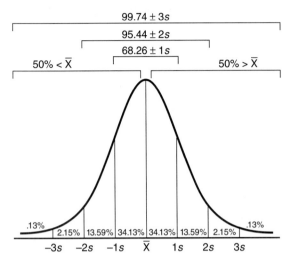

FIGURE 19–2. Percentages of the normal distribution. X̄ = mean; s = standard deviation.

we would estimate that 98% of our measurements would exceed the score of 37.92°; Figure 19–3, *C*, shows that we could expect 68% of our measurements to fall between 57.76° and 97.44°. Clinicians who have a good conceptual understanding of the standard deviation and the probabilities of the normal distribution can understand a great deal about the characteristics of the individuals within a group being studied. In fact, the standard deviation is so fundamental to understanding the literature that one occupational therapy researcher has gone so far as to say that "once the standard deviation is understood, all else follows."[3(p115)] Using the standard deviation to predict the probability of obtaining certain ranges of scores is basic to most of the statistical testing presented in Chapters 20 and 21.

We know from the preceding paragraphs the approximate probability of obtaining scores within 1, 2, and 3 standard deviations of the mean. A table of *z* scores can provide exact probabilities of achieving scores at any level within the distribution. Earlier we calculated that 32° of ROM at 3 weeks postoperatively was 2.30 standard deviations below the mean for patients at

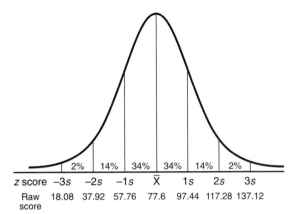

A

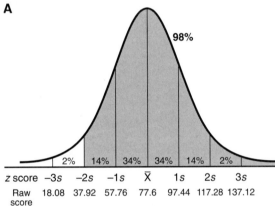

B

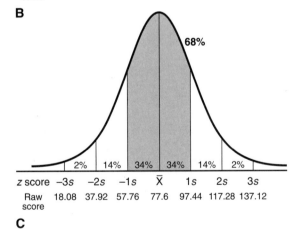

C

FIGURE 19–3. **A,** Percentages of the normal distribution for 3-week range-of-motion scores at Clinic 1. **B,** Shaded area represents approximately 98% of the distribution. **C,** Shaded area represents approximately 68% of the distribution. X̄ = mean; s = standard deviation.

Clinic 1. Without a table, we know only that the probability of obtaining scores outside the second standard deviation is approximately 2%. Consulting a z table tells us the exact probability of obtaining scores that are less than or equal to 2.30 standard deviations below the mean. Appendix B provides a z table.

To identify the z score of 2.30 in Appendix B, look in the far left-hand column for the stem 2.3, and then read across the uppermost row to the leaf .00. The intersection of the row and column gives a value of .011 or, if stated as a percentage, 1.1%. The picture of the normal curve above the table shows that the proportion indicated is either at the upper or lower tail of the curve, depending on whether the z score is positive or negative. Because the curve is symmetric, there is no need for separate tables of positive and negative z scores; researchers simply need to know that the probabilities associated with positive z scores lie in the upper portion of the curve and the probabilities associated with negative z scores lie in the lower portion of the curve. The final column of Table 19–8 gives the probabilities associated with each z score. Readers may wish to use the z table in Appendix B to confirm that they understand how these probabilities were obtained.

■ SAMPLING DISTRIBUTION

To understand statistical testing, it is extremely important to understand sampling distributions. The sampling distribution is a specific type of normal distribution. Imagine that you had access to the entire population of individuals who had total knee arthroplasties in a given year. If we drew a random sample of 10 individuals from this large population and examined their 3-week ROM values, we might get a sample with a mean of 77.6°, as in the example from Clinic 1. If we drew another random sample of 10 individuals, we might get a mean of 98.2°. If we drew another random sample, we might get a mean of 59.1°. Assume that we drew 10 samples and obtained means of 77.6°, 98.2°, 59.1°, 84.5°,

78.9°, 45.6°, 89.5°, 64.3°, 68.7°, and 75.4°. Using each of these mean scores to represent each sample, we can calculate both a mean of the sample means (74.18°) and a standard deviation of the sample means (15.37°).

Table 19–9 shows the calculations that provide this mean and standard deviation. The calculations are the same as those presented in Table 19–8; the only difference is that each score in the distribution in Table 19–9 represents a group rather than an individual, as in Table 19–8. The distribution of the means of several samples drawn from the same population is called a *sampling distribution*. The mean of the sampling distribution is assumed to be the mean of the population. The standard deviation of the sampling distribution is called the *standard error of the mean*, or the SEM. Note that the SEM is also the abbreviation for the standard error of measurement (see Chapter 17). When this

TABLE 19-9	Computation of the Mean, Sample Variance (s^2), and Sample Standard Deviation (s) for the Sampling Distribution of Three-Week Range-of-Motion Scores		
	X	x	x^2
	98.2	24.02	576.96
	89.5	15.32	234.70
	84.5	10.32	106.50
	78.9	4.72	22.28
	77.6	3.42	11.70
	75.4	1.22	1.48
	68.7	– 5.48	30.03
	64.3	– 9.88	97.61
	59.1	– 15.08	227.41
	45.6	– 28.58	816.82
$\Sigma =$	741.8	0	2125.49
$\overline{X} =$	74.18	0	

$$s^2 = \frac{\Sigma x^2}{N-1} = 236.16$$

$$s = 15.37$$

abbreviation is used, it should be made clear whether it refers to the standard error of the mean or the standard error of measurement. The term "error" does not refer to a mistake made by the researcher. Rather, "error" denotes the inevitable differences that are found between a population and the samples that are drawn from the population.

The SEM varies with sample size. When we draw sample sizes of 10, the presence of just one extremely low or high value alters the mean greatly. For example, assume that we have nine scores of 75° and one score of 115°; the mean is 79°, which is 4° away from the modal score of 75°. Do the same to a sample of 100 with 99 scores of 75° and one score of 115°. The mean in this case is 75.4°, which is less than half a degree higher than the majority of scores. Thus, the means of large samples are more stable than means of small samples because they are less influenced by extreme scores. This stability is reflected in the magnitude of the SEM: The SEM of a sampling distribution generated from a large sample is small; the SEM of a sampling distribution generated from a small sample is large.

Researchers usually do not have the time or resources to draw repeated samples from a population to determine the SEM of the resulting sampling distribution. Therefore, the SEM is usually estimated from a single sample drawn for study. As just noted, the sample size greatly affects the variability of mean scores, so the SEM estimation formula takes sample size into account:

$$\text{SEM} = \frac{s}{\sqrt{N}} \qquad \text{(Formula 19–6)}$$

The estimate of the SEM is found by dividing the sample standard deviation (s) by the square root of the number in the sample. This estimated SEM, or one of several mathematical variations, is used in the calculation of many of the statistical tests discussed in Chapters 21 and 22. For our single sample with a mean of 77.6°, a standard deviation of 19.84°, and a sample size of 10, the estimated SEM is $6.27° (19.84/\sqrt{10} = 6.27)$.

Confidence Intervals of the Sampling Distribution

Because the sampling distribution is a normal distribution, we can find the probability of obtaining a sample with a certain range of mean scores by consulting a z table. The procedure is the same as discussed earlier, except that the scores now represent sample means rather than individual scores. Earlier we started with a particular z score and determined the probability of obtaining scores that either equaled or exceeded the selected score. We can also use the z table in reverse by specifying a particular probability in which we are interested and determining the z score that corresponds to that probability. This reverse process is used to determine *confidence intervals* (CIs) about the mean.

Recall that the sample mean of 3-week ROM scores at Clinic 1 is 77.6°, the standard deviation is 19.84°, and the SEM is 6.27°. We recognize that the obtained sample mean is only an estimate of the population mean because of the phenomenon of sampling error. We can use the probabilities of the sampling distribution to identify a range of mean scores that is likely to include the true population mean. If we take the mean score (77.6) and subtract and add one SEM (77.6 − 6.27 = 71.33; 77.6 + 6.27 = 82.87), we get a range of means from 71.33° to 82.87°. From our knowledge of the probabilities of the normal distribution we know that approximately 68% of the scores in a distribution fall within the first standard deviation from the mean. Thus, there is an approximately 68% chance that the true population mean lies somewhere between 71.33° and 82.87°. This is known as the 68% CI.

In practice, researchers usually report a 90%, 95%, or 99% CI. To generate these intervals, we need to determine what z scores correspond to them. For the 90% CI, 10% is excluded—5% (.05) in the upper tail of the distribution and 5% in the lower tail of the distribution. For the 95% and 99% CIs, the percentages excluded in each tail are 2.5% (.025) and 0.5% (.005), respectively.

Refer to the z table in Appendix B to confirm that the z scores that correspond to .05 and .025 are 1.645 and 1.960, respectively. The z table included in this text was selected for its simplicity and conciseness. However, this simplicity is at the expense of some precision in the very low probability ranges. Thus, we cannot determine from the concise z table of Appendix B the exact z score that corresponds to .005. From a more complete z table printed elsewhere, the value is found to be 2.575.[4(p309)] Thus, the desired CI of the mean is determined by adding and subtracting the appropriate number of SEMs to and from the mean. In mathematical notation,

$$90\% \text{ CI} = \overline{X} \pm 1.645 \text{ (SEM)}$$

$$95\% \text{ CI} = \overline{X} \pm 1.960 \text{ (SEM)}$$

$$99\% \text{ CI} = \overline{X} \pm 2.575 \text{ (SEM)}$$

Inserting the values of 77.6° ($\overline{X}$) and 6.27° (SEM), we find the following:

$$90\% \text{ CI} = 67.3° \text{ to } 87.9°$$

$$95\% \text{ CI} = 65.3° \text{ to } 89.9°$$

$$99\% \text{ CI} = 61.4° \text{ to } 93.7°$$

We are 90% confident that the true population mean is somewhere between 67.3° and 87.9°; we are 99% confident that it lies somewhere between 61.4° and 93.7°. The computations given here are for the simplest calculation of a CI for the population mean. CIs can also be calculated for population proportions, for the difference between population proportions, and for the difference between population means.[4(pp123–129)]

■ SIGNIFICANT DIFFERENCE

Researchers often wish to do more than describe their data. They wish to determine whether there are differences between groups who have been exposed to different treatments. The branch of statistics that is used to determine whether, among other things, there are significant differences between groups is known as *inferential statistics*. The theoretical basis of inferential statistics is that population parameters can be inferred from sample statistics. The determination of whether two sample means are significantly different from one another is actually a determination of the likelihood that the two sample means are drawn from populations with the same means. The sampling distribution of the mean is used as the basis for making these inferential statements—it is the link between the observed samples and the theorized population.

When we compare two groups who have received different experimental treatments, we almost always find that there is some difference between the means of the two groups. For example, assume that we wish to determine the effect of continuous passive motion on 3-week ROM in our patients who have had total knee arthroplasty. Assume that the patients at Clinic 1 received continuous passive motion postoperatively and that the patients at Clinic 3 did not. The mean 3-week ROM score for Clinic 1 is 77.6°; for Clinic 3, it is 72.6°. This is a difference of 5.0°. We wonder whether this difference is a true difference between the two groups or chance variation due to sampling error.

If it is highly likely that the difference was due to sampling error, then we conclude that there is *no significant difference* between the two group means. In other words, if sampling errors are a likely explanation for the difference between the means of the groups, then it is likely that the two groups were drawn from populations with the same means. Conversely, if it is highly unlikely that the difference between the groups was the result of sampling errors, then we conclude that there is a *significant difference* between the groups. If sampling error is not a likely explanation for differences between the groups, then it is likely that the two groups come from populations with different means. To determine whether the difference between groups is significant, we test a null hypothesis at a particular alpha level, as described next.

Although the traditional basis for determining statistical differences is presented in the following section, it should be noted that there is a long history of dissatisfaction with this approach to statistical analysis.[5,6] Objections include the need to make all-or-none decisions, the arbitrary nature of conventional levels for determining statistical significance, the sensitivity of results to sample size, and the inability of statistical tests to make value judgments about the clinical importance of statistically significant findings.[6] Despite these objections, significance testing remains the norm for statistical testing, and researchers and readers need to understand the conventions upon which it is based.

Null Hypothesis

The seemingly convoluted language needed to describe the meaning of a statistically significant difference derives from the fact that the statistical hypothesis that is tested is the hypothesis of "no difference." This hypothesis is referred to as the *null hypothesis*, or H_0. The formal null hypothesis for determining whether there are different mean 3-week ROM scores between Clinics 1 and 3 is as follows:

$$H_0: \mu_1 = \mu_3$$

Thus, the null hypothesis is that the population mean for Clinic 1 (μ_1) is equal to the population mean for Clinic 3 (μ_3). For now we will assume that the alternative hypothesis, or H_1, is that the population mean of Clinic 1 is greater than the population mean of Clinic 3:

$$H_1: \mu_1 > \mu_3$$

Alternative hypotheses are addressed later with specific statistical tests. In statistical testing, we determine the probability that the null hypothesis is true. If the probability is sufficiently low, we conclude that the null hypothesis is false, accept the alternative hypothesis, and conclude that there are significant differences between the groups. If the probability that the null hypothesis is true is high, we conclude that

the null hypothesis is true, accept the null hypothesis, and conclude that there are no significant differences between the groups. The clinical importance of any significant differences that are identified cannot be assumed; researchers and readers need to determine the clinical importance of statistical findings in light of clinical knowledge and experience.

Alpha Level

Before conducting a statistical analysis of differences, researchers must determine how much of a probability of drawing an incorrect conclusion they are willing to tolerate. To use null hypothesis terminology, how low is the "sufficiently low" probability needed to detect a significant difference? The conventional level of chance that is tolerated is 5%, or .05. This is referred to as the *alpha* (α) *level*. If a difference in means is significant at the .05 level, this means that 5% of differences of this magnitude would have been the result of chance fluctuations caused by sampling errors. That is, 95% of the time the difference would represent a true difference and 5% of the time the difference would represent sampling error. Occasionally the more stringent level of .01 is used, as is the more permissive level of .10.

There are two twists that occur with alpha levels as they are reported in research. The first is the distinction between the alpha level and the obtained probability; the second is inflation and correction of the alpha level during performance of multiple statistical tests.

The distinction between the alpha level and the obtained probability (p) level is the distinction between what the researcher is willing to accept as chance and what the actual results are. The alpha level is specified before the data analysis is conducted; the probability level is a product of the data analysis. Researchers may set the alpha level at .05, meaning that they are willing to accept a 5% chance that significant findings may actually be the result of sampling error. In studies in which significant differences are found, the actual probability that a given result will occur by chance may be much less than the alpha level set by the researcher.

Assume that the result of a statistical test comparing two group means is that the probability that the difference will occur by chance is .001. This means that in only 1 of 1000 instances would a difference of this magnitude likely be the result of sampling error. Now that computers are available to calculate statistics, such precise probability levels are often reported. Because the obtained probability level of .001 is less than the preset alpha level of .05, the researcher concludes that there is a significant difference between the groups. Does the reporting of the obtained probability level of .001 somehow indicate that the researcher changed the alpha level during the course of the data analysis? No. The reporting of a specific probability level simply indicates to the reader the extent to which the obtained probability was lower or higher than the alpha set by the researcher.

The second twist that is given to an alpha level in a study is called *alpha level inflation.* This occurs when researchers conduct many statistical tests within a given study. Using an alpha level of 5%, we know that the probability that differences occurred by chance is 5% for each test. If we conduct many tests, the overall probability of obtaining chance significant differences increases. This increase is alpha level inflation. When researchers conduct multiple tests, they may correct for alpha level inflation by using a more stringent alpha level for each individual test. They may obtain a more stringent alpha by using, for example, the *Bonferroni adjustment.* This adjustment divides the total alpha level for the experiment, called the *experiment-wise alpha level,* by the number of statistical tests conducted to determine a *test-wise alpha level.*[7(p128)] For example, a researcher may set the experiment-wise alpha level at .05 and conduct 10 tests, each with a test-wise alpha level of .005 (.05/10 = .005). Some researchers consider this adjustment too stringent and compensate by setting a higher experiment-wise alpha level. For example, if a researcher sets the experiment-wise alpha at .15 and conducts seven tests, the adjusted test-wise alpha level would be .0214. Although the Bonferroni adjustment is commonly used, statisticians do not always agree on when to adjust for alpha inflation, nor do they all agree that the Bonferroni adjustment is the best procedure to use when an adjustment is desired.[8,9]

Two articles illustrate somewhat different reasons for using a Bonferroni adjustment. Murray used the adjustment when doing multiple comparisons among four groups of subjects on a variety of spoken language variables.[10] The four groups were those with Huntington's disease (HD), those with Parkinson's disease (PD), and a control group matched to each of the diagnostic groups (CON-HD and CON-PD). In this study, there were three comparisons of interest: HD versus CON-HD, PD versus CON-PD, and HD versus PD. Each statistical test of these differences was conducted at an alpha level of .016 (.05/3 = .016). Mueller and colleagues used a Bonferroni adjustment because of the large number of dependent variables used in their study of functional status after transmetatarsal amputation.[11] One of the measures, the physical performance test, can have a total score as well as be subdivided into eight subscores. Mueller chose to conduct a statistical test on the total score at an alpha level of .05. Then, he conducted eight more tests on the subscores, each at a divided alpha level of .006 (.05/8 = .006).

Statistical analysis requires that the researcher set an alpha level. If the statistical test results in an obtained probability that is less than the predetermined alpha level, the result is deemed statistically significant. Whether a result is statistically significant or not often depends on the way in which the researcher sets the alpha level. Thus, tests of statistical significance do not provide absolute conclusions about the meaning of data. Rather, these tests provide the researcher with information about the probability that the obtained results occurred by chance. The researcher then draws statistical conclusions about whether a statistically significant difference exists. Researchers and readers then need to interpret the statistical conclusions in light of their knowledge of the subject being studied.

Probability Determinants

Three pieces of information are essential to the determination of statistical probabilities: the magnitude of the differences *between* groups (or between levels of the independent variable when there is only one group), variability *within* a group, and sample size. In this section, the effect of each of these determinants is illustrated conceptually, without determination of actual probabilities. Actual probabilities are determined in subsequent chapters when specific statistical tests are discussed.

BETWEEN-GROUPS DIFFERENCE

To illustrate the influence of the size of the difference between two groups, let us compare the differences in mean 3-week ROM scores between Clinics 1 through 3. Clinic 1 has a mean of 77.6°, Clinic 2 a mean of 49.1°, and Clinic 3 a mean of 72.6°. If within-group variability and sample size are held constant, then a larger between-groups difference is associated with a smaller probability that the difference occurred by chance. Thus, there is a relatively low probability that the large 28.5° difference in the 3-week ROM means for Clinics 1 and 2 occurred by chance. Conversely, there is a relatively high probability that the smaller 5.0° difference in the 3-week ROM means for Clinics 1 and 3 did occur by chance.

WITHIN-GROUP VARIABILITY

The second piece of information used to determine the probability that a difference is a true difference is the variability within a group. If the between-groups difference and sample size are held constant, the differences between groups with lower within-group variability have a lower probability of occurring by chance than difference between groups with high within-group variability. Assume that we have two groups of

100 with means of 72.6° and 77.6°. If the groups have high within-group variability—say, standard deviations of 30.0°—curves representing their sampling distributions would look like those drawn in Figure 19–4, *A*. The sampling distributions, which each have an SEM of 3 (30/$\sqrt{100}$ = 3), overlap a great deal.

Because of the overlap in sampling distributions, there is a high probability that the two samples came from populations that have the same mean. Because this probability is high, we conclude that the difference in means occurred

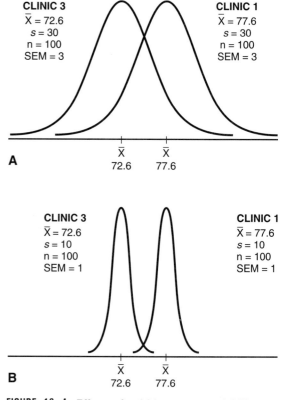

FIGURE 19–4. Effect of within-group variability on the overlap of sampling distributions. **A,** High variability leads to overlap of sampling distributions. **B,** Low variability leads to minimal overlap of sampling distributions. $\bar{X}$ = mean; *s* = standard deviation; *n* = number of subjects; SEM = standard error of the mean.

by chance; that is, the difference between the means of the two groups is not significant.

Contrast Figure 19–4, parts A and B. Figure 19–4, *B,* illustrates the same between-groups difference, 5.0°. However, the within-group variability has been reduced sharply. In this example, each group standard deviation is set at 10.0°, meaning that the SEM is 1° ($10/\sqrt{100} = 1$). With an SEM of only 1°, the two curves overlap very little. Because they do not overlap very much, there is a low probability that the samples could have been drawn from populations with the same mean. Because this probability is low, we can conclude that the difference in means did not occur by chance; that is, the difference between the means of the two groups is a significant one. Even small differences between groups can be statistically significant if the within-group variability is sufficiently low.

EFFECT SIZE

The two pieces of information listed above can be combined into a single concept known as effect size. The effect size is the between-group difference divided by a pooled version of the standard deviations of the groups being compared. Large between-group differences and small within-group variability result in large effect sizes. Small between-group differences and large within-group variability result in small effect sizes. Computing effect size allows the relative magnitude of experimental effects to be compared across variables with different measurement characteristics. Convention has it that an effect size of 0.20 is considered small, 0.50 is considered medium, and 0.80 is considered large when comparing two group means.[12]

SAMPLE SIZE

The third piece of information used to determine the probability that a difference is a true difference is the sample size. We already know that the mean of a large sample is more stable than a mean of a small sample. Assume that we have

two groups of 100, each with a standard deviation of 10.0°, and a mean difference between the groups of 5.0°. Because of the large sample sizes, we are confident that the mean values are stable indicators of the means of the populations from which the samples are drawn. The estimated SEM for each group's sampling distribution is 1.0° ($10/\sqrt{100} = 1$); Figure 19–5, *A,* shows the minimal overlap between the two sampling distributions. This minimal overlap leads us to conclude that it is unlikely that the differences between the two groups are due to chance; in other words, there is a significant difference between the groups.

Now assume that we have two groups of 10 participants each. The mean difference between the groups is the same as the previous example (5.0°), as is the standard deviation of each group (10.0°). Because we know that sample sizes of only 10 are sensitive to extreme values, we know that the mean of a sample of 10 is considerably less stable than a mean from a sample of 100. This is reflected in the calculation of the estimated SEM. With a standard deviation of 10° and a sample size of 10, the SEM becomes 3.16° ($10/\sqrt{10} = 3.16$). Figure 19–5, *B,* shows the curves that correspond to the sampling distributions of our smaller samples. The curves overlap considerably, leading us to conclude that the samples might well have been drawn from populations with the same mean; that is, there is no significant difference between the means of the two groups. Thus, if the sample size is large enough, even small between-groups differences may be statistically significant and, conversely, if the sample size is too small, even large between-groups differences may not be statistically significant.

■ ERRORS

Because researchers determine statistical differences by making probability statements, there is always the possibility that the statistical conclusion has been reached in error. Unfortunately, researchers never know when an error has been

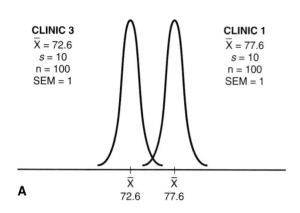

A

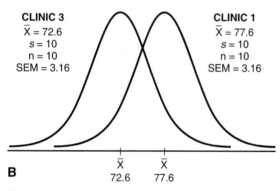

B

FIGURE 19–5. Effect of sample size on the overlap of sampling distributions. **A,** Large sample size leads to low overlap. **B,** Small sample size leads to extensive overlap. $\overline{X}$ = mean; s = standard deviation; n = number of subjects; SEM = standard error of the mean.

made; they only know the probability of making that error. There are two types of statistical errors, labeled simply Type I and Type II. Figure 19–6 shows the difference between them. The columns represent the two possible states of reality: there is or is not a difference between groups. The rows represent the two statistical conclusions that can be drawn: there is or is not a difference between groups. The intersection of the columns and rows creates four different combinations of statistical conclusions and reality. If the statistical conclusion is that there is no difference between groups and there is in fact no

FIGURE 19–6. Type I and Type II errors reflect the relationship between statistical conclusions and reality.

difference, then we have made a correct statistical conclusion. If the statistical conclusion is that there is a difference between groups and this is in fact the case, then we have also come to a correct statistical conclusion.

However, if the statistical conclusion is that there is a difference between groups when in fact there is no difference, then we have come to an erroneous statistical conclusion. This error is called a *Type I error.* The probability of making a Type I error is alpha. Recall that researchers set alpha according to the amount of chance they are willing to tolerate. An alpha level of .05 means that the researcher is willing to accept a 5% chance that significant results occurred by chance. Thus, alpha is the probability that significant results will be found when in fact no significant difference exists. Researchers never know when they have committed a Type I error; they only know the probability that one occurred. If researchers wish to decrease the probability of making a Type I error, they simply reduce alpha.

A *Type II error* occurs when the statistical conclusion is that there is no difference between the groups when in reality there is a difference. The probability of making a Type II error is beta. Beta is related to alpha but is not as easily obtained. Figure 19–7 shows the relationship between alpha and beta.

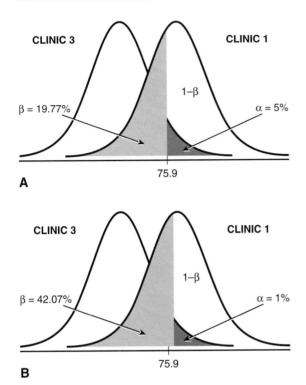

FIGURE 19–7. Relationship between Type I and Type II errors. **A,** α (probability of making a Type I error) is 5% and β (probability of making a Type II error) is 19.77%. **B,** α is 1% and β is 42.07%.

For this example we assume samples of 25 with standard deviations of 10°, giving us an SEM of 2.0° ($10/\sqrt{25}=2$). We also assume that Clinic 3, with a mean of 72.6°, is the standard against which Clinic 1, with a mean of 77.6°, is being compared. Our null hypothesis is that $\mu_1 = \mu_3$. Our alternative hypothesis is that $\mu_1 > \mu_3$. In words, we wish to determine whether the mean of Clinic 1 is significantly greater than the mean of Clinic 3. Alpha is set at 5% in Figure 19–7, *A*.

To determine beta, we first must determine the point on the Clinic 3 curve above which only 5% of the distribution lies. From the z table we find that .05 corresponds to a z score of 1.645. A z score of 1.645 corresponds in this case to a raw score of 75.9° [through algebraic rearrangement, $\overline{X} + (z)(SEM) = X; 72.6 + (1.645)(2) = 75.9$]. Thus, if Clinic 1's mean is greater than 75.9° (1.645 SEM above Clinic 3's mean), it would be considered significantly different from Clinic 3's mean of 72.6 at the 5% level. The dark shading at the upper tail of Clinic 3's sampling distribution corresponds to the alpha level of 5% and is the probability of making a Type I error. This darkly shaded area is sometimes referred to as the *rejection region* because the null hypothesis of no difference between groups would be rejected if a group mean within this area were obtained. Any group mean less than 75.9° would not be identified as statistically different from the group mean of 72.6°.

The entire part of the curve below the rejection region (including the parts that are lightly shaded) is termed the *acceptance region* because the null hypothesis of no difference between groups would be accepted if a group mean within this area were obtained.

Shift your attention now to the lightly shaded lower tail of the sampling distribution of Clinic 1. Using the z table, we can determine the probability of obtaining sample means less than 75.9°, if the population mean was actually 77.6°. To do so, we convert 75.9 to a z score in relation to 77.6: $z = (X - \overline{X})/SEM; (75.9 - 77.6)/2 = -.85$. Using the z table, we find that 19.77% of Clinic 1's sampling distribution will fall below a z score of −.85. This percentage is the probability of making a Type II error. If Clinic 1, in reality, has a mean that is significantly greater than Clinic 3's mean, we would fail to detect this difference almost 20% of the time because of the overlap in the sampling distributions. Almost 20% of Clinic 1's sampling distribution falls within the acceptance region of Clinic 3's sampling distribution.

There is an inverse relationship between the probability of making Type I and II errors. When the probability of one increases, the probability of the other decreases. Figure 19–7, *B*, shows that, for this example, when the probability of making a Type I error is decreased to 1%, the

Type II error increases to 43%. Thus, in setting the alpha level for an experiment, the researcher must find a balance between the likelihood of detecting chance differences (Type I error—alpha) and the likelihood of ignoring important differences (Type II error—beta).

■ POWER

The *power* of a test is the likelihood that it will detect a difference when one exists. Recall that beta was the probability of ignoring an important difference when one existed. The probability of detecting a true difference, or power, is therefore $1 - \beta$, as shown in the Clinic 1 curves in Figure 19–7. Recall that the size of the between-groups difference, the size of the sample, and the variability within the sample are the factors that determine whether significant differences between groups are detected. When the sampling distributions of the groups have minimal overlap, the power of a test is high. Factors that contribute to nonoverlapping sampling distributions are large between-groups differences, small within-group differences, and large sample sizes.

Many authors have shown that power is often lacking in the research of their respective disciplines: medicine,[13] nursing,[14] psychology,[15] occupational therapy,[16] and rehabilitation.[17] This is because between-groups differences are often small, sample sizes are often small, and within-group variability is often large. This lack of statistical power in our literature may mean that promising treatment approaches are not pursued because research has failed to show a significant advantage to the approaches. The power of a given statistical test can be determined by consulting published power tables[12,18] or using power software available commercially or on-line.[19]

Researchers may increase a test's statistical power in four ways. First, they can maximize between-groups differences by carefully controlling extraneous variables and making sure they apply experimental techniques consistently. Note, however, that rigid controls may reduce a study's external validity by making the conditions under which it was conducted very different from the clinical situation to which the researcher wishes to generalize the results.

Second, researchers can reduce within-group variability by studying homogeneous groups of subjects or by using subjects as their own controls in repeated measures designs. Note that these strategies also may reduce external validity by narrowing the group of patients to whom the results can be generalized.

Third, researchers can increase sample size. Increasing sample size does not have the negative impact on external validity that the other two solutions have. However, the increased cost of research with more subjects is an obvious disadvantage to this strategy.

Fourth, researchers can select a more liberal alpha level at which to conduct their statistical tests, for example $p = .10$ or $p = .15$. The obvious problem here is that, unlike the other solutions, this one flies in the face of statistical convention and is unlikely to be acceptable to the scientific community judging the research. The exception to this is research that is clearly exploratory, pilot work designed to determine whether an approach has promise, rather than to provide definitive evidence about the approach.

Power tables or programs can also be used to determine what sample size is needed to achieve a particular level of power. The variables needed to determine sample size requirements are:

- Desired power (the conventional level recommended is .80 or 80%)
- The alpha level that will be used in the research
- An estimate of the size of the between-groups difference that would be considered clinically meaningful
- An estimate of the within-group variability expected

A researcher can obtain estimates of the between-group and within-group values from previous research or from a pilot study. When there is no previous information on which to base these estimates, researchers typically substitute effect sizes, determining whether they wish to have enough power to detect small, medium, or large effects, as previously defined. For example, Clark and colleagues performed an *a priori* power analysis to determine the sample size needed for their study of occupational therapy for independent-living older adults.[20] They found that a sample size of 360 (assuming 20% attrition) would be needed to have 80% power to detect an effect of 0.3 or greater.

■ STATISTICAL CONCLUSION VALIDITY

Readers have previously been introduced to the research design concepts of internal, external, and construct validity (see Chapter 7). The final type of design validity that a researcher must consider when evaluating a research report is statistical conclusion validity. Four threats to statistical conclusion validity, modified from Cook and Campbell, are presented in this section,[21] along with a fifth threat commonly cited in reviews of randomized controlled trials.

Low Power

When statistically insignificant results are reported, readers must ask whether the nonsignificant result is a true indication of no difference or the result of a Type II error. Researchers who give power estimates provide their readers with the probability that their analysis could detect differences and, in doing so, provide information readers need to make a decision about the potential usefulness of further study in the area. The editors of the *Journal of Bone and Joint Surgery,* for example, encourage authors to analyze or discuss power when they report *p* values between .05 and .15.[9]

Whether or not a power analysis is provided, readers should examine nonsignificant results to determine whether any of the nonsignificant changes were in the desired direction or of a clinically important magnitude. If the nonsignificant differences seem clinically useful and the probability of making a Type II error seems high (sample size was small, the within-group variability was large, or an analysis showed less than 80% power), then readers should be cautious about dismissing the results altogether. Studies with promising nonsignificant results should be replicated with more powerful designs.

An example of a study with low power is Palmer and associates' report of the effects of two different types of exercise programs in patients with Parkinson's disease.[22] Seven patients participated in each exercise program. No significant changes were found in measures of rigidity, although some showed nonsignificant changes in the desired direction. A power analysis of this study reveals that it had, at most, a 50% power level.[17] Because the probability of making a Type II error was so high, the nonsignificant findings should not necessarily be taken to mean that exercise was not useful for these patients. A logical next step in investigating the effects of exercise for patients with Parkinson's disease is to replicate this study with a more powerful design.

Lack of Clinical Importance

If the power of a test is sufficiently great, it may detect differences that are so small that they are not clinically meaningful. This occurs when samples are large and groups are homogeneous. Just as readers need to examine the between-groups differences of statistically insignificant results to determine whether there is promise in the results, they must also use their clinical reasoning skills to examine statistically significant between-groups differences to determine whether they are clinically meaningful.

Error Rate Problems

Inflation of alpha when multiple tests are conducted within a study is referred to as an error rate problem because the probability of making a Type I error rises with each additional test. As discussed earlier, some researchers compensate for multiple tests by dividing an experiment-wise alpha among the tests to be conducted. Although division of alpha controls the experiment-wise alpha, it also dramatically reduces the power of each test. Readers must determine whether they believe that researchers who have conducted multiple tests have struck a reasonable balance between controlling alpha and limiting the power of their statistical analyses.

A study of balance function in elderly people illustrates alpha level inflation.[23] In this study, three groups were tested: nonfallers, recent fallers, and remote fallers. Five different measures of balance function were obtained on each of two types of supporting surfaces for each of two types of displacement stimuli. The combination of all these factors produced 20 measures for each subject. In the data analysis, nonfallers were compared with recent fallers, recent fallers were compared with remote fallers, and nonfallers were compared with remote fallers on each of the 20 measures. This yielded a total of 60 different tests of statistical significance. With this many tests, the overall probability that a Type I error was committed was far higher than the .05 level set for each analysis. Statistical techniques that would have permitted comparison of more than two groups or more than one dependent variable simultaneously could have been used to prevent this alpha level inflation; these techniques are presented in Chapters 20 and 21.

Violated Assumptions

Each of the statistical tests that are presented in Chapters 20 through 23 is based on certain assumptions that should be met for the test to be valid. These assumptions include whether the observations were made independently of one another, whether participants were randomly sampled, whether the data were normally distributed, and whether the variance of the data was approximately equal across groups. These assumptions,

and the consequences of violating them, are discussed in detail in Chapters 20 through 23.

Failure to Use Intention-to-Treat Analysis

Contemporary critics of the quality of randomized controlled trials call for an approach to statistical analysis that is referred to as "intention-to-treat" analysis.[24] The historically more common analysis approach can be referred to as "completer" analysis, because only those participants who completed the entire study were included in the data analysis.[6] The problem with the completer approach to statistical analysis is that treatment effects can be greatly overestimated if large numbers of unsuccessful participants drop out of the study. For example, consider a weight loss research study that begins with 200 participants randomized to participate in either a year-long supervised diet and exercise program or a year-long trial of an over-the-counter weight-loss supplement. Twenty participants complete the diet and exercise program with an average weight loss of 20 pounds. Seventy participants complete the supplement program with an average weight loss of 5 pounds. In a traditional completer analysis, the statistical analysis would be run on only those participants who completed the study, and the likely conclusion would be that the diet and exercise program resulted in significantly more weight loss than the supplement program.

In an intention-to-treat analysis, everyone who was entered into the study is included in the final data analysis according to the treatment they were intended to have, whether or not they completed the study. For those individuals who did not complete the study, typically the last data point they provided is used in lieu of an actual ending point.[6,25] In the hypothetical weight loss study, if some individuals came to the first session and never showed up again, their baseline weight would be entered as their final weight. If some individuals participated for 11 of the 12 months, their last weigh-in values would be entered as their final weight. Another approach to determining the missing final data is to follow up with dropouts to obtain the best data possible—perhaps some of the individuals who dropped out of the weight loss study would be willing to come in for a 12-month weigh-in even if they did not participate throughout the year-long program. If we assume that all of the dropouts in the hypothetical weight loss study maintained their baseline weight, an intention-to-treat analysis would show an average weight loss of 4 pounds for the diet and exercise group (400 total pounds lost by the 20 completers + 0 pounds lost by the 80 dropouts = 4 pounds per participant) and an average weight loss of 3.5 pounds for the supplement group (350 total pounds lost by the 70 completers + 0 pounds lost by the 30 dropouts = 3.5 pounds per participant). Compared with the completer analysis, the intention to treat approach shows a very different picture of the relative effectiveness of the two approaches to weight loss.

In an environment that emphasizes research on the effectiveness of clinical treatments, delivered in the context of actual clinical care, intention-to-treat analysis is an important part of capturing the overall effectiveness of treatment for broad groups of patients. In the hypothetical weight loss study, the intention-to-treat analysis tells us that over the course of a year neither the diet and exercise program nor the supplement program resulted in impressive average weight reductions. However, the completer analysis tells us that the diet and exercise program led to substantial average weight reductions for the small subgroup of individuals who persisted with the program. Therefore, despite the contemporary emphasis on intention-to-treat analysis, supplemental completer analysis may be appropriate to document the impact of treatment for those who actually complete the treatment of interest.

■ SUMMARY

All statistical analyses are based on a relatively small set of central concepts. Descriptive statistics are based on the concepts of central tendency (mean, median, or mode) and variability (range, variance, and standard deviation) within a data set. The distribution of many variables forms a bell-shaped curve known as the normal distribution. The percentage of scores that fall within a certain range of the normal distribution is known and can be used to predict the likelihood of obtaining certain scores. The sampling distribution is a special normal distribution that consists of a theoretical distribution of sample means.

Inferential statistical tests use sampling distributions to determine the likelihood that different samples came from populations with the same characteristics. A significant difference between groups indicates that the probability that the samples came from populations with the same characteristics is lower than a predetermined level, alpha, that is set by the researcher. There is always a probability that one of two statistical errors will be made: a Type I error occurs when a significant difference is found when in fact there is no difference; a Type II error occurs when a difference actually exists but is not identified by the test. The power of a test is the probability that it will detect a true difference. The validity of statistical conclusions is threatened by low power, results that are not clinically meaningful, alpha level inflation with multiple tests, violation of statistical assumptions, and failure to use intention-to-treat analysis.

REFERENCES

1. Chottiner S. Statistics: toward a kinder, gentler subject. *J Irreproducible Results*. 1990;35(6):13-15.
2. Ewald FC, Jacobs MA, Miegel RE, Walker PS, Poss R, Sledge CB. Kinematic total knee replacement. *J Bone Joint Surg Am*. 1984;66:1032-1040.
3. Tickle-Degnen L. Where is the individual in statistics? *Am J Occup Ther*. 2003;57:112-115.
4. Elston RC, Johnson WD. *Essentials of Biostatistics*. Philadelphia, Pa: FA Davis Co; 1994.
5. Sterne JA, Smith GD. Sifting the evidence—what's wrong with significance tests? *BMJ*. 2001;322:226-231.
6. Kazdin AE. Statistical methods of data evaluation. In: Kazdin AE, ed. *Research Design in Clinical Psychology*. Boston, Mass: Allyn & Bacon; 2003:436-470.
7. Shott S. *Statistics for Health Professionals*. Philadelphia, Pa: WB Saunders; 1990.

8. Aickin M, Gensler H. Adjusting for multiple testing when reporting research results: the Bonferroni vs Holm methods. *Am J Public Health*. 1996;86:726-727.

9. Senghas RE. Statistics in the *Journal of Bone and Joint Surgery*: suggestions for authors. *J Bone Joint Surg Am*. 1992;74:319-320.

10. Murray LL. Spoken language production in Huntington's and Parkinson's diseases. *J Speech Lang Hearing Res*. 2000;43:1350-1366.

11. Mueller MJ, Salsich GB, Strube MJ. Functional limitations in patients with diabetes and transmetatarsal amputations. *Phys Ther*. 1997;77:937-943.

12. Cohen J. *Statistical Power Analysis for the Behavioral Sciences*. Hillsdale, NJ: Lawrence Erlbaum Associates; 1988.

13. Moher D, Dulberg CS, Wells GA. Statistical power, sample size, and their reporting in randomized controlled trials. *JAMA*. 1994;272:122-124.

14. Polit DF, Sherman RE. Statistical power in nursing research. *Nurs Res*. 1990;39:365-369.

15. Kazantzis N. Power to detect homework effects in psychotherapy outcome research. *J Consult Clin Psychol*. 2000;68:166-170.

16. Ottenbacher KJ, Maas F. How to detect effects: statistical power and evidence-based practice in occupational therapy. *Am J Occup Ther*. 1999;53:181-188.

17. Ottenbacher KJ, Barrett KA. Statistical conclusion validity of rehabilitation research: a quantitative analysis. *Am J Phys Med Rehabil*. 1990;69:102-107.

18. Kraemer HC, Thiemann S. *How Many Subjects? Statistical Power Analysis in Research*. Newbury Park, Calif: Sage Publications; 1987:27.

19. Dupont WD, Plummer WD. *PS: Power and Sample Size*. Available at: *http://mc.vanderbilt.edu/prevmed/ps/ index. htm*. Accessed October 14, 2003.

20. Clark F, Azen SP, Zemke R, et al. Occupational therapy for independent-living older adults. *JAMA*. 1997;278: 1321-1326.

21. Cook T, Campbell D. *Quasi-Experimentation: Design and Analysis Issues for Field Settings*. Chicago, Ill: Rand McNally; 1979.

22. Palmer SS, Mortimer JA, Webster DD, Bistevins R, Dickinson GL. Exercise therapy for Parkinson's disease. *Arch Phys Med Rehabil*. 1986;67:741-745.

23. Ring C, Nayak US, Isaacs B. Balance function in elderly people who have and who have not fallen. *Arch Phys Med Rehabil*. 1988;69:261-264.

24. Moher D, Schulz KF, Altman D, for the CONSORT Group. The CONSORT statement: revised recommendations for improving the quality of reports of parallel-group randomized trials. *JAMA*. 2001;285:1987-1991.

25. Mazumdar S, Liu KS, Houck PR, Reynolds CF. Intent-to-treat analysis for longitudinal clinical trials: coping with the challenge of missing values. *J Psychiatr Res*. 1999;33:87-95.

20

Statistical Analysis of Differences: The Basics

Researchers use statistical tests when they wish to determine whether a significant difference exists between two or more sets of numbers. In this chapter, the general statistical concepts presented in Chapter 19 are applied to specific statistical tests of differences commonly reported in the rehabilitation literature. The distributions most commonly used in statistical testing are presented first, followed by the general assumptions that underlie statistical tests of differences. The sequence of steps common to all statistical tests of differences is then outlined. Finally, specific tests of differences are presented. In this chapter, basic tests using one independent variable are presented. Each is illustrated with an example from the hypothetical knee arthroplasty data set presented in

Chapter 19 as well as an example from the literature. In Chapter 21 more advanced tests using two independent variables are presented, as are a variety of specialized techniques for analyzing differences. In Chapters 22 and 23, statistical tests of relationships among variables are presented.

■ DISTRIBUTIONS FOR ANALYSIS OF DIFFERENCES

In Chapter 19, the rationale behind statistical testing was developed in terms of the standard normal distribution and its z scores. Use of this distribution assumes that the population standard deviation is known. Because the population standard deviation is usually *not* known, we cannot ordinarily use the standard normal distribution and its z scores to draw statistical conclusions from samples. Therefore, researchers conduct most statistical tests using distributions that resemble the normal distribution but are altered somewhat to account for the errors that are made when population parameters are estimated. The three most common distributions used for statistical tests are the t, F, and chi-square (χ^2) distributions, shown in Figure 20–1. Just as we determined the probability of obtaining certain z scores based on the standard normal distribution, we can determine the probability of obtaining certain t, F, and chi-square statistics based on their respective distributions. The exact shapes of the distributions vary with the degrees of freedom associated with the test statistic. The degrees of freedom are calculated in different ways for the different distributions, but in general are related to the number of participants within the study or the number of levels of the independent variable, or both. When test statistics are reported within the literature, they often include a subscript that indicates the degrees of freedom.

t Distribution

The t distribution is a symmetric distribution that is essentially a "flattened" z distribution (see Fig. 20–1, *A*). Compared with the z distribution, a greater proportion of the t distribution is located in the tails and a lesser proportion in the center of the distribution. The z distribution is spread to form the t distribution to account for the errors that are introduced when population parameters are estimated from sample statistics. The shape of a t distribution varies with its degrees of freedom, which is based on sample size. Because estimation of population parameters is more accurate with larger samples, t distributions become more and more similar to z distributions as sample size and degrees of freedom increase.

F Distribution

The F distribution is a distribution of squared t statistics (see Fig. 20–1, *B*). It is asymmetric and, because it is generated from squared scores, consists only of positive values. The actual shape of a particular F distribution depends on two different degrees of freedom—one associated with the number of groups being compared and one associated with the sample size.

Chi-Square Distribution

The chi-square distribution is a distribution of squared z scores (see Fig. 20–1, *C*). As is the case with the t and F distributions, the shape of the chi-square distribution varies with its degrees of freedom.

■ ASSUMPTIONS OF TESTS OF DIFFERENCES

Statistical tests of differences are either parametric or nonparametric. *Parametric tests* are based on specific assumptions about the distribution of populations. They use sample statistics such as the mean, standard deviation, and variance to estimate differences between population parameters. The two major classes of parametric tests are t tests and analyses of variance (ANOVAs).

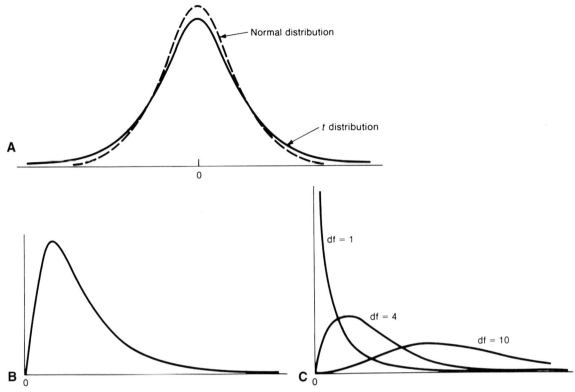

FIGURE 20–1. Distribution of test statistics. **A,** The solid *t* distribution with 5 degrees of freedom (df) compared with the dashed normal distribution. **B,** *F* distribution with 6 and 12 degrees of freedom. **C,** Chi-square distribution with 1, 4, and 10 degrees of freedom. (From Shott S: *Statistics for Health Professionals.* Philadelphia, Pa: WB Saunders; 1990:75, 148, 208.)

Nonparametric tests are not based on specific assumptions about the distribution of populations. They use rank or frequency information to draw conclusions about differences between populations.[1] Parametric tests are usually assumed to be more powerful than nonparametric tests and are often preferred to nonparametric tests, although this has not always proved to be the case with closer scrutiny.[2] However, parametric tests cannot always be used because the assumptions on which they are based are more stringent than the assumptions for nonparametric tests. Two parametric assumptions are commonly accepted: random selection and homogeneity of variance. A third assumption is controversial and relates to the measurement level of the data.

Random Selection from a Normally Distributed Population

The first basic assumption of parametric testing is that the participants are randomly selected from normally distributed populations. However, this assumption may be violated as long as the data sets used in the analysis are relatively normally distributed. Even when the data sets are not normally distributed, statistical researchers have shown that the various statistical tests are *robust,* meaning that they usually still provide an appropriate level of rejection of the null hypothesis. The extent to which a data set is normally distributed may be tested; however, the details are beyond the scope of this text.

When data are extremely nonnormal, one data analysis strategy is to convert, or *transform,* the data mathematically so that they become normally distributed. Squaring, taking the square root of, or calculating a logarithm of raw data are common transformations. Parametric tests can then be conducted on the transformed scores. A second strategy for dealing with nonnormality is to use nonparametric tests, which do not require normally distributed data.

Homogeneity of Variance

The second basic assumption of parametric testing is that the population variances of the groups being tested are equal, or *homogeneous.* Homogeneity of variance may be tested statistically. If homogeneity of variance is tested and the variances of the groups are found to differ significantly, then nonparametric tests must be used. When the sample sizes of the groups being compared are the same, then differences in the variances of the groups become less of a concern.[3] Therefore, researchers generally design their studies to maximize the chance of having equal, or nearly equal, samples sizes across groups.

Level of Measurement

The third, and most controversial, assumption for parametric testing concerns the measurement level of the data. As noted earlier, one distinction between the parametric and nonparametric tests is that the two types of tests are used with different types of data. Nonparametric tests require rankings or frequencies—nominal and ranked ordinal data meet this need, and interval and ratio data can be converted into ranks or grouped into categories to meet this need. Parametric tests require data from which means and variances can be calculated—interval and ratio data clearly meet this need; nominal data clearly do not. The controversy, then, surrounds the use of parametric statistics with ordinal measurements.

The traditional belief that parametric tests can be conducted only with interval or ratio data is no longer considered valid.[4,5(p24)] Although ordinal-scaled variables do not have the property of equal intervals between numerals, the distribution of ordinal data is often approximately normal. As long as the data themselves meet the parametric assumptions, regardless of the origin of the numbers, then parametric tests can be conducted. As is the case with all statistical tests of differences, the researcher must interpret parametric statistical conclusions that are based on ordinal data in light of their clinical or practical implications.

For example, a common type of ordinal measurement used by rehabilitation professionals is a scale of the amount of assistance a patient needs to accomplish various functional tasks. The categories maximal, moderate, minimal, standby, and no assistance could be coded numerically from 1 to 5, with 5 representing no assistance. Assume that four different groups have mean scores of 1.0, 2.0, 4.0, and 5.0 and that these group means have been found to be significantly different from one another. If the researchers believe that the "real" interval between maximal and moderate assistance is greater than the interval between standby and no assistance, they might interpret the difference between the groups with means of 1.0 and 2.0 to be more clinically important than the difference between the groups with means of 4.0 and 5.0. It is reasonable to conduct parametric tests with ordinal data as long as interpretation of the tests accounts for the nature of the ordinal scale.

■ INDEPENDENCE OR DEPENDENCE OF SAMPLES

Another important consideration for either parametric or nonparametric testing concerns whether the different sets of numbers being compared are independent or dependent. Sets are independent when values in one set tell nothing about values in another set. When two or more groups consist of different, unrelated individuals, the observations made about the samples are independent. For example, the 3-week range-of-motion (ROM) scores for patients in Clinics 1 through 3 in our hypothetical knee arthroplasty study are independent of one another. Knowing the 3-week ROM values for patients at Clinic 1 provides us with no information about 3-week ROM values of the different patients being seen at Clinic 2 or Clinic 3.

When the sets of numbers consist of repeated measures on the same individuals, they are said to be dependent. The 3-week, 6-week, and 6-month ROM scores for patients across the three clinics are dependent measures. A patient's 6-week score is expected to be related to the 3-week score. Repeated measures taken on the same individual are not the only type of dependent measures, however. If we compare male and female characteristics by using brother-sister pairs, we have dependent samples. If we study pairs or trios of individuals matched for factors such as income, education, age, height, and weight, then we also have dependent samples.

Different statistical tests are used with independent versus dependent samples, and the assumption of either independence or dependence must not be violated. The researcher must select the correct test according to whether the samples are independent or dependent.

■ STEPS IN THE STATISTICAL TESTING OF DIFFERENCES

The statistical testing of differences can be summarized in 10 basic steps, regardless of the particular test used. A general assumption of these steps is that researchers plan to perform parametric tests and resort to the use of nonparametric tests only if the assumptions for parametric testing are not met. The steps are as follows:

1. State the null and alternative hypotheses in parametric terms.
2. Decide on an alpha level for the test.
3. Determine whether the samples are independent or dependent.
4. Determine whether parametric assumptions are met. If they are not met, revise hypotheses for nonparametric testing.
5. Determine the appropriate statistical test, given the aforementioned information.
6. Calculate the test statistic.
7. Determine the degrees of freedom for the test statistic.
8. Determine the probability of obtaining the calculated test statistic, taking into account the degrees of freedom. Computer statistical packages generate the precise probability of obtaining a given test statistic for the given degrees of freedom.
9. Compare the probability obtained in Step 8 with the alpha level established in Step 2. If the obtained probability is less than the alpha level, the test has identified a statistically significant difference; that is, the null hypothesis is rejected. If the obtained probability is equal to or greater than the alpha level, the test has failed to identify a statistically significant difference; that is, the null hypothesis is not rejected.
10. Evaluate the statistical conclusions in light of clinical knowledge. If the result is statistically significant but the differences between groups do not seem to be important from a clinical perspective, this discrepancy should be discussed. If the result is statistically insignificant but the differences between groups appear clinically important, a power analysis should be conducted and discussed in light of the discrepancy between the statistical and clinical conclusions.

Table 20–1 lists these steps. The first column shows how the steps are implemented when a computer program is used for the statistical analysis, the second column shows how the steps are implemented in the increasingly rare instances when calculators and tables are used to perform the statistical analysis. Steps that are common to both computation methods cross the two columns. The remainder of this chapter illustrates how these 10 steps are implemented for several different statistical tests of differences.

TABLE 20-1	Ten Steps in the Statistical Testing of Differences

Computation Method

Step	Computer Package	Calculator and Tables
1	State hypotheses.	
2	Determine alpha level.	
3	Determine whether samples are independent or dependent.	
4	Run frequency and descriptive programs to determine whether parametric assumptions are met.	Plot frequencies and calculate descriptive statistics to determine whether parametric assumptions are met.
5	Determine appropriate test.	
6	Use appropriate programs to calculate test statistic.	Use appropriate formulas to calculate test statistic.
7	Program calculates the degrees of freedom.	Calculate the degrees of freedom.
8	Program calculates the probability of obtaining the test statistic given the degrees of freedom.	Determine the critical value of the test statistic given the degrees of freedom and predetermined alpha level.
9	Compare the obtained probability with the alpha level to draw statistical conclusion. When the obtained probability is less than alpha, a statistically significant difference has been identified.	Compare the obtained test statistic with the critical value of the test statistic to draw statistical conclusion. When the obtained test statistic is greater than the critical value, a statistically significant difference has been identified.
10	Evaluate the statistical conclusions in light of clinical knowledge.	

■ STATISTICAL ANALYSIS OF DIFFERENCES

The hypothetical total knee arthroplasty data set presented in Chapter 19 is used in the rest of this chapter to illustrate different statistical tests of differences. All the analyses were conducted with SPSS, a statistical package originally known as the Statistical Package for the Social Sciences, but now known only by the initials SPSS.[6] Formulas and computations are included with the first few examples to illustrate how the test statistics are calculated. However, the purpose of this chapter is to enable readers to understand the results of tests, not to perform statistical analyses. Researchers who wish to analyze small data sets by hand can refer to any number of good biostatistical references for the formulas and tables needed to do so.[3,7-11]

The tests presented in this chapter are organized by the type of difference being analyzed, rather than by statistical technique. For each type of difference being analyzed, both a parametric and a nonparametric test are given. Although the number of tests may seem daunting, there are actually only a few basic tests that are varied according to the number of groups being compared, whether the samples are independent or dependent, the nature of the data, and whether parametric assumptions are met. Table 20–2 presents an overview of the tests presented in this chapter.

Differences Between Two Independent Groups

Assume that Clinics 1 and 2 have different postoperative activity protocols for their patients who

TABLE 20-2 Basic Statistical Tests for Analyzing Differences				
	Independent Levels of the Independent Variable		Dependent Levels of the Independent Variable	
Design	*Parametric*	*Nonparametric*	*Parametric*	*Nonparametric*
One independent variable with two levels; dependent variables analyzed one at a time	Independent *t* test	Mann-Whitney (ranks) Wilcoxon rank sum (ranks) Chi-square (frequencies)	Paired-*t* test	Wilcoxon signed rank (ranks) McNemar (frequencies)
One independent variable with two or more levels; dependent variables analyzed one at a time	One-way analysis of variance (ANOVA)	Kruskal-Wallis (ranks) Chi-square (frequencies)	Repeated measures ANOVA	Friedman's ANOVA (ranks)

have had total knee arthroplasty. We wonder whether there are differences in 3-week ROM results between patients at Clinic 1 and Clinic 2. The null and alternative hypotheses that we intend to test are as follows:

$$H_0: \mu_1 = \mu_2$$

$$H_1: \mu_1 \neq \mu_2$$

We set alpha at 5% and determine that we have independent samples because different, unrelated patients make up the samples from the two clinics. Now we have to determine whether our data meet the assumptions for parametric testing. Table 20–3 shows the descriptive statistics and stem-and-leaf plots for the 3-week ROM data for the two groups. The variances, although not identical, are at least of similar magnitude. The ratio of the larger variance to the smaller variance is 1.85, which is less than the 2.0 maximum recommended for meeting the homogeneity-of-variance assumption for the independent *t* test.[9(p117)] The plot for Clinic 1 is negatively *skewed;* that is, it has a long tail of lower numbers. The plot for Clinic 2 looks fairly symmetric. Under these conditions some researchers would proceed with a parametric test, and others would use a nonparametric test because of the

TABLE 20-3 Independent *t* Test

Clinic	1		2	
Data	3	2	2	7
	5	8	3	4
	6	7	4	0579
	8	1478	5	06
	9	225	6	7
			7	6
Mean	$\overline{X}_1 = 77.6$		$\overline{X}_2 = 49.1$	
Variance	$s_1^2 = 393.62$		$s_2^2 = 212.58$	
Standard deviation	$s_1 = 19.84$		$s_2 = 14.58$	

$$t = \frac{\overline{X}_1 - \overline{X}_2}{\left(\sqrt{\dfrac{(n_1 - 1)s_1^2 + (n_2 - 1)s_2^2}{n_1 + n_2 - 2}}\right)\left(\sqrt{\dfrac{1}{n_1} + \dfrac{1}{n_2}}\right)}$$

$$= \frac{28.5}{(17.4)(.447)} = 3.66$$

nonnormal shape of the Clinic 1 data. The parametric test of differences between two independent sample means is the independent *t* test; the nonparametric test is either the Mann-Whitney test or the Wilcoxon rank sum test.

INDEPENDENT *t* TEST

Like most test statistics, the test statistic for the independent *t* test is the ratio of the differences between the groups to the differences within the groups. Conceptually, the difference between the groups, or the numerator, is "explained" by the independent variable. The variance within the groups, or the denominator, is "unexplained" because we don't know what leads to individual differences between subjects. Therefore, the test statistic formula "partitions" the variability in the data set into explained and unexplained variability. When the variability explained by the independent variable is sufficiently large compared with the unexplained variability, the test statistic is large and a statistically significant difference is identified.

The pooled formula for the independent *t* is presented at the bottom of Table 20–3. The numerator is simply the difference between the two sample means. The denominator is a form of a standard error of the mean created by pooling the standard deviations of the samples and dividing by the square root of the pooled sample sizes. When the *t* formula is solved by inserting the values from our example, a value of 3.66 is obtained. A separate variance formula can be used if the difference between the two group variances is too great to permit pooling.[7(p125)] The computer-generated two-tailed probability of obtaining a *t* statistic of 3.66 with 18 degrees of freedom ($n_1 + n_2 - 2$) is .002. Because .002 is less than the predetermined alpha level of .05, we reject the null hypothesis. We conclude that the mean 3-week ROM scores of the populations from which the Clinic 1 and Clinic 2 patients are drawn are significantly different from one another. The difference between the means of the two groups is 28.5°. Because this difference seems clinically important, our statistical and clinical conclusions concur.

In determining our statistical conclusions in the paragraph above, a two-tailed probability was used. The *t* test is one of only a few statistical tests that require the researcher to differentiate between directional and nondirectional

hypotheses before conducting the test. The alternative hypothesis given at the beginning of this section, $\mu_1 \neq \mu_2$, is *nondirectional,* meaning that we are open to the possibility that Clinic 1's mean ROM is either greater than *or* less than Clinic 2's mean ROM. If Clinic 1's mean is greater than Clinic 2's mean, as in our example, the *t* statistic would be positive. If, however, Clinic 2's mean is greater than Clinic 1's mean, the value of *t* would be negative. Because our research hypothesis allows for either a positive or a negative *t,* the probability that *t* will be greater than +3.66 *and* the probability that *t* will be less than −3.66 must both be accounted for. The two-tailed probability of .002 is the sum of the probability that *t* will exceed +3.66 and the probability that *t* will be less than −3.66.

A *directional hypothesis* is used occasionally as the alternative to the null hypothesis. A directional hypothesis specifies which of the means is expected to be greater than the other. Use of a directional hypothesis is justified only if there is existing evidence of the direction of the effect or when only one outcome is of interest to the researcher. Researchers who use a directional hypothesis are interested in only one tail of the *t* distribution. Because the two-tailed probability is the sum of the probabilities in the upper and lower tails of the distribution, the one-tailed probability is determined by dividing the two-tailed probability in half. Thus, for our example, the two-tailed probability of .002 becomes a one-tailed probability of .001.

In this example, both the one- and two-tailed probabilities are so low that both lead to the same statistical conclusion. Imagine, though, if the two-tailed probability for a test was .06. If we set alpha at .05 and conduct a two-tailed test, there is no significant difference between groups. However, if we conduct a one-tailed test, we divide the two-tailed probability in half to get a one-tailed probability of .03. This is less than our alpha level of .05; thus with the one-tailed test we conclude that there is a significant difference between groups. As can be seen, the one-tailed test is more powerful than the two-tailed test. Researchers should not be tempted to abuse this power by conducting one-tailed tests unless they have an appropriate rationale for doing so.

Independent t tests are often used to analyze pretest-posttest designs when there are only two groups and two measurements on each participant. One strategy is to perform an independent t test on the pretest data; if there is no significant difference between groups at pretest, then an independent t test is run on the posttest data to determine whether there was a significant treatment effect. A second strategy is to create gain scores by subtracting the pretest value from the posttest value for each participant. An independent t test is then run on the gain scores to determine whether one group had a significantly greater change than the other. Egger and Miller provide a useful description of different options for analyzing pretest-posttest designs, along with guidelines for making decisions among the options.[12]

An independent t test would typically be summarized in a journal article as follows:

DATA ANALYSIS

An independent t test was used to determine whether there was a significant difference between mean 3-week range-of-motion (ROM) values at Clinics 1 and 2. A two-tailed test was conducted with alpha set at .05.

RESULTS

The mean 3-week ROM at Clinic 1 was 28.5° greater than at Clinic 2; this difference was statistically significant (Table 1).

Table 1. Three-Week Range-of-Motion Difference between Clinics

Clinic	N	$\overline{X}$	s	t	p
1	10	77.6	19.84	3.66	.002
2	10	49.1	14.58		

An independent t test was used by Mueller and colleagues to determine whether there were significant differences between patients with diabetes mellitus and transmetatarsal amputation and a matched control group on a variety of dependent variables.[13] Because the variance on some variables was different between the groups, they used the separate variance version of the independent t test.

MANN-WHITNEY OR WILCOXON RANK SUM TEST

The Mann-Whitney and Wilcoxon rank sum tests are two equivalent tests that are the nonparametric alternatives to the independent t test. If the assumptions for the independent t test are violated, researchers may choose to analyze their data with one of these tests. When nonparametric tests are used, the hypotheses need to be stated in more general terms than the hypotheses for parametric tests.

H_0: The populations from which Clinic 1 and Clinic 2 samples are drawn are identical.

H_1: One population tends to produce larger observations than the other population.[9(p238)]

To perform the Mann-Whitney test, a researcher ranks the scores from the two groups, regardless of original group membership. Table 20–4 shows the ranking of 3-week ROM scores for Clinics 1 and 2. When a number occurs more than once, its ranking is the mean of the multiple ranks it occupies. For example, the two 67s are the 11th and 12th ranked scores in this distribution, so each receives a rank of 11.5. The next-ranked number, 76, receives the rank of 13. The sum of the Clinic 1 ranks is 142.5; the sum of the Clinic 2 ranks is 67.5.

To understand the logic behind the Mann-Whitney, imagine that our two clinics have vastly different scores that do not overlap at all. The Clinic 2 ranks would be 1 through 10, which add up to 55; the Clinic 1 ranks would be 11 through 20, which add up to 155. Now suppose the opposite case, in which the scores are very

TABLE 20–4	**Mann-Whitney or Wilcoxon Rank Sum Test**

	Clinic 1	Clinic 2
	Score (Rank)	*Score (Rank)*
	32 (2)	27 (1)
	58 (10)	34 (3)
	67 (11.5)	40 (4)
	81 (14)	45 (5)
	84 (15)	47 (6)
	87 (16)	49 (7)
	88 (17)	50 (8)
	92 (18.5)	56 (9)
	92 (18.5)	67 (11.5)
	95 (20)	76 (13)
Rank sum	(142.5)	(67.5)

similar. The Clinic 2 scores might get all the odd ranks, which add up to 100; the Clinic 1 scores might get all the even ranks, which add up to 110. When the two samples are similar, their rank sums will be similar. When the samples differ greatly, the rank sums will be very different. The rank sums (67.5 and 142.5) of our two samples of patients with total knee arthroplasty fall between the two extremes of (a) 55 and 155 and (b) 100 and 110. To come to a statistical conclusion, we need to determine the probability of obtaining the rank sums of 67.5 and 142.5 if in fact the populations from which the samples are drawn are identical. To do so, we transform the higher rank sum into a z score and calculate the probability of obtaining that z score.

An alternative form of the Mann-Whitney test uses a U statistic, which is converted into a z score. In this example, the computer-generated z score is 2.84 and the associated two-tailed probability is .0046. We conclude from this that there is a significant difference between the scores from Clinic 1 and the scores from Clinic 2. Given the 28.5° difference in the means and the 37.5° difference in the medians between the clinics, this difference seems clinically important.

Once again, our statistical and clinical conclusions concur.

The results of a Mann-Whitney test might be written up as follows in a journal article:

DATA ANALYSIS

Because the distribution of Clinic 1's range-of-motion (ROM) scores was nonnormal, we chose to analyze differences between the two groups with a nonparametric Mann-Whitney test. The 5% significance level was used for hypothesis testing.

RESULTS

A significant difference between the 3-week ROM scores for the two groups was found. Table 1 shows descriptive measures and rank sums for both groups.

Table 1. Three-Week Range-of-Motion Difference Between Clinics

Clinic	Median	$\overline{X}$	s	Rank Sum*
1	85.5	77.6	19.84	142.5
2	48.0	49.1	14.58	67.5

*Significant at $p < .05$.

Wilcoxon rank sum tests were used by Duncan and associates to determine whether there were significant differences between experimental and control groups on a number of dependent variables.[14] The 20 participants were individuals with stroke who had completed inpatient rehabilitation and were 30 to 90 days post-stroke: 10 received a therapist-supervised home-based exercise program and 10 received usual care. Although the authors do not give an explicit rationale for choosing Wilcoxon rank sum tests, the small number of participants in each group means that it is likely that the normality assumptions required for parametric testing were not met.

CHI-SQUARE TEST OF ASSOCIATION

Assume that we still wish to determine whether there are differences in the 3-week ROM scores of Clinics 1 and 2. However, let us further assume that previous research has shown that the ultimate functional outcome after total knee arthroplasty depends on having regained at least 90° of knee flexion by 3 weeks after surgery. If such evidence existed, we might no longer be interested in the absolute 3-week ROM scores at our clinics. We might instead be interested in the proportion of patients who achieve 90° of knee flexion 3 weeks postoperatively. In this case, we would convert the raw ROM scores into categories: "less than 90°" and "greater than or equal to 90°." Then we would use a chi-square test of association to determine whether the two clinics had similar proportions of patients with and without 90° of knee flexion at 3 weeks postoperatively. A complete chi-square example is presented in the next section on analysis of differences among two or more independent groups.

Differences Between Two or More Independent Groups

If Clinics 1 through 3 all have different postoperative protocols for their patients who have undergone total knee arthroplasty, we might wonder whether there are significant differences in mean 3-week ROM scores among the three clinics. To test this question statistically, we develop the following hypotheses:

H_0: $\mu_1 = \mu_2 = \mu_3$

H_1: At least one of the population means is different from another population mean.

We set alpha at .05 for the analysis. The samples are independent because they consist of different, unrelated participants. The descriptive measures and stem-and-leaf plots for all three clinics are presented in Table 20–5. The scores for both Clinics 1 and 3 appear to be nonnormal; the variances are similar. If we believe that the

TABLE 20–5	Frequencies and Descriptive Statistics for 3-Week Range of Motion at Clinics 1 Through 3		
Clinic	**1**	**2**	**3**
Data		2 7	
	3 2	3 4	3 2
	4	4 0579	4
	5 8	5 06	5 0
	6 7	6 7	6 0
	7	7 6	7
	8 1478		8 111244
	9 225		9 1
$\overline{X}$	77.6	49.1	72.6
s^2	393.62	212.58	357.38
s	19.84	14.58	18.90

parametric assumptions have been met, we test the differences with a one-way ANOVA. If we do not believe that the parametric assumptions have been met, the comparable nonparametric test is the Kruskal-Wallis test. A chi-square test of association can be used to test differences between groups when the dependent variable consists of nominal-level data.

ONE-WAY ANOVA

ANOVA techniques partition the variability in a sample into between-groups and within-group variability. Conceptually, this is the same as the partitioning described for the independent t test, although the F statistic generated within an ANOVA is a squared version of the t statistic. This F ratio is created with between-groups variability as the numerator and within-group variability as the denominator and is distributed as shown in Figure 20–1, B, discussed earlier. Because the F distribution is a squared t distribution, F cannot be negative. This means that all the extreme values for F are in the upper tail of the distribution, eliminating the need to differentiate between one- and two-tailed tests. The ANOVA is a versatile statistical technique, and there are many different variations.[15] All of the ANOVA techniques are based on partitioning variability to create an F ratio that is evaluated against the probabilities of the F distribution.

The ANOVA required in our example is known as a *one-way ANOVA*. "One-way" refers to the fact that only one independent variable is examined. In this case, the independent variable is clinic, and it has three levels—Clinic 1, Clinic 2, and Clinic 3. Table 20–6 shows the calculations needed to determine the F

TABLE 20-6   **One-Way Analysis of Variance Calculations of Sum of Squares Total (SST), Within Group (SSW), and Between Groups (SSB)**

Clinic No.	Raw Score	Deviation from Grand Mean	Deviation²	Deviation from Group Mean	Deviation²
1	32	−34.4	1183.36	−45.6	2079.36
1	58	−8.4	70.56	−19.6	384.16
1	67	.6	.36	−10.6	112.36
1	81	14.6	213.16	3.4	11.56
1	84	17.6	309.76	6.4	40.96
1	87	20.6	424.36	9.4	88.36
1	88	21.6	466.56	10.4	108.16
1	92	25.6	655.36	14.4	207.36
1	92	25.6	655.36	14.4	207.36
1	95	28.6	817.96	17.4	302.76
2	27	−39.4	1552.36	−22.1	488.41
2	34	−32.4	1049.76	−15.1	228.01
2	40	−26.4	696.96	−9.1	82.81
2	45	−21.4	457.96	−4.1	16.81
2	47	−19.4	376.36	−2.1	4.41
2	49	−17.4	302.76	−.1	.01
2	50	−16.4	268.96	.9	.81
2	56	−10.4	108.16	6.9	47.61
2	67	.6	.36	17.9	320.41
2	76	9.6	92.16	26.9	723.61
3	32	−34.4	1183.36	−40.6	1648.36
3	50	−16.4	268.96	−22.6	510.76
3	60	−6.4	40.96	−12.6	158.76
3	81	14.6	213.16	8.4	70.56
3	81	14.6	213.16	8.4	70.56
3	81	14.6	213.16	8.4	70.56
3	82	15.6	243.36	9.4	88.36
3	84	17.6	309.76	11.4	129.96
3	84	17.6	309.76	11.4	129.96
3	91	24.6	605.16	18.4	338.56
Σ			13,303.40 (SST)		8671.70 (SSW)

$SSB = (77.6 - 66.4)^2 (10) + (49.1 - 66.4)^2 (10) + (72.6 - 66.4)^2 (10) = 4631.7$

Note: Clinic 1 mean = 77.6°, Clinic 2 mean = 49.1°, and Clinic 3 mean = 72.6°.

statistic. Although time-consuming, the calculations presented here are not difficult. To compute the F statistic, we must first know the individual group means as well as the grand mean. The *grand mean* is the mean of all of the scores across the groups; for our three samples the grand mean is 66.4°.

The total variability within the data set is determined by calculating the sum of the squared deviations of each individual score from the grand mean. This is called the *total sum of squares* (SST). The SST calculation is shown in the fourth column of Table 20–6. The second column shows the raw scores; the third column, the deviation of each raw score from the grand mean; and the fourth column, the squared deviations. The sum of these squared deviations across all 30 subjects is the SST.

The within-group variability is determined by calculating the sum of the squared deviations of the individual scores from the group mean. This is known as the *within-group sum of squares* (SSW). The second column of Table 20–6 shows the raw scores; the fifth column, the deviations of each raw score from its group mean; and the final column, the squared deviations. The sum of all of the 30 squared deviation scores in the sixth column is the SSW.

The between-groups variability is determined by calculating the sum of the squared deviations of the group means from the grand mean, with each deviation weighted according to sample size. This is known as the *between-groups sum of squares* (SSB) and is shown at the bottom of Table 20–6.

The SST is the sum of the SSB and the SSW. Conceptually, then, the total variability in the sample is partitioned into variability attributable to differences between the groups and variability attributable to differences within each group.

The next step in calculating the F statistic is to divide the SSB and SSW by appropriate degrees of freedom to obtain the mean square between groups (MSB) and the mean square within each group (MSW), respectively. The degrees of

freedom for the SSB is the number of groups minus 1; the degrees of freedom for the SSW is the total number of participants minus the number of groups. The F statistic is the MSB divided by the MSW. Thus, for our example, the MSB is 2315.85:

$$MSB = \frac{SSB}{(groups - 1)} = \frac{4631.7}{2} = 2315.85$$

The MSW is 321.17:

$$MSW = \frac{SSW}{(N - groups)}$$
$$= \frac{8671.7}{27} = 321.17$$

The F statistic is 7.21:

$$F = \frac{MSB}{MSW} = \frac{2315.85}{321.17} = 7.21$$

Large F values indicate differences between the groups are large compared with the differences within groups. Small F values indicate that the differences between groups are small compared with the differences within groups. The computer-generated probability for our F of 7.21 with 2 and 27 degrees of freedom is .0031. Because this is less than our predetermined alpha level of .05, we can conclude that there is at least one significant difference among the three means that were compared.

If a one-way ANOVA does not identify a significant difference among means, then the statistical analysis is complete. If, as in our example, a significant difference is identified, the researcher must complete one more step. Our overall, or *omnibus, F* test tells us that there is a difference among the means. It does not tell us whether Clinic 1 is different from Clinic 2, whether Clinic 2 is different from Clinic 3, or whether Clinic 1 is different from Clinic 3. To determine the sources of the differences identified by the omnibus F, we must make multiple comparisons between pairs of means.

Conceptually, conducting multiple-comparison tests is similar to conducting *t* tests between each pair of means, but with a correction to prevent inflation of the alpha level. A comparison of two means is called a *contrast*. Common multiple-comparison procedures, in order of decreasing power, are as follows:

- Planned orthogonal contrasts
- Newman-Keuls test
- Tukey test
- Bonferroni test
- Scheffé test[8(p386)]

The more powerful tests identify smaller differences between means as significant. Various assumptions must be met for the different multiple-comparison procedures to be valid.

Using a Newman-Keuls procedure on our example, the mean ROM scores for Clinic 1 (77.6°) and Clinic 3 (72.6°) were not found to be significantly different, and the mean ROM score for Clinic 2 (49.1°) was found to differ significantly from the mean ROM scores for both Clinics 1 and 3. From a clinical viewpoint, it seems reasonable to conclude that the 5° difference between Clinics 1 and 3 is not important but the difference of more than 20° between Clinic 2 and Clinics 1 and 3 is.

There are two additional twists to the multiple-comparison procedure: (1) whether the contrasts are planned or post hoc and (2) whether the multiple-comparison results are consistent with the omnibus test.

In *planned contrasts*, the researcher specifies which contrasts are of interest before the statistical test is conducted. If, for some reason, the researcher is not interested in differences between Clinics 2 and 3, then only two comparisons need to be made: Clinic 1 versus Clinic 3 and Clinic 1 versus Clinic 2.

If planned contrasts are not specified in advance, all possible multiple comparisons should be conducted as post hoc tests. As more multiple comparisons are conducted, each contrast becomes more conservative to control for alpha inflation.

Occasionally, the omnibus *F* test identifies a significant difference among the means, but the multiple-comparison procedure fails to locate any significant contrasts. One response to these conflicting results is to believe the multiple-comparison results and conclude that despite the significant *F* there is no significant difference among the means. Another response is to believe the *F*-test results and use progressively less conservative multiple-comparison procedures until the significant difference between means is located. A one-way ANOVA might be reported in the literature as follows:

DATA ANALYSIS

One-way analysis of variance (ANOVA) was used to determine whether there were significant 3-week range-of-motion (ROM) differences among the three clinics. Alpha was set at .05; Newman-Keuls post hoc comparisons were conducted.

RESULTS

Tables 1 and 2 show the descriptive statistics and ANOVA summary for the tests of differences between the 3-week ROM means at the three clinics. The omnibus test identified a significant difference among the means. The post hoc analysis showed that the differences of greater than 20° between Clinic 2 and both Clinics 1 and 3 were significant, but that the 5° difference between Clinics 1 and 3 was not.

Table 1. Three-Week Range of Motion at Clinics 1, 2, and 3

Clinic	N	$\bar{X}$	s
1	10	77.6°	19.8°
2	10	49.1°	14.6°
3	10	72.6°	18.9°

Table 2. Summary of Analysis of Variance for 3-Week Range of Motion at Clinics 1, 2, and 3

Source	Sum of Squares	Degrees of Freedom	Mean Square	F
Between groups	4631.7	2	2315.8	7.21*
Within group	8671.7	27	321.2	
Total	13,303.4	29		

*$p = .0031$.

A one-way ANOVA was used to analyze differences between groups in Murray's study of the differences in spoken language production between individuals with Huntington's disease (HD), Parkinson's disease (PD), and two control groups (one matched to each of the diagnostic groups).[16] The omnibus test identified a significant difference between groups on a number of variables, including total words and mean length of utterances. Multiple comparison tests were performed using planned contrasts and a Bonferroni adjustment of alpha. In this case, there was no reason to compare the two matched control groups, so the researcher only looked for pair-wise differences between the HD group and its control group, the PD group and its control group, and the HD and PD groups.

KRUSKAL-WALLIS TEST

The Kruskal-Wallis test is the nonparametric equivalent of the one-way ANOVA. If the assumptions of the parametric test are not met, the nonparametric test should be performed. The hypotheses for the nonparametric test must be stated in more general terms than the hypotheses for the parametric test:

H_0: The three samples come from populations that are identical.

H_1: At least one of the populations tends to produce larger observations than another population.[9(p241)]

To conduct the Kruskal-Wallis test, a researcher ranks the scores, regardless of group membership. The ranks for each group are then summed and plugged into a formula to generate a Kruskal-Wallis (KW) statistic. The distribution of the KW statistic approximates a chi-square distribution. The computer-generated value of the KW statistic for our example is 11.10; the respective probability is .0039. Because .0039 is less than the alpha level of .05 that we set before conducting the test, we conclude that there is a significant difference somewhere among the groups.

An appropriate multiple-comparison procedure to use when a Kruskal-Wallis test is significant is the Mann-Whitney test with a Bonferroni adjustment of alpha. We have three comparisons to make, and each is tested at an alpha of .017. The probabilities associated with the three Mann-Whitney tests are as follows: For Clinic 1 compared with Clinic 2, $p = .0046$; for Clinic 1 compared with Clinic 3, $p = .2237$; and for Clinic 2 compared with Clinic 3, $p = .0072$. Thus, the multiple comparisons tell us that there is no significant difference between Clinics 1 and 3 and that Clinic 2 is significantly different from both Clinics 1 and 3. In this example, the nonparametric conclusions are the same as the parametric conclusions. The results of a Kruskal-Wallis test might be reported in a journal article as follows:

DATA ANALYSIS

Three-week range-of-motion (ROM) differences among the three clinics were studied with a Kruskal-Wallis (KW) analysis of variance with an alpha level of .05. A nonparametric test was used because the data at Clinics 1 and 3 were not normally distributed. Post hoc comparisons were made with three Mann-Whitney tests. The Bonferroni adjustment was used to set alpha at .017 (.05/3 = .017) for each post hoc comparison to compensate for the alpha level inflation that occurs with multiple tests.

RESULTS

A significant difference among the 3-week ROM scores at the three clinics was found (KW = 11.10, $p = .0039$). Clinics 1 and 3, with medians of 85.5° and 81.0°, respectively, were not significantly different from one another ($p = .2237$). Both were significantly different from Clinic 2, which had a median of 48.0° (for Clinic 1 vs. 2, $p = .0046$; for Clinic 2 vs. 3, $p = .0072$).

Several Kruskal-Wallis tests were used by Rothweiler and colleagues to analyze differences in psychosocial functioning among different age groups of participants with head injury.[17] The independent variable, age, had five levels: 18 to 29 years, 30 to 39 years, 40 to 49 years, 50 to 59 years, and 60+ years. There were several dependent variables: the Glasgow Outcome Scale, postinjury living situation, and postinjury employment status.

CHI-SQUARE TEST OF ASSOCIATION

Assume that we still wish to determine whether there are differences in the 3-week ROM scores of the three clinics. However, let us assume, as we did when the chi-square test was introduced earlier, that previous research has shown that the ultimate functional outcome after total knee arthroplasty depends on having regained at least 90° of knee flexion by 3 weeks postsurgery. In light of such evidence, we might no longer be interested in the absolute 3-week ROM scores at our three clinics. Our interest, instead, would be in the relative proportions of patients with at least 90° of motion across the three clinics. Our hypotheses would be as follows:

H₀: There is no association between the clinic and ROM category proportions.

H₁: There is an association between the clinic and ROM category proportions.

Table 20–7 presents the data in the contingency table format needed to calculate chi-square.

TABLE 20–7	Chi-Square χ^2 Test of Association	
	Three-Week Knee Flexion Range-of-Motion Category	
Clinic No.	**<90°**	**≥90°**
1	7 (8.67)	3 (1.33)
2	10 (8.67)	0 (1.33)
3	9 (8.67)	1 (1.33)
Total	26	4

$$\chi^2 = \Sigma \frac{(O-E)^2}{E} = (.32)+(.20)+(.01)+(2.10)$$
$$+ (.01) + (.08) = 4.04*$$

Note: Values are actual frequencies. Expected frequencies are in parentheses.
*$p = .1327$.

A *contingency table* is simply an array of data organized into a column variable and a row variable. In this table, clinic is the row variable and consists of three levels. ROM category is the column variable and consists of two levels. Calculation of the chi-square statistic is based on differences between observed frequencies and frequencies that would be expected if the null hypothesis were true.

To determine the observed frequencies, we need to examine the raw data and place each participant in the appropriate ROM category. To determine the expected frequencies, we need to determine the distribution of scores if the proportion in each ROM category were equal across the clinics. In our example, 26 of the 30 participants overall have ROM scores less than 90°. If these patients were equally distributed among the clinics, each clinic would be expected to have 8.7 ($26/3 = 8.7$) patients with ROM less than 90°. There are four participants with ROM greater than or equal to 90°. If these four participants were equally distributed among clinics, each clinic would be expected to have 1.3 ($4/3 = 1.3$) participants with ROM greater than or equal to 90°. In this example, the expected frequencies are easy to calculate because there is an equal number of patients in each group. If there are unequal numbers, the expected frequencies are proportionate to the numbers in each group.

An alternative test, the *chi-square test of goodness of fit,* compares the observed frequencies with hypothesized expected frequencies. For example, if we knew of previous research results that indicated that 80% of patients with total knee arthroplasty achieved 90° of motion by 3 weeks postoperatively, then we might test each of our clinic proportions against this hypothesized proportion.

To compute the chi-square statistic, the squared deviation of each expected cell frequency from the observed frequency is divided by the expected frequency for that cell; this is done for every cell, and the values are added together, as shown at the bottom of Table 20–7. If the dependent variable consists of only two categories, then a variation of chi-square called *Fisher's exact test* is sometimes used. If the expected frequencies are below five in a number of the cells of the table, the chi-square statistic is sometimes modified with *Yates's correction.*[8(p288)]

Table 20–7 shows the chi-square calculation for our example. The chi-square of 4.04, with 2 degrees of freedom (the number of columns − 1 × number of rows − 1), is associated with a probability of .1327. Because this probability is higher than the .05 we set as our alpha level, we conclude that there is no significant difference in the proportions of patients in the two ROM categories across the three clinics.

Note that the statistical conclusions of the chi-square analysis differ from those of the ANOVA and Kruskal-Wallis test. The ANOVA, which used all the original values of the data for the analysis, detected a difference among groups. The Kruskal-Wallis test, based on a ranking of the original data, also detected a difference. The chi-square test of association, however, using only nominal data, which eliminated much of the information in the original data set, failed to detect a difference among groups.

In general, if ratio or interval data exist, it is not wise to convert them to a lower measurement

level unless there is a strong theoretical rationale for doing so. Given the hypothetical rationale that was used to set up this chi-square example, we would conclude that patients at all three clinics are likely to have equally poor functional outcomes because of the low proportion of patients at any of the clinics who achieved 90° of motion by 3 weeks postoperatively. Chi-square results might be written up in a journal article as follows:

DATA ANALYSIS

Patients at each clinic were placed into one of two 3-week range-of-motion (ROM) categories. The limited-progress category included those with less than 90° of flexion; the normal-progress category included those with ROM greater than or equal to 90°. The chi-square test of association (alpha = .05) was used to determine whether patients in the two categories were equally distributed across the three clinics.

RESULTS

Chi-square analysis showed no significant difference in the distribution of 3-week ROM categories across the clinics (Table 1).

Table 1. Frequency and Percentage of 3-Week Range-of-Motion Categories across Clinics*

Clinic	<90° Frequency	%	≥90° Frequency	%
1	7	70.0	3	30.0
2	10	100.0	0	0.0
3	9	90.0	1	10.0

*χ_2^2 = 4.04, p = .133.

The chi-square test of association was used by Flynn and colleagues within their study of whether an audible pop is necessary for successful spinal high-velocity thrust manipulation for individuals with low back pain. They used the chi-square test to determine whether there were significant differences in the success rate of manipulation for patients when an audible pop was heard during the manipulation (for those with an audible pop, 14 of 50 patients, or 28%, experienced dramatic improvement) versus patients when an audible pop was not heard during the manipulation (for those without an audible pop, 5 of 21 patients, or 24%, experienced dramatic improvement).[18] The difference between 28% and 24% was not statistically significant.

Differences Between Two Dependent Samples

Suppose that we are interested in whether there is a change in ROM from 3 weeks postoperatively to 6 weeks postoperatively for patients across all three of our clinics. The hypotheses we test are as follows:

H_0: $\mu_{\text{3-week ROM}} = \mu_{\text{6-week ROM}}$

H_1: $\mu_{\text{3-week ROM}} \neq \mu_{\text{6-week ROM}}$

We set the alpha level at .05. In this example, the two levels of the independent variable of interest are dependent—they are repeated measures taken on the same individuals. When determining whether the data are suitable for parametric testing, remember that the relevant data are the differences between the pairs, rather than the raw data. Table 20–8 presents the distributions of the differences for the entire sample. The differences were calculated by subtracting the 3-week ROM values from the 6-week ROM values given in Table 19–2. A positive difference therefore indicates an improvement in ROM over the 3-week time span. The distribution of difference scores is asymmetric, with a greater proportion of scores in the lower end of the range. The parametric test of differences for two dependent samples is the paired-t test. The corresponding nonparametric test is the Wilcoxon signed

rank test. The test of differences between two dependent samples for nominal data is the McNemar test.

PAIRED-t TEST

To calculate the paired-t test, we first determine the difference between each pair of measurements. The mean difference and standard deviation of the differences are calculated, and then the mean is compared with a mean difference of zero. The mean of our example differences is 7.0°; the standard deviation of the differences is 10.03°. We calculate the t statistic for paired samples by dividing the mean difference by the standard error of the mean differences, as shown at the bottom of Table 20–8. The probability associated with the t statistic of 3.82 with 29 degrees of freedom (number of pairs − 1) is .001. Because .001 is less than the alpha level of .05, we conclude that there is a significant difference between 3-week and 6-week ROM scores. Clinically, an average 7.0° difference in motion over 3 weeks seems modest for this population, particularly considering that few patients are even close to achieving the maximal mechanical ROM of their new knee joints. Therefore, the statistical conclusion must be tempered with a statement

TABLE 20–8	Difference Between 6-Week and 3-Week Range-of-Motion Scores Across Clinics
−0	8 7 6 5 4 4 2
0	0 2 3 3 4 4 5 6 7 8 8 9
1	0 1 1 3 4 4 5 7 8
2	9
3	5

Mean of the differences: 7.0°
Standard deviation of the differences: 10.03°

$$t = \frac{\overline{X}_d}{\dfrac{S_d}{\sqrt{n}}} = \frac{7.0}{\dfrac{10.03}{\sqrt{30}}} = 3.82$$

about the relatively small size of the difference. Paired-*t* test results might be reported in a journal article as follows:

DATA ANALYSIS

The difference between 6-week and 3-week range-of-motion (ROM) values was analyzed with a paired-*t* test. A two-tailed test with alpha at .05 was conducted.

RESULTS

The difference between the 6-week and 3-week ROM scores ranged from $-8°$ to $+35°$, with a mean of $7.0°$ and a standard deviation $10.03°$. A positive difference indicates an improvement in ROM score from Week 3 to Week 6. Twenty-two subjects improved in the 3-week time span; eight either did not change or experienced a decrease in ROM. The difference in motion was statistically significant ($t_{29} = 3.82$, $p = .001$).

DISCUSSION

Although the difference in ROM between the 3-week and 6-week measurements was statistically significant, the clinical importance of an average $7.0°$ change over 3 weeks must be questioned, particularly because so few participants were close to the mechanical flexion limits of their prostheses. Because we had anticipated much larger changes, we conclude that the postoperative progress of these participants, although statistically significant, is limited.

Paired-*t* tests were used by Case-Smith to determine whether there were significant differences in handwriting speed and legibility from the beginning of the school year to the end of the school year for a group of children receiving school-based occupational therapy intervention for handwriting.[19]

WILCOXON SIGNED RANK TEST

The Wilcoxon signed rank test is the nonparametric version of the paired-*t* test. The nonparametric hypotheses relate to the median:

> H_0: The difference between the population medians is equal to zero.
>
> H_1: The difference between the population medians is not equal to zero.

To conduct the Wilcoxon signed rank test, we calculate the difference between each pair of numbers. We rank the nonzero differences according to their absolute value and then separate them into the ranks associated with positive and negative differences. If there is no difference from one time to the next, then the sum of the positive ranks should be approximately equal to the sum of the negative ranks. Table 20–9 shows the sums of the positive and negative ranks for this example. As is the case with the Mann-Whitney procedures for analyzing differences between independent samples, the ranked information is transformed into a z score. The computer-generated z score and probability for this example are 3.298 and .001, respectively. This probability being less than our alpha of .05, we conclude that there is a significant difference between 3-week and 6-week ROM.

To determine the clinical importance of the difference, we examine the median of the difference between the two samples. The median difference for this example is $6.5°$. This seems a fairly modest gain for a 3-week period. Once again, we should temper our statistical conclusion with a statement about the relatively small size of the median difference. Wilcoxon signed rank test results might be reported in a journal article as follows:

DATA ANALYSIS

The Wilcoxon signed rank procedure was used to analyze the difference in range-of-motion (ROM) scores from 3 weeks to 6 weeks. This nonparametric test was selected because the distribution of the difference scores was positively skewed and did not meet parametric assumptions. A nondirectional test was performed with alpha set at .05.

RESULTS

The median difference between 3-week and 6-week ROM was 6.5°, with a range from –8° to +35°. A positive difference indicates an improvement over time. This difference was statistically significant ($z = 3.298$, $p = .001$).

DISCUSSION

Although the difference in ROM between the 3-week and 6-week measurements was statistically significant, the clinical importance of a median 6.5° change over 3 weeks must be questioned, particularly because so few participants were close to the mechanical flexion limits of their prostheses. Because we had anticipated much larger changes, we conclude that the postoperative progress of these participants, although statistically significant, is limited.

A Wilcoxon signed rank test was used by Griffin and colleagues to determine whether there was a significant change in hand volume from the time that patients with chronic hand edema entered the clinic to after they rested for 10 minutes with the hand elevated.[20]

McNEMAR TEST

The McNemar test is the nominal-data analogue to the paired-t test and the Wilcoxon signed rank test. It can also be viewed as the dependent samples version of the chi-square test. In fact, a review of rehabilitation research showed that chi-square tests were often used inappropriately for dependent samples when the McNemar test would have been more appropriate.[21] The McNemar test can only be used to analyze 2×2 contingency tables, and thus its usefulness is limited. Suppose we want to determine whether there is a predictable change in ROM from 3 weeks to 6 weeks and are interested not in absolute range scores, but only in whether patients have greater than or less than 90° of motion. Our hypotheses are as follows:

H_0: The proportion of patients with less than 90° of motion at 3 weeks postoperatively

TABLE 20–9	**Wilcoxon Signed Rank Test**		
Difference	Rank by Absolute Value	Positive Difference Rank	Negative Difference Rank
0			
–2	1.5		1.5
2	1.5	1.5	
3	3.5	3.5	
3	3.5	3.5	
–4	6.5		6.5
–4	6.5		6.5
4	6.5	6.5	
4	6.5	6.5	
–5	9.5		9.5
5	9.5	9.5	
–6	11.5		11.5
6	11.5	11.5	
7	13.5	13.5	
–7	13.5		13.5
–8	16		16
8	16	16	
8	16	16	
9	18	18	
10	19	19	
11	20.5	20.5	
11	20.5	20.5	
13	22	22	
14	23.5	23.5	
14	23.5	23.5	
15	25	25	
17	26	26	
18	27	27	
29	28	28	
35	29	29	
Σ signed ranks		370	65

is identical to the proportion of patients with less than 90° of motion at 6 weeks postoperatively.

H_1: The population proportions are not equal at the two time intervals.

To perform the McNemar test, we generate a 2 × 2 table of frequencies, as shown in Table 20–10. Each participant is represented only once in the table. For example, a participant who had less than 90° of motion at 3 weeks and still had less than 90° of motion at 6 weeks is one of the 20 individuals indicated in the upper left corner of the table. If the proportion of patients in each category stays the same from 3 weeks to 6 weeks, we would expect that (1) some patients will not change categories (upper left and lower right cells) and (2) the number of patients who change categories will be evenly distributed between those moving from less than to greater than 90° and those moving from greater than to less than 90° (lower left and upper right cells). Table 20–10 shows that 23 patients did not change ROM categories, six improved from less than to greater than 90°, and only one had a decline in motion from greater than to less than 90°.

The probability of such an occurrence, if in fact there is no difference in proportions, is .1250, as generated by the computer program. Thus, we conclude that the change in proportions from 3 weeks to 6 weeks is not significant. Clinically, a change of categories in only seven of 30 patients seems to indicate minimal effectiveness of the intervention over the 3-week time span. Thus, the statistical conclusion of an insignificant difference in proportions concurs with our clinical impression. Our McNemar test might be reported in a journal article as follows:

DATA ANALYSIS

To determine whether there was a significant change in range of motion (ROM) from 3 weeks to 6 weeks postoperatively, we compared the proportion of patients with less than 90° of motion (limited progress) or greater than or equal to 90° of motion (normal progress) at 3 weeks and 6 weeks. Because the 3-week and 6-week categories are repeated measures, we made the comparison with a McNemar test, setting alpha at .05.

RESULTS

Twenty-three of 30 participants did not change ROM categories over the time span studied: 20 had limited motion at both occasions, and 3 had acceptable ROM at both occasions. Of the 7 participants who changed ROM categories over the 3-week time span, 6 moved from the limited- to the normal-progress category, and 1 moved from the normal- to the limited-progress category. This change in proportions was not statistically significant ($p = .1250$).

A McNemar test was used by Calkins and colleagues to analyze differences in perceptions of patient and physician communication about postdischarge treatment plans.[22] The McNemar test identified a significant difference, with almost all the physicians believing that patients understood when to resume normal activities after discharge, although only about half of the patients thought they understood postdischarge treatment.

Differences Between Two or More Dependent Samples

We wish now to determine whether patients show a pattern of ROM improvement from 3 weeks

TABLE 20–10 **McNemar Test**		
	Six-Week Range of Motion	
Three-Week Range of Motion	**Limited Progress (<90°)**	**Normal Progress (≥90°)**
Limited progress (<90°)	20	6
Normal progress (≥90°)	1	3

TABLE 20-11	Stem-and-Leaf Displays of Range-of-Motion Data at Three Times		
Stem	**Week 3**	**Week 6**	**Month 6**
2	7		
3	224		
4	0579	06	
5	0068	0568	
6	077	033577	5
7	6	0018	8
8	1111244478	00555	0345
9	1225	000004555	00555558
10			00000345555556
11			00

postoperatively, to 6 weeks postoperatively, to 6 months postoperatively. Our hypotheses for such a question are as follows:

H_0: $\mu_{\text{3-week ROM}} = \mu_{\text{6-week ROM}} = \mu_{\text{6-month ROM}}$

H_1: At least one population mean does not equal another population mean.

We set alpha at .05. The samples are dependent because each participant is measured three times. Table 20–11 shows the stem-and-leaf displays for the ROM scores at all three time periods; none is symmetric. Additional assumptions about the variances and covariances of the measures must be met, but a full discussion of these is beyond the scope of this text. The parametric test of differences between more than two dependent means is the repeated measures ANOVA. The corresponding nonparametric test is Friedman's ANOVA.

REPEATED MEASURES ANOVA

Just as the one-way ANOVA is the extension of the independent t test from two groups to more than two groups, the repeated measures ANOVA is the extension of the paired-t test to more than two dependent samples. There are three different approaches to a repeated measures ANOVA:

multivariate, univariate, and adjusted univariate. The assumptions for the univariate approach are more stringent than those for the multivariate approach; statistical packages provide a test (Mauchly test of sphericity) of the assumptions to guide researchers in deciding which approach to use.[9(p169)] The univariate approach is similar to the one-way ANOVA and is discussed here.

Recall the procedure used for the paired-t test. We started with a group of subjects with ROM scores ranging from 32° to 95°. To determine the test statistic, we calculated the difference between the 3-week and 6-week measures. Taking the difference of the paired scores effectively eliminated the widespread variability between participants in the sample and allowed us to focus on the changes within participants with time. Like the paired-t test, the repeated measures ANOVA mathematically eliminates between-subjects variability to focus the analysis on within-subject variability.

Recall that the one-way ANOVA partitioned the variability in the data set into between-groups and within-group categories. The univariate repeated measures ANOVA first partitions the variability in the data set into *between-subjects* and *within-subject* categories. The within-subject variability is then subdivided into between-treatments and error (or residual) components (Table 20–12). Two F ratios can be generated from a repeated measures ANOVA: One is the ratio of between-subjects to within-subject variability; the other is the ratio of between-treatments to residual variability. The first ratio is sometimes reported but is not relevant to the research question we are addressing here. A significant between-subjects F ratio would merely tell us that there is substantial variability between individual participants, and a nonsignificant between-subjects F ratio would tell us that participants are fairly homogeneous. Neither result is relevant to the question of whether there are differences between *treatments*. Thus, the between-treatments F ratio is the one that is relevant to our research question. It is the ratio of the between-treatments variability to the variability that is left after the variability due to differences between

TABLE 20-12	Summary of a Repeated Measures Analysis of Variance				
Source	**Sum of Squares**	**Degrees of Freedom**	**Mean Square**	**F**	**p**
Between subjects	20,710.46	29	714.15	2.23	.0047
Within subject	19,244.67	60	320.74		
Between treatments	14,709.42	2	7354.71	94.06	.0001
Residual	4535.24	58	78.19		
Total	39,955.12	89			

participants is removed. Thus, the variability that makes up the denominator of the *F* ratio is called the *residual*. It is also referred to as *error* because this represents random differences in participants due to sampling errors.

If a repeated measures ANOVA identifies a significant difference among the means, the next step is to make multiple comparisons between pairs of means to determine which time frames are significantly different from one another. The multiple-comparison procedures for repeated measures must be based on assumptions of dependence between the pairs being compared. Maxwell recommends the use of paired-*t* tests with a Bonferroni adjustment of alpha.[23]

In our example, a significant difference between treatments was identified: $F_{2,58} = 94.06$, $p = .0001$. Three paired-*t* tests are used as the multiple comparisons to determine where the differences lie. Because three comparisons are needed, the overall alpha level of .05 becomes .017 (.05/3 = .017). The results of the paired-*t* tests are as follows: For 3-week versus 6-week scores, $t_{29} = 3.83$, $p = .001$; for 3-week versus 6-month scores, $t_{29} = 10.38$, $p = .000$; and for 6-week versus 6-month scores, $t_{29} = 11.51$, $p = .000$. (Note that the probability is never actually zero, but in this case it is low enough that it can be rounded off to zero.)

To determine the clinical relevance of these differences, we need to examine the means for the different time periods: 3 weeks—66.4°, 6 weeks—73.4°, and 6 months—96.4°. As noted previously, the average 7.0° difference between weeks 3 and 6 seems small, but the 23.0° difference between week 6 and month 6 seems highly

important. A repeated measures ANOVA might be reported in the literature as follows:

DATA ANALYSIS

Differences in range-of-motion (ROM) scores at the three time periods were analyzed with a univariate approach to repeated measures analysis of variance since the Mauchly test of sphericity showed that the required assumptions were met ($p = .642$). Post hoc comparisons were made with paired-*t* tests. The alpha level for the ANOVA was set at .05; the Bonferroni correction was used to set alpha at .017 for each of the multiple comparisons.

RESULTS

The means and standard deviations for ROM scores at 3 weeks, 6 weeks, and 6 months, respectively, are 66.4° ± 21.4°, 73.4° ± 17.3°, and 96.4° ± 10.5°. Repeated measures ANOVA demonstrated a significant difference among the means, $F_{2,58} = 94.06$, $p = .000$. All three means were significantly different from one another at $p = .001$.

A repeated measures ANOVA was used by Schaechter and colleagues to examine differences in motor recovery at four different times (baseline, immediately postintervention, 2 weeks postintervention, and 6 months postintervention) in a group of individuals with stroke who received constraint-induced movement therapy.[24]

FRIEDMAN'S ANOVA

Friedman's ANOVA is the nonparametric equivalent of the repeated measures ANOVA. Hypotheses are as follows:

H_0: All possible rankings of the observations for any subject are equally likely.

H_1: At least one population tends to produce larger observations than another population.[9(p245)]

Calculation is based on rankings of the repeated measures for each participant. Two different formulas can be used to calculate either a Friedman's F or a Friedman's chi-square. The computer-generated chi-square for the differences in ROM at 3 weeks, 6 weeks, and 6 months postoperatively is 48.75, and the associated probability is .0000. Because .0000 is less than our preset alpha of .05, we conclude that at least one time frame is different from another. An appropriate nonparametric multiple-comparison procedure is the Wilcoxon signed rank test with a Bonferroni adjustment of the alpha level for each test. All three multiple comparisons show significant differences: For 3-week ROM versus 6-week ROM, $p = .001$; for 3-week ROM versus 6-month ROM, $p = .000$; and for 6-week ROM versus 6-month ROM, $p = .000$. Thus, for this example, the nonparametric and parametric results agree. These results might be written in a journal article as follows:

DATA ANALYSIS

Friedman's analysis of variance (ANOVA) was used to assess the differences in range of motion (ROM) 3 weeks, 6 weeks, and 6 months postoperatively. This nonparametric test was chosen because the distribution of scores at each time was not normal. Alpha was set at .05 for Friedman's ANOVA. Multiple comparisons were conducted between the paired time frames with Wilcoxon signed rank procedures with alpha set at .017 (.05/3 tests = .017) to compensate for alpha inflation with multiple testing.

RESULTS

The median ROM scores for each time frame are as follows: 3 weeks, 71.5°; 6 weeks, 74.5°; and 6 months, 100.0°. The Friedman's ANOVA revealed a significant difference among the groups, $\chi^2 = 48.75$, $p = .0000$; the post hoc analysis showed that all three groups were significantly different from one another at $p = .001$.

A Friedman's ANOVA was used by MacKean and associates to determine whether there was a significant difference in rankings of ankle orthoses during performance of a battery of basketball skills tests.[25]

■ SUMMARY

Statistical testing of differences between samples is based on 10 steps: (1) stating the hypotheses; (2) deciding on the alpha level; (3) examining the frequency distribution and descriptive statistics to determine whether the assumptions for parametric testing are met; (4) determining whether samples are independent or dependent; (5) determining the appropriate test; (6) using the appropriate software or formulas to determine the value of a test statistic; (7) determining the degrees of freedom; (8) determining the probability of obtaining the test statistic for the given degrees of freedom if the null hypothesis is true; (9) evaluating the obtained probability against the alpha level to draw a statistical conclusion; and (10) evaluating the statistical conclusions in light of clinical knowledge.

The independent t, Mann-Whitney or Wilcoxon rank sum, and chi-square tests are used to evaluate differences between two independent samples; the one-way ANOVA, Kruskal-Wallis, and chi-square tests can be used for two or more independent samples. The paired-t, Wilcoxon signed rank, and McNemar tests are used to evaluate differences between two dependent samples; the repeated measures ANOVA and Friedman's ANOVA can be used for two or more dependent samples.

REFERENCES

1. Siegel S, Castellan NJ. *Nonparametric Statistics for the Behavioral Sciences.* 2nd ed. New York, NY: McGraw-Hill; 1988.
2. Fitzgerald S, Dimitrov D, Rumrill P. The basics of nonparametric statistics. *Work.* 2001;16:287-292.
3. Dawson-Saunders B, Trapp RG. *Basic and Clinical Biostatistics.* 3rd ed. Norwalk, Conn: Appleton & Lange; 2000.
4. Gaito J. Measurement scales and statistics: resurgence of an old misconception. *Psychol Bull.* 1980;87:564-567.
5. Nunnally JC, Bernstein IH. *Psychometric Theory.* 3rd ed. New York, NY: McGraw-Hill; 1994.
6. SPSS Inc. Available at: *www.spss.com.* Accessed April 30, 2004.
7. Munro BH. *Statistical Methods for Health Care Research.* 3rd ed. Philadelphia, Pa: JB Lippincott; 1997.
8. Glass GV, Hopkins KD. *Statistical Methods in Education and Psychology.* 2nd ed. Englewood Cliffs: Prentice-Hall; 1984.
9. Shott S. *Statistics for Health Professionals.* Philadelphia, Pa: WB Saunders; 1990.
10. Polit DF. *Data Analysis and Statistics for Nursing Research.* Stamford, Conn: Appleton & Lange; 1996.
11. Elston RC, Johnson WD. *Essentials of Biostatistics.* Philadelphia, Pa: FA Davis; 1994.
12. Egger MJ, Miller JR. Testing for experimental effects in the pretest-posttest design. *Nurs Res.* 1984;33:306-312.
13. Mueller MJ, Salsich GB, Strube MJ. Functional limitations in patients with diabetes and transmetatarsal amputations. *Phys Ther.* 1997;77:937-943.
14. Duncan P, Richards L, Wallace D, et al. A randomized, controlled pilot study of a home-based exercise program for individuals with mild and moderate stroke. *Stroke.* 1998;29:2055-2060.
15. Fitzgerald SM, Rumrill P, Hart RC. Using analysis of variance (ANOVA) in rehabilitation research investigations. *Work.* 2000;15:61-65.
16. Murray LL. Spoken language production in Huntington's and Parkinson's diseases. *J Speech Lang Hearing Res.* 2000;43:1350-1366.
17. Rothweiler B, Temkin NR, Dikmen SS. Aging effect on psychosocial outcome in traumatic brain injury. *Arch Phys Med Rehabil.* 1998;79:881-887.
18. Flynn TW, Fritz JM, Wainner RS, Whitman JM. The audible pop is not necessary for successful spinal high-velocity thrust manipulation in individuals with low back pain. *Arch Phys Med Rehabil.* 2003;84:1057-1060.
19. Case-Smith J. Effectiveness of school-based occupational therapy intervention on handwriting. *Am J Occup Ther.* 2002;56:17-25.
20. Griffin JW, Newsome LS, Stralka SW, Wright PE. Reduction of chronic posttraumatic hand edema: a comparison of high voltage pulsed current, intermittent pneumatic compression, and placebo treatments. *Phys Ther.* 1990;70:279-286.
21. Ottenbacher KJ. The chi-square test: its use in rehabilitation research. *Arch Phys Med Rehabil.* 1995;76:678-681.
22. Calkins DR, Davis RB, Reiley P, et al. Patient-physician communication at hospital discharge and patients' understanding of the postdischarge treatment plan. *Arch Intern Med.* 1997;157:1026-1030.
23. Maxwell SE. Pairwise multiple comparisons in repeated measures designs. *J Educ Stat.* 1980;5:269-287.
24. Schaechter JD, Kraft E, Hilliard TS, et al. Motor recovery and cortical reorganization after constraint-induced movement therapy in stroke patients: a preliminary study. *Neurorehabil Neural Repair.* 2002;16:326-338.
25. MacKean LC, Bell G, Burnham RS. Prophylactic ankle bracing vs. taping: effects on functional performance in female basketball players. *J Orthop Sports Phys Ther.* 1995;22:77-81.

21

Statistical Analysis of Differences: Advanced and Special Techniques

Advanced ANOVA Techniques
Differences Between More Than
One Independent Variable
Between-Subjects Two-Way ANOVA
Mixed-Design Two-Way ANOVA
Differences Across Several
Dependent Variables
Effect of Removing an Intervening
Variable
Analysis of Single-System Designs
Celeration Line Analysis
Level, Trend, and Slope Analysis
Two Standard Deviation Band
Analysis
C Statistic

Survival Analysis
Survival Curves
Differences Between Survival
Curves
**Hypothesis Testing with
Confidence Intervals**
Review of Traditional Hypothesis
Testing
Foundations for Confidence
Interval Testing
Interpretation and Examples
Power Analysis
Power Analysis—Design Phase
Power Analysis—Analysis Phase
Summary

The analyses presented in Chapter 20 provide broad coverage of the most commonly reported statistical tests of differences. Readers will, however, find articles of interest that include a variety of advanced or special data analysis techniques. It seems likely that the use of these advanced techniques will increase because the widespread availability of sophisticated statistical analysis software eliminates the computational burden of these techniques. This chapter provides an overview of these more advanced or specialized techniques. First, the following advanced analysis of variance (ANOVA) techniques are covered: factorial ANOVA and the

important concept of interaction (including between-subjects and mixed-design models), multivariate ANOVA (MANOVA), and analysis of covariance (ANCOVA). Second, four specialized techniques for analyzing single-system data are presented: celeration lines; analysis of level, trend, and slope; the two standard deviation band approach; and the C statistic. Third, the concept of survival analysis and determining differences between survival curves are introduced. Fourth, the use of confidence intervals for hypothesis testing is discussed. Finally, the related concepts of power analysis and effect size are presented.

ADVANCED ANOVA TECHNIQUES

From Chapter 20 we know that ANOVA is a powerful statistical technique that can be used to evaluate differences among two or more independent or dependent groups by partitioning the variance in the data set in different ways. The same general process can be extended to analyze differences between more than one independent variable at a time, between more than one dependent variable simultaneously, and when it is desirable to mathematically remove the impact of an intervening variable.

Differences Between More Than One Independent Variable

There are several instances in which researchers wish to determine the impact of more than one independent variable on a dependent variable. Different forms of advanced ANOVA techniques are used for such analysis, depending on the nature of the independent variables selected for analysis. Using the data set presented in Chapter 19, we might wish to know whether there are differences in 3-week range-of-motion (ROM) values between clinics and between the sexes. This particular question involves two between-subjects factors, meaning that neither factor consists of repeated measures on the same participants. A different research question is whether ROM differences between clinics (a between-subjects factor) are consistent across time (a repeated, within-subject factor). The first research question is analyzed with a two-factor ANOVA for two between-subjects factors; the second is analyzed with a two-factor ANOVA for one between-subjects and one within-subject factor. The second analysis is sometimes referred to as a mixed-design ANOVA.

Whenever we examine the influence of more than one independent variable on a dependent variable, we must also examine whether there is an *interaction* between the independent variables. In the between-subjects example, the interaction question is whether the responses of men and women to treatment depend on the clinic at which they are treated. In the mixed design, the interaction question is whether changes across time are consistent across the clinics. Each of these two variations on two-factor ANOVA is discussed subsequently.

BETWEEN-SUBJECTS TWO-WAY ANOVA

The statistical hypotheses for the between-subjects two-way ANOVA are as follows:

H_0: There is no interaction between clinic and sex.

H_I: There is an interaction between clinic and sex.

H_0: $\mu_{C1} = \mu_{C2} = \mu_{C3}$

H_C: At least one clinic population mean is different from another clinic population mean.

H_0: $\mu_W = \mu_M$

H_S: The population mean for women is different from the population mean for men.

There are null and alternative hypotheses for the interaction between clinic and sex, for the main effect of clinic, and for the main effect of sex. The overall alpha level is set at .05. This particular test is known as a two-way or two-factor ANOVA because two independent variables are examined. It can also be described as a 3 × 2 ANOVA, describing the number of levels of each of the factors. Three- and four-way ANOVAs are also possible. Table 21–1 shows the data, and Table 21–2 summarizes the ANOVA for this example.

Because interpretation of two-way ANOVAs depends on the interaction result, let's examine the interaction first. The F ratio for interaction (the Clinic × Sex row in Table 21–2) is only .070, and the probability is .932. Because the probability exceeds the .05 alpha level we set prior to the analysis, we conclude that there is no interaction between sex and clinic. This means that men and women respond the same across the clinics. Interactions can be interpreted best if the cell means are graphed as shown in Figure 21–1.

Note that although the means for men and women are different, the pattern of response is the same across clinics: Both men and women do best at Clinic 1, slightly worse at Clinic 3, and the worst at Clinic 2. The nearly parallel lines between the means of the men and women across clinics provide a visual picture of what is meant by no interaction.

Because no interaction has been identified, we now examine the main effects for clinic and sex. The main effect for clinic is determined by comparing the means of all subjects at each clinic, regardless of whether they are men or women. The main effect for sex is calculated by determining the sum of squares for men and women, regardless of the clinic at which they are treated. Analysis of the main effects depends on the assumption that the factors do not interact and that therefore each factor can be examined independently, without concern for the other factors. In this example, the main effects for both clinic and sex are significant: $F_{2,24} = 9.96$, $p = .001$, and $F_{1,24} = 13.16$, $p = .001$, respectively (see Table 21–2). Because the sex variable has only two levels, we do not need to conduct post hoc testing to locate the difference. Because the clinic variable has three levels, multiple comparisons are needed, as described in the one-way ANOVA example in Chapter 20.

When an interaction is present, the data analysis generally proceeds differently. To illustrate this, the data presented previously have been altered to create a significant interaction between clinic and sex. Table 21–3 shows the new data, Table 21–4 summarizes the ANOVA, and Figure 21–2 shows the modified graph of the cell means. The lines in Figure 21–2 are not parallel, indicating an interaction. Although women do better than men at Clinics 2 and 3, men do better than women at Clinic 1.

When a significant interaction is present, the main effects for the individual variables are often difficult to interpret. For example, although Table 21–4 indicates that the main effect for clinic is significant, it would be erroneous for us to make any general statements about differences between clinics because these differences are not uniform across men and women. Likewise, the main effect for sex would lead us to conclude that there are

TABLE 21-1	Three-Week Range-of-Motion Data for Two-Factor Between-Subjects Analysis of Variance

| Clinic | Sex | |
	Men	Women
1	32, 67, 92, 87, 58	95, 92, 88, 84, 81
	$\overline{X}_{1M} = 67.2$	$\overline{X}_{1W} = 88.0$
2	34, 56, 45, 27, 40	76, 49, 47, 50, 67
	$\overline{X}_{2M} = 40.4$	$\overline{X}_{2W} = 57.8$
3	32, 50, 60, 84, 81	81, 84, 81, 82, 91
	$\overline{X}_{3M} = 61.4$	$\overline{X}_{3W} = 83.8$

TABLE 21-2	Summary of a Two-Factor Between-Subjects Analysis of Variance

Source	Sum of Squares	Degrees of Freedom	Mean Square	F	p
Clinic	4631.66	2	2315.83	9.963	.001
Sex	3060.30	1	3060.30	13.165	.001
Clinic × Sex	32.60	2	16.30	.070	.932
Residual	5578.80	24	232.45		
Total	13,303.36	29			

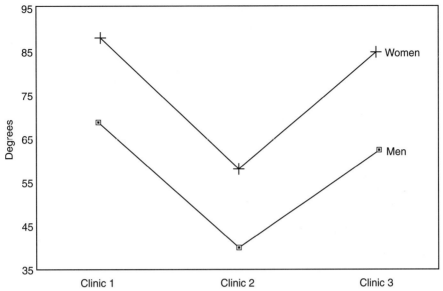

FIGURE 21–1. Parallel lines indicate no interaction between clinic and sex.

TABLE 21-3	Three-Week Range-of-Motion Data for Two-Factor Analysis of Variance Revealing an Interaction

	Sex	
Clinic	**Men**	**Women**
1	95, 92, 87, 92, 88 $\overline{X}_{1M} = 90.8$	32, 67, 58, 84, 81 $\overline{X}_{1W} = 64.4$
2	34, 56, 45, 27, 40 $\overline{X}_{2M} = 40.4$	76, 49, 47, 50, 67 $\overline{X}_{2W} = 57.8$
3	32, 50, 60, 84, 81 $\overline{X}_{3M} = 61.4$	81, 84, 81, 82, 91 $\overline{X}_{3W} = 83.8$

main effect is one in which the differences among the levels of one factor are assessed separately for each level of the other factor. In this example, there are significant differences between clinics for the men and for the women (see Table 21–4). These results might be summarized in a journal article as follows:

DATA ANALYSIS

A two-way analysis of variance was used to determine whether there were significant differences between clinics and sexes for 3-week range of motion and whether there was a significant interaction between clinic and sex. Identification of a significant interaction led to further analysis of a simple main effect for clinic and post hoc analysis of significant simple main effects with the Newman-Keuls procedure. Alpha was set at .05 for each analysis.

RESULTS

As illustrated in Figure 21–2, there was a significant interaction between clinic and sex

no differences between men and women. However, it is clear that there are differences between the sexes at each clinic—the opposite directions of these differences cancel out any main effect and erroneously make it appear that there are no differences between the sexes.

When a significant interaction is identified, the researcher typically analyzes simple main effects, rather than overall main effects. A simple

($F_{2,24}$ = 8.794, p = .001). For both the men and the women the simple main effect of clinic was significant, as shown in Table 21–4. Post hoc analysis revealed that all clinics were significantly different for the men, whereas only Clinics 2 and 3 were significantly different for the women.

An example of a two-factor ANOVA can be found in Magalhaes and colleagues' study of differences in bilateral motor coordination on three different tasks based on age and sex.[1] The age variable had five levels: 5, 6, 7, 8, and 9 years old. The sex variable had two levels: boys and girls. In this study, no interactions were found, so the main effects were interpreted for each of the analyses.

MIXED-DESIGN TWO-WAY ANOVA

We are now interested in determining whether there are differences in ROM across the three clinics and across the three times that measurements

TABLE 21-4 **Summary of a Two-Factor Analysis of Variance Revealing an Interaction with Simple Main Effects for Clinic within Sex**

Source	Sum of Squares	Degrees of Freedom	Mean Square	F	p
Clinic	4631.66	2	2315.83	11.301	.000
Sex	149.63	1	149.63	.730	.401
Clinic × Sex	3604.06	2	1802.03	8.794	.001
Clinic within sex (Women)	1826.53	2	913.27	4.457	.023
Clinic within sex (Men)	6409.20	2	3204.60	15.639	.000
Residual	4918.00	24	204.91		
Total	13,303.36	29			

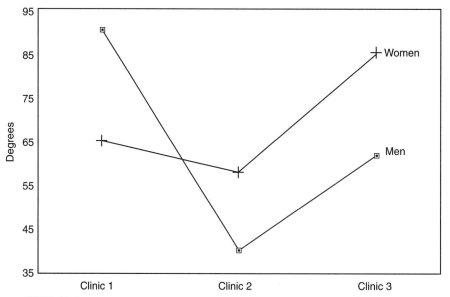

FIGURE 21–2. Nonparallel lines indicate an interaction between clinic and sex.

are taken: 3 weeks, 6 weeks, and 6 months. Clinic is a between-subjects factor because different participants are measured at each clinic. Time is a within-participant factor because ROM measures are repeated on each of the participants across the time intervals in the study. The hypotheses for our test are as follows:

H_0: There is no interaction between clinic and time.

H_1: There is an interaction between clinic and time.

H_0: $\mu_{C1} = \mu_{C2} = \mu_{C3}$

H_C: At least one clinic population mean is different from another clinic population mean.

H_0: $\mu_{3\text{-week ROM}} = \mu_{6\text{-week ROM}} = \mu_{6\text{-month ROM}}$

H_T: At least one time population mean is different from another time population mean.

Interpretation of a mixed-design ANOVA follows the same sequence of analysis as the two-factor, between-subjects ANOVA. Table 21–5 presents the means for our example, and Table 21–6

presents the *F* ratios and *p* levels associated with each comparison. As shown in Figure 21–3, there is no interaction between clinic and time. This indicates that all the clinics had the same pattern of change across time. Because there is no interaction, the main effects for clinic and time are examined, and there is a significant effect for each. Post hoc analysis shows that all three clinics are significantly different from one another and that all three time periods are significantly different from one another.

The mixed-design ANOVA is frequently used to analyze pretest-posttest control group designs. In the simplest design, there is a treatment factor with two levels (treatment group and control group) and a time factor with two levels (pretest and posttest). The ideal results for such a study would be for the two groups to be essentially the same at the pretest, the control group to remain unchanged at posttest, and the treatment group to be improved considerably at posttest. Figure 21–4 shows a graph of these ideal results. A significant interaction is illustrated—the treatment group responded differently over time than did the control group. Thus, when a mixed-design two-factor ANOVA is used to analyze a pretest-posttest design, the research question is answered by examining the interaction between the group factor and the time factor. These results might be summarized in a journal article as follows:

DATA ANALYSIS

A 3 × 3 analysis of variance with one between-subjects factor (clinic) and one within-subject factor (time) was used to analyze differences between range-of-motion (ROM) means at an

TABLE 21–5	Mean Range of Motion over Time at Clinics 1 Through 3		
Clinic	*Three Weeks*	*Six Weeks*	*Six Months*
1	77.6°	78.9°	100.0°
2	49.1°	58.6°	85.8°
3	72.6°	82.8°	103.3°

TABLE 21–6	Summary of Two-Factor Mixed Design Analysis of Variance				
Source	*Sum of Squares*	*Degrees of Freedom*	*Mean Square*	*F*	*p*
Clinic	9138.76	2	4569.38	10.66	.000
Error	11,571.70	27	428.58		
Time	10,709.42	2	7354.71	100.89	.000
Clinic × Time	598.64	4	149.66	2.05	.100
Error	3936.60	54	72.90		

alpha level of .05. Post hoc comparisons were made for the clinic factor, with Newman-Keuls tests at alpha = .05, and for the time factor, with paired-*t* tests at alpha = .017.

RESULTS

The mean ROM for each group at each point in time is presented in Table 21–5. There was no significant interaction between clinic and

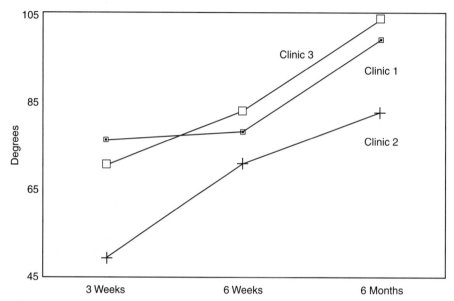

FIGURE 21–3. Nearly parallel lines indicate no interaction between clinic and time.

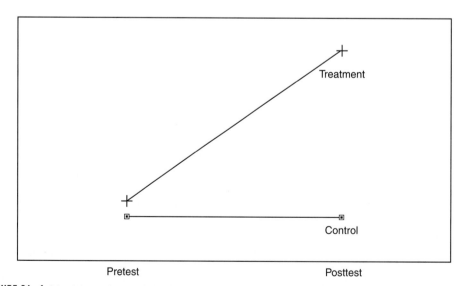

FIGURE 21–4. Ideal pretest–posttest results. The two groups are almost equal at pretest, the control group does not change at posttest, and the treatment group shows significant improvement at posttest. The nonparallel lines indicate a significant interaction between group and time.

time ($F_{4,54}$ = 2.05, p = .100). There were significant main effects for both clinic ($F_{2,27}$ = 10.66, p = .000), and time ($F_{2,54}$ = 100.89, p = .000). Overall means for Clinic 1 (85.5°) and Clinic 3 (86.2°) were not significantly different; Clinic 2's mean (64.5°) was significantly different from those of Clinics 1 and 3. Means for all three time periods were significantly different from one another (3-week mean = 66.4°, 6-week mean = 73.4°, and 6-month mean = 96.4°).

A mixed-design two-factor ANOVA was used by Binder and colleagues[2] to test the effect of exercise training (two levels: exercise and control) and time (four levels: baseline, 3 months, 6 months, and 9 months) on physical performance, peak oxygen consumption, and activities of daily living. The interaction between group and time was significant, indicating a difference in response over time for the two groups. The researchers then explored differences between groups at each time. On the physical performance variable, for example, they found no difference between exercise groups at baseline and increasingly large differences between groups at the 3-month, 6-month, and 9-month assessments.

Differences Across Several Dependent Variables

Researchers are often interested in the effects of their treatments on several different dependent variables. In our sample data set, we are now interested in whether several 6-month outcomes are different between clinics: ROM, knee extensor strength, knee flexor strength, and gait velocity. One analysis approach is to run a one-way ANOVA for each dependent variable. There are two potential problems with this approach. The first is the alpha level inflation that results from conducting multiple tests. The second is the possibility that although no single variable exhibits significant differences across clinics, small, consistent differences across several dependent

variables are present. Because an ANOVA can handle only one dependent variable at a time, a cumulative effect over several dependent variables would be undetected.

Multivariate procedures solve these problems by analyzing several dependent variables simultaneously. Multivariate analyses should not be confused with multifactor analyses: The former analyze several *dependent* variables simultaneously; the latter analyze several *independent* variables simultaneously. Although the mathematical basis for multivariate testing of differences is beyond the scope of this text, the interpretation of multivariate results is simply an extension of what has already been learned about ANOVA procedures.

A multivariate analysis of variance (MANOVA) uses an omnibus test to determine whether there are significant differences on the factor of interest (in our case, clinic) when the dependent variables of interest are combined mathematically. The multivariate test statistic used most frequently is Wilks' lambda, although several others are often reported by computer statistical packages. Wilks' lambda is usually converted to an estimated F statistic, and the probability of this estimated F is determined to test the null hypothesis.[3]

If the omnibus F level is significant, then a univariate ANOVA is conducted for each dependent variable to determine where among the dependent variables the differences lie. Once the dependent variables that are significantly different are identified, multiple-comparison procedures can be conducted to determine which levels of the independent variable are different on the dependent variables for which significant differences have been identified. However, just as an ANOVA can produce inconsistent findings between the omnibus and multiple comparison procedures, so too can a MANOVA yield inconsistent findings between the omnibus multivariate test and the univariate tests on each dependent variable.

In the total knee arthroplasty example, the omnibus F is 3.53 and is significant at the .003 level. Table 21–7 presents univariate and post

TABLE 21-7	Multivariate Analysis of Variance for Four Dependent Variables							
Dependent Variable	**Independent Variable**			**Statistic**		**Multiple Comparisons**		
	Clinic 1	**Clinic 2**	**Clinic 3**	**F**	**p**	**1/2**	**1/3**	**2/3**
Six-month range of motion (°)	100.0	85.8	103.3	15.63	.000	*		*
Extension torque (N·m)	135.8	105.4	142.2	4.90	.015	*		*
Flexion torque (N·m)	81.8	62.6	84.1	5.12	.013	*		*
Gait velocity (cm/s)	144.0	107.6	145.6	8.25	.002	*		*

Note: Asterisk indicates a significant difference between the means of the indicated pair of clinics.

hoc results for each of the dependent variables. This analysis might be reported in a journal article as follows:

DATA ANALYSIS

Differences in 6-month status across clinics were examined with a multivariate analysis of variance (MANOVA) for the following dependent variables: 6-month range of motion, extension torque, flexion torque, and gait velocity. Univariate F tests with Newman-Keuls post hoc analyses were conducted to determine the sources of any difference identified by the MANOVA.

RESULTS

The multivariate F of 3.53 was significant at the .003 level. Table 21–7 shows the mean for each dependent variable for each clinic, the F and p values for the test for differences across clinics for each dependent variable, and an indication of which multiple comparisons showed significant differences between clinics. All four dependent variables were significantly different across clinics. In addition, all four dependent variables showed the same pattern of pairwise differences among clinics: None of the dependent variable means

were significantly different between Clinics 1 and 3; all were significantly different between Clinics 1 and 2 and between Clinics 2 and 3.

A MANOVA was used by Worrell and colleagues to analyze their study of health outcomes in participants with patellofemoral pain.[4] One research question was whether there were significant differences in outcomes across the four treatment years included within the study (1993 through 1996). The outcomes that were measured included self-rated global function, a functional score, satisfaction, and stress. Rather than performing four separate ANOVAs—one each for each of the dependent variables—Worrell and colleagues analyzed all of the dependent variables simultaneously with a MANOVA technique. They found significant differences among years for all of the dependent variables combined. Having found this overall difference, they then searched for specific differences among years for the individual dependent variables.

Effect of Removing an Intervening Variable

In our examples thus far we have identified significant differences between clinics. However, scrutiny of patient characteristics at the three clinics shows that Clinic 2 has a patient population that is much older ($\overline{X}$ = 81.0 years) than the patients at Clinic 1 ($\overline{X}$ = 55.8 years) and Clinic 3 ($\overline{X}$ = 69.8 years). If younger patients tend to gain ROM faster than older patients, perhaps the age difference between the clinics, rather than differences in the quality of care, explains the difference in early ROM results.

A procedure known as *analysis of covariance* (ANCOVA) uses the overall relationship between a dependent variable and an intervening variable, or *covariate,* to adjust the dependent variable scores in light of the covariate scores. For example, let us reexamine the differences between clinics on the 3-week ROM variable by using age as a covariate. In our example, there is a strong negative correlation between age and 3-week ROM; that is, younger patients tend to have higher scores, and older patients tend to have lower scores (Figure 21–5).

An ANCOVA essentially takes each participant's 3-week ROM score and adjusts it to a predicted value as if the participant's age was the same as the mean age of the sample. In our total sample of 30 patients, the mean age is 68.8 years. Thus, the 3-week ROM scores of participants who are younger than 68.8 years are reduced and those of participants who are older than 68.8 years are increased. Once this mathematical adjustment has taken place, an ANOVA is run on the adjusted data. Figure 21–6 shows this adjustment graphically. The ANCOVA is summarized in Table 21–8. Once age is accounted for, the differences between the groups disappear—the *F* value of 1.88 is not significant (*p* = .173).

The preceding example used a patient characteristic (age) as the covariate. Another typical use of an ANCOVA is to test for differences between posttest scores using pretest scores as covariates. If pretest scores between groups are significantly different, as is common in clinical research when random assignment to groups has not been possible, then posttest scores can be adjusted to mathematically eliminate the pretest differences.[5,6] However, it is preferable to have equivalent

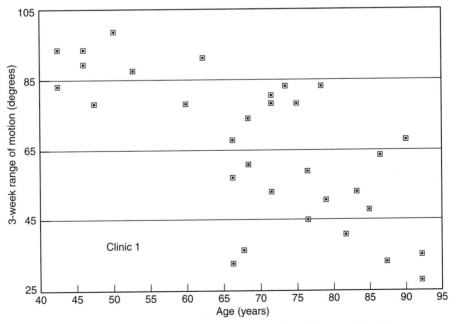

FIGURE 21–5. Relationship between age and 3-week range of motion.

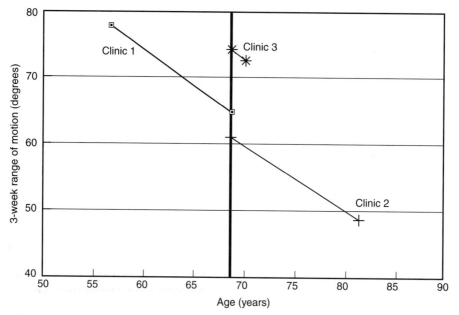

FIGURE 21–6. Analysis of covariance with age as the covariate. Original group means are adjusted to predicted values as if the mean age of each group is equal to the overall mean age of 68.8 years, represented by the vertical line.

TABLE 21-8	Analysis of Covariance of 3-Week Range of Motion (ROM)		

Clinic	Mean Age (yr)	Actual 3-Week ROM	Adjusted 3-Week ROM*
1	55.8	77.6°	64.54°
2	81.0	49.1°	61.22°
3	69.8	72.6°	73.53°

*No significant differences among clinics, $F_{2,26} = 1.88$, $p = .173$.

DATA ANALYSIS

An analysis of covariance was used to determine whether there were significant differences between clinics once the effect of participant age was removed. Alpha was set at .05.

RESULTS

Table 21–8 shows the mean values for age, actual 3-week range of motion (ROM), and adjusted 3-week ROM across the three clinics. The difference among the adjusted means was not statistically significant.

The first ANCOVA example from the literature shows the use of extraneous variables as covariates. Wolfson and colleagues studied the impact of balance and strength training for older adults, followed by group Tai Chi instruction to maintain any gains experienced during the

groups at the start of the study, because there are any number of assumptions that must be met before an ANCOVA can be used legitimately. The ANCOVA results in the total knee arthroplasty example might be reported in a journal article as follows:

balance and strength training phase of the study.[7] They studied four different groups: those receiving balance and strength training, those receiving just balance training, those receiving just strength training, and a control group that received neither training. All of the participants received the maintenance group Tai Chi instruction. The variables measured within the study were a battery of balance tests, strength tests, and usual gait velocity. Because these variables may vary by age and gender, the researchers used ANCOVA to adjust for differences in age and gender mix among the four groups.

A second ANCOVA example illustrates the use of a pretest score as the covariate. Flynn and associates used this kind of ANCOVA in their study of whether an audible pop is necessary for a manipulation to be successful.[8] Dependent variables were a pain rating scale, lumbopelvic range of motion, and scores on the Oswestry Disability Questionnaire, all measured before manipulation and at a follow-up visit 2 to 4 days after the manipulation. Because it was impossible to randomize which patients would experience an audible pop while receiving the manipulation, the chance that the two groups (those with and those without an audible pop during manipulation) would be different at baseline was a real possibility. Therefore, ANCOVA was used to adjust each participant's posttest values in light of his or her pretest values.

■ ANALYSIS OF SINGLE-SYSTEM DESIGNS

Thus far, most of our analyses have examined group differences by making inferences to the populations from which the groups were drawn. This approach is not satisfactory for single-system designs, in which our interest is in whether an individual has changed over time. Assume that a patient has extremely limited ROM 10 weeks after total knee arthroplasty. After treating the patient for 10 weeks with manual stretching and exercise, the therapist decides that more drastic measures are needed and implements a new treatment for 10 weeks, which has the results shown in

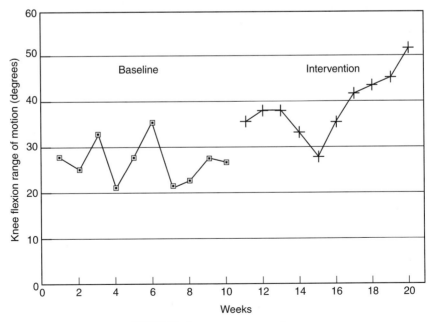

FIGURE 21–7. Single-system data.

Figure 21–7. It appears that the new treatment results in an improvement over the baseline, but is there any way to express this more quantitatively? There are, in fact, many different techniques that can be used to analyze single-system data.[9-13] Readers are referred to these references for specific calculation details and for discussion of when to use which of the analyses. In this chapter, four of the more commonly used techniques are summarized: celeration line analysis; analysis of level, trend, and slope; the two standard deviation band analysis approach; and the C statistic.

Celeration Line Analysis

In celeration line analysis, a researcher compares data in different phases by generating a line or lines based on the median of subsets of data in each phase (Figure 21–8). To determine the celeration line through the baseline data, the researcher splits the data in half and splits each half in half again. The median of each of the halves is plotted on vertical lines (the points in Fig. 21–8 represent these two medians). A line is drawn through these two points and is extended into the intervention area. The number of data points in the intervention phase and the number exceeding the celeration line are counted. The probability of having a certain proportion of scores above the celeration line can be generated from a table based on the binomial distribution.[12(p184)] The table indicates that in a one-tailed test at an alpha level of .05, nine or 10 intervention-phase numbers must be above the celeration line for a significant difference to have occurred. Because all 10 intervention-phase points are above the celeration line, we can conclude that significant improvement occurred during the treatment phase. A basic assumption of the celeration line approach is that the baseline data do not exhibit serial dependency, a phenomenon associated with the ability to predict the next point from the previous point.[12(p170)]

A sample analysis with celeration lines is presented in the next section. In the literature,

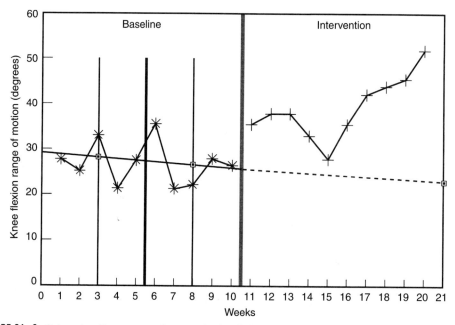

FIGURE 21–8. Celeration line approach to analysis of single-system data. The celeration line determined for the baseline phase *(solid line)* is extrapolated into the intervention phase *(dotted line).*

Goodman and Bazyk used extended celeration lines to analyze the effects of a thumb splint on hand function for a child with cerebral palsy.[14]

Level, Trend, and Slope Analysis

In addition to the results related to the extended celeration line, observation or quantification of changes in level, trend, and slope of the data may facilitate the description of the patterns seen across time (Figure 21–9). To evaluate these changes, a researcher may calculate a celeration line for each phase of the study or may use these concepts to guide their visual analysis of the data.

Level is the difference between the numerical value of observations in one phase and the numerical value of observations in a subsequent phase. A change in level is quantified by calculating the difference between the end of one celeration line and the beginning of the celeration line in the subsequent phase. There is a difference of +4° in level between the baseline and intervention phases of our example.

Trend is the direction of change in the pattern of results. In our example there has been a reversal of the trend: It was downward in the baseline phase and is upward in the intervention phase. Trend can be quantified by calculating the slopes of the lines. *Slope* is the amount that the Y value changes for each unit change in X. To calculate slope, we select two data points on the celeration line. The slope is the difference between the two Y values divided by the difference between the X values. In our example, the data points used to generate the baseline celeration line are (3, 28) and (8, 27). The slope is calculated as follows: $(27 - 28)/(8 - 3) = -1/5 = -0.2$. This means that, on average, the patient loses 0.2° of motion each week during the baseline phase. The slope of the intervention-phase celeration line is calculated similarly and is +1.8. On average, the patient gained 1.8° of

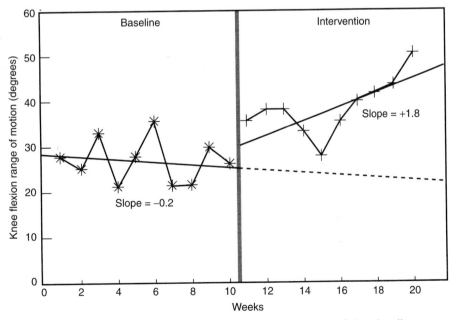

FIGURE 21–9. Level, trend, and slope analysis of single-system data. Celeration lines are calculated for each phase. There is a 4° level change, indicated by the intersections of the celeration lines in each phase with the vertical line separating the phases. There is a change in trend from downward to upward and a change in slope from –0.2 to +1.8.

motion each week in the intervention phase. Thus, not only does the trend reversal indicate a positive treatment effect, but the difference in the magnitude of the slopes also indicates that treatment led to a fairly rapid improvement in ROM in the intervention phase compared with the baseline phase. The results of this example analysis might be reported in a journal article as follows:

DATA ANALYSIS

Celeration lines for the baseline and intervention phases were developed using the split-middle approach. In addition, differences between phases were described through calculation of trend, slope, and level changes from phase to phase. To determine whether the difference between the baseline and intervention phase was statistically significant, we extended the celeration line for the baseline phase into the intervention phase and evaluated the distribution of scores above and below the line in the intervention phase against a tabled value based on binomial probabilities. Alpha was set at .05.

RESULTS

Figure 21–9 shows the data and celeration lines for each phase of the study. The baseline trend was downward and the intervention trend upward, as indicated by the slopes of –0.2 and +1.8, respectively. The change in level, or the extent of discontinuity between the celeration lines where they intersect the vertical line separating the two phases, was +4°. All 10 data points in the intervention phase fall above the extended baseline celeration line; this indicates a statistically significant treatment effect at $p = .05$.

Visual analysis of trend and slope was part of the data analysis strategy of Cadenhead and colleagues as they examined the effect of passive ROM exercises on lower-extremity ROM of adults with cerebral palsy.[15]

Two Standard Deviation Band Analysis

A third way to analyze single-system data is to calculate the mean and standard deviation of the baseline points. Using this information, a horizontal line representing the mean is drawn across the baseline and intervention phases that are being compared. Two other horizontal lines are drawn in at two standard deviations above and below the mean. The area between the two new lines is the "two standard deviation (2-SD)" band. This band represents the "likely" scores for the patient if there is no change as a result of the treatment. If there is a change, one would expect that several scores during the intervention phase would fall outside of the 2-SD band. In fact, Ottenbacher, citing earlier authors, indicates that a general rule of thumb is that when two successive points fall outside of the 2-SD band a statistically significant (at an alpha of .05) difference has been detected between the baseline and intervention points.[12(p188)] Figure 21–10 shows that the 2-SD band method of analysis leads to the conclusion that a significant different does exist between the baseline and intervention scores. The results of this example analysis might be reported in a journal article as follows:

DATA ANALYSIS

The two standard deviation (2-SD) band analysis technique was used to determine whether there was a significant difference between baseline and intervention scores. The mean and standard deviation of the baseline data were calculated and a 2-SD band around the baseline data was plotted across both the baseline and intervention phases

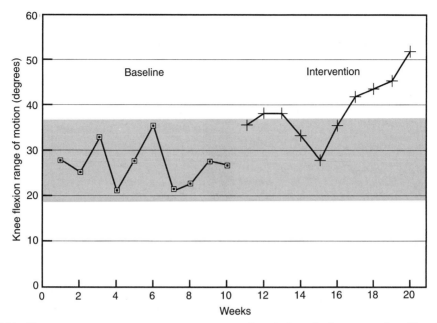

FIGURE 21–10. Two standard deviation band method of analyzing single-system data. The shaded band shows 2 standard deviations above and below the mean of the baseline data.

(see Fig. 21–10). Our statistical decision rule was that a significant difference between baseline and intervention phases would be identified if two successive intervention points fell outside the 2-SD band.[11(p188)]

RESULTS

Figure 21–10 shows that more than two successive intervention points fell outside the 2-SD band, indicating a statistically significant difference between the baseline and intervention phases.

The 2-SD band method was used by Miller to analyze her study of outcomes after body-weight–supported treadmill and overground walking training in a patient after cerebrovascular accident.[16] Significant differences were found between phases for several variables including the Berg Balance Scale and the 6-minute walk.

C Statistic

The C statistic is a data analysis method thought to be particularly appropriate for small data sets and for data sets with serial dependency.[10] The logic of the C statistic is similar to that of analysis of variance—the sum of squared deviation scores related to the treatment effect are divided by the sum of squared deviation scores related to the baseline. Nourbakhsh and Ottenbacher[10] provide instructions for calculating the C statistic, which can be interpreted with a normal probability table such as the one in Appendix B. The C statistic was used as part of the data analysis strategy of Cadenhead and colleagues as they examined the effect of passive ROM exercises on lower-extremity ROM of adults with cerebral palsy.[15]

■ SURVIVAL ANALYSIS

Survival analysis, as its name implies, is a mathematical tool that was initially used to analyze the changing proportion of survivors over time after some naturally occurring initial event (e.g., survival after stroke) or after some manipulation (e.g., survival after heart transplant surgery). Just as the outcomes movement in health care research, discussed in Chapter 15, has led to widespread use of dependent variables other than mortality, there is now expanded use of survival analysis for outcomes other than death.

Survival Curves

The basic elements needed for survival analysis are two defined events that form the basis for a survival curve: the event that qualifies a patient for inclusion in the analysis and the event that removes the patient from the analysis. In classic survival analysis, for example, a patient would enter the analysis when he or she received a heart transplant and exit the analysis when he or she died. With contemporary survival analysis, the exit event might be one of many outcomes other than death: failure of a prosthetic joint replacement, resumption of independent ambulation after surgery, admission to an extended care facility, return to a health care practitioner for further consultation for a condition presumed to be resolved, return to sport following injury, or loss of a job following successful placement after completion of a work conditioning program. The exit event may be negative or positive as long as it separates the proportion of individuals who have not yet experienced the event from those who have.

Determining the proportion of patients who have and have not experienced the exit event across time is easier to conceptualize than it is to actually calculate. First, the calculations depend on whether a new proportion is calculated at specified time intervals (actuarial or life table analysis) or each time a patient changes status (Kaplan-Meier analysis).[17(pp188-209)] Second, the calculations depend on the handling of subjects who are lost to follow-up or who must leave the study because of an event other than the specified exit event. For example, assume that the exit

event is admission to an extended care facility after returning home following an intensive poststroke rehabilitation program. Researchers need to know how to account for patients who die shortly after completing the rehabilitation program but who remained independent in their homes until their death. Computation details and information about the use of statistical analysis programs for survival analysis are beyond the scope of this text but can be found in other resources.[17(pp188-209)]

Differences Between Survival Curves

Although researchers may be interested in a single survival curve for participants who have experienced a single event or procedure, they are often more interested in whether there is a significant difference in survival curves for participants who have experienced different events or procedures. Hoenig and associates[18] made such a comparison when they sought to determine whether there were differences in the timing of ambulation after surgical repair of a hip fracture, based on the timing of the surgical repair (early, defined as within 2 days of hospital admission, versus late) and the frequency of physical and occupational therapy (high frequency, defined as more than five sessions per week, versus low frequency). Readers can refer to Chapter 15 and Figure 15–2 for a more complete presentation of their findings.

There are several statistical methods, each using different mathematical principles, that can be used to compare survival curves.[17(pp196-203)] The Wilcoxon rank sum test, introduced in Chapter 20, can be used to determine differences in the survival time ranking between two groups. The log-rank test, sometimes referred to with the addition of either or both the Cox and Mantel names, uses chi-square test principles, also introduced in Chapter 20, to compare the observed survivors in each group with the expected survivors based on the combined groups. The Mantel-Haenszel test uses odds ratios, introduced in Chapter 14, to compare the odds of survival for both groups. A final type of test for differences in survival is known as a proportional hazards, or Cox regression, model.[17(p221)] This model is based on regression analysis techniques, which are presented in Chapters 22 and 23. Clearly, additional details about these methods are beyond the scope of this text. However, readers should take from this brief discussion two central ideas. First, the array of tests and the varied naming conventions make it difficult for even sophisticated readers to make judgments about the appropriateness of the test chosen. Second, despite the wide variety of tests of differences between survival curves, all of the tests rest on the basic statistical foundations presented elsewhere in this text.

■ HYPOTHESIS TESTING WITH CONFIDENCE INTERVALS

Up to this point, the process of testing differences between groups or levels has been presented in terms of comparisons between an obtained probability level (p) and a predetermined probability of error set by the researcher, the alpha (α) level. Recall that the determinants of the p value in any statistical test of differences are (1) the size of the difference in the dependent variable between levels of the independent variable, (2) the amount of variability on the dependent variable within levels of the independent variable, and (3) the sample size. In traditional hypothesis testing these factors are used within a specific formula for a statistic such as t or F. The t or F value is calculated and computerized statistical analysis programs are used to determine the probability (p) associated with the calculated value of t or F. If this p value is less than the preset alpha level, then a statistically significant finding has been identified.

Critics of this traditional approach note that the emphasis on p and alpha levels leads to "lazy thinking"[19(p746)] because each decision about the meaningfulness of data is reduced to a dichotomy of "significant" versus "nonsignificant."

Put into terms of the steps of statistical analysis that were presented in Chapter 20, these critics believe that an emphasis on p values leads many researchers to stop the analysis process with Step 9 (comparing the obtained probability with the alpha level to draw a statistical conclusion) instead of proceeding to the final Step 10 (evaluating the statistical conclusions in light of clinical knowledge). These critics believe that presentation of statistical results in the form of confidence intervals rather than p values facilitates the higher level of evaluation that they believe is important to the proper interpretation of research results.

Review of Traditional Hypothesis Testing

Understanding the basis of the argument for using confidence intervals for hypothesis testing requires revisiting of some of the statistical principles originally introduced in Chapter 19. Readers who have difficulty following the greatly abbreviated discussion of these principles should review the appropriate sections of Chapters 19 and 20.

Recall that the mean is a sample statistic. Furthermore, sample statistics are not precise values in and of themselves; rather, they are estimates of population parameters. As estimates, sample means contain a certain amount of error. The magnitude of this error depends on the variability within the data and the size of the sample. Specifically, this error is known as the standard error of the mean (SEM) and can be calculated for each group by dividing the group's standard deviation by the square root of the size of the group. *Confidence intervals* (CIs) around the mean can be computed by adding and subtracting standard errors to and from the mean. The error that the researcher is willing to tolerate is based on the number of standard deviations above and below the mean that are included in the confidence interval. With large groups of normally distributed data, adding and subtracting 1.645 SEMs yields a 90% CI; 1.96 SEMs yields a 95% CI; and 2.576 SEMs yields a 99% CI.

Earlier, an independent t test was used to compare the 3-week ROM values between Clinic 1 ($\overline{X}$ = 77.6°, s = 19.84) and Clinic 2 ($\overline{X}$ = 49.1°, s = 14.58). The independent t formula, presented in Table 20–3, is the difference between the means divided by the standard error of the difference between the means (t = 28.5/7.78 = 3.66). The computer-generated probability of obtaining this t value was .002, which was less than the preset alpha of .05, so a statistically significant difference was identified.

Foundations for Confidence Interval Testing

As noted in the previous section, in traditional hypothesis testing we compute a probability and reach our statistical conclusion when we compare the obtained p to a preset alpha level. In hypothesis testing with confidence intervals, we calculate a confidence interval for the difference of interest and reach our statistical conclusion by determining whether the confidence interval includes the value that corresponds to the null hypothesis. For most purposes this value is zero ("0") because the null hypothesis proposes that there will be "no difference" between groups. If the confidence interval contains "0," then we conclude that there is no statistically significant difference between groups. If the confidence interval does not contain "0," then we conclude that there is a statistically significant difference between groups. When using confidence intervals to determine the significance of odds ratios and relative risk ratios, a significant difference is identified when the interval does not contain the number one ("1"). This is because a ratio of "1" means that the risks for the groups being compared are equal.

Using confidence intervals for hypothesis testing means that the concept of confidence intervals for each group must be extended to the concept of a confidence interval for the difference between groups. Doing so involves rearranging the mathematical concepts of the t test.[19(p749)] The general confidence interval

formula for the difference between two independent group means is:

CI = (difference between the means) ± (appropriate multiplier) (standard error of the difference)

For this example, the computations given in Chapter 20 (see Table 20–3) give two of the three values needed for computing the confidence interval:

CI = 28.5 ± (appropriate multiplier) (7.78)

The third value cannot be determined directly from the information in this text, because it depends on access to a complete t table, commonly found in texts solely devoted to statistics. However, the conceptual basis for this value can be identified easily. Recall that when determining the confidence interval for a single, normally distributed group, the appropriate multiplier for a 95% confidence interval, based on the normal z distribution, was 1.96. Furthermore, recall that the t distribution is a slightly flattened z distribution. The appropriate multiplier for a 95% confidence interval for the difference between two means is based on the t distribution rather than the z distribution, and is slightly further toward the tail of the distribution at 2.101. Inserting 2.101 into our formula, we find that the 95% confidence interval for the difference between these two means is 12.15° to 44.85°:

95% CI = 28.5 ± (2.101) (7.78)

95% CI = 28.5 ± 16.35

95% CI = 12.15 to 44.85

Because this confidence interval does not contain "0," we conclude that there is a significant difference between the means of Clinics 1 and 2. This statistical conclusion matches the conclusion we reached with the independent t test in Chapter 20. This is not surprising in that the two methods depend on algebraic rearrangement of the same formula. Sim and Reid recommend that confidence intervals be used (1) when sample statistics are used as estimates of population parameters; (2) in addition to or instead of the results of hypothesis testing; (3) as a means to assess the clinical importance of research results; (4) with adjusted confidence levels when multiple intervals are calculated (the equivalent to controlling for alpha inflation); and (5) when reporting the results of individual studies that are included within meta-analyses.[20]

Interpretation and Examples

With the traditional method, the reader is tempted to believe that in our hypothetical example the "true" difference between the means is 28.5° and that the difference between the means is "really" significant because the p value of .002 is so much less than the alpha of .05. With the confidence interval presentation, the reader is reminded that 28.5° is only an estimate of a difference between the means. The confidence interval tells us that there is a 95% chance that the population difference in mean 3-week ROM values is between approximately 12° and approximately 45°. With this information the researcher or reader has a sound basis on which to judge the clinical importance of the finding.

Van der Windt and colleagues used confidence intervals to supplement their traditional hypothesis testing in a study of the effectiveness of corticosteroid injections versus physical therapy for treatment of painful stiff shoulders.[21] For example, they found a difference of 31% in success rates between groups: 77% of patients treated with the corticosteroid injections were "successes" at 7 weeks compared with only 46% of those treated with physical therapy. The confidence interval for this difference in percentage was 14% to 48%. Because this interval does not contain "0," it corresponds to a statistically significant difference in percentage of treatment successes between groups after 7 weeks of treatment. Prencipe and coworkers used confidence intervals to test the significance of the

odds ratio for dementia in elderly, community-dwelling individuals with and without stroke.[22] The odds ratio for dementia was 5.8 with a 95% confidence interval from 3.1 to 10.8. Since this interval does not contain "1," the authors concluded that there was a significant increase in the odds of dementia for individuals who have had stroke compared with those without stroke. Furthermore, there is a 95% chance that the population of individuals with stroke is 3.1 to 10.8 times more likely to have dementia compared with the population of individuals without stroke.

■ POWER ANALYSIS

Power is the ability of a statistical test to detect a difference when it exists, as discussed in Chapter 19. Maximizing power within a research design involves (1) maximizing the size of the difference in the dependent variable between levels of the independent variable, (2) minimizing the amount of variability on the dependent variable within levels of the independent variable, and (3) maximizing the sample size. In addition, the alpha level selected by the researcher influences power, with higher power associated with larger alpha levels. Power analysis is used at two very different points in the research process: in the design phase and after the analysis phase. Texts[23,24] and computer software[25] can be used to conduct a power analysis at either time.

Power Analysis—Design Phase

During the design phase of a research project power analysis is used to help the researcher design a study that has "enough" power, typically 80%, to detect differences that exist. To do so, the researchers could estimate the size of the between-group difference that they would consider to be important, the variability they would expect to see within the groups being studied, and the sample size that is reasonable given the constraints of the research setting. From this information a "dry run" statistical analysis can be done and the power of the analysis can be calculated. If the power is less than 80%, then the researchers need to reconsider some of the elements of the design. Could treatment be extended to maximize the chance of a large between-group difference? Could a more homogeneous group of subjects be studied to minimize the within-group variability? Could another clinic be involved to increase the sample size?

In the preceding paragraph, the between-group difference, within-group variability, and sample size were given and the power was calculated based on those givens. When power analysis is used in the design phase of a study, however, it is usually run in "reverse." Rather than solving for "power," researchers usually specify power at 80% and solve for one of the other factors that they can control. Because the nature of the treatment and the characteristics of the subjects are often dictated by the research question, sample size is generally seen to be the most controllable factor related to power. Therefore, power analysis in the design phase is most often used to help estimate the sample size for the study.

When power analysis is used to estimate sample size, researchers must specify their desired power level, as well as the anticipated between-group differences and within-group variability. In practice, estimating these two factors may be difficult, particularly in topic areas for which little previous research exists. When this is the case, researchers may use the concept of *effect size* to help them plan their sample sizes. The effect size is a ratio of the difference between the means to the pooled standard deviation of the groups being compared. For a comparison of two group means, an effect size of .20 is considered small, .50 is considered medium, and .80 is considered large.[23] Using these conventions, researchers who do not have reliable estimates of the between-group differences and within-group variability can determine what sample sizes would be required to detect effect sizes that would be considered small, medium, and large.

Without going into computational details, for power of 80% and an alpha level of .05, the sample size requirements for a two-sample independent *t* test can be shown to be 25 per group to detect a large effect of .80, 63 per group to detect a medium effect of .50, and 392 per group to detect a small effect of .20.[24] This means that a total of 50, 126, or 784 participants would be required to detect large, medium, and small effects, respectively. Of 100 rehabilitation studies reviewed by Ottenbacher and Barrett,[26] the maximum number of participants in a study was 126. In addition, 76 of the 100 studies had fewer than 50 participants. If we assume that all 100 studies were two-group studies, this means that none of the 100 studies had enough participants to detect a small effect, only one could detect a medium effect, and only 23 studies could detect a large effect. Clearly, rehabilitation researchers who use group designs should work to design more powerful studies.

Power Analysis—Analysis Phase

The second use of power analysis is to compute the power of a statistical test after it has failed to identify a statistically significant difference. When a difference is not identified, the researcher and the reader wonder whether a correct conclusion has been reached or whether a Type II error has been committed. A correct conclusion is assured when the finding of no difference between the samples corresponds with the reality of no difference between the populations from which the samples were drawn. A Type II error is committed when the finding of no difference between the samples is at odds with a true difference between the populations. Because the entire populations are generally not available for study, researchers never know whether they are correct or whether they have committed a Type II error. The probability of making a Type II error is known as beta, or β (power is 1 − β). Because of this relationship between power and Type II errors, low probabilities of Type II errors are associated with high power values. Power may be expressed as a percentage by moving the decimal two places to the right. By convention, 80% power is desirable. As noted earlier, rehabilitation research often lacks power. Thus, lack of power, or a Type II error, is often a likely explanation for a nonsignificant result in rehabilitation research. Editorial policies for journals may require that researchers present power analyses in the face of nonsignificant findings.[27,28] Murray[29] used power analysis in the analysis phase of her study of spoken language production in Huntington's and Parkinson's diseases, noting that the study had 75% power to detect large effect sizes, but only 30% power to detect medium effect sizes.

■ SUMMARY

Basic ANOVA techniques can be extended to factorial ANOVA (analyzing more than one independent variable simultaneously, including between-subjects and mixed-design models), multivariate ANOVA, or MANOVA (analyzing more than one dependent variable simultaneously), and analysis of covariance, or ANCOVA (removing the effect of an intervening variable). Four specialized techniques for analyzing single-system data are presented. Celeration line analysis extrapolates a baseline celeration line into the treatment phase and determines whether the distribution of data points in the treatment phase reflects a significant difference. Level, trend, and slope analysis compares the characteristics of the celeration lines from different phases of the study. Two standard deviation band analysis compares actual values in the treatment phase with values that would be expected if there was no difference between treatment and baseline phases. The C statistic uses logic similar to ANOVA to compare baseline and treatment phases. Actuarial and Kaplan-Meier survival analysis methods are used to determine the proportion of patients who have and have not experienced a defined event at different points in time. Differences in survival curves can be determined by Wilcoxon rank sum, log rank, Mantel-Haenszel, and proportional

hazards methods. Some researchers prefer to present their statistical findings in terms of confidence intervals rather than p values. Doing so involves algebraic rearrangements of traditional hypothesis testing formulas. Power analysis can be used in the design phase of a study to determine the sample size needed to detect different effect sizes or used in the analysis phase to look for possible explanations of nonsignificant findings.

REFERENCES

1. Magalhaes LC, Koomar JA, Cermak SA. Bilateral motor coordination in 5- to 9-year-old children: a pilot study. *Am J Occup Ther.* 1989;43:437-443.
2. Binder EF, Schechtman KB, Ehsani AA, et al. Effects of exercise training on frailty in community-dwelling older adults: results of a randomized, controlled trial. *J Am Geriatr Soc.* 2002;50:1921-1928.
3. Tabachnick BG, Fidell LS. *Using Multivariate Statistics.* 4th ed. New York, NY: Harper & Row; 2000.
4. Worrell TW, Guenin J, Huse L, et al. Health outcomes in subjects with patellofemoral pain. *J Rehabil Outcomes Meas.* 1998;2(4):10-19.
5. Egger MJ, Miller JR. Testing for experimental effects in the pretest-posttest design. *Nurs Res.* 1984;33:306-312.
6. Dimitrov DM, Rumrill PD. Pretest-posttest designs and measurement of change. *Work.* 2003;20:159-165.
7. Wolfson L, Whipple R, Derby C, et al. Balance and strength training in older adults: intervention gains and Tai Chi maintenance. *J Am Geriatr Soc.* 1996;44:497-506.
8. Flynn TW, Fritz JM, Wainner RS, Whitman JM. The audible pop is not necessary for successful spinal high-velocity thrust manipulation in individuals with low back pain. *Arch Phys Med Rehabil.* 2003;84:1057-1060.
9. Ottenbacher KJ. Analysis of data in idiographic research. *Am J Phys Med Rehabil.* 1992;71:202-208.
10. Nourbakhsh MR, Ottenbacher KJ. The statistical analysis of single-subject data: a comparative examination. *Phys Ther.* 1994;74:768-776.
11. Bobrovitz CD, Ottenbacher KJ. Comparison of visual inspection and statistical analysis of single-subject data in rehabilitation research. *Am J Phys Med Rehabil.* 1998; 77:94-102.
12. Ottenbacher KJ. *Evaluating Clinical Change: Strategies for Occupational and Physical Therapists.* Baltimore, Md: Williams & Wilkins; 1986.
13. Reboussin DM, Morgan TM. Statistical considerations in the use and analysis of single-subject designs. *Med Sci Sports Exerc.* 1996;28:639-644.
14. Goodman G, Bazyk S. The effects of a short thumb opponens splint on hand function in cerebral palsy: a single-subject study. *Am J Occup Ther.* 1991;45:726-731.

15. Cadenhead SL, McEwen IR, Thompson DM. Effect of passive range of motion exercise on lower-extremity goniometric measurement of adults with cerebral palsy: a single-subject design. *Phys Ther.* 2002;82:658-669.

16. Miller EW. Body weight supported treadmill and overground training in a patient post cerebrovascular accident. *Neurorehabilitation.* 2001;16:155-163.

17. Dawson-Saunders B, Trapp RG. *Basic and Clinical Biostatistics.* 2nd ed. Norwalk, Conn: Appleton & Lange; 1994.

18. Hoenig H, Rubenstein LV, Sloane R, Horner R, Kahn K. What is the role of timing in the surgical and rehabilitative care of community-dwelling older persons with acute hip fracture? *Arch Intern Med.* 1997;157:513-520.

19. Gardner MJ, Altman DG. Confidence intervals rather than *P* values: estimation rather than hypothesis testing. *BMJ.* 1986;292:746-750.

20. Sim J, Reid N. Statistical inference by confidence intervals: issues of interpretation and utilization. *Phys Ther.* 1999;79: 186-195.

21. van der Windt DA, Koes BW, Deville W, Boeke AJP, de Jong BA, Bouter LM. Effectiveness of corticosteroid injections versus physiotherapy for treatment of painful stiff shoulder in primary care: randomised trial. *BMJ.* 1998;317:1292-1296.

22. Prencipe M, Ferretti C, Casini AR, Santini M, Giubilei F, Culasso F. Stroke, disability, and dementia: results of a population survey. *Stroke.* 1997;28:531-536.

23. Cohen J. *Statistical Power Analysis for the Behavioral Sciences.* 2nd ed. Hillsdale, NJ: Lawrence Erlbaum Associates; 1988.

24. Polit DF. *Data Analysis and Statistics for Nursing Research.* Stamford, Conn: Appleton & Lange; 1996.

25. Dupont WD, Plummer WD. *PS: Power and Sample Size.* Available at: *http://mc.vanderbilt.edu/prevmed/ps/index.htm.* Accessed October 14, 2003.

26. Ottenbacher KJ, Barrett KA. Statistical conclusion validity of rehabilitation research: a quantitative analysis. *Am J Phys Med Rehabil.* 1990;69:102-107.

27. Senghas RE. Statistics in the Journal of Bone and Joint Surgery: suggestions for authors. *J Bone Joint Surg Am.* 1992;74:319-320.

28. *Information for authors (Arch Phys Med Rehabil).* Available at: *http://www2.archives-pmr.org.* Accessed January 11, 2004.

29. Murray LL. Spoken language production in Huntington's and Parkinson's diseases. *J Speech Lang Hearing Res.* 2000;43:1350-1366.

22

Statistical Analysis of Relationships: The Basics

Researchers often wish to know the extent to which variables are related to one another. For example, Powers and colleagues studied the relationship between lower extremity muscle force and gait characteristics for individuals with transtibial amputations.[1] This is an example of the use of relationship analysis to determine the extent to which different concepts, in this case muscle force and gait characteristics, are related to one another. Analysis of relationships is not always between different concepts but may be between different conditions under which a single concept is measured. In reliability studies, relationship analysis is used to determine the relationship between repeated measurements of scores taken across time or by different practitioners. For example, Beaton and colleagues[2] examined the test-retest reliability of the self-reported Disabilities of the Arm, Shoulder, and Hand outcome measure by having individuals with upper limb problems complete the questionnaire twice within 5 days, and Nussbaum and Downes[3] examined the reliability of a pressure-pain algometer by using two measurers, each taking three measurements on 3 different days.

Relationship analysis studies are generally nonexperimental, with the researcher observing different phenomena rather than manipulating groups of subjects, as is done in experimental studies. Recall from Chapters 20 and 21 that the analysis of differences centers on determining whether there are mean differences between groups or between repeated administrations of a test to a single group. In contrast, the analysis of relationships centers on determining the *association* between scores on two or more variables that are available for each individual in a single group.

This chapter introduces the major ways in which relationships among variables are analyzed. As in Chapters 20 and 21, the purpose of this chapter is not to enable readers to conduct their own statistical analyses, but rather to enable them to understand relationship analysis as it is presented in the rehabilitation literature. Simple correlation and linear regression are presented in this chapter. The more advanced topics of multiple and logistic regression techniques, discriminant analysis, the uses of relationship analysis for documenting reliability, and factor analysis are discussed in Chapter 23.

■ CORRELATION

When two variables are correlated, the value an individual exhibits on one variable is related to the value he or she exhibits on another variable. The magnitude and direction of the relationship between variables are expressed mathematically as a correlation coefficient. The presence of relationships among variables does not enable researchers to draw causal inferences about the variables: Correlation is not causation. For example, although there is an obvious relationship between the amount of corn grown in a particular locale and the flatness of the land on which it is grown, reasonable people do not conclude that growing corn causes the land to become flat.[4]

This section begins with calculation of the most frequently used correlation coefficient, the

Pearson product moment correlation. This is followed by discussion of alternative correlation coefficients, the assumptions that underlie correlation coefficients, the ways in which correlation coefficients are interpreted, and examples of the use of correlation from the literature.

Calculation of the Pearson Product Moment Correlation

Calculation of the Pearson product moment correlation is mathematically tedious, although relatively simple conceptually: The Pearson product moment correlation, or r, is the average of the cross-products of the z scores for the X and Y variables. In mathematical notation,

$$r = \frac{\Sigma z_x z_y}{N}$$

Suppose we are interested in determining the extent of the relationship between a functional variable such as gait velocity and a physical impairment variable such as knee flexion range of motion (ROM) in patients who have undergone total knee arthroplasty. Table 22–1 shows the calculation of the correlation between 6-month

| TABLE 22–1 | Calculation of Pearson r: Relationship Between Six-Month Range of Motion and Gait Velocity at Clinic 1 |

Subject	X	x	Y	y	Z_x	Z_y	$z_x z_y$
01	100	0	165	21	0.00	1.13	0.00
02	85	−15	100	−44	−2.24	−2.37	5.31
03	100	0	130	−14	0.00	−0.75	0.00
04	105	5	170	26	0.75	1.40	1.05
05	105	5	150	6	0.75	0.32	0.24
06	95	−5	135	−9	−0.75	−0.48	0.36
07	110	10	153	9	1.49	0.48	0.72
08	100	0	145	1	0.00	0.05	0.00
09	95	−5	147	3	−0.75	0.16	−0.12
10	105	5	145	1	0.75	0.05	0.04
Σ	1000.0		1440.0				7.6
N	10.0		10.0				10.0
Mean	100.0		144.0				$r = .76$
σ	6.71		18.60				

ROM and gait velocity in patients at Clinic 1. In the calculation of the Pearson r value, either variable may be designated X or Y, and neither is considered independent or dependent. The X and Y scores for each subject are converted to z scores, and the product of zx and zy (called the *crossproduct*) is determined for each participant. The mean of the crossproducts is the Pearson product moment correlation coefficient.

The values that r may take range from -1.0 to $+1.0$. A correlation coefficient of -1.0 indicates a perfect negative, or inverse, relationship: A higher value on one variable is associated with a lower value on the other variable. A correlation coefficient of $+1.0$ indicates a perfect positive, or direct, relationship; a higher value on one variable is associated with a higher value on the other variable. In this example, $r = .76$, indicating a fairly strong direct relationship between the two variables. Figure 22–1 shows a scatterplot of the 10 pairs of scores. They fall rather loosely around an imaginary diagonal line running from the bottom left corner of the graph to the top right corner. This indicates that, as ROM scores increase, so do gait velocity values.

Researchers often collect many variables within a single study and are interested in which of the variables are most related to one another. When a researcher calculates many correlation coefficients in a study, he or she usually displays them in a correlation matrix, as shown in Table 22–2. In this table, all the variables of interest are listed as both columns and rows, and the correlation between each pair of variables is presented at the intersection of the row and column of interest. For example, the Pearson r between flexion torque and extension torque is .9524 and can be found in two places on the table (the intersection of Row 2 and Column 3 and the intersection of Row 3 and Column 2). A full correlation matrix like this includes redundant information because each correlation coefficient between two different variables is listed twice. It also includes unnecessary information because the correlation between each variable and itself is known (1.000), and these correlations form the diagonal. In articles, therefore, most researchers display only the nonredundant portion of the correlation matrix, which lies either above or below the diagonal.

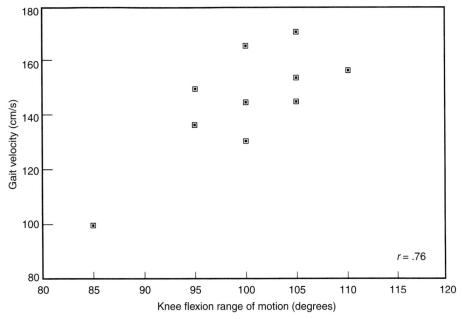

FIGURE 22–1. Relationship between 6-month knee flexion range of motion and gait velocity.

TABLE 22-2 Correlation Matrix for Six-Month Variables

	Range of Motion	Flexion Torque	Extension Torque	Gait Velocity
Range of motion	1.0000	.5610	.5947	.6399
Flexion torque	.5610	1.0000	.9524	.8921
Extension torque	.5947	.9524	1.0000	.9014
Gait velocity	.6399	.8921	.9014	1.0000

Alternative Correlation Coefficients

Correlation coefficients other than the Pearson product moment correlation have been developed for a variety of uses beyond that of quantifying the degree of relationship between two interval or ratio variables. Several are listed in Chapter 17, where correlation is introduced as a concept related to measurement theory, and Table 22-3 lists the characteristics of several additional correlation measures.

Spearman's rho (ρ) and Kendall's tau (τ) correlations are designed for use when both variables are ranked. The point-biserial correlation is used with one continuous and one dichotomous variable. The Spearman rho and point-biserial formulas are simply shortcut versions of the Pearson r.[5(pp237,238)] Correlation coefficients for use with nominal data are the phi (φ),Cramer's V, and kappa (κ) coefficients. Phi is another shortcut version of the Pearson r, applicable when both variables are dichotomous, such as in determining the relationship between sex and the answer to a yes-or-no question.[5(p237)] Cramer's V is used when there are two categorical variables. Kappa, discussed in more detail in Chapter 23, is a reliability coefficient that can be used when nominal variables consist of more than two categories.

Correlation coefficients for more than two variables are also available. The *intraclass* correlation coefficients (ICCs), discussed more fully in Chapter 23, are a family of reliability coefficients that can be used when two or more repeated measures have been collected. *Kappa* can also be used with more than two nominal repeated measures. *Partial* correlation is used to assess the relationship between two variables with the effect of a third variable eliminated. *Multiple* correlation is used to assess the variability shared by

TABLE 22-3 Characteristics of Different Correlation Coefficients

Coefficient	Characteristics
Pearson product moment correlation	Two continuous variables
Spearman's rho (ρ)	Two ranked variables; shortcut calculation of Pearson
Point biserial	One continuous variable, one dichotomous variable
Kendall's tau (τ)	Two ranked variables
Phi (ϕ)	Two dichotomous variables; shortcut calculation of Pearson
Cramer's V	Two categorical variables
Kappa (κ)	Two or more nominal variables with two or more categories; a reliability coefficient
Intraclass correlation	Two or more continuous variables; a reliability coefficient
Partial correlation	Two variables, with effects of a third held constant
Multiple correlation	More than two variables
Canonical correlation	Two sets of variables

three or more variables. *Canonical* correlation is a technique for assessing the relationships between two sets of variables.

Assumptions of the Correlation Coefficients

Calculation of the Pearson product moment and related correlation coefficients depends on three major assumptions. First, the relationships between variables are assumed to be *linear*. Analysis of a scatterplot of the data must show that the relationship forms a straight line. Curvilinear relationships (those that do not follow a straight line) may be analyzed, but this requires more advanced techniques than are discussed in this text. Figure 22–2 shows the scatterplot of our hypothetical total knee arthroplasty data showing the relationship between age and a new variable, length of acute care hospital stay postoperatively. There is an obvious relationship between variables, but it is not linear. Both the

young and very old patients have short lengths of stay, possibly because younger adults reach their ROM goals quickly and older adults are transferred to a skilled nursing facility for continued rehabilitation. Those of intermediate age stay in the hospital somewhat longer, presumably to achieve their ROM goals in the acute care hospital, without transfer to a skilled nursing facility. The Pearson *r* for this relationship is .3502, indicating a minimal degree of linear relationship between these two variables. If researchers rely solely on Pearson *r* values to guide their conclusions, they may mistakenly conclude that no relationship exists when in fact a strong *nonlinear* relationship exists.

The second assumption is *homoscedasticity*. As shown in Figure 22–3, *A,* homoscedasticity means that for each value of one variable, the other variable has equal variability. Nonhomoscedasticity is illustrated in Figure 22–3, *B.* Because the calculation of Pearson *r* is based on *z* scores, whose calculation in turn depends on standard deviations for each variable, widely varying variances

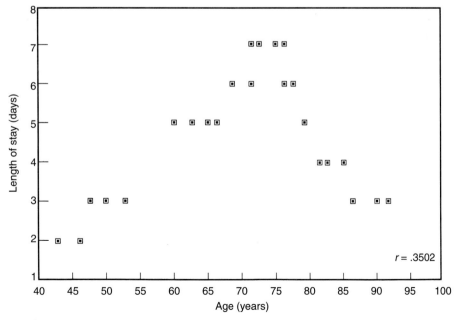

FIGURE 22–2. Relationship between age and length of stay. There is a strong nonlinear relationship between the two variables. The low *r* value is deceptive because it is designed to detect linear relationships only.

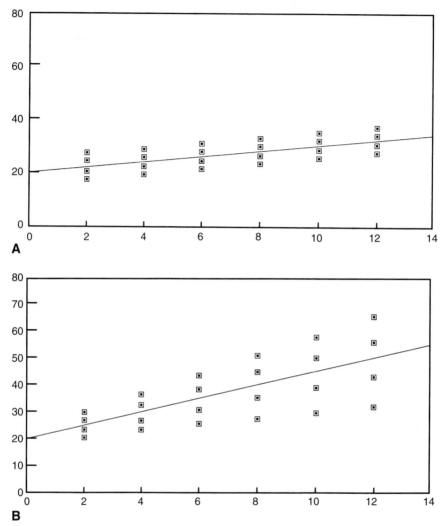

FIGURE 22–3. A, Example of homoscedasticity; the Y values are equally variable at each level of X.
B, Example of nonhomoscedasticity; the Y values are not equally variable at each level of X.

at different levels will distort the calculated value of *r*.

The third assumption is that both variables have enough *variability* to demonstrate a relationship. If either or both variables have a restricted range, then the correlation coefficient will be artificially low and uninterpretable. Figure 22–4, *A,* shows the scatterplot of Clinic 3's data for 6-month ROM and gait velocity. There appears to be little relationship between the two, because the data cluster in the top right corner

of the graph and the Pearson *r* is −.2673. However, the range of ROM values is very restricted, with all participants showing close to full ROM of their prosthetic knees.

Figure 22–4, *B,* shows the scatterplot of 6-month ROM and gait velocity for the entire sample of 30 patients. In this example each variable takes a fairly wide range of values, and the relationship between 6-month ROM and gait velocity is obvious. The Pearson *r* for this set of data is .6399. Thus, the restricted-range data

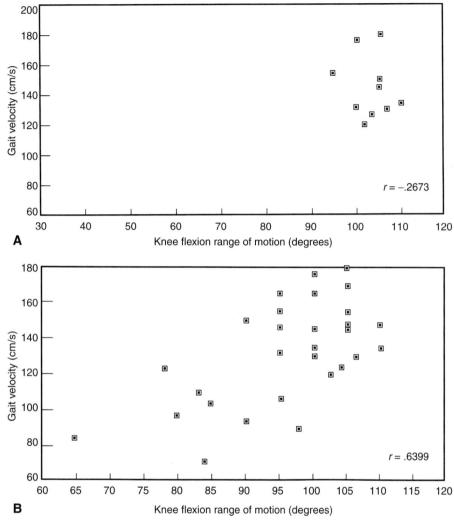

FIGURE 22–4. A, Restricted range of the X variable results in a low correlation coefficient. **B,** The addition of a broader range of X values reveals a pattern that was not apparent in A.

yielded a correlation coefficient that was different in both magnitude and direction from the coefficient calculated on data with a greater range of values. Restricted range issues may be present in just about any study in which relationships among variables are examined within a highly selected group of individuals such as elite athletes, students enrolled in health professions programs, or children who are identified as having marked developmental delays.

Interpretation of Correlation Coefficients

Correlation coefficients are interpreted in four major ways: (1) the strength of the coefficient itself; (2) the variance shared by the two variables, as calculated by the coefficient of determination; (3) the statistical significance of the correlation coefficient; and (4) the confidence intervals about the correlation coefficient. Regardless of which method is chosen, the interpretation should not be extrapolated beyond the range of the data used to generate the correlation coefficient.

STRENGTH OF THE COEFFICIENT

The first way to interpret the coefficient is to examine the strength of the relationship, which is independent of the direction (direct or inverse) of the relationship. This method of interpretation is exemplified by Munro's descriptive terms for the strength of correlation coefficients[5(p235)]:

.00–.25	Little, if any correlation
.26–.49	Low correlation
.50–.69	Moderate correlation
.70–.89	High correlation
.90–1.00	Very high correlation

Such a system of descriptors assumes that the meaningfulness of a correlation is the same regardless of the context in which it is used. This assumption is not necessarily valid. For example, if one is determining the reliability of a strength measure from one day to the next, an r of .70 may be considered unacceptably low for the purpose of documenting day-to-day changes in status. However, if one is determining the relationship between abstract constructs such as self-esteem and motivation that are difficult to measure, then a correlation of .50 may be considered very strong.

VARIANCE SHARED BY THE TWO VARIABLES

The second way to evaluate the importance of the correlation coefficient is to calculate what is called the *coefficient of determination*. The coefficient of determination, r^2, is the square of the correlation coefficient, r. The coefficient of determination is an indication of the percentage of variance that is shared by the two variables. For the relationship between 6-month ROM and gait velocity at Clinic 1 (see Table 22–1), the coefficient of determination is approximately .58 ($.76^2 = .5776$). This means that 58% of the variability within one variable can be accounted for by the other variable. The remaining 42% of the variability is due to variables not yet considered, perhaps height, leg length, pain, age, or sex. Using the coefficient of determination, we find, for example, that a "high" correlation coefficient of .70 accounts for only 49% of the variance among the variables, and a "low" correlation of .30 accounts for an even lower 9% of the variance between the variables.

STATISTICAL SIGNIFICANCE OF THE COEFFICIENT

The third method of interpreting correlation coefficients is to statistically determine whether the coefficient calculated is significantly different from zero. In other words, we determine the probability that the calculated correlation coefficient would have occurred by chance if in fact there was no relationship between the variables. A special form of a t test is used to determine this probability. The problem with this approach is that very weak correlations may be statistically different from zero even though they are not very meaningful. This is particularly likely to occur with large samples. For example, Alexander and associates studied the relationship between different components of stroke rehabilitation and health outcomes in 152 individuals and found a statistically significant correlation of .174 between the number of sessions of speech and language therapy and general health at 3 months after stroke.[6] Although statistically significant, a correlation of this magnitude probably does not describe a clinically meaningful relationship.

CONFIDENCE INTERVALS AROUND THE COEFFICIENT

The fourth way to determine the meaningfulness of a correlation coefficient is to calculate a confidence interval about the correlation coefficient. To do so, a researcher converts the r values into z scores, calculates confidence intervals with the z scores, and transforms the z-score intervals back into a range of r scores. Using steps outlined by Munro, the 95% confidence interval for an *r* of .76 for 6-month ROM and gait velocity at Clinic 1 is .17 to .94.[5(pp236,237)] The confidence interval is very large because the sample is small (n = 10) and does not permit accurate estimation. Using the same procedures, the 95% confidence interval for the same *r* calculated for a sample of 100 participants is approximately .65 to .83, a far smaller interval. As is the case for the confidence intervals calculated in the analysis of differences, larger samples permit more accurate estimation of true population values.

LIMITS OF INTERPRETATION

A consideration common to all four interpretation methods is that the interpretation of correlation coefficients should not extend beyond the range of the original data. For example, Figure 22–5 shows the fairly strong relationship between the 6-month ROM and gait velocity data (asterisks). The line showing the trend of the data is extrapolated to a ROM of 0°. At this ROM, the trend line indicates that the gait velocity would be estimated to be approximately *negative* 38 cm/s, an impossible figure! Rather than being a linear relationship throughout the ROM, it is likely that the relationship becomes curvilinear as ROM becomes closer to 0° with gait velocity bottoming out at some low level (crosses). Knowing that the relationship between ROM and gait velocity is strong and linear in the top half of the usual values does not permit us to extrapolate these conclusions to values outside the ranges encountered in the original data collection. A full interpretation of the correlation between 6-month ROM and gait velocity might be written in a journal article as follows:

DATA ANALYSIS

A Pearson product moment correlation (*r*) was used to quantify the relationship between 6-month range of motion (ROM) and gait velocity for

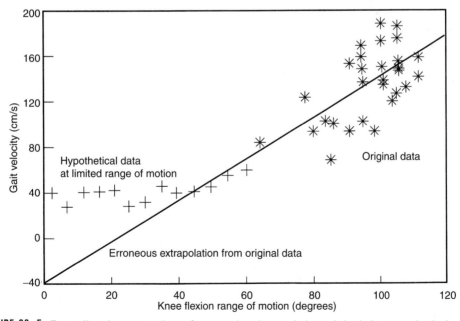

FIGURE 22–5. Extending interpretation of regression beyond the original data results in invalid conclusions. Original data *(asterisks)* extrapolated past the X and Y values predict that patients with no flexion range of motion will have a negative gait velocity. Crosses indicate the more likely relationship between the two variables in their lower ranges.

the sample of 30 participants. Interpretation of the coefficient was through significance testing at the 5% level, calculation of r^2, and construction of a 95% confidence interval around the correlation coefficient.

RESULTS

The Pearson r between 6-month ROM and gait velocity was .6399. This was significantly different from zero at a level of $p < .01$. The coefficient of determination (r^2) was .41, indicating that about 40% of the variability in gait velocity can be attributed to differences in 6-month ROM. The 95% confidence interval for r was .365 to .812.

DISCUSSION

The moderate correlation of approximately .64 between 6-month ROM and gait velocity seems important clinically because it provides evidence that those patients with less physical impairment (i.e., those with good ROM) also have less functional disability, as measured by gait velocity. The confidence interval for r is large, because of the moderate sample size within this study. Based on the strength of the correlation found in this study, we recommend further data collection on a larger sample to provide a more accurate estimation of the true relationship between these two variables.

Literature Examples

Powers and colleagues studied the relationship of muscle force and gait characteristics of individuals with transtibial amputation.[1] They examined the strength of seven different lower extremity muscle groups (bilateral hip extensors, bilateral hip abductors, bilateral knee extensors, and unilateral ankle plantar flexors) for three different gait characteristics (velocity, cadence,

and stride length) at two walking speeds (free and fast). They calculated 42 Pearson product moment correlation coefficients within their study: there was a coefficient for each muscle group correlated with each of the gait characteristics for each speed. The importance of each correlation was evaluated by testing it for statistical significance and calculating the coefficient of determination to see how much of the variability in one variable could be accounted for by the other variable. To simplify the reporting of results, p values and coefficients of determination were reported for only those correlation coefficients that were found to be statistically different from zero.

Alexander and colleagues studied the relationships between different components of stroke rehabilitation and health outcomes.[6] They chose to present an extensive correlation matrix showing the relationships between six measures of rehabilitation inputs (number of sessions of physical therapy, occupational therapy, speech and language therapy, dietetics, podiatry, and community nursing) and 27 measures of outcomes (nine measures, each taken at 1 month, 3 months, and 6 months after stroke). The importance of the various correlations in the study was evaluated by determining the statistical significance of the correlations and by discussing the pattern of significance seen across the variables.

The alternate correlation coefficient, Cramer's V, was used by Harter and associates[7] to document the relationship between instrumented and manual Lachman ligament laxity testing. They interpreted the V coefficient of .27 with significance testing, finding that the relationship between the two types of laxity testing was not significant.

■ LINEAR REGRESSION

Correlational techniques, as discussed earlier, are used to describe the relationships among two or more variables. When the researcher's purpose extends beyond description of relationships to include prediction of future characteristics from previously collected data, then the statistical analysis extends from correlation to regression techniques.

Suppose we wish to predict a patient's eventual gait velocity on the basis of an early post-operative indicator such as 3-week ROM. The Pearson product moment correlation between these two variables is .5545, indicating a moderate degree of correlation in which 31% of the variability in gait velocity ($r^2 = .3075$) can be accounted for by variability in 3-week ROM. Unlike correlation techniques, regression techniques require that variables be defined as independent or dependent. In this example, the independent variable is 3-week ROM and is used to predict the dependent variable, gait velocity.

Figure 22–6 shows a scatterplot of 3-week ROM and gait velocity scores, with a line showing the best fit between these two variables. This line is generated by using the data to solve the general equation for a straight line:

$$Y = bX + a$$

where b is the slope of the line and a is the intercept (i.e., the Y value at the point at which

the line intersects the Y axis). The slope, b, is found by multiplying the Pearson r value by the ratio of the standard deviation of Y to the standard deviation of X: $[b = r(s_y/s_x)]$. The intercept, a, is found by subtracting the product of the slope and the mean of X from the mean of Y: $(a = \overline{Y} - \overline{X}b)$. As with most statistical analyses today, computer programs can generate regression equations quickly and easily without the need for hand calculations. The formula for the regression line of gait velocity on 3-week ROM is $Y = 0.75X + 82.56$. Although this equation defines the best-fitting line through the data, most of the points do not fall precisely on the line. The vertical distance from each point to the line is known as the *residual,* and the mean of the residuals is zero. The standard deviation of the residuals is known as the *standard error of the estimate* (SEE).

Once the regression equation is generated, it can be used to predict the gait velocity of future patients by solving for Y (gait velocity) on the basis of the patient's X (3-week ROM) score. For example, suppose that a patient has 70° of

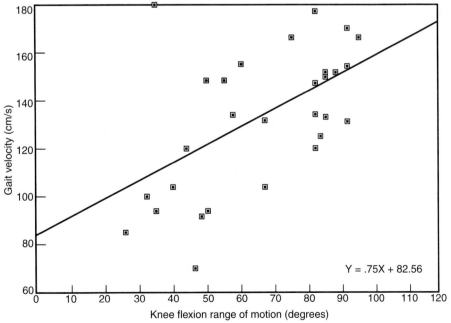

FIGURE 22–6. Regression of gait velocity on 3-week knee flexion range of motion.

ROM 3 weeks postoperatively. The predicted gait velocity for this patient is 135.06 cm/s [0.75(70) + 82.56 = 135.06]. Because we know that this prediction is unlikely to be precise, we can provide additional useful information by generating a confidence interval around the predicted value. The confidence interval around the predicted value is created by using the SEE. A 95% confidence interval, for example, is created by adding and subtracting 1.96 SEEs from the regression line, as shown graphically in Figure 22–7. In this example, the SEE generated by the computer is 24.54 cm/s and the 95% confidence interval would be found by adding and subtracting 48.09 cm/s to and from the predicted Y value. For patients with 3-week ROM of 70°, we therefore are 95% certain that their gait velocity at 6 months will be between 86.96 and 183.16 cm/s. Ideally, the dependent variable is highly correlated with the independent variable, resulting in small residuals, a small SEE, and a more precise prediction.

The statistical significance of a regression equation is usually determined with an F test to evaluate whether r^2, the amount of variance in Y predicted by X, is significantly different from zero. As is the case with statistical testing of the correlation coefficient using a t test, r^2 may be statistically different from zero without being terribly meaningful. In our example, the r^2 of .3075 is significantly different from zero at $p = .0015$. Despite this statistical significance, we know that the 95% confidence interval for predicting a single score is quite large and may not allow for clinically useful prediction. For instance, the gait velocity needed to cross most streets safely is approximately 130 cm/s.[8] The range of the confidence interval is great enough that for most patients we could not predict whether their eventual velocity would enable them to be community ambulators. This reflects the fact that there is only a moderate correlation between the two variables in question.

In practice, then, this regression equation would not likely be perceived to be very useful, and the researchers would search for additional independent variables that would allow for more

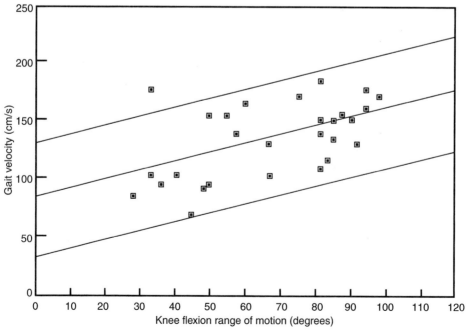

FIGURE 22–7. Ninety-five percent confidence intervals around the predicted gait velocity.

precise prediction of the dependent variable. When more than one variable is used to predict another variable, the simple linear regression technique is extended to multiple regression, as discussed in Chapter 23.

■ SUMMARY

Relationship analysis studies are generally non-experimental, with the researcher observing different phenomena rather than manipulating groups of participants. The magnitude and direction of relationships between variables are expressed mathematically as Pearson product moment correlations or a variety of alternative correlation coefficients. Assumptions for use of the correlation coefficients include linearity, homoscedasticity, and an adequate range of values for each variable. Correlation coefficients are interpreted in several ways: by the strength of the coefficient itself, by the coefficient of determination, by the statistical significance of the correlation coefficient, and by confidence intervals about the correlation coefficient. When the researcher's purpose extends beyond description of relationships to include prediction, then the

statistical analysis extends from correlation to regression techniques.

REFERENCES

1. Powers CM, Boyd LA, Fontaine CA, Perry J. The influence of lower-extremity muscle force on gait characteristics in individuals with below-knee amputations secondary to vascular disease. *Phys Ther.* 1996;76:369-377.
2. Beaton DE, Katz JN, Fossel AH, Wright JG, Tarasuk V, Bombardier C. Measuring the whole or the parts? Validity, reliability, and responsiveness of the Disabilities of the Arm, Shoulder, and Hand outcome measure in different regions of the upper extremity. *J Hand Ther.* 2001;14:128-146.
3. Nussbaum EL, Downes L. Reliability of clinical pressure-pain algometric measurements obtained on consecutive days. *Phys Ther.* 1998;78:160-169.
4. Swartz HM, Flood AB. The corntinental theory of flat and depressed areas: on the relationship between corn and topography. *J Irreproducible Results.* 1990;35(5):16-17, 19.
5. Munro BH. *Statistical Methods for Health Care Research.* 4th ed. Philadelphia, Pa: JB Lippincott; 2000.
6. Alexander H, Bugge C, Hagen S. What is the association between the different components of stroke rehabilitation and health outcomes? *Clin Rehabil.* 2001;15:207-215.
7. Harter RD, Osternig LA, Singer KM, Cord SA. A comparison of instrumented and manual Lachman test results in anterior cruciate ligament-reconstructed knees. *Athl Train.* 1990;25:330-334.
8. Lerner-Frankiel MB, Vargas S, Brown M, Krusell L, Schoneberger W. Functional community ambulation: what are your criteria? *Clin Manage Phys Ther.* 1986;6(2):12-15.

23

Statistical Analysis of Relationships: Advanced and Special Techniques

Chapter 22 introduced basic correlation and regression techniques by emphasizing bivariate procedures, that is, those in which just two variables are involved. In addition, the techniques presented in Chapter 22 were used to analyze relationships between distinctly different variables such as age and gait velocity. In this chapter, which covers more advanced correlation and regression techniques, these basic concepts are extended in two ways. First, specialized reliability correlation coefficients, in which repeated measures of the same variable are analyzed, are examined. Second, procedures that examine the complex interrelationships among many variables are introduced. These procedures include multiple regression, logistic

regression, discriminant analysis, and factor analysis.

■ RELIABILITY ANALYSIS

A specialized type of relationship analysis is used to assess the reliability of a measure. As discussed in Chapter 17, there are two major classes of reliability measures: those that document relative reliability and those that document absolute reliability. It is the measures of relative reliability that depend on correlational techniques. In some instances, the correlational technique does not provide all of the desired reliability information, and regression or difference analysis techniques are used to supplement the correlational technique. Three techniques used for reliability analysis are presented here: the Pearson product moment correlation with regression and difference analysis extensions, the intraclass correlation coefficients, and the kappa correlations.

Pearson Product Moment Correlation with Extensions

The discussion of reliability coefficients begins with the Pearson product moment correlation coefficient, not because it is an ideal reliability coefficient (it is not), but because it is familiar. The fact that extensions to the Pearson correlation coefficient are needed to make it an acceptable reliability coefficient suggests that researchers might do better with correlations that are specifically designed to quantify reliability.[1] The central problem with the Pearson product moment correlation as a reliability coefficient is that it is only a measure of relative reliability: A high, positive Pearson value indicates that high scores on one measure are associated with high scores on another measure and that low scores on one measure are associated with low scores on another measure. When we compare two different variables, such as 3-week range-of-motion (ROM)

and gait velocity, the strength of the relationship is the only information we desire, so the Pearson correlation is ideal.

When comparing paired measurements for the purpose of determining their reliability, however, we are concerned with both the relationship between the two measures and the magnitude of the differences between the two measures. These two forms of reliability are called *relative reliability* and *absolute reliability* (also *association* and *concordance*), respectively. Alone, the Pearson product moment correlation (introduced in Chapter 22) is not a complete tool for documenting reliability because it assesses association and not concordance.

There are three strategies used by researchers to supplement the information gained from the Pearson correlation coefficient: paired-*t* test, slope and intercept documentation, and determination of the standard error of measurement. They are all demonstrated in this section using a data sample representing repeated measures of 3-week ROM made by Therapists A and B at Clinic 3, as shown in Table 23–1. Therapist B consistently rates participants higher than Therapist A—in fact, an average of 10.8° higher. The participant who scores highest for Therapist A also scores highest for Therapist B, even though the actual ROM scores differ based on

TABLE 23–1	Reliability Data for 3-Week Range-of-Motion Measurements by Therapists A and B		
Subject	Therapist A	Therapist B	Difference (B – A)
1	32	38	6
2	50	64	14
3	60	73	13
4	84	90	6
5	81	87	6
6	81	93	12
7	84	94	10
8	81	98	17
9	82	98	16
10	91	99	8
Σ	726.0	834.0	108.0
$\overline{X}$	72.6	83.4	10.8

which therapist took the measure. Thus, the relative reliability is high, with a Pearson r of .977. However, to assume that the scores are interchangeable would clearly be incorrect given the 10.8° difference between therapist, measures.

The first way to extend the reliability analysis beyond the Pearson measure of relative reliability is to conduct a paired-t test on the data. For our data, t is 8.11, with an associated probability of .000. This means that there is a very small chance that the difference between therapists' scores occurred by chance, so we conclude that there is a significant difference between the scores of Therapist A and Therapist B. The scores from the two therapists are highly associated but lack concordance.

The second way to extend the reliability analysis beyond the Pearson measure is to generate a regression equation for the data and document the slope and intercept. If a measure is absolutely reliable, the slope will be close to 1.0 and the intercept will be close to 0.0.[2] In Figure 23–1, the dotted line represents perfect concordance between the two repeated measures,

with a slope of 1.0 and an intercept of zero. The solid line represents a proportionate bias on the part of Rater 2. The intercept is still zero, but the slope exceeds 1.0. In Figure 23–2, the dotted line again represents perfect concordance between the two repeated measures, with a slope of 1.0 and an intercept of zero. The solid line represents an additive bias on the part of Rater 2, with scores consistently 5 points higher than those of Rater 1. The slope of this regression line is still 1.0, but the intercept is now 5.0. For the Therapist A and B data, the slope is 1.0156 and the intercept is 9.666, as shown in Figure 23–3. This indicates the presence of a largely additive bias on the part of one of the therapists.

The third way to add to the usefulness of the Pearson product moment correlation for documenting reliability is to also report the standard error of measurement for the paired data. Using the formula presented in Chapter 17, we find that the standard error of measurement for this data is 2.96, meaning that a 95% confidence interval for two repeated measurements would be ±8.2° ($\sqrt{2} \times$ 2.96 × 1.96), permitting us to be 95% confident

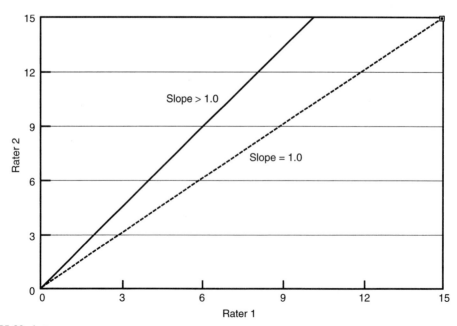

FIGURE 23–1. Proportionate bias between raters is revealed by a slope greater than 1.0. The dotted line represents perfect agreement with a slope of 1.0 and an intercept of 0.0.

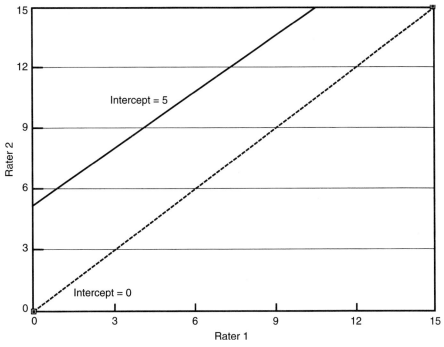

FIGURE 23–2. Additive bias between raters is revealed by an intercept equal to 5.0. The dotted line represents perfect agreement with a slope of 1.0 and an intercept of 0.0.

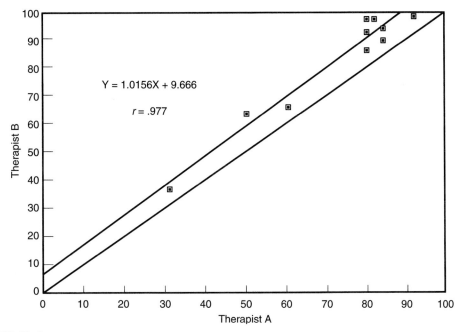

FIGURE 23–3. Bias between Therapist A and Therapist B. There is almost no proportionate bias (slope = 1.0156), but there is a large additive bias (intercept = 9.666°).

that repeated measures would fall within 8.2° of one another. The results of an extended Pearson reliability analysis might be written up as follows:

DATA ANALYSIS

To assess the association between the two therapists' scores, the Pearson product moment correlation was calculated. The concordance of the scores was assessed by calculation of the slope and intercept of the regression equation of one therapist's scores on the other, determination of the standard error of measurement (SEM), and calculation of a paired-t test.

RESULTS

The Pearson r was found to be .977, indicating a high degree of association between the scores of the two therapists. However, the slope was 1.02 and the intercept was 9.67. The 95% confidence interval for the SEM was 8.2°. The paired-t test revealed that the 10.8° mean difference between therapist scores was statistically significant at the .000 level.

DISCUSSION

Despite the high degree of association between the measures taken by Therapist A and Therapist B, the absolute difference between scores means that the absolute interrater reliability is too low for the measures of the two therapists to be considered interchangeable.

Readers should recognize that researchers would probably not use all three extensions in a single study. Any one of these extensions in this case would be sufficient to cast doubt on the absolute reliability of the measures. This example also illustrates that the Pearson correlation alone is not an acceptable way to measure reliability, a point that is reinforced in Hyde's analysis of psychometric standards for outcomes measures used in audiological rehabilitation.[3]

Intraclass Correlation Coefficients

The intraclass correlation coefficients (ICCs) are a family of coefficients that allow comparison of two or more repeated measures. The technique depends on repeated measures analysis of variance (ANOVA). There are at least six different ICC formulas, and the issue of which one to use in a particular calculation has generated considerable confusion.[4] Table 23–2 provides two of the formulas and indications for their use, based on the work of Shrout and Fleiss.[5] In addition to being able to handle more than two repeated measures, the ICC is thought to be a better measure than the Pearson r because it accounts for absolute as well as relative reliability. However, because they take into account "level" differences, but are not true measures of concordance,[2] researchers who report reliability on the basis of an ICC should still report the results of an absolute reliability indicator such as the SEM[1] or the repeated measures ANOVA.

For our example of the interrater reliability between Therapists A and B at Clinic 3, the ICC (2,1) may be most appropriate because the two therapists in question were selected from a larger group of therapists at the clinic, both measured each patient, and the results are to be generalized to other randomly selected judges rather than just applied to the two therapists in question. Table 23–3 shows the ICC (2,1) calculation to be .854. This is less than the .977 that was calculated with the Pearson product moment correlation, but it still would generally be interpreted to be a fairly high level of correlation. Thus, it is useful to examine the results of a repeated measures ANOVA, which shows that there is a significant difference between the measures of the two therapists, $F_{1,9} = 65.7$, $p = .000$. Using the repeated measures ANOVA results with an ICC is analogous to using a paired-t test to extend the results of a Pearson product moment correlation reliability analysis.

Although this example of an ICC used only two raters to compare the results with those found with the Pearson product moment correlation analysis in the previous section, the ICC, like the

ANOVA it is based on, extends easily to accommodate more than two raters. When only two raters are present, the researcher has a choice between the Pearson and an ICC; when three or more raters measure each participant, an ICC must be used.

Watkins and associates studied intertester reliability of measurements of knee ROM.[6] Fourteen different raters were involved in the study, with each participant being measured by a randomly selected pair of raters. The ICC (1,1) they used for analysis seems appropriate for their design, in which raters for each participant were selected randomly.

Beaton and colleagues used the ICC (2,1) formula to determine test-retest reliability of the Disabilities of the Arm, Shoulder, and Hand (DASH) outcome measure.[7] The reported ICC of

---

TABLE 23-2 Calculations of Intraclass Correlation Coefficients (ICCs)

Source of Variation	Degrees of Freedom	Mean Square (MS)
Between subjects	$N^* - 1$	Between subjects (BMS)
Within subject	$N(K^\dagger - 1)$	Within subject (WMS)
Between judges	$K - 1$	Between judges (JMS)
Error	$(N - 1)(K - 1)$	Error (EMS)

Formula	Appropriate Use
$ICC(1,1) = \dfrac{BMS - WMS}{BMS + (K - 1)WMS}$	Each subject is rated by different randomly selected judges.
$ICC(2,1) = \dfrac{BMS - EMS}{BMS + (K - 1)EMS + \dfrac{K(JMS - EMS)}{N}}$	Each subject is rated by the same randomly selected judges.

*Subjects.
†Judges.

TABLE 23-3 ICC (2,1) Calculation for 3-Week Range of Motion for Therapists A and B

Source of Variation	Degrees of Freedom	Mean Square (MS)	F	p
Between subjects	9	734.78 (BMS)		
Within subject	10	66.30 (WMS)		
Between judges	1	583.20 (JMS)	65.7	.000
Error	9	8.87 (EMS)		

$$ICC(2,1) = \frac{BMS - EMS}{BMS + (K - 1)EMS + \dfrac{K^*(JMS - EMS)}{N^\dagger}}$$

$$ICC(2,1) = \frac{734.78 - 8.87}{734.78 + (2 - 1)8.87 + \dfrac{(2)(583.20 - 8.87)}{10}} = .854$$

*Judges.
†Subjects.

.96, along with an SEM of 4.6 DASH points on a 100-point scale, led to their conclusion that test-retest reliability of the DASH is acceptable for individuals with upper limb problems and that the 95% minimally detectable change for two repeated measures of the DASH is 12.75 points ($4.6 \times 1.96 \times \sqrt{2} = 12.75$).

Kappa

Kappa is a reliability coefficient designed for use with nominal data. Suppose that we wanted to determine whether Therapists A and B at Clinic 3 agreed with each other on the stair-climbing ability of their patients. Table 23–4 shows the cross-tabulation of the data of Therapists A and B. For 6 of the 10 patients, the therapists gave identical scores. For 4 of the 10 patients, the therapists differed by one category. The simplest way to express the degree of concordance between the therapists' observations is to calculate

the percentage of patients on whose ability the two therapists agreed completely. For this example, the agreement is 60%. However, because there are only a few nominal categories, there is a high probability that some of the agreements occurred by chance. The kappa correlation coefficient adjusts the agreement percentage to account for chance agreements, as shown in the formula at the bottom of Table 23–4.[8] The kappa for this example is .3939.

Kappa can also be weighted to account for the seriousness of the discrepancy.[9] Consider one disagreement in which one rater scores the patient as a 5 in stair climbing (reciprocal, no railing) and the other scores the patient as a 4 (reciprocal, with rail). Contrast this with a disagreement between a 4 and a 3 (one at a time, with or without rail). Some might believe that disagreement on the use of a rail is a less serious reliability problem than disagreement about whether the patient can maneuver the stairs reciprocally. A weighted kappa allows the

TABLE 23-4	Kappa Correlation Calculation				

	Therapist A				
Therapist B	**5**	**4**	**3**	**2**	**Total**
5	2 (.20) [.12]	1			3 (.30)
4	2	3 (.30) [.20]			5 (.50)
3			1 (.10) [.02]		1 (.10)
2			1		1 (.10)
Total	4 (.40)	4 (.40)	2 (.20)		10 (1.0)

$$\kappa = \frac{p_0 - p_c}{1 - p_c} = \frac{.60 - .34}{1 - .34} = .3939$$

p_0 = sum of the observed probabilities in perfect agreement = .60
p_c = sum of the chance probabilities for perfect agreement = .34

Note: Numbers are the number of observations in the cell. Numbers in parentheses are the proportion of observations in the cell. Numbers in brackets are the proportion of observations expected by chance in the cell. The proportion expected by chance is calculated by multiplying the marginal proportion (total row or column) for the corresponding row and column.

researcher to establish different weights for different disagreements. In addition to occurring in weighted and nonweighted forms, kappa can be extended to more than two raters.[10]

Van Dillen and colleagues studied the reliability of physical examination items used for classification of patients with low back pain.[11] Many of the items required patients to report whether their symptoms were the same, decreased, or increased in response to a particular movement. Other items described alignment and movement, scoring the items as "yes" or "no" based on whether a patient exhibited the various alignment or movement patterns. Because these scoring systems are nominal, the authors used kappa to determine reliability. For the symptom behavior items the agreement percentage ranged from 98% to 100% and the corresponding kappas ranged from .87 to 1.00. For the alignment and movement variables the agreement percentage ranged from 55% to 100% and the corresponding kappas ranged from .00 to .78. Landis and Koch described the strength of agreement of kappa to be slight for kappas between .00 and .20, fair for kappas between .21 and .40, moderate for between .41 and .60, substantial between .61 and .80, and almost perfect for .81 to 1.00.[12] According to these descriptors, Van Dillen and colleagues found almost perfect correlations for the symptom behavior items, but wide variation in the strengths of agreement (from slight to substantial) for the alignment and movement variables.

■ MULTIPLE REGRESSION

Multiple regression techniques are designed to analyze complex relationships among many different variables. The classic use of multiple regression uses numerical independent variables to predict a numerical dependent variable.[13(p213-222)] With the development of large databases containing many cases and many different variables, multiple regression strategies are more feasible than ever, but no less difficult to implement

effectively.[14] In the small data set used throughout this text, gait velocity is a continuous numerical variable that is appropriate for analysis with multiple regression. Many of the independent variables we might use to generate a multiple regression equation would also be numerical variables such as age, height, leg length, and weight. In addition to these variables, however, we might also wish to include some nominal independent variables such as gender (male, female) or postoperative complications (yes, no). Even though multiple regression techniques were designed for use with numerical variables, they can accommodate nominal independent variables if a different number is assigned to each of the nominal levels. For example, the presence of a postoperative complication might be entered as a "1" whereas the absence of a complication would be entered as a "0." This process of assigning arbitrary numbers to nominal independent variables is called *dummy coding*.

In Chapter 22, simple linear regression was used to predict 6-month gait velocity (the dependent variable) from 3-week ROM of patients after total knee arthroplasty. A regression equation was calculated, but it was not very precise, with 3-week ROM accounting for only 31% of the variability in gait velocity. Clearly, there are factors other than 3-week ROM that must account for the gait velocity of these patients.

Because the prediction of gait velocity from 3-week ROM is not precise enough to be useful clinically, the next logical step is to add an additional variable or variables to the equation to determine whether the prediction can be made more precise. For example, suppose we add patients' age to the equation. The general prediction equation for multiple regression is

$$Y = b_1 X_1 + b_2 X_2 + b_i X_i + a$$

For each independent variable there is a corresponding slope, which is referred to in multiple regression as a *b-weight*. For the entire equation there is one intercept, which is referred to as the *constant*. The computer-generated regression equation for 3-week ROM and age as predictors of gait velocity is

$$(velocity) = .04 \ (3\text{-week ROM}) - 1.41 \ (age) + 227.04$$

A 65-year-old patient with 70° of motion 3 weeks postoperatively would be predicted to have a gait velocity of 138.19 cm/s 6 months postoperatively:

$$.04 \ (70) - 1.41 \ (65) + 227.04 = 138.19$$

The raw regression coefficient for age can be interpreted as follows: If ROM is held constant, for each 1-year increase in age, the velocity prediction decreases by 1.41 cm/s. If age is held constant, for each 1° increase in ROM, the velocity prediction increases by only .04 cm/s.

The correlation between all the independent variables and the dependent variable in a multiple regression equation is represented by R, to distinguish it from r, the correlation between the two variables in a simple linear regression equation. For this equation, the multiple correlation, R, is .77483 and the R^2 is .55477. This means that the combination of 3-week ROM and age accounts for 55% of the variability in gait velocity. Recall that 3-week ROM alone accounted for only 31% of the variability in gait velocity. The addition of age to the equation has greatly improved its predictability.

Variable Entry in Multiple Regression

When performing a multiple regression, researchers often specify various decision rules to guide the computer in generating the regression equation. The rules are generally constructed so that the method of variable entry maximizes the accuracy of predictions while minimizing the number of variables in the equation. Variables are retained in the equation if they improve the R^2 by a

specified amount or if they are associated with a probability of some specified amount.

In a forward regression strategy, a researcher adds one variable at a time and stops when additional variables do not contribute the preset amount. In a backward regression strategy, the researcher begins with all the possible variables of interest in the equation and deletes them one at a time if their presence does not contribute the preset amount. A stepwise regression strategy combines forward and backward procedures to generate the equation. If any of these strategies were used in our example, the age variable would be entered first and the 3-week ROM variable would not be entered because it contributes so little beyond that of age. For example, the R^2 associated with age alone is .55432; for age and 3-week ROM combined, it is only .55477, an increase of only .00045. This means that the addition of 3-week ROM to the equation adds only .045% of additional predictability for gait velocity. Clinically, this means that, if our interest is primarily in predicting gait velocity, we can eliminate the possibly inconvenient and expensive measurement of 3-week ROM and substitute the inexpensive, easily obtained age value.

Interpretation of the Multiple Regression Equation

The meaningfulness of the multiple regression equation can be assessed in several ways. First, an F test of R^2 can be conducted to determine whether it is significantly different from zero. For our example, the computer-generated significance of the F test is .0000, indicating that there is a very low probability that the R^2 of .55477 was obtained by chance.

The second way to assess the meaningfulness of a multiple regression equation is to generate a confidence interval. The computer-generated standard error of the estimate (SEE) for the multiple regression equation is 20.03 cm/s, and a 95% confidence interval would add and subtract 39.27 cm/s to the predicted Y value

[±1.96 (SEE)]. Thus, we could be 95% certain that our 65-year-old patient with 70° of knee flexion 3 weeks postoperatively would have a 6-month gait velocity of 98.92 to 177.46 cm/s. Recall that the 95% confidence interval for the simple regression of gait velocity on ROM was 86.96 to 183.16 cm/s, as presented in Chapter 22. Because a greater proportion of the variability in gait velocity is accounted for by the multiple regression compared with the simple regression, this multiple regression interval is somewhat narrower than the simple regression interval.

A third way to evaluate the regression equation is to determine the relative contribution of each of the variables to the equation. This can be done by either conducting a t test of the contribution of each variable or dividing the R^2 into the components attributable to each variable. This division is done through beta (β)-weights, which are standardized versions of b-weights. The beta-weight for each variable is multiplied by the correlation coefficient between that variable and the dependent variable. For our example, the mathematical notation is

$$R^2 = (\beta_{\text{3-week ROM}}) (r_{\text{3-week ROM, velocity}}) + (\beta_{\text{age}}) (r_{\text{age, velocity}})$$

Using computer-generated beta-weights and correlation coefficients, we find the following:

$$.5547 = (.0305) (.5545) + (-.7224) (-.7445)$$
$$= .0169 + .5378$$

This means that of the 55% of the variability in gait velocity predicted by the equation, almost 54% is due to the relationship between age and gait velocity and less than 2% is due to the relationship between 3-week ROM and velocity. The t tests of the contribution of variables yield significance levels of .8711 for 3-week ROM and .0006 for age. Both the division of R^2 and the t tests indicate that age is a much more important predictor of gait velocity than is 3-week ROM.

Recall that in the simple linear regression of gait velocity on 3-week ROM, the ROM variable

accounted for approximately 31% of the variability in gait scores. How is it that it now accounts for only 2% of that variability? The answer can be found in an examination of the interrelationships among all three variables. The Venn diagrams in Figure 23–4 illustrate this principle. Independently, 3-week ROM accounts for about 31% of the variability in gait velocity, as shown in Figure 23–4, A. Independently, age accounts for about 55% of the variability in gait velocity, as shown in Figure 23–4, B. In addition, age and 3-week ROM are highly related, with one variable accounting for approximately 53% ($r_{\text{age, 3-week ROM}}$ = −.7253) of the variability in the other, as shown in Figure 23–4, C. When all three are examined together, almost all of the variability in velocity that is accounted for by 3-week ROM is also accounted for by the relationship between age and velocity. Thus, in the regression of gait velocity on both age and 3-week ROM, the latter assumes much less importance than when it is the sole variable used to predict gait velocity.

With the availability of computer-based statistical packages, it is deceptively easy to run multiple regression analyses. However, factors that influence the validity of multiple regression procedures include the extent of multicollinearity (high levels of correlation among the predictor variables, which is undesirable), cross-validation of the regression equation with a second sample of participants or with random subsets of the original sample, adequate sample size, and how outlying data points are handled.[15]

The results of this multiple regression analysis might be written up in a journal article as follows:

DATA ANALYSIS

Simple linear regression of gait velocity on 3-week range of motion (ROM) was used initially to test whether early ROM status could be used to predict eventual function as measured by gait velocity. Multiple regression was used to add the variable of age to the prediction equation when 3-week ROM proved to be an inadequate

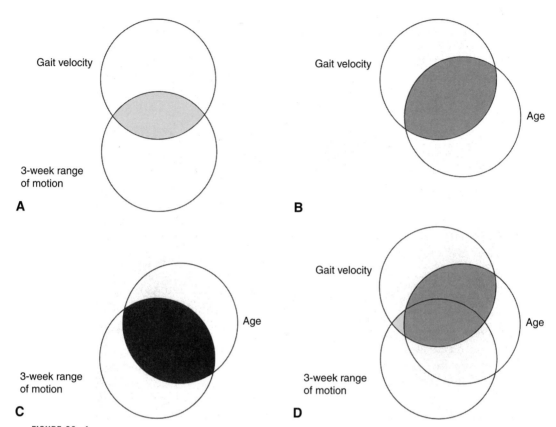

FIGURE 23–4. **A,** Relationship between gait velocity and 3-week range of motion. **B,** Relationship between gait velocity and age. **C,** Relationship between 3-week range of motion and age. **D,** Relationship of both age and 3-week range of motion to gait velocity. Most of the variability in gait velocity accounted for by 3-week range of motion is also accounted for by age.

independent predictor. The significance of each variable was determined with a *t* test, the significance of R^2 was determined with an *F* test, and alpha was set at .05. In addition, confidence intervals around the predicted Y value were generated.

RESULTS

For the simple regression of gait velocity on 3-week ROM, *r* was only .5545. Although significantly different from zero (*p* = .0015), this means that only 30.75% of the variance in gait velocity was accounted for by 3-week ROM. The 95% confidence interval around the predicted gait

velocity score for a given individual would require that 48.09 cm/s be added to and subtracted from the predicted score.

To enhance predictability, a multiple regression equation was developed to predict gait velocity from both 3-week ROM and age. The equation developed from the two predictor variables was: Velocity = .04 (3-week ROM) − 1.41 (age) + 227.04. The R^2 for this equation was .5547 and was significant at *p* = .0000. The contribution of age was .5378 and was significant at *p* = .0006; the contribution of 3-week ROM was only .0169 and was not significant at *p* = .8711. For this equation, the

95% confidence interval around the predicted gait velocity score for a given individual would require that 39.27 cm/s be added to and subtracted from the predicted score.

DISCUSSION

The simple regression of gait velocity on 3-week ROM did not confirm the clinical observation that early ROM status is a good predictor of eventual gait outcome. When age was added to the equation, prediction of gait velocity improved. However, the very strong relationship between age and gait velocity meant that the contribution of 3-week ROM to prediction of gait velocity became insignificant when age was included in the equation. Thus, for this group of patients, eventual gait velocity can be predicted almost as well by age alone as by the combination of age and 3-week ROM.

Literature Examples

Andrews and associates used stepwise multiple regression to develop prediction equations for muscle force for dominant and nondominant sides.[16] The independent variables they used for these predictions were gender, weight, and age. Because gender is a nominal variable, dummy codes (0 = male, 1 = female) were assigned so that it could be included in the analysis. The multiple R^2 associated with the different muscle groups ranged from .389 for ankle dorsiflexion on the nondominant side to .770 for shoulder medial rotation on the nondominant side. Thus, they found that they could predict between 39% and 77% of the variability in muscle force based on these three easily collected variables (gender, weight, and age).

Goverover and Hinojosa used multiple regression to predict instrumental activities of daily living (IADL) performance based on categorization and deductive reasoning abilities

for adults with brain injury. They developed several different regression models to determine how well different combinations of age, education, categorization, and deductive reasoning variables predicted performance on IADLs.[17]

■ LOGISTIC REGRESSION

Multiple regression procedures, as described previously, can provide useful information for predicting numerical dependent variables. However, therapists are often interested in predicting dichotomous outcomes, such as whether or not a patient achieves independence or whether or not a patient returns home following rehabilitation. For example, we might be interested in determining what factors predict the need for an assistive device 6 months after total knee arthroplasty.

Rationale for Logistic Regression

Using the data set originally presented in Chapter 19, we find that almost 100% of patients in their 40s and 50s, 57% in their 60s, 22% in their 70s, and 0% in their 80s and 90s are independent in gait without an assistive device. Figure 23–5 illustrates these data conceptually with a smoothed line representing the approximate relationship between age and use of gait devices 6 months after total knee arthroplasty. It is obvious that the relationship between these two factors is not linear. Rather, it remains at a high level in the younger age ranges, drops off rapidly for the intermediate ages, and then bottoms out at a low level for the older age ranges.

This S-shaped curve is typical of the relationship between a dichotomous variable and a continuous variable. Because the relationship is nonlinear, standard linear correlation and regression techniques are not appropriate and techniques that use logarithmic and exponential transformations of the data are used instead.[18(p255)] The general technique that is used to predict dichotomous outcomes from

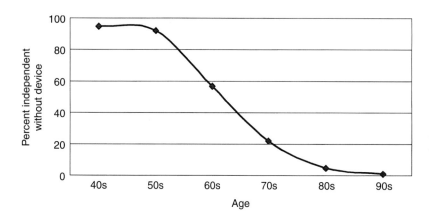

FIGURE 23–5. Graph illustrates the nonlinear, S-shaped curve that describes the relationship between a continuous variable (age) and a dichotomous variable (independence without an assistive device).

numerical independent variables is called *logistic regression*.

Literature Examples

In the rehabilitation literature, logistic regression has been used to examine the factors that predict falls among the elderly. Because of the complex mathematical transformations involved in logistic regression, the presentation of results can be confusing and a full discussion is beyond the scope of this text. However, readers should know that there are two common ways of presenting the results of logistic regression: with odds ratios for the variables within the logistic regression equation or by presenting the equation itself.

For example, Berg and associates used logistic regression to determine the extent to which a variety of factors could predict multiple falls versus single or no falls (over a 12-month period of time) in a group of elderly individuals.[19] The analysis showed that Berg Balance Scale scores, a history of falls in the 3 months before the initiation of the study, and visual problems were significant predictors of fall status during the study. By reporting the odds ratios associated with each independent variable and the dependent variable of fall status, the authors showed that individuals with a history of falls in the past 3 months were 5.75 times as likely to have multiple falls as those without such a history and individuals with visual problems were 2.80 times

as likely to have multiple falls as those without visual problems. The odds ratio for the Berg Balance Scale scores, .90, was less than 1.0, indicating an inverse relationship. That is, individuals with lower Berg Balance Scale scores were more likely to sustain multiple falls.

Shumway-Cook and her colleagues also used logistic regression to analyze the relationships among falls and a variety of other factors.[20] Rather than presenting their results as odds ratios, they chose to provide readers with the actual logistic regression equation and with some sample predictions from the equations. By doing so, they help readers get past the complex equation that results from any logistic regression to see the implications of the equation. They showed that solving the equation for an individual without a history of imbalance and a Berg Balance Scale score of 54 would result in a prediction of a 5% probability of falling. They also solved their equation for an individual with a history of imbalance and a Berg Balance Scale score of 42 to show a predicted 91% probability of falling.

■ DISCRIMINANT ANALYSIS

Discriminant analysis is a procedure in which multiple predictor variables are used to place individuals into groups. Essentially, it is a backward MANOVA procedure. Recall that MANOVA uses a grouping factor to examine differences on multiple dependent variables at the same time. For example, MANOVA might be used to determine whether boys and girls differ on the combined communication variables of vocabulary, mean length of utterance, grammatically complete utterances, and complex sentences. In contrast, discriminant analysis uses the set of combined communication variables from each participant to predict whether each is a boy or a girl. Knowing which participants are, in fact, boys and girls, allows the researchers to document the proportion of participants who were classified correctly by the discriminant analysis. A data set that produces a MANOVA identifying significant differences between boys and girls on the combined communication variables would produce a discriminant analysis with a high proportion of correct classifications.

Woodford-Rogers and colleagues used discriminant analysis to predict the anterior cruciate ligament (ACL) injury status of male high school and college football players and female high school and college gymnasts and basketball players based on measures of navicular drop, calcaneal alignment, and anterior knee joint laxity.[21] ACL injury status was predicted correctly for 71.4% of football players and 87.5% of gymnasts and basketball players, suggesting a role for these biomechanical variables in ACL injury, particularly in women.

In another study, Rogers and Case-Smith used handwriting speed and legibility to predict whether students would be fast or slow keyboarders.[22] If handwriting difficulties predict slow keyboarding, then using keyboarding as an alternative way for students with handwriting difficulties to complete school assignments might not be as effective as hoped. The handwriting variables correctly categorized students as fast or slow keyboarders in 71.1% of cases. However, for those not correctly classified, some with handwriting difficulties were actually fast keyboarders (rather than slow keyboarders as predicted). This suggests that at least some students with handwriting difficulties can develop keyboarding skills that may facilitate written work in school.

■ FACTOR ANALYSIS

Factor analysis is a tool whereby correlational techniques are used to discover which of many variables cluster together as a related unit, separate from other, unrelated clusters. It is a data reduction technique in which many variables are grouped into a smaller number of related groups.

Factor analysis is generally done for one of three reasons: test development, theory development, or theory testing. In test development, factor analysis is often used to help reduce a great number of items into a smaller number. Factor analysis groups items that are related to one another, and the test developer can then select certain questions from each factor for inclusion in the final version of the test. In theory development, factor analysis is used to examine the underlying structure of a set of variables about which the researcher has not developed a conceptual framework. The factors that emerge are then examined and named by the researcher, who then develops hypotheses about interrelationships among the factors. In theory testing, items thought to be representative of certain constructs are factor analyzed to determine whether the items load as hypothesized.

In our sample data set, 12 different pieces of data are recorded for each patient at 6 months postoperatively:

One ROM measure

Two muscle strength measures

Four deformity measures

Four activities of daily living (ADL) measures

One gait velocity measure

A theoretical grouping of these variables might be according to changes in body structure and function and disability, as defined in the World Health Organization's International Classification of Functioning, Disability, and Health.[23] The bodily change variables relate to abnormal structures and would include the ROM measure, the strength measures, and the deformity measures. The disability variables relate to abnormal performance of activities and in this example would include the ADL measures and gait velocity. Researchers might hypothesize that if bodily changes and disability are truly different constructs, then a factor analysis of the 12 variables would yield one factor that consists of the bodily change variables and one factor that consists of the disability variables.

Factor Analysis Steps

The result of a factor analysis of these 12 variables is presented here. The mathematical basis of factor analysis has been presented well by others and is therefore omitted so that emphasis may be placed on interpretation rather than calculation.[24] In brief, the steps in a factor analysis are as follows:

1. A group of variables is analyzed for interrelationships.
2. The number of important underlying factors is determined by reviewing eigenvalues associated with each factor.
3. Factors are extracted.

4. The factor solution is rotated to maximize differences between the factors.
5. Rotated factor loadings are examined to determine a simple structure.
6. The resulting factors are interpreted.

Let's examine these steps in sequence for the twelve 6-month variables. First, a correlation matrix is developed, as shown in Table 23–5. In this example, the matrix has been set up so that the theorized bodily change and disability variables are close to one another. If we examine the last five columns of the matrix, which consists of the theorized disability variables, we find that they are all fairly highly correlated with the ROM and strength variables (Rows 1 through 3) and with the other disability variables (Rows 8 through 11). They are minimally correlated with the deformity variables (Rows 4 through 7). Although we can visually detect some patterns within the relationships among variables, the matrix is far too complex for simple visual analysis; hence, there is need for a mathematical tool like factor analysis.

The second step of a factor analysis is to determine the number of factors in the solution. Initially, the variables in the factor analysis

TABLE 23–5				Correlation Matrix for 12-Variable Factor Analysis							
	F	**E**	**DFC**	**DVV**	**DML**	**DAP**	**V**	**ADW**	**AAD**	**ASC**	**ARC**
M6R	.56	.59	−.17	−.23	.11	−.15	.63	.68	.70	.71	.65
F		.95	−.19	.19	.04	−.05	.89	.72	.69	.75	.81
E			−.13	.24	.03	−.09	.90	.70	.65	.75	.79
DFC				.46	.45	.14	−.22	−.34	−.26	−.21	−.24
DVV					.27	−.01	.17	−.10	−.19	−.01	.02
DML						.45	−.07	−.16	−.10	−.12	.02
DAP							−.17	−.06	.02	−.17	.12
V								.80	.75	.82	.85
ADW									.83	.78	.81
AAD										.83	.81
ASC											.82

M6R, 6-month range of motion; *F*, flexion torque; *E*, extension torque; *DFC*, deformity-flexion contracture; *DVV*, deformity–varus/valgus angulation; *DML*, deformity–mediolateral instability; *DAP*, deformity–anteroposterior in ability; *V*, gait velocity; *ADW*, activities of daily living (ADL)–distance walked; *AAD*, ADL–assistive device; *ASC*, ADL–stair climbing; *ARC*, ADL–rising from chair.

problem are used to create the same number of factors. Each factor has an associated eigenvalue, which is related to the percentage of variability within the data set that can be accounted for by the factor. Some factors will account for very little variance and are therefore eliminated from the analysis. One convention for determining the number of factors in the solution is that only factors with eigenvalues of greater than 1.0 are retained. Another method is the scree method, which examines the pattern of eigenvalues graphically.[24(p635)] When a researcher is testing a theory, the number of factors he or she retains may simply be the number of theorized factors.

The factor analysis of our 12 variables shows that three factors had eigenvalues greater than 1.0; the scree method would retain either two or three factors, and our theoretical model predicted two factors. For the purpose of this example, then, two factors are selected for extraction, the third step in factor analysis. Terms that describe different extraction techniques are *principal components extraction, image factoring,* and *alpha factoring,* among others.

The fourth step in factor analysis is to rotate the factors. In essence, rotation can be thought of as resetting the zero point within the factor analysis. Doing so maximizes the appearance of differences between factors. Terms that describe different types of rotation techniques are *orthogonal, oblique, varimax,* and *quartimax,* among others. Once rotation has occurred, one speaks in terms of "factor loadings" rather than "correlation." A factor loading is essentially the correlation between each variable within a factor and the entire factor. Table 23–6 shows the rotated factor loadings determined by the factor analysis.

The fifth step in factor analysis is to determine, if possible, a simple structure for the factors. A simple structure is developed when each variable is associated with only one factor. To determine a simple structure, the researcher decides to retain in each factor only those variables that loaded above some arbitrary point, often .30. In our example, if factor loadings

above .30 are retained, the flexion contracture variable remains in both factors because its loading on Factor I is –.305 and its loading on Factor II is .71. Thus, to obtain a simple structure for this analysis, we need to adopt a more restrictive criterion for variable retention. If we adopt a criterion of .35, then a simple structure is created.

The final step in factor analysis is to name and interpret the factors. This is done according to the variables that were retained in each factor and is highly subjective. Researchers often name the factors in a manner consistent with the theoretical underpinnings of the study. Factor II in our solution consists of the four deformity variables and could be named "Changes in Body Structure." This name lets the reader know that Factor II consists of a subgroup of the hypothesized construct of bodily change. Factor I is more difficult to name, because it consists of a combination of functional, strength, and ROM variables. A name consistent with the theoretical

TABLE 23–6	Rotated Factor Loadings	
Variable	**Factor I**	**Factor II**
V	.94	.10
ARC	.92	.12
ASC	.91	–.03
ADW	.89	–.12
F	.89	.20
E	.88	.24
AAD	.88	–.09
M6R	.76	–.05
DML	–.07	.77
DFC	–.30	.71
DVV	–.00	.71
DAP	–.10	.44
% of variance accounted for	53.7	16.6

V, Gait velocity; *ARC,* activities of daily living (ADL)–rising from chair; *ASC,* ADL–stair climbing; *ADW,* ADL–distance walked; *F,* flexion torque; *E,* extension torque; *AAD,* ADL–assistive device; *M6R,* 6-month range of motion; *DML,* deformity–mediolateral instability; *DFC,* deformity–flexion contracture; *DVV,* deformity–varus/valgus angulation; and *DAP,* deformity–anteroposterior instability.

underpinnings would be "Changes in Body Function and Disability." Table 23–7, a modified version of Table 23–6, illustrates how a simple structure with named factors might be presented. Once the factors are named, the implications of the factors are discussed by the researcher. The following is the interpretation of this factor analysis as it might be written in a journal article:

DATA ANALYSIS

Factor analysis with principal components extraction and orthogonal varimax rotation was used to test whether variables loaded as predicted on two theorized factors described in the International Classification of Functioning, Disability, and Health (ICF). A simple structure was developed by including in each factor only those variables with rotated factor loadings higher than .35.

RESULTS

Table 23–7 shows the rotated factor loadings for the two-factor solution. The first factor included all the activities of daily living (ADL) variables, as well as the gait velocity, range of motion (ROM), and torque variables. The second factor included all the deformity variables. Factor I was labeled "Changes in Body Function and Disability" and accounted for 53.7% of the variance; Factor II was labeled "Changes in Body Structure" and accounted for 16.6% of the variance.

DISCUSSION

Our results do not fully support the hypothesized distinction between body changes and disability because some of the body change variables loaded with the disability variables. However, the body change variables did split among the two factors according to the structure and function dimensions described in the ICF. The structural, that is, anatomical, body change variables (the four measures of deformity) all loaded together and were separate from the other eight variables. This indicates that the actual anatomical alignment of the knees was not highly associated with eventual functional recovery. The variables that are more representative of physiological function than anatomical structure (flexion and extension torque and flexion ROM) loaded with the disability variables of ADL status and gait velocity. These results suggest that the constructs of body changes and disability, as defined within the ICF, are not completely valid for patients who have had total knee arthroplasty. However, the fact that body function and body structure variables loaded within different factors supports the notion that these two types of body changes represent distinct different underlying constructs.

TABLE 23-7	**Rotated Factor Loadings**	
	Factor	
Variable	**Changes in Body Function and Disability**	**Changes in Body Structure**
Gait velocity	.94	
ADL–rising from chair	.92	
ADL–stair climbing	.91	
ADL–distance walked	.89	
Flexion torque	.89	
Extension torque	.88	
ADL–assistive device	.88	
Six-month range of motion	.76	
Deformity–mediolateral instability		.77
Deformity–flexion contracture		.71
Deformity–varus/ valgus angulation		.71
Deformity–anteroposterior instability		.44

ADL, Activities of daily living.

Literature Examples

Jarus and Poremba used factor analysis to determine what factors might underlie a wide range of hand evaluation items.[25] Their analysis identified four factors, which they named "Pinch," "Grasp," "Target Accuracy," and "Activities of Daily Living." The authors believed that this set of factors could be used as the basis for developing a battery of hand function tests that would be more comprehensive than existing tests, none of which include items from all four factors.

A different example is Mulligan's use of factor analysis to test a theoretical model of sensory integration dysfunction.[26] The hypothesized model predicted that the different subtests of the Sensory Integration and Praxis Tests (SIPT) would cluster into five separate latent variables. A complex analysis that tested various factor analytic models led the author to conclude that a model with one generalized variable and four latent variables fit that data better than the originally hypothesized model.

■ SUMMARY

Advanced and special relationship analysis techniques are used to analyze more than two variables simultaneously or to analyze repeated measures of the same variable. Specialized reliability correlation coefficients, in which repeated measures of the same variable are analyzed, include the Pearson product moment correlation with extensions to evaluate the slope and intercept of an associated regression line; intraclass correlation coefficients based on analysis of variance techniques; and kappa, which is used with nominal data. Multiple regression is used to predict a numerical dependent variable from many different independent variables. Logistic regression is used to predict a nominal dependent variable from many different independent variables. Discriminant analysis uses a set of predictor variables to place individuals into groups. Factor analysis is a correlational technique that is used to determine which of many variables cluster

together as a related unit separate from other, unrelated clusters.

REFERENCES

1. Rankin G, Stokes M. Reliability of assessment tools in rehabilitation: an illustration of appropriate statistical analysis. *Clin Rehabil.* 1998;12:187-199.
2. Delitto A, Strube MJ. Reliability in the clinical setting. *Research Section Newsletter.* 1991;24(1):2-8.
3. Hyde ML. Reasonable psychometric standards for self-report outcomes measures in audiological rehabilitation. *Ear Hear.* 2000;21:24S-36S.
4. Müller R, Büttner P. A critical discussion of intraclass correlation coefficients. *Stat Med.* 1994;13:2465-2476.
5. Shrout PE, Fleiss JL. Intraclass correlations: uses in assessing rater reliability. *Psychol Bull.* 1979;86:420-428.
6. Watkins MA, Riddle DL, Lamb RL, Personius WJ. Reliability of goniometric measurements and visual estimates of knee range of motion obtained in a clinical setting. *Phys Ther.* 1991;71:90-97.
7. Beaton DE, Katz JN, Fossel AH, Wright JG, Tarasuk V, Bombardier C. Measuring the whole or the parts? Validity, reliability, and responsiveness of the Disabilities of the Arm, Shoulder, and Hand outcome measure in different regions of the upper extremity. *J Hand Ther.* 2001;14:128-146.
8. Cohen J. A coefficient of agreement for nominal scales. *Educ Psychol Measur.* 1960;20: 37-46.
9. Cohen J. Weighted kappa: nominal scale agreement with provision for scaled disagreement or partial credit. *Psychol Bull.* 1968;70:213-220.
10. Fleiss JL. Measuring nominal scale agreement among many raters. *Psychol Bull.* 1971;76:378-382.
11. Van Dillen LR, Sahrmann SA, Norton BJ, et al. Reliability of physical examination items used for classification of patients with low back pain. *Phys Ther.* 1998;78: 979-988.
12. Landis JR, Koch GG. The measurement of observer agreement for categorical data. *Biometrics.* 1977;33: 159-174.
13. Dawson-Saunders B, Trapp RG. *Basic and Clinical Biostatistics.* 3rd ed. Norwalk, Conn: Appleton & Lange; 2000.
14. Nick TG, Hardin JM. Quantitative research series—regression modeling strategies: an illustrative case study from medical rehabilitation outcomes research. *Am J Occup Ther.* 1999;53:459-470.
15. Dimitrov D, Fitzgerald S, Rumrill P. Multiple regression in rehabilitation research. *Work.* 2000;15:209-215.
16. Andrews AW, Thomas MW, Bohannon RW. Normative values for isometric muscle force measurements obtained with hand-held dynamometers. *Phys Ther.* 1996;76:248-259.
17. Goverover Y, Hinojosa J. Categorization and deductive reasoning: predictors of instrumental activities of daily

living performance in adults with brain injury. *Am J Occup Ther.* 2002;56:509-516.

18. Elston RC, Johnson WD. *Essentials of Biostatistics.* Philadelphia, Pa: FA Davis; 1994.

19. Berg KO, Wood-Dauphinee SL, Williams JI, Maki B. Measuring balance in the elderly: validation of an instrument. *Can J Public Health.* 1992;83(suppl 2): S7-S11.

20. Shumway-Cook A, Baldwin M, Polissar NL, Gruber W. Predicting the probability of falls in community-dwelling older adults. *Phys Ther.* 1997;77:812-819.

21. Woodford-Rogers B, Cyphert L, Denegar CR. Risk factors for anterior cruciate ligament injury in high school and college athletes. *J Athl Train.* 1994;29:343-346.

22. Rogers J, Case-Smith J. Relationships between handwriting and keyboarding performance of sixth-grade students. *Am J Occup Ther.* 2002;56:34-39.

23. World Health Organization. *International Classification of Functioning, Disability, and Health.* Available at: *www.who.int/classification/icf.* Accessed October 27, 2003.

24. Tabachnick BG, Fidell LS. *Using Multivariate Statistics.* 4th ed. New York, NY: Harper & Row; 2000.

25. Jarus T, Poremba R. Hand function evaluation: a factor analysis study. *Am J Occup Ther.* 1993;47:439-443.

26. Mulligan S. Patterns of sensory integration dysfunction. *Am J Occup Ther.* 1998;52:819-828.

Being a Consumer

Locating the Literature

Regular reading of the rehabilitation literature is an essential activity for all rehabilitation professionals, an important hedge against professional obsolescence. In a world where the volume of information is increasing at a rapid rate, clinicians need to learn how to gain access to the wealth of available information. Equally important, they must also learn how to sift through the information to identify and use manageable amounts of high-quality information. This chapter will help clinicians learn to use a wide array

of contemporary tools to locate literature relevant to their practice.

First, broad categories of information and literature are defined. Then, strategies for performing a focused, short-term literature search and for maintaining an ongoing search of the literature for material related to a topic of interest are presented. Finally, suggestions are given for obtaining copies of literature items using both library and Internet resources. Readers should recognize that they may need to modify the strategies in this chapter in response to the rapid pace of technological change in library and information services.

Throughout the chapter, different search strategies are illustrated with a sample search of the literature on the use of continuous passive motion (CPM) in patients who have undergone total knee arthroplasty (TKA). CPM is a mechanical device that alternately moves the knee into flexion and extension. It may be used up to 24 hours a day in the several days following total knee replacement and is designed to promote rapid return of knee motion after surgery.

TYPES OF INFORMATION

The basic goal of any literature review is to discover what is known about a certain topic. Accomplishing this goal depends on at least four types of information about the topic: theory, facts, opinions, and methods. Some references provide primarily one type of information; others contain many different types of information. The rehabilitation clinician who is interested in treating patients with CPM will likely want to know (1) theories about how CPM works; (2) factual information about protocols and results from other clinics; (3) opinions of therapists and surgeons about future directions for the clinical use of CPM; and (4) methods that others have used to measure the results of CPM use. A researcher planning a study in the area of CPM use after TKA needs to (1) place the topic of CPM into a conceptual, theoretical context; (2) know the facts of previous investigations of CPM; (3) understand the opinions of other researchers about important areas still in need of study; and (4) be familiar with the methods others have used to measure and analyze data in previous studies.

TYPES OF PROFESSIONAL LITERATURE

The literature is divided broadly into primary and secondary sources. *Primary sources* are those in which the authors are providing the original report of research they have conducted. Commonly encountered primary sources include journal articles describing original research, theses and dissertations, and conference abstracts and proceedings. *Secondary sources* of information are those in which the authors summarize their own work or the work of others. Book chapters and journal articles that review the literature are considered secondary sources. Secondary sources are useful because they organize the literature for the reader and provide a ready list of primary sources on the topic of interest.

In the past, secondary sources of information were often viewed as less important than primary sources, and researchers and clinicians alike were encouraged to always go to the primary source for their information. In today's world, with the explosion of information in all areas, including rehabilitation research, review articles have gained new respect as a practical way for clinicians to update their knowledge regularly. For researchers, review articles can serve the important function of concisely summarizing gaps in the literature of interest and suggesting areas for further research. While both clinicians and researchers can profitably use the secondary literature, both groups will likely wish to follow up with readings in the primary literature. Clinicians will probably seek out just a few primary articles from a literature review, selecting those that appear to have the most relevance to the particular types of patients they see or the settings in which they work. Researchers tend to seek out many primary articles, selecting those that have the most potential to influence the work they plan to undertake.

FOCUSED LITERATURE SEARCH

Rehabilitation practitioners often need to conduct focused literature searches to help them plan care for individual patients, evaluate existing programs, or develop research proposals.

The focused search is conducted over a short period of time to meet a specific information need. In addition to their own books and journals collected over the years, practitioners initiating such a literature search have an array of tools and strategies at their disposal. Five different categories of search tools are described in this section: library holdings, single-journal indexes or databases, electronic bibliographic databases, dissertation and thesis databases, and conference papers and proceedings databases. In addition, several ways to use identified sources to find other citations are presented.

Practitioners who use a library should also make use of a human resource: their librarian. Librarians are educated in the art and science of retrieving information, and practitioners should not hesitate to ask for their assistance as they plan and implement their literature searches. One of my colleagues advises students to use the "30-minute rule"—if you work on your own for 30 minutes without finding the resources you need, seek out a librarian for assistance.

Finding Library Holdings

Library holdings are typically accessed through an on-line catalog that indexes books, conference proceedings published as books, audiovisual materials, dissertations and theses, and the titles of journals held by the library. This on-line catalog is accessible at the library and may be accessible from any location through an Internet connection. In addition, as is discussed later, many libraries subscribe to databases that also provide access to reference material available at other libraries.

Finding works of interest within the catalog is straightforward when users know the name of the author or the title of the work they wish to use. When specific authors or titles are not known, the user identifies works of interest by using either subject heading or keyword searches. Users need to know the distinction between subject headings and keywords so that they can take full advantage of the characteristics of each method of searching a card catalog.

KEYWORD SEARCHES

The collections of libraries with electronic catalogs can be searched by *keywords,* meaning any words that are found in the catalog's record of each volume. For example, in a recent search of an Indianapolis library, "continuous passive motion" was entered in a keyword search. The use of this keyword yielded a very valuable book authored by Robert Salter, one of the founding researchers in the area of CPM.[1] For this part of the sample search the keyword, or "free-text," method of searching led directly to a useful reference.

The problem with exclusive searching by keywords, however, is that there is limited control of synonyms. TKA procedures might be referred to as "total knee arthroplasty," "total knee replacement," and "artificial knee." In this sample search "artificial knee" as a keyword was entered and nine references were identified; however, only one reference was from the 2000s. A researcher using only this keyword search would conclude—erroneously—that the library held few contemporary references about total knee replacement.

An additional problem with keyword searches is that the specified words are not searched in context. This means that there are often false "hits" of references that are not relevant to the topic at hand. However, if at least one relevant reference is identified, the library user can review the complete record of that reference to find the subject headings under which it is indexed. One of the real strengths of keyword searching is that it can be an efficient route into a subject heading search.

SUBJECT HEADING SEARCHES

Library materials are organized by subject headings provided by the Library of Congress (Library of Congress Subject Headings) or the National Library of Medicine (Medical Subject Headings, or MeSH). Using subject headings for searches is known as "controlled vocabulary searching" because only specific words or phrases are recognized as subject headings. Although catalogs have cross-referencing systems to help users who search under nonstandard subject headings, valuable information is often missed by users who do not find the correct subject headings for their topic. A thesaurus of these subject headings should be available in the library, typically on-line, to help the practitioner determine the terms under which the desired information is likely to be found.

In the sample search, two examples illustrate the advantages and disadvantages of subject heading searches. Using an outdated term, "artificial knee," as a subject heading (rather than as a keyword) yielded no matches and the alternate subject headings that were suggested all involved prosthetic limb replacements for individuals with lower limb amputation rather than total knee arthroplasty for individuals with otherwise intact limbs. In this case, the subject heading search yielded much less information than the keyword search of the same term. However, if the researcher goes to the detailed record of the best of the references identified in the keyword search, he or she would find that the proper subject heading is "total knee replacement." A subject heading search with "total knee replacement" yielded 14 references, with six from the 2000s. To avoid coming to a premature conclusion that a library does not hold the desired resources when an initial search strategy is not fruitful, users should conduct both subject heading and keyword searches, consult the thesaurus of subject headings if available, or seek assistance from a reference librarian.

SAMPLE SEARCH RESULTS

Searching the catalog of a particular library is limited in that the sources revealed are only as good as the collection of the library. However, even identification of a few key resources may lead to many others by examination of the references contained in each source. Table 24–1 shows how the identification of relevant chapters[2-4] in only two recent books[5,6] led to 27 unique citations related to use of CPM after TKA. Of these 27 references, a good starting point for a researcher would be the seven sources cited

TABLE 24–1	**Use of Catalog of Library Holdings to Identify Literature Related to Continuous Passive Motion in Patients After Total Knee Arthroplasty**

Resource 1—Chapter within a Book:
Gotlin RS, Becker EA. Rehabilitation. In: Scuderi GR, Tria AJ, eds. *Surgical Techniques in Total Knee Arthroplasty*. New York, NY: Springer-Verlag; 2002:651-679.[2]
Relevant references: 11

Resource 2—Chapter within a Book:
Rorabeck CH, Howell GED. Range of motion after total knee replacement can best be obtained using a CPM machine: pro. In: Laskin RS, ed. *Controversies in Total Knee Replacement*. Oxford, UK: Oxford University Press; 2001.[3]
Relevant references: 19

Resource 3—Chapter within a Book:
Ward SR, Longjohn DB, Dorr LD. Range of motion after total knee replacement can best be obtained using a CPM machine: con. In: Laskin RS, ed. *Controversies in Total Knee Replacement*. Oxford, UK: Oxford University Press; 2001.[4]
Relevant references: 4

Reference Summary:
27 unique journal article references (seven references were cited in more than one chapter) 5 published between 1995 and 1999, 11 between 1990 and 1994, 11 in 1989 or earlier

within two of the book chapters or the five most recent references. One obvious limitation to using library books to identify relevant primary references is that the references identified can be no more recent than the books that cite them. In this example, the books were published in 2001 and 2002 and the most recent relevant article cited was published in 1998.

HOLDINGS AT OTHER LIBRARIES

Recognizing that any one library is unlikely to hold all the desired resources, practitioners may expand their searches beyond the library walls to see what is available on a particular topic anywhere in the world. One way to do this is by searching, library-by-library, the on-line catalogs to which you can gain access through the Internet or through your home library. A more efficient way is to use a specific database, WorldCat, to simultaneously search for records of any type of material cataloged by libraries that are members of the Online Computer Library Center (OCLC). For example, searching WorldCat for English-language books on total knee replacement yielded 76 records. Each of the records includes a list of those libraries that hold the publication. With this information, the reference librarian at the home library can work with the patron to obtain an interlibrary loan of the desired item. Because a WorldCat search includes the home library collection as well as all the participating libraries, some researchers never even search the home library collection separately, preferring to let a single WorldCat search identify both local and distant resources.

Using Single-Journal Indexes or Databases

Many professionals receive one or more journals regularly either as a benefit of belonging to a professional association or by subscribing to a journal of particular interest. One's own journals are a convenient starting point for a literature search. Many journals publish an annual subject and author index in the last issue of each volume. Thus, readers with an interest in a particular topic can easily identify any pertinent citations from the journals in their own collection. Even if a professional decides not to retain all the journals he or she receives, this ready source of citations can be maintained by keeping the annual indexes from each journal. Alternatively, many journals maintain a website with a searchable database of contents. If, for example, I remember reading an article about continuous passive motion after total knee replacement in the *Archives of Physical Medicine*

and Rehabilitation, I might choose to go directly to this journal's website to search for the article. For this example, a search of the *Archives of Physical Medicine and Rehabilitation* website (www2.archives-pmr.org) for "continuous passive motion" and "total knee replacement" yielded four citations, including three articles and one conference presentation.

Using Electronic Bibliographic Databases

References to articles in many journals, and, increasingly, the full text of the articles themselves, can be found by using various databases. Although most of these databases exist in hard copy as well as CD-ROM or on-line formats, the emphasis in this chapter is on searching the databases electronically. Not long ago, most computer searches of the literature were performed by librarians from keywords supplied by patrons. Today, most computerized databases are user-friendly and designed to be used by the patrons themselves. Several common steps should be taken when searching an electronic database.[7]

SEARCH STEPS

First, the practitioner defines the information need. For the sample search, the need might be defined by the following question: What is known about the effect of continuous passive motion on recovery after total knee arthroplasty?

Second, the practitioner breaks the need into components. For the sample search, the two main components are "continuous passive motion" and "total knee arthroplasty."

Third, the practitioner identifies synonyms for each concept. As was the case with library catalog searching, users can choose to search by subject heading or by keyword. Many databases include subject headings at the bottom of each reference. This enables a person to start with a keyword search and use the information provided to refine the search by using standardized subject headings.

Fourth, the practitioner constructs logical relationships among the concepts, using the terms "AND," "OR," and "NOT." Figure 24–1 shows the relationships that are defined by the use of these terms. The use of "AND" narrows a search. In our example, searching for "continuous passive motion" AND "total knee arthroplasty" would yield only those articles containing both concepts. Another way of narrowing a search is to specify a "NOT" term. In our example, if we were not interested in TKA done for those with rheumatoid arthritis we could modify our search to look for "total knee arthroplasty" NOT "rheumatoid arthritis." This command lops off a portion of the search that is not of interest to the researcher. In contrast, the use of "OR" broadens a search to include articles that include at least one of the specified terms.

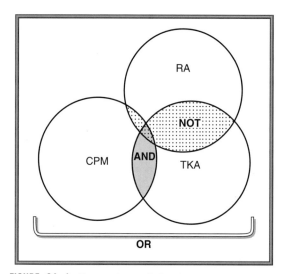

FIGURE 24–1. Illustration of Boolean relationships. Specifying "continuous passive motion (CPM) OR total knee arthroplasty (TKA)" would result in retrieval of articles in both circles, including the shaded intersection of both circles. Adding the command "NOT rheumatoid arthritis (RA)" would result in the elimination of all the stippled areas in the figure. Specifying "CPM AND TKA" would result in retrieval of articles in the shaded intersection of the two circles, including the stippled, shaded area. Specifying "CPM AND TKA NOT RA" would result in retrieval of articles in the shaded intersection, excluding the stippled, shaded region.

If we were interested in reviewing articles documenting the use of CPM after anterior cruciate ligament reconstruction as well as after TKA, then we could specify the surgery term as "total knee arthroplasty" OR "anterior cruciate ligament reconstruction." The "AND," "OR," and "NOT" terms are known as Boolean operators, after a 19th-century logician named George Boole.[8]

Fifth, the practitioner may limit the search according to certain variables offered by the database. Common limits relate to "language" and "year of publication." For example, many researchers in the United States restrict their searches to English language journals and to articles published in a certain time frame. A clinician planning a new program may search the last 3 years of the database; a researcher who wishes to trace the history of a particular procedure may search 20 or more years of a database.

Rehabilitation professionals need to consider several potential databases: MEDLINE, EMBASE, *Cumulative Index of Nursing and Allied Health Literature* (CINAHL), PsycINFO, ERIC, and SPORTDiscus. The literature of the different rehabilitation professions may be found in different databases. For example, a mapping of the literature of selected health professions found that for physical therapy most of the relevant citations would be found with a combined MEDLINE and CINAHL search.[9] In contrast, a combined search of MEDLINE and PsycINFO would be more comprehensive for speech-language pathology.[10]

All of these databases are widely available in medical school libraries and the libraries of institutions with rehabilitation programs. The databases are supplied to libraries through various vendors or platforms, so the looks and features of the database vary from library to library, but the contents remain the same. Individual access to each of these databases is also available, as noted later in the chapter. Table 24–2 shows which of several journals of interest to rehabilitation professionals are indexed in several of the databases. The databases provide complete indexing of some of the journals and selective indexing of

TABLE 24-2 Databases That Index Representative Journals of Interest to Rehabilitation Professionals*

Journal	MEDLINE	EMBASE	CINAHL	PsycINFO	ERIC
American Journal of Audiology	✓	✓	✓		
American Journal of Occupational Therapy	✓		✓	✓	
American Journal of Physical Medicine and Rehabilitation	✓	✓	✓		
American Journal of Speech-Language Pathology	✓		✓	✓	
American Journal of Sports Medicine	✓	✓	✓		
Archives of Physical Medicine and Rehabilitation	✓	✓	✓		
Australian Journal of Physiotherapy	✓	✓	✓		
British Journal of Sports Medicine	✓	✓	✓		
Canadian Journal of Occupational Therapy		✓	✓	✓	✓
Clinical Biomechanics	✓	✓	✓		
Clinics in Sports Medicine	✓	✓	✓		
Developmental Medicine and Child Neurology	✓	✓	✓	✓	
International Journal of Language and Communication Disorders	✓	✓	✓	✓	
Journal of Allied Health	✓		✓		✓
Journal of Athletic Training	✓	✓	✓	✓	✓
Journal of Child Language	✓		✓	✓	✓
Journal of Hand Therapy	✓	✓	✓		
Journal of Musculoskeletal Medicine			✓		
Journal of Occupational Rehabilitation	✓	✓	✓	✓	
Journal of Orthopaedic and Sports Physical Therapy	✓	✓	✓		
Journal of Physical Therapy Education			✓		
Journal of Rehabilitation Research and Development	✓	✓	✓		
Journal of Speech, Language, and Hearing Research		✓	✓	✓	✓
JPO: Journal of Prosthetics and Orthotics			✓		
Language and Communication	✓			✓	✓
Language and Speech	✓		✓	✓	✓
Language, Speech, and Hearing Services in Schools			✓	✓	✓
Medicine and Science in Sports and Exercise	✓	✓	✓	✓	✓
Occupational Therapy International	✓	✓	✓		
Orthopaedic Physical Therapy Clinics of North America		✓	✓		
Pediatric Physical Therapy		✓	✓		
Physical and Occupational Therapy in Geriatrics	✓	✓	✓	✓	
Physical and Occupational Therapy in Pediatrics	✓	✓	✓		
Physical Medicine and Rehabilitation Clinics of North America	✓	✓	✓		
Physical Therapy	✓	✓	✓		
Physician and Sportsmedicine	✓	✓	✓		✓
Physiotherapy	✓	✓	✓		
Physiotherapy Canada			✓		
Physiotherapy Research International	✓		✓		
Prosthetics and Orthotics International	✓	✓			
Spine	✓	✓	✓		
Work: A Journal of Prevention, Assessment, and Rehabilitation	✓		✓	✓	

*From on-line journal lists for MEDLINE *(see http://www.nlm.nih.gov)*, CINAHL *(see http://www.cinahl.com)*, ERIC *(see http://www.eric.ed.gov)*, and PsycINFO (see *http://www.apa.org/psychinfo/about/covlist.htm*), accessed December 29, 2003, and *EMBASE List of Journals Indexed.* Amsterdam, The Netherlands: Elsevier; 2003.

other journals. This means that, even though two databases include a particular journal, different articles from the journal may be selected for inclusion in each of the databases. Because of the irregular overlapping of coverage among databases, users who wish to be as comprehensive as possible should search several databases. Even though many of the same articles are identified by different databases, each database typically identifies unique resources not identified by others.

MEDLINE

MEDLINE is a comprehensive medically oriented on-line database compiled by the National Library of Medicine. The entries in the database are indexed according to the medical subject headings (MeSH) of the National Library of Medicine. In addition to its widespread availability in academic libraries, free MEDLINE access, in a

format known as PubMed, is available to anyone with an Internet connection (http://www.nlm. nih.gov). The steps to and results of the sample search, done through MEDLINE, are shown in Table 24–3. Nine relevant articles were identified,[11-19] four of which were also identified by the CINAHL search (discussed subsequently).[11,13,16,19] Other searches in areas for which MEDLINE is not the ideal database would not be as fruitful. For example, a search for English language articles from 2000 through 2003 about "Parkinson's disease" and "speech-language pathology" yielded three citations, only two of which appeared to be relevant to the desired topic.

EMBASE

EMBASE is a proprietary database that combines MEDLINE with additional resources, particularly in biomedical research and pharmacology.[20] Available by subscription, most users gain access

---

TABLE 24–3 **Comparison of MEDLINE and CINAHL Searches**

SEARCH STRATEGY

		Number of Articles	
Steps	Terms or Limits	MEDLINE	CINAHL
Step 1	Continuous passive motion (CPM)	289	77
Step 2	Total knee arthroplasty (TKA)	2640	188
Step 3	CPM AND TKA	48	16
Step 4	LIMIT TO English	43	15
Step 5	LIMIT TO Publication Years 2000–2003	9	4

SEARCH RESULTS

Primary Author	Source, Date	MEDLINE	CINAHL
Milne S[11]	Cochrane Library, 2003	✓	✓
Chiu[12]	J Orthop Surg, 2002	✓	
Davies[13]	Can J Surg, 2003	✓	✓
Chelly[14]	J Arthroplasty, 2001	✓	
Lau[15]	J Arthroplasty, 2001	✓	
Beaupre[16]	Phys Ther, 2001	✓	✓
Lachiewicz[17]	Clin Orthop, 2001	✓	
MacDonald[18]	Clin Orthop, 2000	✓	
Chen[19]	Am J Phys Med Rehabil, 2000	✓	✓

to this database through an academic library or an employer subscription.

CUMULATIVE INDEX OF NURSING AND ALLIED HEALTH LITERATURE

CINAHL was developed in 1956 to meet the needs of nonphysician health care practitioners. As illustrated in Table 24–2, many of the journals of interest to nurses and other health professionals are not indexed in MEDLINE. CINAHL provides a means to gain access to these journals. For example, in late 2003, the *Canadian Journal of Occupational Therapy,* the *Journal of Speech, Language, and Hearing Research,* and *Pediatric Physical Therapy* were not indexed in MEDLINE but were indexed in CINAHL. In addition to journals, CINAHL indexes books of interest to nurses and other health professionals and nursing dissertations. The CINAHL indexing terms are based on MeSH, but provide for greater specificity in the terms related to each profession represented in the index. Libraries that serve health professionals generally subscribe to CINAHL. It is also available on-line by subscription to individual users. In 2003, rates ranged from as low as approximately $40 for about 15 hours of use per year to $700 for 400 hours of use (http://www.cinahl.com).[21] Table 24–3 shows the steps to and results of the CINAHL search of the sample topic of CPM after TKA. Four relevant articles were identified,[11,13,16,19] all of which also happened to be identified in the MEDLINE search. For this particular topic, which has good coverage in MEDLINE, the CINAHL search did not result in any additional resources. For the "Parkinson's disease" and "speech-language pathology" search reported earlier, CINAHL identified 10 resources, eight of which were not identified in the previous MEDLINE search, illustrating the need to use multiple databases to ensure the comprehensiveness of a search.

PSYCINFO

This database, which is produced by the American Psychological Association, provides extensive coverage of journals in psychology and related disciplines, as well as some book chapters, dissertations, and various university and government reports (http://www.apa.org/psycinfo/products/psycinfo.html). Most academic libraries and large employers with psychology services purchase an institutional subscription to PsycINFO. For those who do not have access to an institutional subscription of PsycINFO, individual access in 2003 could be obtained for approximately $12 per day for nonmembers of the American Psychological Association and for between $99 and $299 per year for members.[22]

ERIC

The Educational Resource Information Center (ERIC) is a large database of education-related documents and articles. Funded by the United States Department of Education, it offers free database access to anyone with an Internet connection (http://www.eric.ed.gov). Like MEDLINE, it can also be accessed through different interfaces available in academic libraries. Rehabilitation professionals who interface with the educational system through school-based services, physical education, and sports may find ERIC to be a good source of information on relevant topics.

SPORTDISCUS

SPORTDiscus is a large sport, fitness, and sports medicine bibliographic database (http://www.sportdiscus.com). Based in Canada, it includes journal citations as well as book references, and access to relevant theses and dissertations. Many academic libraries and sports-related employers purchase institutional subscriptions to the database; in 2003, individuals could gain access for around $10 per day or $50 per month.[23]

Finding Dissertations and Theses

The research that students undertake as a requirement for completion of a master's or doctoral degree often is not published in the literature or is published several years after the master's thesis or doctoral dissertation has been filed with the university where the degree was completed. There are two effective ways to retrieve information on dissertations and theses. The first is to use the WorldCat database. Because dissertations and theses are generally held in the library of the institution offering the degree, and because most academic libraries participate in OCLC, this means that dissertation and thesis titles can be retrieved in a search of WorldCat. One master's thesis relevant to the sample search was identified by searching the years 2002 and 2003 using the terms "continuous passive motion" and "total knee arthroplasty."[24]

The second method is to search *Dissertation Abstracts.* Most doctoral programs and some master's degree programs require that students file a copy of the thesis or dissertation for inclusion in *Dissertation Abstracts.* The full database is available through an institutional subscription and the most recent 2 years are available on-line without a fee (http://wwwlib.umi.com/dissertations). A computer search of *Dissertation Abstracts* for 2002 and 2003 identified one master's thesis related to continuous passive motion use in total knee arthroplasty.[25] Abstracts and excerpts of identified theses and dissertations can be printed from *Dissertation Abstracts* and copies of most of the full documents can be purchased on-line. Access through *Dissertation Abstracts* is important in that many libraries at the universities where a thesis or dissertation was completed are unwilling to loan out what is often their only hard copy of the document.

Finding Conference Proceedings

As with dissertations and theses, research papers presented at conferences may not make it to the journal literature for several years, if at all. Access to abstracts of papers presented at conferences can often be obtained by reviewing the conference website or the conference issue of journals of a particular society or association.

One such conference presentation, a poster presentation at the 2003 American Congress of Rehabilitation Medicine Annual Assembly, was identified by a search of the website for the *Archives of Physical Medicine and Rehabilitation.*[26]

A broader source of conference proceedings is the *Index of Scientific and Technical Proceedings* (ISTP), which indexes published work from selected conferences. The database is organized by conference sponsor, location, paper authors, geographical location of the authors, and organizational affiliation of the authors. Depending on one's interest and the information available, any of these items of information might be the starting point of a search of conference proceedings. Using a CD-ROM version of the ISTP, two publications on continuous passive motion that were based on conference presentations were identified: one by Beaupre and associates[16] presented at the 63rd Annual Scientific Meeting of the American College of Rheumatology in Boston, Massachusetts, in 1999 and another by Yashar and colleagues[27] presented at the Combined Meeting of the Knee Society and the American Association of Hip and Knee Surgeons in San Francisco, California, in 1997. Both were redundant citations of papers already identified through other means, indicating that the search is nearly complete.

Using Single Articles

In addition to the five search tools just described, a single relevant journal article citation can be used in several different ways to identify other sources of information. It is possible to use a single article to work backward, forward, and sideways through the literature.[8(p108)] To work backward, one examines the reference list of the article and identifies relevant citations. This strategy can also be used with the reference lists of book chapters, conference proceedings, and dissertations and theses. The disadvantage of using this strategy is that it identifies only citations that are older than the source itself.

SCIENCE CITATION INDEX

Working forward through the literature from a single article, or from an influential author, can be accomplished with hard copy or electronic versions of the *Science Citation Index*. This index lists sources that have used a particular article as a reference or cited particular authors. A key citation or author is used to begin the forward search. For the sample search, we will use Salter as an author of interest because his work on CPM has been cited in many of the articles we have identified thus far in our CPM literature search. One of his articles, a 1989 review of the biological concept of continuous passive motion,[28] would likely be cited by researchers publishing results about continuous passive motion. A search of the *Science Citation Index* showed that this article of Salter's was cited in 39 other articles. Of these, two were relevant to our search about continuous passive motion and total knee arthroplasty.

RELATED RECORD SEARCHING

There are two ways of working sideways through the literature based on a single article. "Working sideways" means identifying additional citations that are contemporary to the original article. The first way is to call up the MEDLINE or CINAHL citation for the article and determine the subject headings under which it is indexed. Use of these terms in a new search is likely to yield related articles. The second way to work sideways takes advantage of "related-record" searching in some of the electronic databases. The PubMed interface for MEDLINE, for example, uses a complex algorithm to identify articles that are related in some way to a single article identified by the user. The algorithm includes things like shared title words, shared references, and shared subject headings. Doing a related-record search of the Chen and colleagues' paper[19] cited earlier yielded 337 related records in MEDLINE. Because they are arranged in order of relatedness, it is easy to scan down the list to determine the most relevant of the related citations.

Relationships Among Search Tools

Figure 24–2 summarizes the way in which the search tools and single-article strategies interrelate. Search tools, represented by the outer circle, are used to identify literature items. The literature items, represented as the inner circle, can then be used to identify other literature items. Practitioners conducting literature searches frequently use several strategies to identify all the literature of interest. When the citations identified by these different strategies become redundant, then the searcher can be confident that the most important references have been found.

■ ONGOING LITERATURE SEARCH

Regular consumers of the literature generally have developed strategies that enable them to identify articles of interest on a routine basis. Because of the enormous volume of clinical literature, practitioners must accept that they cannot remain up-to-date in all areas of their profession. Thus, the first element of an ongoing search strategy is to identify the specific topics in which one is most interested. Once these topics are selected, the basic strategies used for ongoing searches are single-journal contents scanning, multiple-journal contents scanning, evidence-based review databases, and focused database scanning.

Scanning Single Journals

The journals that arrive in a professional's mailbox each month can be a tremendous asset to the regular literature consumer. The most obvious resources in each journal are the articles in each issue. For a broadly ranging area such as rehabilitation, general interest journals such as *Archives of Physical Medicine and Rehabilitation, Physical Therapy,* or *American Journal of Occupational Therapy* may contain relatively

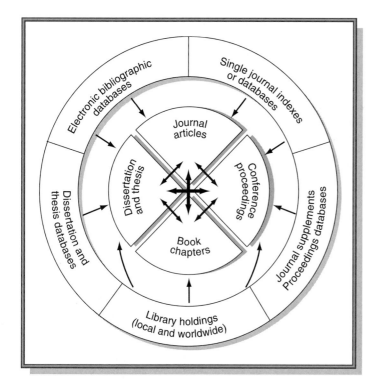

FIGURE 24–2. Relationship among search tools and types of professional literature. The search tools shown in the outer circle are used to identify relevant citations of the different literature types, as noted by the arrows. Once a citation is identified, its reference list can be used to identify other citations, as noted by the arrows between the pieces of the inner circle. For journal articles, additional tools such as citation indexes and related record searches can be used to identify other relevant sources.

few articles within the particular interest area of a professional. However, the regular reader of the literature should not limit his or her scanning to the articles portion of the journal's table of contents. Many journals publish book reviews and abstracts of relevant articles published in other journals. Both of these sections of the journal can point the reader to areas of interest not addressed in a given issue.

Scanning Contents of Multiple Journals

Scanning the table of contents of several journals of interest is a second excellent way of keeping up with the literature outside the journals that one receives personally. Some libraries even provide a service in which the tables of contents of requested journals are sent to patrons when the journal arrives each month. This allows the consumer to scan the contents conveniently,

marking for later review any articles that seem of interest. Literature consumers new to contents scanning may select a fairly large number of journals for initial scanning and reduce the number as it becomes apparent over time which journals most frequently publish articles in their area of interest. For those without a library table of contents service, the websites of journals of interest can be bookmarked for regular review of journal contents.

Another way to scan new journal tables of contents is provided by a weekly publication called *Current Contents*. Different versions of this publication, such as *Current Contents: Life Sciences* or *Current Contents: Clinical Medicine*, compile and publish tables of contents from journals relevant to the version. This tool exists in hard copy and electronic formats, with institutional and individual subscription rates. *Current Contents: Clinical Medicine* contains many journals of interest to rehabilitation professionals including *American Journal of Physical*

Medicine and Rehabilitation, American Journal of Sports Medicine, British Medical Journal, Cleft Palate-Craniofacial Journal, Clinical Neurology and Neurosurgery, Clinics in Sports Medicine, Developmental Medicine and Child Neurology, Geriatrics, Hand Clinics, Journal of Bone and Joint Surgery, Journal of Orthopaedic and Sports Physical Therapy, Journal of Rehabilitation Research and Development, Physical Therapy, and *Spine,* to name a few of the approximately 1000 titles that are listed.[29]

Searching Evidence-Based Review Databases

Several reference products not only inform the practitioner of new articles but also provide commentary or rate the quality of articles to assist the practitioner in assessing the potential value of the literature.

The Cochrane Library is an electronic collection of evidence-based reviews of health care research. Each review employs a systematic search of literature on the topic, with expert synthesis across sources of information. Subscribers, including many medical and academic libraries, have access to a searchable database of reviews and the full text of reviews. In addition, relevant Cochrane reviews are indexed in the major bibliographic databases. For example, the previous MEDLINE search on "continuous passive motion" and "total knee arthroplasty" yielded a 2003 review of the topic.[11]

The *ACP (American College of Physicians) Journal Club,* produced in paper and electronic formats (http://www.acpjc.org) six times annually, uses stringent review methods to select articles for inclusion and provides commentary to help practitioners make "evidence-based" decisions about patient care. Although the topics included in the publication are based on the information needs of physicians, reviews of interest to a broad range of rehabilitation providers are published. For example, looking from 2000 to 2003, there were two reviews in this journal related to total knee arthroplasty;

both focused on use of various pharmacological agents for prevention of deep vein thrombosis after surgery.

PEDro is a physiotherapy evidence database based at the School of Physiotherapy at the University of Sydney in Australia. Full, free access to PEDro is available on the Internet (http://www.pedro.fhs.usyd.edu.au). This database includes clinical trials, systematic reviews, and practice guidelines in physical therapy. The trials are rated with a 10-item checklist (the PEDro scale) to help readers assess the quality of the trial. A search of PEDro identified one Cochrane review and 17 clinical trials related to use of continuous passive motion after total knee arthroplasty. Quality scores of the trials ranged from 3/10 to 8/10. With this information, a clinician interested in this topic could focus his or her initial efforts on reading the review and a few of the highest quality trials.

OTseeker is a parallel project developed at the University of Queensland and the University of Western Sydney in Australia.[30] Like PEDro, full, free access to OTseeker is available on the Internet (http://www.otseeker.com) and the database includes clinical trials and systematic reviews relevant to occupational therapy practice. A search of OTseeker on "continuous passive motion" identified two systematic reviews and six articles about continuous passive motion, mostly related to treatment of limited motion in the hand.

A final evidenced-based review tool, Hooked on Evidence, is a relatively new initiative of the American Physical Therapy Association (http://www.apta.org/hookedonevidence/index.cfm). Volunteers, usually members of the association, extract and verify information from articles about physical therapy interventions. The abstracted variables include a variety of indicators of quality, such as research design, allocation methods, and the level of researcher and participant masking. Members of the association have full access to the database, including its search features.[31] Searches of this database can yield a set of highly focused articles. For example, a search of "continuous passive motion" and "total knee" yielded five relevant citations. A search of a database such as this is not expected to provide comprehensive results, but the citations that are identified are accompanied by more information about design and validity than is typically available from reading the abstracts of articles that are provided by the electronic bibliographic databases.

Scanning Electronic Bibliographic Databases

Regular scanning of relevant databases can be accomplished through regular in-person or on-line visits to the library, with individual subscriptions to various affordable databases described in the chapter, and with use of information that is freely available through the Internet. Some of the databases have automatic alert features that notify users when new articles that meet user-specific criteria have been added to the database.

Professionals who have made a commitment to remaining up to date in focused areas can do so easily by scanning the contents of journals to which they subscribe, by reviewing the tables of contents of selected journals of interest, by using evidence-based review databases, and by periodically conducting searches of electronic bibliographic databases.

■ OBTAINING LITERATURE ITEMS

Obtaining literature items quickly and efficiently is no longer dependent on the quality of the collection at one's home library. If one's local library does not have a desired item, it can generally be obtained through interlibrary loan or a full text retrieval system. If these strategies are not successful, some low-technology strategies may work, include requesting a reprint from the author, purchasing the journal from the publisher, or using one's network of professional colleagues.

Interlibrary loan arrangements give the patron of one library access to the resources of many other libraries. The patron requests the item, and the librarian uses a computer network to determine the libraries that have the item. When a journal article is requested, the lending library usually furnishes a photocopy, often for a fee to cover photocopying and mailing. This fee may or may not be passed on to the patron.

A growing number of journals make the full text of articles available, either through the database subscription held by the library, with a link from an Internet database, or from the journal's website. Some journals provide this service free to anyone with Internet access, some provide free electronic access to members of the association that publishes the journal or for those who subscribe to the journal, and some charge a fee per article or for a period of time (such as 30-day electronic access to a journal or a family of journals).

Reprints were a common form of journal article transmission until the advent of the photocopier. The system still exists, although it is not used frequently. Authors can usually request reprints of their articles, for a fee, at the time of publication. If they order the reprints they will have a ready supply to mail out if they receive requests. Today, many authors do not buy their own reprints because they realize that interested readers will simply photocopy the item themselves or will obtain it through one of the many other ways of getting a journal article. Some authors of articles published in obscure journals are willing to mail or fax a photocopy of an article if the requesting party is able to convince them that their efforts to obtain the article through other means were unsuccessful. Students of mine who were doing a comprehensive literature review were able to obtain a particularly elusive source by faxing the author in Australia. Back issues of journals can often be purchased from the publisher. If requests for an item through interlibrary loan and full-text retrieval systems have been unsuccessful, and if the author cannot be located, the most expedient way to obtain the citation may be to purchase the entire issue. This is a particularly good solution if the issue is a "special focus" issue containing many articles of interest. If a potentially important citation still eludes you, turn to your network of professional colleagues for assistance. Colleagues with an interest in the topic may have the needed article and are often willing to share their resources to foster the growth of others with that interest.

■ SUMMARY

Literature searches are undertaken to obtain information about the theory, facts, opinions, and methods related to a particular area within a discipline. Primary literature sources include original journal articles, dissertations and theses, and conference proceedings. Literature search tools include catalogs of library holdings, single-journal indexes and databases, electronic bibliographic databases, dissertation and thesis abstract databases, and conference proceedings databases. Regular readers of the literature identify articles of interest by scanning the tables of contents of one or more journals, by using evidence-based review databases, and by regular searching of electronic bibliographic databases. Once identified, literature items can be obtained through local library holdings, interlibrary loans, full text retrieval, requests to authors, purchase from the publisher, or one's network of colleagues.

REFERENCES

1. Salter RB. *Continuous Passive Motion (CPM): A Biological Concept for the Healing and Regeneration of Articular Cartilage, Ligaments, and Tendons: From Origination to Research to Clinical Applications.* Baltimore, Md: Williams & Wilkins; 1993.
2. Gotlin RS, Becker EA. Rehabilitation. In: Scuderi GR, Tria AJ, eds. *Surgical Techniques in Total Knee Arthroplasty.* New York, NY: Springer-Verlag; 2002:651-679.
3. Rorabeck CH, Howell GED. Range of motion after total knee replacement can best be obtained using a CPM machine: pro. In: Laskin RS, ed. *Controversies in Total Knee Replacement.* Oxford, UK: Oxford University Press; 2001.
4. Ward SR, Longjohn DB, Dorr LD. Range of motion after total knee replacement can best be obtained using a CPM machine: con. In: Laskin RS, ed. *Controversies in Total Knee Replacement.* Oxford, UK: Oxford University Press; 2001.
5. Scuderi GR, Tria AJ, eds. *Surgical Techniques in Total Knee Arthroplasty.* New York, NY: Springer-Verlag; 2002.
6. Laskin RS, ed. *Controversies in Total Knee Replacement.* Oxford, UK: Oxford University Press; 2001.
7. Duffel P. Constructing a search strategy. *CINAHLnews.* 1995;14(4):1-2.
8. Mann T. *The Oxford Guide to Library Research.* New York, NY: Oxford University Press; 1998.
9. Wakiji EM. Mapping the literature of physical therapy. *Bull Med Libr Assoc.* 1997;85:284-288.
10. Slater LG. Mapping the literature of speech-language pathology. *Bull Med Libr Assoc.* 1997;85:297-302.
11. Milne S, Brosseau L, Robinson V, et al. Continuous passive motion following total knee arthroplasty (Cochrane Review). The Cochrane Library. Chichester, UK: John Wiley & Sons; 2003: Issue 4.
12. Chiu KY, Ng TP, Tang WM, Yau WP. Review article: knee flexion after total knee arthroplasty. *J Orthop Surg.* 2002;10:194-202.
13. Davies DM, Johnston DW, Beaupre LA, Lier DA. Effect of adjunctive range-of-motion therapy after primary total knee arthroplasty on the use of health services after hospital discharge. *Can J Surg.* 2003;46:30-36.
14. Chelly JE, Greger J, Gebhard R, et al. Continuous femoral blocks improve recovery and outcome of patients undergoing total knee arthroplasty. *J Arthroplasty.* 2001;16: 436-445.
15. Lau SK, Chiu KY. Use of continuous passive motion after total knee arthroplasty. *J Arthroplasty.* 2001;16:336-339.
16. Beaupre LA, Davies DM, Jones CA, Cinats JG. Exercise combined with continuous passive motion or slider board therapy compared with exercise only: a randomized controlled trial of patients following total knee arthroplasty. *Phys Ther.* 2001;81:1029-1037.
17. Lachiewicz PF. The role of continuous passive motion after total knee arthroplasty. *Clin Orthop.* 2000;380:144-150.
18. MacDonald SJ, Bourne RB, Rorabeck CH, McCalden RW, Kramer J, Vaz M. Prospective randomized clinical trial of continuous passive motion after total knee arthroplasty. *Clin Orthop.* 2000;380:30-35.
19. Chen B, Zimmerman JR, Soulen L, DeLisa JA. Continuous passive motion after total knee arthroplasty: a prospective study. *Am J Phys Med Rehabil.* 2000;79:421-426.
20. *EMBASE List of Journals Indexed.* Amsterdam, The Netherlands: Elsevier; 2003.
21. CINAHL general information. Available at: http://www.cinahl.com/cdirect/cdirectinfo.htm. Accessed January 2, 2004.
22. PsycINFO database information. Available at: http://www.apa.org/psycinfo/products/psycinfo.html. Accessed December 31, 2003.
23. SIRCDetective. Available at: http://www.sircdetective.com/. Accessed December 30, 2003.

24. Norton E, Pedersen J. *Continuous Passive Motion Post Total Knee Arthroplasty: Effects on Range of Motion and Length of Hospital Stay* [master's thesis]. Forest Grove, Or: Pacific University; 2003.

25. Gustus TJ. *Acute Total Knee Arthroplasty Outcomes: Exercise and Continuous Passive Motion* [master's thesis]. Boston, Mass: Massachusetts General Hospital Institute of Health Professions; 2002.

26. Denis M, Moffet H, Caron F, Ouellet D, Paquet J, Nolet L. Comparative efficacy of 3 in-hospital rehabilitation programs on knee flexion after total knee arthroplasty: a randomized controlled trial (conference abstract). *Arch Phys Med Rehabil.* 2003;84:A6.

27. Yashar AA, Venn-Watson E, Welsh T, Colwell CW, Lotke P. Continuous passive motion with accelerated flexion after total knee arthroplasty. *Clin Orthop.* 1997;345:38-43.

28. Salter RB. The biological concept of continuous passive motion in synovial joints—the first 18 years of basic research and its clinical application. *Clin Orthop.* 1989; 242:12-25.

29. Institute for Scientific Information. *ISI master journal list.* Available at: http://www.isinet.com. Accessed January 2, 2004.

30. Bennett S, Hoffmann T, McCluskey A, McKenna K, Strong J, Tooth L. Introducing OTseeker (occupational therapy systematic evaluation of evidence): a new evidence database for occupational therapists. *Am J Occup Ther.* 2003;57:635-638.

31. Scalzitti D. Happy birthday to Hooked on Evidence. *PT Magazine.* 2003;11(9):56-58.

Evaluating Evidence One Article at a Time

Evidence-based practice is a major force in health care practice in the twenty-first century. Influenced by the same forces that advanced the emergence of the outcomes movement (Chapter 15) in the 1990s, evidence-based practice requires that clinicians use the literature of their professions to guide practice. A common definition of evidence-based medicine is that it is "the integration of best research evidence with clinical expertise and patient values."[1(p1)] Thus, evidence-based practice does not demand that practitioners be ruled by research evidence; rather, it requires that they *integrate* research evidence with their own clinical experiences and the values of their patients or clients. To effectively integrate research evidence, practitioners must evaluate research reports critically before applying the results to

401

practice. Such evaluation requires that practitioners apply the principles from the first 23 chapters of this text to the articles they are reading. This chapter provides a number of frameworks for doing so. First, the elements of a research article and a few general rules-of-thumb for discussing published research are listed. Then, generic frameworks for the evaluation of original research articles and review articles are outlined. Next, a more structured approach to evaluation of research according to the clinical issue at hand is presented. Approaches that evaluate levels of evidence are also outlined. Finally, some scoring systems specific to the evaluation of randomized controlled trials are presented.

■ ELEMENTS OF A RESEARCH ARTICLE

Table 25–1 lists and describes the elements of a research article. The components encountered first are the journal article title and abstract. Following these is the body of the article, which typically consists of introduction, methods, results, discussion, conclusions, and reference sections. Several sections may contain tables, which consist

TABLE 25–1 Elements of a Research Article

Element	Characteristics
Title	Is concise, yet descriptive. Identifies major variables studied. Provides clues about whether the purpose of the research is description, relationship analysis, or difference analysis through use of phrases such as "characteristics of," "relationship between," or "effects of," respectively.
Abstract	Briefly summarizes research purpose, methods, and results. Depending on journal, is usually 150–300 words. Does not include summary of related literature or significant discussion of the limitations and implications of the research.
Introduction	Sets the stage for the presentation of the research. Usually does *not* have a heading; sometimes is subdivided into Problem, Purpose, or Literature Review sections. Whether subdivided or not, defines the broad problem that underlies the study, states the specific purposes of the study, and places the problem and purposes into the theoretical context of previous work. Often presents research hypotheses. Occasionally contains tables or figures.
Method	Describes the conduct of the study. Usually is subdivided into Subjects, Instruments, Procedures, and Data Analysis sections. Often refers to methods or procedures used by others as the basis for the present study. Often contains figures showing equipment used.
Results	Presents the results without comment on their meaning. Often is subdivided into sections corresponding to the variables studied. Is often brief because much of the information is contained in tables and figures.
Discussion	Presents the authors' interpretation of their results, along with their assessment of study limitations and directions for future research. Often refers to previous work that is related to the findings of the study. May be subdivided into Limitations, Clinical Relevance, and Future Research sections.
Conclusions	Concisely restates the important findings of the research. Presents a conclusion for each individual purpose outlined in the introduction.
References	Lists references cited in the text of the article. Is followed occasionally by a bibliography that lists relevant work that is not cited in the article.
Appendix	If included, follows the references. Typically includes survey instruments or detailed treatment protocols.

of rows and columns of numbers or words; figures may also be included, which include photographs, diagrams, graphs, or other visual displays that illustrate important concepts or results within the study. Occasionally an article contains an appendix of information that may be useful to readers but is too detailed for inclusion in the body of the report.

■ GUIDELINES FOR DISCUSSING PUBLISHED RESEARCH

Readers who discuss their reviews in writing or through oral presentation to others should follow three basic style guidelines:

1. Discuss the study in the past tense.
2. Clearly distinguish between your own opinions and those of the authors.
3. Qualify generalizations so they are not erroneously attributed.

Table 25–2 presents examples of inappropriate and appropriate wording in the context of some actual articles[2,3] to illustrate each of the three stylistic guidelines.

■ GENERIC EVALUATION OF ORIGINAL RESEARCH STUDIES

Single reports of original research should be evaluated from two major perspectives: trustworthiness and utility. *Trustworthiness* relates to whether sources of invalidity have been controlled as well as is practical, whether authors openly acknowledge the limitations of the study, and whether the conclusions drawn are defensible in light of the methods used in the study. In Chapters 7 and 19, more than 20 sources of invalidity within research studies are identified. Armed with a list of these potential problems, readers of the research literature can easily become overly critical and conclude that all studies are hopelessly flawed and offer nothing of value to the practitioner. However, as we have seen in Chapters 7 and 19, there are no perfect studies because of the reciprocal nature of many of the threats to validity. In many instances, when a researcher controls one source of invalidity, another one rears its ugly head. Thus, there is no absolute standard of trustworthiness to which every study can be held. However, because

TABLE 25-2 Style Guidelines for Writing about Published Research	
Inappropriate Wording	*Appropriate Wording*
Chiarello and colleagues state that there is no difference in outcome between patients who receive short-duration CPM versus long-duration CPM.[2] (This wording implies that the authors still hold this belief.)	Chiarello and colleagues found no differences in outcome between patients who received short-duration CPM versus long-duration CPM.[2] (This wording makes it clear that the authors' statements relate to the particular study under discussion.)
Use of CPM after total knee arthroplasty decreases the need for postoperative manipulation under anesthesia. (This wording does not make it clear whether this is the conclusion of the review author or the author of the study.)	Based on their research, Ververeli and colleagues concluded that CPM after total knee arthroplasty decreased the need for postoperative manipulation under anesthesia.[3] (This wording clearly attributes the statement to the study authors.)
Patients with greater knee range of motion have better functional outcomes after surgery. (This wording implies that this relationship between range of motion and functional outcome is well established.)	Therapists and surgeons often assume that patients with greater knee range of motion have better functional outcomes after surgery. (This wording makes it clear that the relationship between range of motion and functional outcome is an unsubstantiated assumption.)

trustworthiness focuses on the design and interpretation of studies themselves, different readers can be expected to identify common areas of concern related to the trustworthiness of a study.

In contrast, the *utility* of a study relates to the usefulness of its results to a particular practitioner. Unlike the assessment of trustworthiness, the assessment of utility may vary widely among readers. The results of a well-controlled study of a narrowly defined patient population may be highly trustworthy, but of low utility to a practitioner who sees a different patient population. Conversely, a first study of a given phenomenon may be very useful to a particular practitioner even if it suffers from several methodological flaws.

When evaluating the literature, readers must balance legitimate criticisms with a realistic sense of the compromises that all researchers must make in designing and implementing a study. Several authors have presented guidelines for evaluating the research literature.[4-8] In fact, many different scales and checklists have been developed to aid readers in evaluating the literature,[9,10] and some are presented later in the chapter. In addition, examples of research evaluations by experienced consumers of the literature can be found as commentaries to published reports in several journals.[11] Although different evaluators of the literature structure their commentaries differently, they all assess the same basic aspects of research articles.

In this section, a six-step generic sequence for evaluating the literature is presented to help novice evaluators structure their critiques. The first steps emphasize classification and description of the research in order to place it in the larger context of research as a vast and varied enterprise. The middle steps emphasize identification of threats to the validity of the research. The final steps involve assessing the place the research has in both the existing literature and one's own practice. Appendix C provides a set of questions to help readers structure their critiques. Because of the great variety of research designs and analyses that appear in the published literature, readers should recognize that the questions need to be applied thoughtfully and selectively, because they are neither exhaustive nor universally applicable.

In addition, readers need to move from merely answering the questions to interpreting the implications of the answers in the context of each study they review. For example, one of the questions in Appendix C is "Was the independent variable implemented in a laboratory-like or clinic-like setting?" In one study, a tightly controlled, laboratory-like setting might be exactly what is needed to establish the effectiveness of a particular technique under ideal conditions. In another study of a phenomenon for which effectiveness is already well established, looser, clinic-like control might be exactly what is needed to establish whether the technique still works when the vagaries of actual clinical practice apply. Thus, merely answering the question of "laboratory-like" versus "clinic-like" control of the independent variable does not tell the reader whether the control was appropriate. Rather, the reader, having determined the level of control, then needs to evaluate whether that level of control was appropriate for the study at hand.

To further assist readers embarking on a review of a study, a written critique of Gose's investigation of continuous passive motion (CPM) for patients after total knee arthroplasty (TKA) is provided as an example. The example is developed step by step as each of the six critique steps is presented. This article was selected for review because its design and its publication date (1987) provide many opportunities to illustrate the various control and validity issues addressed in this text. The abstract of Gose's report reads:

The purpose of this study was to evaluate the effects of adding three 1-hour sessions of continuous passive motion (CPM) each day to the entire postoperative program of patients who received a total knee replacement (TKR). A retrospective chart review was completed for 55 patients (8 with bilateral involvement, totalling 63 knees) who received a TKR between 1981 and 1984. The data analysis compared the following variables for 32 patients who received CPM and 23 patients who received no CPM: the length of hospital stay (LOS), the number of postoperative days (PODs) before discharge, the frequency of postoperative complications, and the knee range of motion at discharge. The CPM groups showed significant decreases in the frequency of complication ($p < .05$), the LOS

(p <.01), and in the number of PODs (p <.001). No difference was demonstrated in the ROM of the two groups. These results support the use of postoperative applications of CPM, but not as strongly as those reported from studies that used longer periods of CPM. Further research is indicated to delineate the minimum dosage of CPM needed to obtain the maximum beneficial effects.[12(p39)]

Step 1: Classify the Research and Variables

Classification of the research and variables provides an immediate sense of where the individual piece of research belongs in the literature. The information needed to classify the research is found in the abstract, introduction, and methods sections of a journal article. If the reviewer determines that the research is experimental, then it should come as no surprise if the authors make causal statements about their results; if the reviewer determines that the research is nonexperimental, then the reader's expectations about causal statements should change. If the dependent variables of interest are range-of-motion (ROM) measures, then the reviewer should expect clean, easily understood results; if the dependent measures relate to patterns of interaction between therapists and patients, then the reviewer should expect complexity and depth. We might summarize this first evaluative step for Gose's CPM study as follows:

Gose's study of the effects of continuous passive motion (CPM) on rehabilitation after total knee arthroplasty is an example of a retrospective analysis of differences between groups. The study had one independent variable, treatment, with two levels: usual postoperative therapy and postoperative therapy supplemented with CPM. The type of treatment received by each participant was not actively manipulated, but rather was apparently determined by physician prescription.

There were five dependent variables: total length of stay in the acute care hospital, number of postoperative days in the acute care hospital,

frequency of postoperative complications, knee flexion range of motion (ROM) at discharge, and knee extension ROM at discharge. All data were gathered through retrospective chart review.

Step 2: Compare Purposes and Conclusions

Any piece of research needs to be assessed in light of the contribution it was designed to make to the profession. It is not fair to fault a study for not accomplishing a purpose that it was never designed to meet. Before reading the methods, results, and discussion sections of an article, it is often useful to compare the purposes, which may be found in the introduction, and the conclusions. This comparison serves two purposes. First, it provides an indication of whether or not the study is internally consistent. Purposes without conclusions, or conclusions without purposes, should alert the reader to look for the points at which the study strays from its original intent.

Knowing the study conclusions also provides guidance for the critique of the methods, results, and discussion. If the conclusions indicate that statistically significant relationships or differences were identified, then the reader knows to evaluate the remainder of the article with an eye to how well the researcher controlled for alternative explanations for the results and whether the statistical results are clinically important. If the conclusions do not indicate any statistically significant results, then the reader knows to evaluate the study with respect to power and the clinical importance of the results. With regard to Gose's study, we might write up this second step of our critique as follows:

The purpose of this study was clearly stated at the end of the introduction section of the paper: to compare the effects of adding three 1-hour daily sessions of CPM to a postoperative total knee arthroplasty rehabilitation program. The effects measured related to both the physical status of the patient (flexion and extension ROM and frequency of complications) and the cost-effectiveness of care (total length of stay and length of postoperative stay).

The conclusions were consistent with the purpose. There were significant differences between the CPM and non-CPM groups for three of the five dependent measures: length of stay, number of days of postoperative hospitalization, and frequency of postoperative complications. There were no significant differences between groups on the two ROM variables, knee flexion and extension.

Step 3: Describe Design and Control Elements

In the third step of the evaluation process, the reviewer completes the description of the study elements and begins to make judgments about the adequacy of the research design. The design of the study is identified so that the sequence of measurement and manipulation (if present) is clear to the reader of the review. This identification can be done in any of the three ways introduced earlier in Chapters 6 and 9:

- Making a diagram of the design
- Using symbols such as Campbell and Stanley's Os and Xs
- Using descriptive terms

The research design alone does not indicate the trustworthiness of the study. For example, a "strong" design such as a pretest-posttest control-group design may not yield trustworthy information if the independent variable is not implemented consistently for participants in the treatment group. Thus, a critical reader of the literature needs to determine both the design of the study and the level of control the researchers exerted over implementation of the independent variable, selection and assignment of participants, extraneous variables related to the setting or participants, measurement, and information.

The third step in our review of Gose's CPM study can be written as follows:

As noted previously, data for this study were collected retrospectively, with group membership determined by the postoperative rehabilitation program each patient happened to have undergone. This study was therefore of a nonexperimental, ex post facto nature with nonequivalent treatment and control groups. Because all dependent variables were collected at the completion of either rehabilitation program, the study followed a posttest-only design.

The nonexperimental, retrospective nature of data collection means that many design control elements were absent. The implementation of the independent variable took place in the hospital setting and would be expected to vary accordingly. The author did not indicate the proportion of patients who received all of the intended CPM sessions. Because he later discussed how the intended dosage of CPM in this study differs from that reported in other studies, it seems important to know whether the actual dosage received by the patients was equal to, greater than, or less than the intended dosage.

The selection and assignment of participants to groups were accomplished through chart review to determine, first, whether participants met general inclusion criteria and, second, whether they had undergone traditional or CPM-added rehabilitation. The basic inclusion criteria were having undergone a total knee arthroplasty between 1981 and 1984 at one hospital, having had ROM values recorded at admission and discharge, and having accomplished certain rehabilitation tasks by postoperative days (PODs) 2 and 7. These criteria mean that patients with complications severe enough to impede the rehabilitation process were excluded from the study. Thus, the frequency of postoperative complications indicated in this study was likely less than the number of actual complications that occur after total knee arthroplasty.

Assignment of participants to group was accomplished simply by identification of which type of rehabilitation they had undergone. The author did not indicate what factors might have led one patient to receive CPM-added rehabilitation and another patient to receive traditional rehabilitation. If, for example, certain surgeons prescribed CPM-added rehabilitation and others prescribed traditional rehabilitation, then the effects of the type of rehabilitation would be confounded by the surgeon.

If the traditional rehabilitation group had their surgery and rehabilitation in 1981 and 1982 and the CPM-added group received care in 1983 and 1984, then the effects of type of rehabilitation would be confounded with any general changes in surgical technique, knee prosthesis design, hospital staffing patterns, and the like that may have differed between the two time periods.

Because of the retrospective design, extraneous variables such as disease severity and medication received postoperatively were not controlled. In addition, there was no control over ROM measurements taken and no indication of how many different therapists recorded ROM values in the study.

Step 4: Identify Threats to Validity

Once the type of research has been defined, the purposes and conclusions reviewed, and the design and control elements outlined, the reviewer is able to examine the threats to the validity of the study. This step involves not only assessing the threats to validity but also evaluating the extent to which the authors identify the study's limitations themselves.

As described in Chapter 7, the threats to validity can be divided into construct, internal, statistical conclusion, and external validity. Any study should be assessed for construct and external validity, asking "Do the ideas that undergird the study make sense?" and "To whom and under what conditions can the results of the study by applied?" Studies that use statistical tools should be assessed for statistical conclusion validity, asking "Were statistical tools used appropriately within this study?" Studies that have one or more independent variables and analyze differences between or within groups should be assessed for internal validity, asking "Is the independent variable the most plausible explanation for differences between or within groups?" Our analysis of all four types of validity for Gose's CPM study might be written as follows:

CONSTRUCT VALIDITY CONCERNS

The major construct validity concerns in Gose's study are construct underrepresentation and interaction of different treatments. The variables studied were a combination of cost-effectiveness variables related to length of stay and patient-oriented variables such as frequency of complications and knee ROM. These variables did not, however, represent a full range of outcomes for patients after total knee arthroplasty. It would have been nice if functional measures such as ambulation or stair-climbing ability had been measured. Presumably, this information would have been as available from the medical record as the ROM data were. In addition to underrepresentation of the dependent variables, the author acknowledged that the independent variable was also underrepresented: the dosage of CPM in this study was low compared with the dosage in other studies. A more complete, prospective study would assess several different dosages of CPM to determine the minimum level needed to obtain desired results.

The interaction of different treatments is always a concern with a retrospective study such as this one. We have no way of knowing, for example, whether the CPM treatments, which were administered by nursing staff, consisted of mechanical application of the unit with minimal interpersonal contact between nurse and patient or took the form of relaxed interchanges that provided an opportunity for education and discussion. If the latter was the case, then this study may have actually been assessing the effects of a combined program of CPM, education, and attention, rather than the isolated addition of CPM to the treatment regimen. The author acknowledged the possibility that differences between groups may be related to factors other than the use of CPM.

INTERNAL VALIDITY CONCERNS

The major internal validity concerns in this study are assignment, mortality, diffusion of treatment, compensatory equalization of treatments, and compensatory rivalry or resentful demoralization of participants. Very little information was given about why a particular patient received either the CPM-added rehabilitation or the non-CPM regimen. As noted earlier, if group membership was confounded with surgeon or time frame, it would be difficult to conclude that differences between groups were related solely to the differences in their rehabilitation regimens.

Regarding the threat of mortality to internal validity, we have no way of knowing how many potential participants in each group were not included in the study because they developed serious complications that prevented them from meeting the inclusion criteria of supervised ambulation on POD 2 and progressive ambulation by POD 7.

A third threat to internal validity comes from having patients from both groups being treated at the same time. It is plausible that members of each group were hospital roommates, and if the roommate in the CPM group extolled the virtues of this new device, perhaps the roommate in the non-CPM group compensated by moving her knee more frequently. If the therapists believed that CPM was beneficial, they could have become upset when some physicians did not prescribe it and compensated by increasing the number of ROM repetitions they included for their patients who were not receiving CPM. Because the author did not clearly indicate whether the two regimens were in effect simultaneously or sequentially, we cannot speculate about the likelihood that these internal validity threats actually occurred.

STATISTICAL CONCLUSION VALIDITY CONCERNS

No concerns about statistical conclusion validity seem warranted. The sample sizes were reasonable (32 and 23); there was only one statistical test performed per dependent variable; the homogeneity of variance assumptions seem to have been met; the statistically significant results seem clinically important (e.g., the CPM group had an average postoperative length of stay approximately 3.5 days shorter than the non-CPM group); and the statistically insignificant results seem clinically unimportant (the difference in the mean ROM values between groups was only $1.0°$ for both knee flexion and extension).

EXTERNAL VALIDITY CONCERNS

The external validity of the study is strong in some areas and weak in others. The participants seem representative of typical patients who received total knee arthroplasties in the 1980s: elderly women with osteoarthritis. However, the average age of patients receiving total knee arthroplasty continues to move downward and today it is not uncommon to have individuals in their 40s and 50s undergo the procedure. If individuals who choose total knee arthroplasty at younger ages are both healthier and more active than older adults who received the procedure in the past and more highly committed to returning to active lifestyles, they may have similarly short lengths of stay and low levels of complications regardless of whether CPM is used.

External validity is strengthened, ironically, by the relatively low dosage of CPM provided in this study. At the time the study was done, typical CPM protocols called for many hours per day—often up to 20 hours per day—of CPM. Although 3 hours of CPM per day seemed like a very low dosage at the time of the study, lower daily doses or fewer numbers of days of CPM are more common in contemporary reports. Therefore, compared with other studies of CPM administered in the early 1980s, this study has a dosage per day that more closely matches protocols in use today.

External validity is limited, however, by the dramatic changes in length of stay for almost all diagnoses and surgical procedures during the last 20 years. Although the CPM group's length of stay was significantly less in this study than the non-CPM group's, both lengths of stay (mean of 16.4 and 20.0 days, respectively) were much longer than is typical today, irrespective of the nature of the rehabilitation regimen. This means that although the daily dosage of CPM may match contemporary protocols, the total dosage of CPM given across the hospital stay may be greater than typical in today's short-stay environment.

Step 5: Place the Study in the Context of Other Research

In the fifth and sixth steps of evaluation, the reviewer assesses the utility of the research. First, the reviewer determines how much new information the study adds to what is already known about a topic. Even though only a single study is being critiqued, the question of utility cannot be answered in isolation. For example, if a treatment has consistently been shown to be effective in tightly controlled settings with high internal validity, another well-controlled study may not add much to our knowledge about that treatment. In such a case, what is needed is a study conducted in a realistic clinical setting, where control is difficult. Similarly, a small one-group study of a previously unstudied area might be an important addition to the physical therapy literature, whereas the same design applied to a well-studied topic may add little.

The best assessments of context are made by reviewers who have extensive knowledge of the literature on the topic. Knowledgeable reviewers can assess whether the authors of a research report have adequately reviewed and interpreted the literature they cite. Reviewers without this knowledge must rely on the authors' descriptions of the literature. Our review of the place Gose's CPM study has in the literature might be written as follows:

Despite the previously noted limitations of Gose's study, this work played an important role in the evolution of CPM from a 20-hour-per-day treatment modality to a modality that is used in varying dosages. The author indicated that previous studies of 20-hour-per-day CPM protocols found shorter lengths of stay, lower frequencies of postoperative complications, and greater early knee ROM in CPM groups compared with non-CPM groups. This study provided preliminary evidence that a low dosage of CPM could reduce the length of stay and frequency of complications in a typical group of older osteoarthritic patients receiving total knee replacement. Interestingly, there is still no consensus on appropriate dosage, as noted by the authors of a recent meta-analysis of 14 randomized controlled trials of CPM after total knee arthroplasty.[13]

Step 6: Evaluate the Personal Utility of the Study

As the final step in any research critique, the reviewer determines whether the study has meaning for his or her own practice. Whereas the determination of the trustworthiness of a research article will be somewhat consistent across reviewers, the question of personal utility will be answered differently by different reviewers. Hypothetically, we might write our assessment of the personal utility of Gose's CPM study as follows:

The results of this study have some potential application for the setting in which we work. In our setting, we follow an 8- to 10-hour-a-day regimen of CPM with excellent early ROM and relatively short stays. However, for those patients who cannot sleep well with the CPM unit on, this means that they are in the CPM unit during many of their waking hours. We believe that these patients stay in bed too much and are unable to give adequate attention to the development of effective quadriceps femoris muscle power and the development of more functional skills such as walking at a relatively normal velocity and for longer distances.

Although this study provides only partial support for the effectiveness of a low dosage of CPM, its findings are consistent with a more recent report that found no difference between a low-dosage protocol and a high-dosage protocol.[2] On the basis of the results of these studies, as well as our own dissatisfaction with some aspects of high

dosages of CPM, we plan to implement and assess a trial of medium to low dosages of CPM in our patients who have had total knee arthroplasty.

The evaluation of personal utility is a very concrete way to conclude a review of a single research study. This ending is a reminder that the first five evaluative steps are not mere intellectual exercises, but are the means by which each reader decides whether and how to use the results of a study within his or her own practice.

◼ GENERIC EVALUATION OF REVIEW ARTICLES

Review articles provide practitioners with a time-efficient way of remaining up-to-date in areas of importance to their practice. In fact, the authors of the *Users' Guide to the Medical Literature,* a series of articles appearing in *JAMA* beginning in 1993, and now compiled into a book,[14] recognize the importance of review articles and go so far as to recommend that "resolving a clinical problem begins with a search for a valid overview or practice guideline as the most efficient method of deciding on the best patient care."[15(p2097)] Having made this statement, though, they then indicate that clinicians need help in differentiating good reviews from poor reviews. This section of the chapter provides guidelines to help rehabilitation practitioners make such judgments about review articles. Although there are mathematical ways to synthesize the results of several related studies (see Chapters 11 and 26 for additional information on meta-analysis), the focus in this section is on the conceptual synthesis that is presented in many review articles. The series of points to consider has been compiled from several different resources.[8,16-18]

Step 1: Assess the Clarity of the Review Question

Readers should assess the clarity of the question being posed within the review. Well-formulated questions that can help direct practice should generally address (1) the type of exposure (to a risk factor, an intervention, or a diagnostic test); (2) the outcome of interest; (3) the type of person being studied; and (4) the comparison against which the exposure is being compared.[17] An example that illustrates these four areas is found in van der Heijden and colleagues' systematic review of randomized controlled trials (RCTs) of physiotherapy for patients with soft-tissue shoulder disorders.[19] Within the body of the article the type of exposure (different forms of physiotherapy), the outcomes of interest (success rates, pain reduction, functional status, mobility, and need for drugs or surgery), the type of person being studied (those with soft-tissue shoulder disorders; studies reporting on individuals after mastectomy or fracture were excluded, as were studies reporting on shoulder pain with hemiplegia or rheumatoid arthritis), and the comparison groups (some compared various forms of physiotherapy, some compared physiotherapy with placebo treatment, and some compared physiotherapy with other interventions such as drug or injection therapies).

Step 2: Evaluate the Article Identification and Selection Strategies

The reader should determine whether the method used to identify articles was comprehensive and whether the criteria used to select articles for review were appropriate. The process of identifying articles should be as comprehensive as possible, using the strategies identified in Chapter 24 or by other authors[17,20] and proceeding until new strategies yield only redundant studies. The search strategy should be documented clearly so that the reader has a clear sense of the time span of the review, the search terms used, and the databases that were accessed. Once a pool of articles is identified, the reviewers must cull those articles that include the information needed to answer the question posed by the review. In the study of physiotherapy for

soft tissue shoulder disorders, the authors of the review reported that their search strategy yielded 47 articles that met five initial criteria: patients had shoulder pain; treatments were randomly allocated; at least one treatment included physiotherapy; outcomes included success rate, pain, mobility, or functional status; and results were published prior to January 1996. Of these 47 articles, 24 were excluded from the review because the shoulder pain was not related to soft tissue and three were excluded because they represented multiple reports of the same data. Thus, 20 papers were ultimately included in the review.[19] Because the authors carefully reported their identification and selection process, readers are in a position to judge the completeness and appropriateness of the articles selected for review. Without this information, readers are left to wonder about the criteria used by the review author in selecting articles on which to report.

Step 3: Determine How the Authors Assess Validity of the Studies

The reader should determine whether and how the review authors assessed the validity of each of the studies within the review. In the study of soft tissue shoulder disorders, the authors compared each trial against eight validity criteria: selection criteria, assignment procedures, similarity of groups at baseline, withdrawals from treatment, missing values, presence of additional interventions, masked application of the intervention, and masked assessment of the outcome.[19] Readers can have a higher level of confidence in reviews in which two or more individuals have reviewed each study independently, with a process for resolving disagreements between reviewers.[8]

Step 4: Evaluate the Results Against the Strength of the Evidence

Readers should determine whether the results of the individual studies are evaluated against the strength of the evidence in those studies as well as in closely related studies. This generally means that the articles are not discussed in an article-by-article fashion (i.e., the reviews do not read as follows: Brown found x, Smith found y, Johnson found z). Rather, the articles are discussed topic by topic, and any single article may be referred to in several different sections of the review. For example, in van der Heijden and associates' systematic review of physiotherapy for soft-tissue shoulder disorders, the findings were grouped first by the type of intervention and then by the findings of those studies that were thought to have sufficiently high levels of validity.[19] For example, they first identified six studies that evaluated the effect of ultrasound against various alternatives and judged that four of the six studies had acceptable validity. They then summarized the findings from those four studies, one of which compared ultrasound to cold therapy. Later, they evaluated the effect of cold therapy against various alternatives—one of which was obviously ultrasound. Thus, the one study comparing ultrasound and cold therapy was cited at least twice—once during the discussion of the effectiveness of ultrasound and once with the discussion of the effectiveness of cold therapy.

Step 5: Evaluate the Personal Utility of the Review

Readers should evaluate the discussion and conclusions sections of the review to determine whether this information is consistent with the findings in the review and whether it has applications to their own practice. As was the case with the evaluation of a single study, readers must place the results of the review within the context of their own practices to determine the usefulness of the information.

■ STRUCTURED EVALUATION BY CLINICAL RESEARCH ISSUES

Recognizing the wide variety of types of research, some authors have developed more structured evaluation and application systems for different types of articles. One of the most widely used frameworks is the one developed by Sackett and colleagues.[21] In this framework, studies are classified according to the clinical issue being addressed: diagnosis and screening, prognosis, therapy, and harm. The study is then evaluated by working through a series of questions specific to the clinical issue at hand. In general, readers are first asked to determine whether the study results are valid. If they are, readers are then asked to consider the importance of the results. If the results are found to be both valid and important, then readers are asked to consider whether they can be applied to the patient at hand.

Box 25–1 presents a simplified version of Sackett and colleague's questions for studies related to therapy, meaning any health care intervention. These questions should seem familiar, as they generally relate to concepts of design, control, and validity that have been presented in detail in early chapters of this text.

Box 25–2 presents a simplified version of Sackett and colleagues' questions related to diagnosis, screening, prognosis, and harm. Background information about this kind of research is discussed in Chapter 14, Epidemiology. Readers of this literature are encouraged to go to Sackett and colleagues' text for more detail[22-24] or to go to any number of excellent general or discipline-specific evidence-based websites that feature similar information:

- Centre for Health Evidence (Canada): http://www.cche.net
- Occupational Therapy Evidence-Based Practice Research Group (McMaster University, Canada): http://www-fhs.mcmaster.ca/rehab/ebp
- Centre for Evidence-Based Medicine (University of Toronto, Canada): http://cebm.utoronto.ca
- Resource Guide for Evidence-Based Practice (University of Alberta, Canada): http://www.library.ualberta.ca/subjects/evidence/guide/index.cfm

Web searches of "evidence-based practice" or "evidence-based practice" *and* "rehabilitation"

BOX 25-1

Structured Questions for Articles about Therapy

Are the results of this individual study valid?

Was the assignment of patients to treatment randomized?

Was follow-up sufficiently long and complete?

Were all patients analyzed in the groups to which they were randomized?

Were patients and clinicians masked to the treatment?

Were groups treated equally, apart from the therapy?

Were the groups similar at the start of the study?

Are the results important?

What is the magnitude of the treatment effect?

How precise is the estimate of the treatment effect?

Are the results applicable to our patient?

Is our patient so different from those in the study that the results do not apply?

Is the treatment feasible in our setting?

What are our patient's potential benefits and harms from the treatment?

What are our patient's values and expectations related to the treatment we are offering?

Modified from Sackett DL, Straus SE, Richardson WS, Rosenberg W, Haynes RB. Therapy. In: *Evidence-Based Medicine: How to Practice and Teach EBM.* 2nd ed. Edinburgh, UK: Churchill Livingstone; 2000:105-153.

(or a specific rehabilitation discipline) will yield many useful resources.

■ EVALUATION OF LEVELS OF EVIDENCE

Another approach to the evaluation of single articles is to determine the "level of evidence" represented within the study. Once again, the work of Sackett and colleagues is a common framework used in level of evidence approaches.[24] Table 25–3 presents a modified version of their levels of evidence. Four different

types of research designs involving patients are represented, in the following order from the highest to lowest level: RCTs, cohort designs, case-control designs, and case series. Information about these different types of research can be found in Chapters 9, 11, and 12 of this text. Each of these levels is divided into an "a" and "b" sublevel, with the "a" sublevel representing a systematic review of several studies at that level and the "b" sublevel representing a report of an individual study at that level or a poor-quality report of a study with a higher level design. A fifth, and lowest, level is reserved for expert opinion without critical appraisal or reports of basic science research that is not applied to patients in a clinical context. Although the Sackett and colleagues' framework for levels of evidence is cited frequently, readers should be aware that other, similar frameworks exist.[25]

One of the criticisms of taking a level-of-evidence approach to the literature is that readers may simply identify the designs of studies, without looking further to determine the quality of the research within the level, as noted by Ciccone: "Some people treat levels of evidence like a poker game in which an RCT beats two cohort studies. That is not always true in evidence-based practice. Studies from lower levels may be better for your purposes or they may be better in terms of the quality of the study."[26(p48)]

Another criticism of the level-of-evidence approach is that it places RCTs at the top of the hierarchy, without critically addressing the limitations imposed by the controlled manipulation that is required within an RCT. As is discussed in the chapter on outcomes research (Chapter 15), the outcomes movement developed in part because of the sense that RCTs were limited because they could not often capture the complexity of the clinical environment. A quote from that chapter, by Kane, is repeated here:

> If the practice of medicine (including rehabilitation) is to become more empiric, it will have to rely on epidemiological methods. Although some may urge the primacy of randomized clinical trials as the only path to true enlightenment, such a position is untenable for several reasons. First, the

Structured Questions for Articles About Diagnosis, Screening, Prognosis, and Harm

Diagnosis

Is evidence about a diagnostic test valid?
  Was there an independent, masked comparison with a reference standard?
  Was the diagnostic test evaluated in an appropriate spectrum of patients?
  Was the reference standard applied uniformly?
  Was the test validated in a second group of patients?
Does the test accurately distinguish patients who do and do not have the disorder?
  What are the sensitivity, specificity, and likelihood ratios?
  Are multilevel likelihood ratios used?
Can I apply this test to a specific patient?
  Is the test available, affordable, accurate, and precise in our setting?
  Can we generate a sensible pretest probability for the patient?
  Will resulting posttest probabilities affect the management of our patient?

Screening

Does early diagnosis lead to improved survival or quality of life?
Are early diagnosed patients willing to participate in treatment?
Is the time and energy it will take to confirm the diagnosis and provide care well spent?
Do the frequency and severity of the condition warrant the effort and expenditure of screening?

Prognosis

Is the evidence about prognosis valid?
  Was a representative sample of patients assembled at a common point early in the course of the disease?
  Was patient follow-up sufficiently long and complete?
  Were objective outcome criteria applied in a masked fashion?
  If done, was subgroup analysis adjusted and validated appropriately?
Is the evidence about prognosis important?
  How likely are the outcomes over time?
  How precise are the prognostic estimates?
Can we apply this prognostic evidence to our patients?
  Are study patients similar to our own?
  Will this evidence have an impact on our conclusions about what to tell our patients?

Harm

Are the results of this harm study valid?
Were groups similar in ways other than exposure to the potentially harmful agent?
Were exposures and outcomes measured in the same way in both groups?
Was the follow-up sufficiently long for the outcome to have occurred?
Is there strong evidence of causation from the exposure?
What is the magnitude of the association between exposure and outcome?
Can this evidence of harm be applied to our patient?
  Is our patient so different from those in the study that the results do not apply?
  How are risks and benefits balanced for this patient?
  What are our patient's preferences, concerns, and expectations from this treatment?
  What alternative treatments are available?

Modified from Sackett DL, Straus SE, Richardson WS, Rosenberg W, Haynes RB. *Evidence-Based Medicine: How to Practice and Teach EBM.* 2nd ed. Edinburgh, UK: Churchill Livingstone; 2000.

TABLE 25-3 Level of Evidence	
Level	**Characteristics**
1a	Systematic review of randomized controlled trials, with homogeneity*
1b	Individual randomized controlled trial with narrow confidence intervals (representing large sample sizes or low variability of participants within groups)
2a	Systematic review of cohort studies, with homogeneity*
2b	Individual cohort study or low-quality randomized controlled trial
3a	Systematic review of case-control studies, with homogeneity*
3b	Individual case-control study
4	Case series and poor-quality cohort and case-control studies
5	Expert opinion without critical appraisal or based on physiology or bench research

Modified from Sackett DL, Straus SE, Richardson WS, Rosenberg W, Haynes RB. Guidelines. In: *Evidence-Based Medicine: How to Practice and Teach EBM*. 2nd ed. Edinburgh, UK: Churchill Livingstone; 2000:169-182.
*Homogeneity refers to the extent to which confidence intervals from individual studies overlap in a meta-analysis; see Chapter 26 for a more detailed discussion of homogeneity in meta-analysis.

exclusivity of most trials is so great that the results are difficult to extrapolate to practice. Such trials may be the source of clinically important truths, but these findings will have to be bent and shaped to fit most clinical situations. Second, researchers do not have the time or resources to conduct enough trials to guide all practice. Instead, we need a more balanced strategy that combines targeted trials with well-organized analysis of carefully recorded clinical practice.[27(pJS22)]

An approach to levels of evidence that bridges the RCT-versus-outcomes research debate is that of the Medical Research Council (London) (MRC), which presents a continuum-of-evidence model for studying complex interventions to improve health, including rehabilitation interventions that may involve substantial biopsychosocial elements, training of family members, and behavior modification (Figure 25–1).[28] The beauty of this approach is that it captures the dynamic nature of the research endeavor, differentiates among research designs in a way that highlights the importance of RCTs, and acknowledges the role that pragmatic outcomes research should play once definitive RCTs have been completed.

In Chapter 9, research on the technique of body-weight–supported treadmill training for individuals with locomotor disabilities was presented to illustrate how a body of evidence develops across time. This literature is now presented in the context of both Sackett and colleagues' levels of evidence and the MRC framework. Some of the earliest literature about this technique documented the responses in men without locomotor disabilities,[29] corresponding to Sackett and colleagues' Level 5 and the MRC preclinical phase. Next, researchers published the results of nonrandomized trials of small numbers of individuals with spastic paretic gait that determined the impact of treadmill training with or without body weight support on gait patterns,[30,31] corresponding to Sackett and colleagues' Levels 3b and 4b and doing the MRC modeling work needed before exploratory studies could be undertaken. More recently, RCTs comparing body-weight–supported treadmill training to traditional gait training have been published,[32,33] representing Sackett and colleagues' Levels 2b and the MRC exploratory phase (none had the characteristics needed to qualify as 1b or definitive). Finally, a recent systematic review article synthesized the growing body of evidence about body-weight–supported treadmill training,[34] corresponding, at best, to Sackett and colleagues' Level 2a (the studies reviewed and the findings of the review did not meet the criteria for Level 1a).

The conclusion from this systematic review was that there was little evidence to justify the addition of body-weight–supported treadmill training to the routine practice of rehabilitation after stroke. Based on the findings of this review,

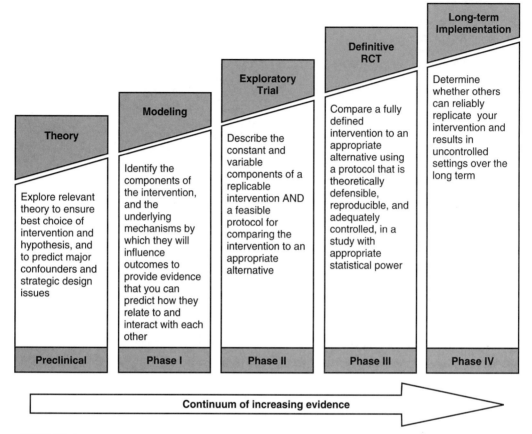

FIGURE 25–1. Medical Research Council's Continuum of Increasing Evidence. From Medical Research Council; London, UK. Available at: http://www.mrc.ac.uk/pdf-mrc_cpr.pdf.

authors critical of the growing clinical enthusiasm for adding body-weight–supported treadmill training to stroke rehabilitation programs expressed concern that this change in practice is "'evidence-tinged' at best."[35(p599)]

The levels-of-evidence approach to evaluation of research studies is attractive, in part because of its apparent simplicity. On the surface, assigning a level of evidence requires only a cursory examination of each article to determine the study design. However, a more careful reading of the work on levels of evidence shows that determining the appropriate level of evidence represented by a given piece of research requires both an assessment of the quality of the work as well as the identification of the research design. The tools

identified in the next section of this chapter can help readers make such quality distinctions.

■ EVALUATION OF RANDOMIZED CONTROLLED TRIALS

A final approach to the evaluation of original research involves assigning a quality score to the study. Typically, this is done for RCTs and reflects an important step beyond merely identifying the level of evidence of a study. Although many scoring systems exist,[9,10] two scoring systems for RCTs are described here, the Jadad 5-point scale[36(p14)] and the PEDro/OTseeker 10-point scale.[37] The Jadad scale has been evaluated for reliability by several authors with conflicting results.[38-41] The single published report of the reliability of the PEDro scale concluded that the reliability of consensus judgments of the total PEDro scale is acceptable.[42]

Table 25–4 shows the criteria and scoring for both the PEDro and Jadad scales. This table shows that the information that contributes to

each score is similar, with both scales including scored criteria related to random allocation, masking of participants and researchers, and retention of participants within the study. In addition, the PEDro scale allocates points for proper use of statistical tools. Operational definitions for each PEDro criterion can be found at the PEDro website (http://www.pedro.fhs.usyd.edu.au/scale_item.

TABLE 25-4 Scales for Scoring the Quality of Randomized Controlled Trials

RESEARCH CONCEPT	PEDro Scale*	Jadad Scale†
Eligibility	1. Eligibility criteria were specified. Not scored.	
Random Allocation and Its Impact on Baseline Characteristics	2. Subjects were randomly allocated to groups (in a crossover study, subjects were randomly allocated to an order in which treatments were received). No = 0, Yes = 1. 3. Allocation was concealed. No = 0, Yes = 1. 4. The groups were similar at baseline regarding the most important prognostic indicators. No = 0, Yes = 1.	1. Was the study described as randomized? No = 0, Yes = 1. Give 1 additional point if method of randomization was appropriate. Deduct 1 point if method of randomization was inappropriate.
Masking of Participants, Clinicians, and Researchers	5. There was blinding of all subjects. No = 0, Yes = 1. 6. There was blinding of all therapists who administered the therapy. No = 0, Yes = 1. 7. There was blinding of all assessors who measured at least one key outcome. No = 0, Yes = 1.	2. Was the study described as double blind? No = 0, Yes = 1. Give 1 additional point if method of blinding was appropriate. Deduct 1 point if method of blinding was inappropriate.
Retention of Participants	8. Measures of at least one key outcome were obtained from more than 85% of the subjects initially allocated to groups. No = 0, Yes = 1. 9. All subjects for whom outcome measures were available received the treatment or control condition as allocated or, where this was not the case, data for at least one key outcome was analyzed by "intention to treat." No = 0, Yes = 1.	3. Was there a description of withdrawals and drop outs? No = 0, Yes = 1
Use of Statistical Tools	10. The results of between-group statistical comparisons are reported for at least one key outcome. No = 0, Yes = 1. 11. The study provides both point measures and measures of variability for at least one key outcome. No = 0, Yes = 1.	
TOTAL POSSIBLE	10 points	5 points

*PEDro scale. Available at: http://www.pedro.fhs.usyd.edu.au/scale_items.html. Accessed January 3, 2004.
†Jadad AR. Chapter 4: Assessing the quality of RCTs: why, what, how, and by whom? *Randomised Controlled Trials*. London: BMJ Publishing Group; 1998. Available at http://www.bmjpg.com/rct/chapter4.html. Accessed October 24, 2003.

TABLE 25–5 PEDro Scoring of Selected Randomized Controlled Trials in Rehabilitation

Primary Author/ Study Characteristics	Chin A Paw[43]*	Clark[44]†	Kraemer[45]	Mancini[46]	Nilsson[33]*	Perry[47]†	Purdy[48]†
Year	2001	1997	2001	2003	2001	1999	1987
Participant characteristics or diagnosis	Independent living frail older adults	Independent living older adults	Healthy women exposed to maximal eccentric exercise	Older adults with Parkinson's disease and drooling	Older adults with hemiparesis after stroke	Adults with bipolar disorder	Children with Down syndrome
Intervention	Exercise and/or enriched foods	Occupational therapy	Compression therapy	Botulinum toxin	Body-weight-supported treadmill training	Patient education	Oral-motor treatment or behavioral modification
PEDro Scale Scores							
Random allocation	Y	Y	Y	Y	Y	Y	Y
Concealed allocation	Y	N	N	N	Y	Y	N
Baseline similarity	Y	N	Y	Y	Y	Y	N
Participant masking	N	N	N	Y	N	N	N
Clinician masking	N	N	N	Y	N	N	N
Assessor masking	N	Y	N	Y	Y	Y	Y
High retention	N	N	Y	Y	Y	Y	N
Intention to treat	N	Y	Y	Y	N	Y	N
Between-group comparisons	Y	Y	Y	Y	Y	Y	N
Point and variability	Y	Y	Y	N	Y	Y	Y
Total	5	5	6	8	7	8	3

*Rating from PEDro.
†Rating from OTseeker.

html) or in an appendix to Maher and associates' report on PEDro scale reliability.[42]

Maher and associates also reported on the base rate at which the various PEDro scale items were found in the trials they reviewed. Random allocation was present in about 96% of trials, groups were similar at baseline in about 63%, but in only 19% was the allocation concealed from the person determining participant eligibility for the trial. Assessors were masked in about 42% of trials, but the participant was masked in only about 6% and the clinician in only about 4% of trials. The low levels of participant and clinician masking is to be expected given the interactive, participative nature of many rehabilitation interventions. About 66% of trials had less than 15% of participants drop out of the study, but only about 15% of trials used an intention-to-treat analysis to manage the dropouts. About 93% of trials made between-groups statistical comparisons and about 88% provided both point measures and variability data. Table 25–5 shows the use of the PEDro score to rate the quality of a sample of RCTs in rehabilitation.

■ SUMMARY

The major elements of a research article are the title; abstract; introduction, methods, results, discussion, conclusions, and references sections; and, sometimes, an appendix. When discussing previously published work, reviewers should use the past tense and should make clear whether statements are their own or the opinions of the authors whose study they are reviewing. Reviewers of single studies should classify the research and its variables, compare the purposes and conclusions, outline the design and control elements, determine the threats to the validity of the study, place the study in the context of previous work, and assess the study's utility for their personal practice. Evaluators of review articles should assess the clarity of the review question, evaluate the article identification and selection strategies, determine how the authors assess the validity of the studies, evaluate the results against the strength of the evidence, and evaluate the personal utility of the review. Other methods of evaluating research articles include using structured evaluation checklists for different types of research, evaluating the level of evidence generated by a study, and by using scoring systems developed for RCTs.

REFERENCES

1. Sackett DL, Straus SE, Richardson WS, Rosenberg W, Haynes RB. *Evidence-Based Medicine: How to Practice and Teach EBM.* 2nd ed. Edinburgh, UK: Churchill Livingstone; 2000.
2. Chiarello CM, Gundersen L, O'Halloran T. The effect of continuous passive motion duration and increment on range of motion in total knee arthroplasty patients. *J Orthop Sports Phys Ther.* 1997;25:119-127.
3. Ververeli PA, Sutton DC, Hearn SL, Booth RE, Hozack WJ, Rothman RR. Continuous passive motion after total knee arthroplasty: analysis of costs and benefits. *Clin Orthop.* 1995;321:208-215.
4. Riegelman RK, Hirsch RP. *Studying a Study and Testing a Test: How to Read the Health Science Literature.* 4th ed. Boston, Mass: Little, Brown & Co; 1999.
5. Chalmers TC, Smith H, Blackburn B, et al. A method for assessing the quality of a randomized control trial. *Control Clin Trials.* 1981;2:31-49.
6. Guyatt GH, Sackett DL, Cook DJ, for the Evidence-Based Medicine Working Group. Users' guides to the medical literature. II: How to use an article about therapy or prevention. A: Are the results of the study valid? *JAMA.* 1993;270:2598-2601.
7. Guyatt GH, Sackett DL, Cook DJ, for the Evidence-Based Medicine Working Group. Users' guides to the medical literature. II: How to use an article about therapy or prevention. B: What were the results and will they help me in caring for my patients? *JAMA.* 1994;271:59-63.
8. Meade MO, Richardson WS. Selecting and appraising studies for a systematic review. *Ann Intern Med.* 1997;127:531-537.
9. Moher D, Jadad AR, Nichol G, Penman M, Tugwell P, Walsh S. Assessing the quality of randomized controlled trials: an annotated bibliography of scales and checklists. *Control Clin Trials.* 1995;16:62-73.
10. Verhagen AP, de Vet HCW, de Bie RA, et al. The art of quality assessment of RCTs included in systematic reviews. *J Clin Epidemiol.* 2001;54:651-654.
11. Rothstein JM. Commenting on commentaries [editor's note]. *Phys Ther.* 1991;71:431-432.
12. Gose JC. Continuous passive motion in the postoperative treatment of patients with total knee replacement: a retrospective study. *Phys Ther.* 1987;67:39-42.

13. Milne S, Brosseau L, Robinson V, et al. Continuous passive motion following total knee arthroplasty (Cochrane Review). *The Cochrane Library.* Chichester, UK: John Wiley & Sons; 2003: Issue 4.

14. Guyatt GH, Rennie D, ed. *Users' Guides to the Medical Literature: Essentials of Evidence-Based Clinical Practice.* Chicago, Ill: American Medical Association; 2002

15. Guyatt GH, Rennie D. Users' guides to the medical literature [editorial]. *JAMA.* 1993;270:2096-2097.

16. Oxman AD, Sackett DL, Guyatt GH. Users' guides to the medical literature: I. How to get started. *JAMA.* 1993; 270:2093-2095.

17. Counsell C. Formulating questions and locating primary studies for inclusion in systematic reviews. *Ann Intern Med.* 1997;127:380-387.

18. Shaughnessy AF, Slawson DC. Getting the most from review articles: a guide for readers and writers. *Am Fam Physician.* 1997;55:2155-2160.

19. van der Heijden GJMG, van der Windt DAWM, de Winter AF. Physiotherapy for patients with soft tissue shoulder disorders: a systematic review of randomised clinical trials. *BMJ.* 1997;315:25-30.

20. Dickersin K, Scherer R, Lefebvre C. Identifying relevant studies for systematic reviews. *BMJ.* 1994;309: 1286-1291.

21. Sackett DL, Straus SE, Richardson WS, Rosenberg W, Haynes RB. Guidelines. *Evidence-Based Medicine: How to Practice and Teach EBM.* 2nd ed. Edinburgh, UK: Churchill Livingstone; 2000:169-182.

22. Sackett DL, Straus SE, Richardson WS, Rosenberg W, Haynes RB. Diagnosis and screening. *Evidence-Based Medicine: How to Practice and Teach EBM.* 2nd ed. Edinburgh, UK: Churchill Livingstone; 2000:67-93.

23. Sackett DL, Straus SE, Richardson WS, Rosenberg W, Haynes RB. Prognosis. *Evidence-Based Medicine: How to Practice and Teach EBM.* 2nd ed. Edinburgh, UK: Churchill Livingstone; 2000:95-103.

24. Sackett DL, Straus SE, Richardson WS, Rosenberg W, Haynes RB. Harm. *Evidence-Based Medicine: How to Practice and Teach EBM.* 2nd ed. Edinburgh: Churchill Livingstone; 2000:155-168.

25. Law M, Philip I. Evaluating the evidence. In: Law M, ed. *Evidence-Based Rehabilitation: A Guide to Practice.* Thorofare, NJ: Slack; 2002:97-107.

26. Glatos S. Evidence is not created equal: a discussion of levels of evidence. *PT Magazine.* 2003;11(10): 42-49,52.

27. Kane RL. Improving outcomes in rehabilitation: a call to arms (and legs). *Med Care.* 1997;35(suppl):JS21-JS27.

28. Medical Research Council. *A Framework for Development and Evaluation of RCTs for Complex Interventions to Improve Health.* Available at: http://www.mrc.ac.uk/pdf-mrc_cpr.pdf. Accessed January 5, 2004.

29. Finch L, Barbeau H, Arsenault B. Influence of body weight support on normal human gait: development of a gait retraining strategy. *Phys Ther.* 1991;71:842-855.

30. Visintin M, Barbeau H. The effects of parallel bars, body weight support and speed on the modulation of the locomotor pattern of spastic paretic gait: a preliminary communication. *Paraplegia.* 1994;32:540-553.

31. Waagfjord J, Levangie P, Certo CM. Effects of treadmill training on gait in a hemiparetic patient. *Phys Ther.* 1990;70:549-558.

32. Visintin M, Barbeau H, Korner-Bitensky N, Mayo N. A new approach to retrain gait in stroke patients through body weight support and treadmill stimulation. *Stroke.* 1998;29:1122-1128.

33. Nilsson L, Carlsson J, Danielsson A, et al. Walking training of patients with hemiparesis at an early stage after stroke: a comparison of walking training on a treadmill with body weight support and walking training on the ground. *Clin Rehabil.* 2001;15:515-527.

34. Manning C, Pomeroy VM. The effectiveness of treadmill retraining on the gait of hemiparetic stroke patients: a systematic review of current evidence. *Physiotherapy.* 2003; 89:337-349.

35. Pomeroy VM, Tallis RC. Avoiding the menace of evidenced-tinged neuro-rehabilitation. *Physiotherapy.* 2003; 89:595-601.

36. Jadad AR. Chapter 4: Assessing the quality of RCTs: why, what, how, and by whom? *Randomised Controlled Trials.* London: BMJ Publishing Group; 1998. Available at www.bmjpg.com/rct/chapter4.html. Accessed October 24, 2003.

37. *PEDro scale.* Available at: http://www.pedro.fhs.usyd.au/scale_item.html. Accessed January 3, 2004.

38. Bhandari M, Richards RR, Sprague S, Schemitsch EH. Quality in the reporting of randomized trials in surgery: is the Jadad scale reliable? *Control Clin Trials.* 2001; 22:687-688.

39. Clark HD, Wells GA, Huet C, et al. Assessing the quality of randomized trials: reliability of the Jadad scale. *Control Clin Trials.* 1999;20:448-452.

40. Oremus M, Wolfson C, Perrault A, et al. Interrater reliability of the modified Jadad quality scale for systematic reviews of Alzheimer's disease drug trials. *Dement Geriatr Cogn Disord.* 2001;12:232-236.

41. Jadad AR, Moore RA, Carroll D, et al. Assessing the quality of reports on randomized clinical trials: is blinding necessary? *Control Clin Trials.* 1996;17:1-12.

42. Maher CG, Sherrington C, Herbert RD, Moseley AM, Elkins M. Reliability of the PEDro scale for rating the quality of randomized controlled trials. *Phys Ther.* 2003; 83:713-721.

43. Chin A Paw MJM, de Jong N, Schouten EG, Hiddink GJ, Kok FJ. Physical exercise and/or enriched foods for functional improvement in frail, independently living elderly: a randomized controlled trial. *Arch Phys Med Rehabil.* 2001;82:811-817.

44. Clark F, Azen SP, Zemke R, et al. Occupational therapy for independent-living older adults: a randomized controlled trial. *JAMA.* 1997;278:1321-1326.

45. Kraemer WJ, Bush JA, Wickham RB, et al. Influence of compression therapy on symptoms following soft tissue injury from maximal eccentric exercise. *J Orthop Sports Phys Ther*. 2001;31:282-290.

46. Mancini F, Zangaglia R, Cristina S, et al. Double-blind, placebo-controlled study to evaluate the efficacy and safety of botulinum toxin type A in the treatment of drooling in parkinsonism. *Mov Disord*. 2003;18:685-688.

47. Perry A, Tarrier N, Morriss R, McCarthy E, Limb K. Randomised controlled trial of efficacy of teaching patients with bipolar disorder to identify early symptoms of relapse and obtain treatment. *BMJ*. 1999;318:149-153.

48. Purdy AH, Deitz JC, Harris SR. Efficacy of two treatment approaches to reduce tongue protrusion of children with Down syndrome. *Dev Med Child Neurol*. 1987;29: 469-476.

Synthesizing Bodies of Evidence

Learning to evaluate research evidence one study at a time is a necessary, but not sufficient, skill for evidence-based practitioners. Because single studies, by themselves, rarely provide definitive answers to guide practice, clinicians must base their work on the aggregate evidence available about a given issue. Sometimes the aggregate evidence needed to answer a clinical question may be available in published reviews completed by other clinicians or researchers or in published guidelines promulgated by various private or government agencies committed to improving the use of evidence in health care.[1,2] Other times the evidence needed to answer a clinical question may not have been aggregated by others and clinicians need to synthesize the literature themselves. This chapter outlines reasons for synthesizing the literature, defines three approaches to synthesizing the literature, and provides guidance for conducting a systematic review of the literature, including preparation for the review, review methods, and ways of reporting on systematic reviews.

■ REASONS TO SYNTHESIZE THE LITERATURE

Aggregating evidence to guide practice is one of the most important reasons for synthesizing the literature, but it is not the only reason to do so. Fink, in her text on conducting research literature reviews,[3] outlines five additional reasons for synthesizing the literature: (1) developing research proposals required for academic degrees, (2) developing proposals required to apply for external research funding, (3) identifying research methods, (4) identifying experts in a given topic area, and (5) identifying funding sources in a given area. For all these reasons, the ability to synthesize the literature is an essential skill for rehabilitation professionals. Looking across a rehabilitation career, the same professional may need to synthesize the literature to fulfill academic requirements as a student, to guide practice as a clinician, to identify possible consultants for a new program as a service administrator, and to obtain funding for research as an academician.

■ WAYS TO SYNTHESIZE THE LITERATURE

There are three general approaches to synthesizing research results across several different studies: narrative reviews, systematic reviews without meta-analysis, and systematic reviews with meta-analysis.[4-6] Definitions and characteristics of each approach are presented, with examples from the rehabilitation literature.

Narrative Reviews

Narrative reviews of the literature are often characterized by their limitations, as noted in this humorous quote presented earlier in Chapter 11:

> A common method of integrating several studies with inconsistent findings is to carp on the design

or analysis deficiencies of all but a few studies—those remaining frequently being one's own work or that of one's students and friends—and then advance the one or two "acceptable" studies as the truth of the matter.[7(p7)]

In the past, narrative reviews were the norm and guidelines for conducting literature searches focused on developing a conceptual understanding of the topic of interest.[8] Narrative reviews rarely provide detailed methods about how the review was conducted, typically do not have independent evaluation of articles by more than one rater, and do not generally include formal evaluation or scoring of the studies. In format, they often read more like book chapters than research articles. Narrative reviews often summarize the reviewed studies in series—Jones found this, Brown found that, Smith found something else altogether—rather than integrating information across the studies.

Although largely replaced by systematic reviews as a means of aggregating evidence to apply to practice, there are still valid reasons to undertake narrative reviews of the literature. Take, for example, Hesse and colleagues' narrative review about treadmill training with partial body weight support after stroke.[9] The purpose of this review appeared to be to provide practitioners with a broad base of information about body-weight–supported treadmill training (BWSTT). Thus, their review provided an overview of the motor learning theory and physiological basis for BWSTT, a description of current and emerging technical aspects of BWSTT, and a narrative summary of the clinical literature about BWSTT.

Another time to conduct a narrative review is when the literature in an area is sparse, yet diverse. For example, Geertzen and colleagues undertook a review of the literature on rehabilitation after lower limb amputation.[10] They identified 24 articles for inclusion in the review, but these articles covered so many different themes (from functional outcomes to phantom pain and skin problems) and appeared to represent such a wide array of research designs that it would be difficult to apply the more uniform criteria typical of systematic reviews.

Similarly, Sommers and colleagues undertook a review and critical analysis of treatment research related to articulation and phonological disorders.[11] Their interest was in evaluating research methods across two decades rather than in aggregating evidence about the effectiveness of treatment for articulation and phonological disorders. Indeed, if they had tried to conduct a systematic review of treatment effectiveness, they would have had difficulty given the wide variety of designs they identified and the limited information they found about participant characteristics and extent and duration of treatment.

Narrative write-ups of reviews are also the norm in research and grant proposals and in the introductory sections of research papers. Space is often limited in these formats and so the written literature review highlights only the information needed to "build a case" for the study at hand—even when the researchers have been more systematic in gathering and evaluating evidence on the topic.

Systematic Reviews without Meta-analysis

Systematic reviews, which require documented search strategies and explicit inclusion and exclusion criteria for studies used in the review, reduce the sorts of biases noted in the quote in the above section. Although some systematic reviews include statistical pooling of results across studies (meta-analysis, discussed in the next section), many do not. In some cases, review authors simply do not have the statistical expertise needed to conduct a meta-analysis; in other instances, the body of literature consists of such varied designs and diverse types of data presentation and analysis that statistical pooling of data is not feasible.

Bilney and colleagues conducted a systematic review of literature to determine the effectiveness of physiotherapy, occupational therapy, and speech pathology for people with Huntington's disease.[12] Their work exhibits the characteristics typical of a systematic review

without meta-analysis: research article format, a documented search strategy, explicit rules for including and excluding studies from the review, independent data extraction by two reviewers, formal ratings of study quality, and results that are presented in tables that summarize important information from each study.

Systematic Reviews with Meta-analysis

Systematic reviews with meta-analysis are differentiated from other reviews by their meta-analytic component. Meta-analysis is the analysis of analyses (in the same way that meta-theory, introduced in Chapter 2, is theorizing about theory). The basic concept behind meta-analysis is that the size of the differences between treatment groups (the effect size) is mathematically standardized so that it can be pooled across studies with different, but conceptually related, dependent variables. Recent examples in the rehabilitation literature include two meta-analyses that synthesize the evidence about the effectiveness of occupational therapy and physical therapy for treating persons with Parkinson's disease[13,14] and a meta-analysis on treatment of aphasia.[15]

Having outlined the three general ways of synthesizing the literature, the remainder of this chapter provides more detail on how to conduct a systematic review of the literature, with or without meta-analysis. The methodology of systematic reviews is designed to produce a review that is systematic, explicit, and reproducible.[3] Two important resources provided most of the methodological details for this section: Fink's book on conducting research literature reviews[3] and Law and Philip's chapter on systematically reviewing the evidence.[16] Brief examples based on several studies of continuous passive motion (CPM) use after total knee arthroplasty (TKA) are given to illustrate some of the steps.[17-23] Figure 26–1 reproduces Fink's overview of the steps in conducting a systematic review of the literature.[3(p190)]

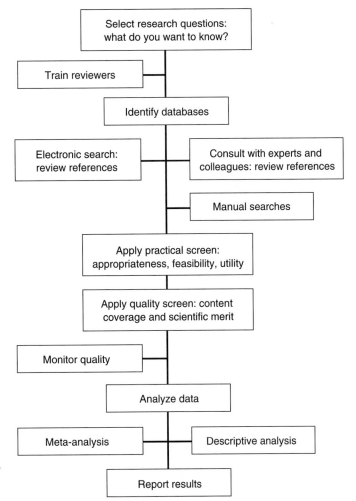

FIGURE 26–1. An overview of the systematic literature review process.
From Fink A. *Conducting Research Literature Reviews: From Paper to the Internet.* Thousand Oaks, Calif: SAGE Publications; 1998:190.

■ PREPARING FOR A SYSTEMATIC REVIEW

Three preparatory steps need to be completed before a systematic review can be undertaken: (1) determining the purpose of the review, (2) identifying literature for potential inclusion in the review, and (3) selecting studies for inclusion.

Determine the Purpose of the Review

Just as any research that involves the collection of new data should have a clearly stated purpose, so should a systematic review of the literature. Common items that might be specified in a purpose statement include participant characteristics and diagnoses, intervention characteristics, and dependent variables of interest. The specificity of the purpose statement should match the body of literature that is expected to be identified for the review. For example, the purpose statement for Bilney and colleagues' review of therapy effectiveness in Huntington's disease is relatively broad:

> To assist physiotherapists, occupational therapists, speech pathologists, and rehabilitation physicians to effectively treat people with Huntington's disease by providing a review and critical evaluation of the evidence on therapy outcomes.[12(p12)]

Contrast this general objective with the far more specific objective of Milne and colleagues' meta-analysis on CPM following TKA:

> The aim of this meta-analysis is to determine the effectiveness of CPM following knee arthroplasty. We will compare CPM to standard physiotherapy treatments done on patients after a total knee arthroplasty. Standard physiotherapy treatment consisted of any combination of the following interventions: range of motion (ROM) exercises, muscle strengthening exercises (isometric, dynamic), functional exercises, gait training, immobilization and ice. The outcome measures of interest for the meta-analysis were active and passive knee ROM, length of hospital stay, pain, knee swelling, fixed flexion deformity and quadriceps strength at end of treatment and during follow-up.[24(p2)]

Although Figure 26–1 implies that determining the research question occurs as the first step of the process, in my experience the initial statement of the research question is merely a draft question that is revised and refined as the literature search is undertaken and studies are selected for inclusion in the review. Imagine that Bilney and colleagues started their review hoping to determine the effect of rehabilitation therapies on quality of life in individuals with Huntington's disease. Once they rooted around in the literature they would have discovered that few studies used quality of life measures—and they would need to either abandon the review or revise their purpose to include a broader range of dependent variables. Likewise, imagine

that Milne and colleagues had not specified their interest in comparing CPM to standard care. On review of the literature, they would discover a large number of studies of CPM following TKA, some of which compared different CPM protocols to one another—requiring that they either examine several different comparisons or limit their purpose to comparing CPM to standard care.

Identify the Literature

Using the techniques outlined in Chapter 24, the researcher must identify a relatively complete set of articles on the topic for possible inclusion in the review. Typically this begins with a search of one or more electronic bibliographic databases. Because a systematic review needs to be explicit and reproducible, the researchers must carefully document the final search strategy used to identify articles for possible inclusion. Of course, most researchers will "play around" in the electronic databases to see what is yielded from different combinations of terms and different limitations on searches—these exploratory searches need not be documented. However, once a set of search terms and limits (such as the years included in the review, the language of articles) is set, researchers should re-run their searches to obtain a definitive set of articles for possible inclusion in the review.

Select Studies for Inclusion

Once a set of articles for possible inclusion in the review is identified, the researchers need to determine which articles are relevant to the question at hand. For example, assume that the electronic database searches yield 100 unique articles for possible inclusion in a review that compares standard care plus CPM to standard care following TKA.

The next step is to review the article abstracts to ensure that each article is a report of original research, that the participants have undergone

TKA, and that at least one of the comparisons in the article is between standard care plus CPM and standard care. Perhaps 25 articles will be review articles or "how-we-do-it" articles, 16 will compare various CPM protocols to one another, and four will be "false hits" with participants who have undergone anterior cruciate ligament reconstruction, leaving 55 articles for possible inclusion in the review. Because this is still a relatively large number of articles of varying quality, perhaps the researchers will decide to eliminate any study that includes fewer than 20 participants per group or that uses nonexperimental, retrospective methods. After reviewing the abstracts of the 55 remaining articles, this might reduce the number of articles for possible inclusion to a manageable 35. The researchers would obtain hard copies of those 35 articles, using the various strategies presented in Chapter 24. After the hard copies of the selected studies are obtained, they should be reviewed to ensure that they meet the specified criteria—in some instances, the abstract will not have included enough information to make this determination; in others, the abstract will have misrepresented the particulars of the study.

Once a hard copy review confirms that an article meets the study criteria, its reference list should be reviewed to identify other potential studies that meet the inclusion criteria but were missed by the electronic searches. Some reviewers supplement this strategy with "hand searching" of journals expected to be good sources of articles on the topic and with consultation with experts to determine whether they know of relevant studies, particularly unpublished studies, that have been missed.

To enhance the reproducibility of the systematic review, two or more reviewers should independently determine which of the 100 initial articles to eliminate from the review and independently determine whether to add any additional articles through citation checking or hand searching. Discrepancies in eliminated or added articles would be resolved by discussion among the reviewers or by consultation with another reviewer who serves as a referee. For our hypothetical search, assume that two additional studies

are identified through citation checking, leaving a core of 37 articles to use in the next phase of the review.

Systematic reviews are always vulnerable to the criticism that the search strategies were incomplete, that the authors selected the wrong set of studies from those identified, and that publication bias could have had an impact on the review conclusions. To guard against these criticisms, authors should use comprehensive search strategies that extend beyond electronic bibliographic databases, should use more than one researcher to select studies, should make their inclusion and exclusion criteria explicit, and should attempt to include information from relevant unpublished studies. The issue with publication bias is the possibility that a higher proportion of studies favorable to the intervention being studied are published than are those unfavorable to the intervention, either because journal editors prefer to publish positive results or because authors more often submit positive results for publication. At minimum, authors should address the possibility of publication bias in their narrative. In meta-analysis, authors may also address the possibility of publication bias with a variety of analytic techniques.[3,15]

■ SYNTHESIZING THE LITERATURE

Having identified the core of 37 articles for the review, the next task is to undertake the intellectual task of identifying, organizing, and synthesizing the results across studies. Six steps can guide this process: (1) identifying important characteristics of individual studies, (2) determining the quality of the individual studies, (3) identifying important constructs across the studies, (4) making descriptive comparisons across studies, (5) pooling statistical information across studies if a meta-analysis is being done, and (6) specifying problems in need of further study. It is useful to create a database for the review, much as one would do for a study of original research. The rows of the database are the included studies and the columns are the variables related to each study.

Identify Important Characteristics of Individual Studies

Typically the first step of a systematic review is "getting to know" each of the studies within the review. Important characteristics of each study are extracted, including items such as primary author, publication date, total number of participants, design features, independent variables, dependent measures, and summary results. Table 26–1 shows the individual characteristics that might be recorded for a subset of articles included for a systematic review of CPM use following TKA.

Determine the Quality of the Individual Studies

Many systematic reviews include a formal evaluation of quality, typically a level-of-evidence approach if the study designs vary widely, or a scoring approach if the review is limited to randomized controlled trials. For example, Bilney and colleagues identified the levels of evidence represented by each study in their review of therapy outcomes for Huntington's disease[12] and de Goede and associates scored the trials in their review of the effects of physical therapy for Parkinson's disease,[14] using a tool similar to those presented in Chapter 25. Table 26–2 shows how quality scoring might be presented for the randomized controlled trials included in a review of CPM after TKA. In this example, the quality scores are uniform and the item scores are similar, so there would be little reason to place more or less weight on particular studies based on their methodological rigor. Narrative validity analysis, as presented in Chapter 25, is also important to undertake—even randomized controlled trials with high scores for their design may have implementation flaws that limit their usefulness as a source of evidence. For example,

if there was a rigorous randomized controlled trial from 1990 that identified shorter lengths of stay for patients who used CPM after TKA, these results would need to be interpreted in light of the much shorter stays typical of contemporary practice.

Identify Important Constructs Across Studies

In this phase of the review, the constructs and variables that undergird the studies become the focus, rather than the individual studies. By doing so, as in Table 26–3, it becomes clear, for example, that knee ROM is a dependent variable for all of the studies in the review, but that edema is a dependent variable in only two of them. Likewise, it is clear that there are more data to answer a question about the impact of CPM at discharge (seven studies) than there are at 1 year postoperatively (three studies).

Make Descriptive Comparisons Across Studies

Once each study has been examined independently, the reviewer compares results across the studies. In this hypothetical review of CPM after TKA, we see that several investigators have examined the impact of CPM on length of stay. Of the four authors who address this issue, Gose[20] found shorter lengths of stay with low-dose CPM added to usual care, and the other three researchers (Basso,[21] Yashar,[22] and MacDonald[17]) found no differences in length of stay between those receiving usual care or various types of CPM in addition to usual care. Having identified an inconsistent finding, the task of the review author is to examine this conflicting evidence carefully to determine whether there are differences among the studies that might explain the contradictory results. In this case, the only significant finding is in one of the older studies and the one with the weakest design (the retrospective chart review).

| TABLE 26-1 | Characteristics of Included Studies |

Primary Author	Publication Year	Design	Total N	Comparison Groups	Dependent Variables	Major Results
Chen[18]	2000	RCT	51	Usual care Usual care + CPM	Knee ROM Edema	No differences between groups
MacDonald[17]	2000	RCT	120	Usual care Usual care + 0-50° CPM Usual care + 70-110° CPM	Knee ROM Functional score Pain Length of stay	No differences between groups
Chiarello[19]	1997	RCT	45	Usual care control group Short-duration, set progression CPM Short-duration, as tolerated progression CPM Long-duration, set progression CPM Long-duration, as tolerated progression CPM	Knee ROM	No differences between groups
Pope[23]	1997	RCT	57	Usual care Usual care + 0-40° CPM Usual care + 0-70° CPM	Knee ROM Functional score Pain Complications	No long-term differences between groups
Yashar[22]	1997	RCT	210	Usual care + 0-30° CPM Usual care + 70-100° CPM	Knee ROM Functional score Pain Length of stay Complications	Few long-term differences between groups
Basso[21]	1987	Successive cohorts	23	Usual care + high-dose CPM Usual care + low-dose CPM	Knee ROM Edema Pain Length of stay	No differences between groups
Gose[20]	1987	Retrospective chart review	55	Usual care Usual care + low-dose CPM	Knee ROM Length of stay Complications	No ROM differences between groups CPM group had shorter length of stay and fewer complications

CPM, Continuous passive motion; *ROM*, range of motion.

TABLE 26-2	Quality Scores (PEDro Scale)* of Randomized Controlled Trials Included in the Review				
Primary Author	Chen[18]	MacDonald[17]	Chiarello[19]	Pope[23]	Yashar[22]
Year	2000	2000	1997	1997	1997
Random allocation	Y	Y	Y	Y	Y
Concealed allocation	N	N	N	N	N
Baseline similarity	Y	Y	Y	Y	Y
Participant masking	N	N	N	N	N
Clinician masking	N	N	N	N	N
Assessor masking	Y	Y	N	N	Y
High retention	N	N	Y	Y	Y
Intention to treat	N	N	N	N	N
Between-group comparisons	Y	Y	Y	Y	Y
Point and variability	Y	Y	Y	Y	N
TOTAL	5	5	5	5	5

*http://www.pedro.fhs.usyd.edu.au/scale_item.html.

The review conclusion would likely be that there is no contemporary evidence that use of CPM leads to reduced length of stay after TKA. Similar comparisons across studies would be made for each of the factors of interest within the review.

Pool Statistical Data Across Studies

When there are enough studies, with enough comparisons in common, and with enough statistical detail, then statistical synthesis of studies can be accomplished through meta-analysis. The details needed to implement a meta-analysis are beyond the scope of this text, but readers are referred to a number of excellent articles, texts, and websites for further information.[7,25-33] Many reviewers who undertake a meta-analysis work with statisticians who have expertise in this specialized branch of statistics.

The central concepts that undergird meta-analysis are (1) the use of confidence intervals for hypothesis testing and (2) the pooling of effects across studies. In traditional hypothesis testing, a probability is computed and a statistical conclusion is reached when the obtained p value is compared with a preset alpha level (see Chapter 19). In hypothesis testing with confidence intervals, a confidence interval is

calculated for the difference of interest and a statistical conclusion is reached by determining whether the confidence interval includes the value that corresponds to the null hypothesis (see Chapter 21). In a meta-analysis, the results of each of the studies are converted to confidence intervals, allowing all of the studies to be evaluated against a common indicator of "no difference," even when the variables used within the different studies are not the same. After confidence intervals are calculated for each study for a given comparison, the results are pooled, weighting by sample size, to obtain a single value. This value, with an associated confidence interval, represents the aggregate effect across the reviewed studies.

For most purposes, the null hypothesis is represented by the value zero ("0") because the null hypothesis proposes that there will be "no difference" between groups. If the confidence interval contains "0," then it is concluded that there is no statistically significant difference between groups. If the confidence interval does not contain "0," then it is concluded that there is a statistically significant difference between groups. When using confidence intervals to determine the significance of odds ratios and relative risk ratios, a significant difference is identified when the interval does not contain the

TABLE 26-3 Selected Constructs in Studies in the Review	
Constructs	**Primary Author and Year of Publication***
Design Elements	
Group assignment	
Nonrandom	Gose–1987, Basso–1987
Random	Pope–1995, Yashar–1997, Chiarello–1997, Chen–2000, MacDonald–2000
Group comparisons	
Usual care vs usual care + CPM	Gose–1987, Chen–2000
Usual care vs usual care + different CPM protocols	Chiarello–1997, Pope–1997, MacDonald–2000
Usual care + different CPM protocols	Basso–1997, Yashar–1997
Implementation of CPM	
Dosage	
20+ hours/day	Basso–1987, Pope–1997, Yashar–1997, MacDonald–2000
10 hours/day	Chiarello–1997
3-6 hours/day	Basso–1987, Gose–1987, Chiarello–1997, Chen–2000
Initial CPM ROM	
Not specified	Basso–1987, Chiarello–1997, Chen–2000
0° to 30°-50°	Gose–1987, Pope–1997, Yashar–1997, MacDonald–2000
0° to 60°-70°	Pope–1997
70° to 100°-110°	Yashar–1997, MacDonald–2000
Outcomes	
Knee ROM	Basso–1987, Gose–1987, Chiarello–1997, Pope–1997, Yashar–1997, Chen–2000, MacDonald–2000
Functional score	Pope–1997, Yashar–1997, MacDonald–2000
Complications	Gose–1987, Yashar–1997, Pope–1997
Pain	Basso–1987, Yashar–1997, Pope–1997, MacDonald–2000
Edema	Basso–1987, Chen–2000
Length of stay	Basso–1987, Gose–1987, Yashar–1997, MacDonald–2000
Follow-up	
Hospital discharge	Basso–1987, Gose–1987, Chiarello–1997, Yashar–1997, Pope–1997, MacDonald–2000, Chen–2000
One-year postoperative	Yashar–1997, Pope–1997, MacDonald–2000

*References associated with each cited article are as follows: Basso,[21] Chen,[18] Chiarello,[19] Gose,[20] MacDonald,[17] Pope,[23] and Yashar.[22]

number one ("1"). This is because a ratio of "1" means that the risks for the groups being compared are equal.

The mathematical complexities of meta-analysis are often elegantly summarized in a "forest plot." In fact, the central part of the logo for the Cochrane Collaboration is a stylized forest plot for a meta-analysis, reproduced as Figure 26–2. The vertical line represents "no

difference" between comparison groups, and we will assume that values to the left of the line favor treatment (perhaps this is a meta-analysis of seven studies of a popular weight loss program and values to the left represent weight loss) and values to the right of the line favor the control condition. The seven horizontal lines represent the seven different studies. The first and sixth studies in the meta-analysis demonstrate

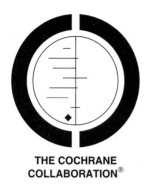

**THE COCHRANE
COLLABORATION®**

FIGURE 26–2. Logo of the Cochrane Collaboration, depicting a stylized forest plot of meta-analysis results.

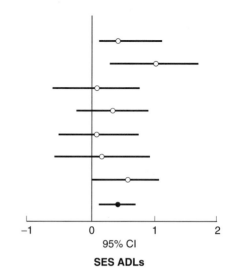

SES ADLs

FIGURE 26–3. Forest plot showing significant impact of therapy on activities of daily living (ADLs) for individuals with Parkinson's disease. Visual analysis shows that the trials are homogeneous and the summary effect size (SES) is significant.
From de Goede CJT, Keus SHJ, Kwakkel G, Wagenaar RC. The effects of physical therapy in Parkinson's disease: a research synthesis. *Arch Phys Med Rehabil.* 2001;82: 509-515.

significant weight loss because their confidence intervals do not encompass the "no difference" point. The second, third, and fifth studies tend toward the weight loss side of the plot, but do not represent significant differences because they encompass the "no difference" point. The fourth and seventh studies do not show significant differences and tend toward the "no difference" point. The diamond at the bottom of the plot represents the pooled effect across all of the studies. The vertical axis of the diamond gives the mean pooled effect and the horizontal axis gives the confidence interval for the pooled effect. The conclusion from the Cochrane Collaboration forest plot is that the program results in modest weight losses when considered across these seven studies.

In an actual meta-analysis, many separate analyses may be done. For example, in our hypothetical review of CPM after TKA (assuming more than the seven studies that are presented in tables throughout this chapter), we might calculate pooled effects for the comparison between usual care and CPM for each of five different dependent variables and then do an additional five analyses for the comparison between long-duration and short-duration CPM. For example, Figure 26–3 illustrates a forest plot from de Goede and colleague's meta-analysis of therapy effects in Parkinson's disease, showing the results of one of the four analyses that were

done for different dependent variables (activities of daily living, walking speed, stride length, and neurological signs).

One of the major statistical concerns about meta-analysis revolves around the concept of whether the different study results are homogeneous or heterogeneous. Homogeneity is desirable and "means that the results of each individual trial are mathematically compatible with the results of any of the others."[32] When the individual confidence intervals that are plotted on a forest plot overlap, then the trials are said to be homogeneous. Conversely, when some lines do not overlap with any other lines, the trials are said to be heterogeneous, and they are often thought to represent different clinical populations of interest. More formal testing for heterogeneity is often done with a chi-square test. Heterogeneity can be managed by "correcting" for covariates such as age, by doing separate meta-analyses for different clinical subgroups, or with a variety of other statistical maneuvers that require the assistance of a skilled meta-analyst.

Specify Problems That Need Further Study

Just as original research studies lead to recommendations for further study, the results of systematic reviews with or without meta-analysis generally suggest areas for further study. For some variables, the review may demonstrate consistent, rigorous results that can be considered definitive. For other variables, the review may reveal inconsistencies in the literature that need further study, may identify gaps in the literature that require more study, or may reveal methodological limitations of the literature that need to be rectified with more rigorous studies. For the actual meta-analysis on CPM after TKA, Milne and colleagues[24] found improvements in active knee flexion and analgesic use and reduced length of stay and need for manipulation under anesthesia with CPM and physical therapy compared with physical therapy alone. They concluded that CPM combined with physical therapy "may" be beneficial but noted that the potential benefits need to be weighed against the inconvenience and cost of CPM. Furthermore, they concluded that more research is needed to determine whether there are differences in effectiveness with different durations and intensities of CPM intervention. Note that these actual meta-analysis results are different from what might be concluded from the incomplete, hypothetical review presented in Tables 26–1 to 26–3, supporting the need to use complete, systematic methods to synthesize the literature.

■ REPORTING ON SYSTEMATIC REVIEWS

Reports of systematic reviews follow the format typical of a research article, with introduction,

methods, results, and discussion sections. Reporting issues unique to systematic reviews are highlighted, including those specific to meta-analyses.[34]

Describing Review Methods

The methods section of a systematic review needs to be explicit and reproducible. This means that it is important to provide detailed information on search strategies, on how studies were selected for inclusion, and on how data were extracted from the studies. The possibility of publication bias should be addressed in the narrative or with analytic techniques if a meta-analysis was performed. If, as is good practice, more than one reviewer independently selected studies and extracted data, information about the interrater reliability of the raters needs to be provided. In addition, the method for resolving any inconsistencies between raters needs to be specified. If a meta-analysis was done, a data analysis section with statistical information needs to be included, including information about the homogeneity of the trials.

Any systematic review needs to include a listing of studies that were included in the review. Sometimes this is done in a separate table or appendix, other times the study citations are simply included in the reference list of the paper. Sometimes authors will also include a table or appendix of excluded studies so that readers can evaluate the results of the selection process used in the review.

Presenting Review Results

A typical systematic review tabulates basic information from each step of the synthesis. Tables 26–1, 26–2, and 26–3 are typical of the tables that would be included in a published report of a systematic review. Results of meta-analyses can be presented in tables, but they are often also presented in forest plots similar to those in Figures 26–2 and 26–3.

■ SUMMARY

Synthesis of the literature is needed for evidence-based practice, developing research proposals, and identifying research methods, experts, and funding sources in a given area. There are three general approaches to synthesizing research results across several different studies: (1) narrative review, (2) systematic review without meta-analysis, and (3) systematic review with meta-analysis. Narrative reviews, although the norm in the past, are being replaced by systematic reviews, which are designed to be systematic, explicit, and reproducible. When enough studies in a review meet certain mathematical requirements, a systematic review with meta-analysis may be done to pool results across many studies. Systematic reviews require a clearly stated purpose, a comprehensive search strategy, and clearly stated inclusion and exclusion criteria. Synthesis steps in a systematic review include identifying important characteristics of each study, determining the quality of each study, identifying important constructs across studies, making descriptive or statistical comparisons across studies, and specifying problems that need further study. Reports of systematic reviews follow the format of a traditional research article, with explicit methods, tabulations of information from each step of the synthesis, and, when appropriate, tables or forest plots of meta-analytic results.

REFERENCES

1. Ilott I. Challenging the rhetoric and reality: only an individual and systemic approach will work for evidence-based occupational therapy. *Am J Occup Ther.* 2003;57: 351-354.
2. Lieberman D, Scheer J. AOTA's evidence-based literature review project: an overview. *Am J Occup Ther.* 2002;56: 344-349.
3. Fink A. *Conducting Research Literature Reviews: From Paper to the Internet.* Thousand Oaks, Calif: SAGE Publications; 1998.
4. Victor N. "The challenge of meta-analysis": discussion. Indications and contraindications for meta-analysis. *J Clin Epidemiol.* 1995;48:5-8.
5. Finney DJ. A statistician looks at meta-analysis. *J Clin Epidemiol.* 1995;48:87-103.
6. Pogue J, Yusurf S. Overcoming the limitations of current meta-analysis of randomised controlled trials. *Lancet.* 1998;351:47-52.
7. Glass GV. Primary, secondary and meta-analysis of research. *Educ Res.* 1976;5:3-9.
8. Findley TW. Research in physical medicine and rehabilitation. II. The conceptual review of the literature or how to read more articles than you ever want to see in your entire life. *Am J Phys Med Rehabil.* 1989;68:97-102.
9. Hesse S, Werner C, von Frankenberg S, Bardeleben A. Treadmill training with partial body weight support after stroke. *Phys Med Rehabil Clin N Am.* 2003;14: S111-S123.
10. Geertzen JHB, Martina JD, Rietman HS. Lower limb amputation. Part 2: rehabilitation—a 10 year literature review. *Prosthet Orthot Int.* 2001;25:14-20.
11. Sommers RK, Logsdon BS, Wright JM. A review and critical analysis of treatment research related to articulation and phonological disorders. *J Commun Disord.* 1992;25:3-22.
12. Bilney B, Morris ME, Perry A. Effectiveness of physiotherapy, occupational therapy, and speech pathology for people with Huntington's disease: a systematic review. *Neurorehabil Neural Repair.* 2003;17:12-24.
13. Murphy S, Tickle-Degnen L. The effectiveness of occupational therapy-related treatments for persons with Parkinson's disease: a meta-analytic review. *Am J Occup Ther.* 2001;55:385-392.
14. de Goede CJT, Keus SHJ, Kwakkel G, Wagenaar RC. The effects of physical therapy in Parkinson's disease: a research synthesis. *Arch Phys Med Rehabil.* 2001;82: 509-515.
15. Robey RR. A meta-analysis of clinical outcomes in the treatment of aphasia. *J Speech Lang Hear Res.* 1998;41: 172-187.
16. Law M, Philip I. Systematically reviewing the evidence. In: Law M, ed. *Evidence-Based Rehabilitation: A Guide to Practice.* Thorofare, NJ: Slack; 2002:97-107.
17. MacDonald SJ, Bourne RB, Rorabeck CH, McCalden RW, Kramer J, Vaz M. Prospective randomized clinical trial of continuous passive motion after total knee arthroplasty. *Clin Orthop.* 2000;380:30-35.
18. Chen B, Zimmerman JR, Soulen L, DeLisa JA. Continuous passive motion after total knee arthroplasty: a prospective study. *Am J Phys Med Rehabil.* 2000;79: 421-426.
19. Chiarello CM, Gundersen L, O'Halloran T. The effect of continuous passive motion duration and increment on range of motion in total knee arthroplasty patients. *J Orthop Sports Phys Ther.* 1997;25:119-127.
20. Gose JC. Continuous passive motion in the postoperative treatment of patients with total knee replacement: a retrospective study. *Phys Ther.* 1987;67:39-42.
21. Basso DM, Knapp L. Comparison of two continuous passive motion protocols for patients with total knee implants. *Phys Ther.* 1987;67:360-363.

22. Yashar AA, Venn-Watson E, Welsh T, Colwell CW, Lotke P. Continuous passive motion with accelerated flexion after total knee arthroplasty. *Clin Orthop.* 1997; 345:38-43.

23. Pope RO, Corcoran S, McCaul K, Howie DW. Continuous passive motion after primary total knee arthroplasty: does it offer any benefits? *J Bone Joint Surg Br.* 1997;79: 914-917.

24. Milne S, Brosseau L, Robinson V, et al. Continuous passive motion following total knee arthroplasty (Cochrane Review). *The Cochrane Library.* Chichester, UK: John Wiley & Sons; 2003:Issue 4.

25. Lipsey MW, Wilson DB. *Practical Meta-analysis.* Thousand Oaks, Calif: SAGE Publications; 2000.

26. Hunter JE, Schmidt FL. *Methods of Meta-analysis: Correction Error and Bias in Research Findings.* 2nd ed. Thousand Oaks, Calif: SAGE Publications; 2004.

27. Rosenthal R. *Meta-Analytic Procedures for Social Research.* Newbury Park, Calif: SAGE Publications; 1991.

28. Petiti DM. *Meta-analysis, Decision-Analysis, and Cost-Effectiveness Analysis.* Oxford: Oxford University Press; 1994.

29. Geller NL, Proschan M. Meta-analysis of clinical trials: a consumer's guide. *J Biopharm Stat.* 1996;6:377-394.

30. Basu A. *How to Conduct a Meta-analysis.* Available at: *http://www.pitt.edu/~super1/lecture/lec1171/001.htm.* Accessed January 6, 2004.

31. *Comprehensive Meta-Analysis.* Available at: *http://www.meta-analysis.com.* Accessed January 5, 2004.

32. Greenhalgh T. How to read a paper: papers that summarize other papers. Systematic reviews and meta-analyses. *BMJ.* 1997;315:672-675.

33. Sutton AJ, Abrams KR, Jones DR. An illustrated guide to the methods of meta-analysis. *J Eval Clin Pract.* 2001;7:135-148.

34. Stroup DF, Thacker SB, Olson CM, Glass RM, Hutwagner L. Characteristics of meta-analyses related to acceptance for publication in a medical journal. *J Clin Epidemiol.* 2001;54:655-660.

Implementing Research

Implementing a Research Project

Although the primary purpose of this text is to provide readers with the knowledge they need to use research evidence in practice, some readers will want to extend that knowledge by implementing projects of their own. The final two chapters of this text, then, are designed to provide practitioners with some "nuts and bolts" guidance about implementing research and disseminating the results of that research (Chapter 28). However, research is rarely an individual venture—most studies are undertaken by multiple authors who provide different types of expertise to the project. Individuals beginning a research program are encouraged to identify mentors and colleagues who can provide the diverse array of skills needed to mount a successful project, as suggested in Whyte's "scientific autobiography," which sheds light on the complex way in which research agendas in rehabilitation grow and develop.[1]

This chapter first identifies three preliminary steps that must be completed before any data are collected: (1) a research plan, or proposal, must be prepared and submitted for approval through appropriate academic or administrative channels; (2) the researchers must seek the approval of human or animal subject protection committees, if appropriate; and (3) the researchers must secure the funds needed to implement the study. Next, the chapter presents guidelines for implementing all phases of a research project, from participant selection to data analysis. Methods of obtaining participants are discussed first, followed by the development and use of research instrumentation. Tips for managing data collection and recording are then presented, and the chapter ends with suggestions for data analysis, including guidelines for using computer statistical programs and statistical consultants.

■ PROPOSAL PREPARATION

The research proposal is a blueprint for the conduct of a research study. The proposal is also the mechanism by which the researcher sells the study idea to those individuals who are in a position to approve and fund it. Thus, the proposal must be written in a fashion that makes the purpose and methods of the study intelligible to those outside the researcher's sphere of interest. In this section of the chapter, general guidelines for proposal preparation are given, followed by specific suggestions related to each basic element of a research proposal. Detailed suggestions for proposal preparation have been provided by others.[2,3]

General Proposal Guidelines

Ideas with merit may never get to the implementation stage if the proposal does not meet the technical standards of the agency to which it is submitted, if the language is confusing, or if the appearance of the document makes it difficult to read. Thus, researchers need to prepare their proposal in the format, style, and appearance preferred by the agency to which they are submitting it. Whether one is submitting the proposal to a doctoral dissertation committee, to an institutional review board for assessment of whether the proposal contains adequate safeguards for the human participants involved in the research, or to a foundation for funding, there will be guidelines to follow for preparation of the proposal. If there is a page limit, do not exceed it. If you are required to submit one original and three copies, do not submit an original and two copies. If the proposal must be in someone's office by a certain date, do not simply mail the proposal on that date. In short, follow the directions of the group to whom the proposal will be submitted. The proposal may need to be modified to meet different needs at different times. The format that students must use for the proposal they submit to their research advisors will likely differ from the format required for submission of the proposal to the human participants review committee, and the format required for foundation funding will probably differ from the other two formats.

The proposal must be well organized and contain clear, concise language appropriate for the individuals who will be reviewing it. A proposal submitted to one's academic advisors can be written with the assumption that the audience has basic knowledge of the area of study; a proposal submitted to a family-run philanthropic foundation must be written so that lay individuals can grasp the essential elements and importance of the proposal. The appearance of the document must both invite the reader and convey the investigator's competence. Misspellings convey the message that the proposal writer does not pay attention to details and may make the reviewer wonder whether adequate attention would be paid to the details of the research. Cramped type, narrow margins, draft-quality print, and poor photocopying all make the document difficult to read. Attractive documents have a good balance between text and white space, achieved through adequate margins, lots of headings for skimming, and numbered or bulleted lists.

Elements of the Research Proposal

In many ways, the elements of a research proposal are similar to those of a research article. In fact, a good proposal can serve as the outline for the first draft of a research article. Box 27–1 outlines the typical sections of a proposal.

TITLE

The proposal title should be concise yet precise, and should mention the most important variables under study. When seeking funding for a study, researchers may include in the title of their study words similar to those listed as priorities by the funding agency. For example, if an agency lists the funding of research related to Down syndrome as one of its priorities, researchers studying children with hypotonia (including some with Down syndrome) might do well to title their proposal "Assessment of Children with Down Syndrome and Other Hypotonic Conditions" rather than "Assessment of Children with Hypotonia."

INVESTIGATORS

The names, credentials, and institutional affiliations of the investigators should be given. If cooperating institutions with whom the researchers are

---

BOX 27–1

Components of a Research Proposal

Title
  Key words
  Variables of interest
Investigators
  Names and credentials
  Affiliation
  Curricula vitae in appendix
Abstract
Problem
  Based in the work of the profession
  Backed up with literature
Purposes
  Specific objectives of the study
  Researcher hypotheses about results
Methods
  Subject selection and assignment
    Procedures
    Provisions for confidentiality
  Procedures
    Justified by literature
    Detailed enough to assess benefits and risks
    Qualifications of investigators or others to
      perform procedures
    Provisions for protection of participants during
      testing or treatment
    Reference to informed consent form in
      appendix, if appropriate

Data analysis
  Based on best-case scenario
  May include contingency plans
References
Dissemination
  Conferences at which presentations may be given
  Journal to which results will be submitted first
  Other means by which results may be
    disseminated to the communities of interest
Budget
  Personnel, salaries, and benefits
  Supplies
  Equipment
  Mailing, printing, etc.
  Participant stipends
  Data analysis
  Presentation and publication preparation
  Presentation travel
Work plan
  All phases, from implementation to dissemination
Appendices
  Curricula vitae of investigators
  Informed consent form
  Very detailed procedures

not formally affiliated will be involved in the research, they should be specified here. A curriculum vita, or scholar's resumé, of each investigator is often included in an appendix to the proposal.

PROBLEM STATEMENT

The problem statement in a research proposal is generated and placed in the context of related literature. A persuasive paragraph or two are needed to convince the prospective sponsors of the study's importance, perhaps using the "given, however, therefore" framework presented in Chapter 4. The problems need to be consistent with the goals and mission of the institution at which the research will be performed and with the purposes for which an agency is making funds available.

PURPOSES

The purposes section of a proposal enumerates how the problem will be approached in the study. If there are several purposes, they should be listed in a logical sequence according to factors such as importance, underlying concepts, or timing. The format of the purposes varies depending on the type of research being proposed. For example, if the research is exploratory in nature, the purposes may take the form of broad questions, as in the following statement:

The purpose of this study is to answer four questions:

1. To what extent do health professions students feel isolated from the clinical environment during their first year of study?
2. What difficulties do newly licensed clinicians experience in making the transition from student to professional?
3. Does participation in a program in which students are matched with clinician advisors decrease feelings of isolation from the clinic?

4. Does participation in the clinician advisor program ease the transition from student to professional?

If the research is in a more developed area, then more formalized research hypotheses may be appropriate.

METHODS

The methods section of a research proposal should include information on participant selection, procedures, and data analysis. Description of the sample must include the source of participants for the study; the sample size anticipated; the methods of assigning participants to groups, if appropriate; and the means by which the informed consent of the participants will be obtained, if appropriate. A copy of the informed consent document should be included as an appendix to the proposal (guidelines for writing informed consent statements are presented later in this chapter).

Procedures should be discussed in detail, with reference to the literature that provides justification for the choice of procedures. Any independent and dependent variables should be clearly defined. The means by which extraneous variables are controlled should be noted, and the reasons for leaving any extraneous variables uncontrolled should be given.

The data analysis procedures in the proposal are usually based on a best-case scenario, but may include contingency plans for nonnormal data or if the number of anticipated participants does not materialize. There should be a data analysis element for every research hypothesis or question. If statistical consultants have been used to develop the data analysis section of the proposal or will be available to assist with data analysis, this should be indicated here.

DISSEMINATION

Readers of the proposal will want to know how the researchers will disseminate the study findings. Conference presentation and journal article publications are the most common means of dissemination (see Chapter 28).

BUDGET

There are costs associated with any research project. If a project is self-funded by the researcher or internally funded by an organization, these costs are frequently hidden because the individuals doing the research are donating their time or the institution in which the research is being conducted simply does not actually calculate the loss of revenue from the decreased clinical productivity of the individuals involved. Externally funded projects require detailed budgets that account for both the direct and indirect costs of the research. Direct costs include equipment, supplies, computers, salaries and benefits of individuals working on the project, and the like. Indirect costs include administrative costs, overhead, and salaries and benefits of individuals peripherally involved with the study. See the Funding section of this chapter for more detailed information on developing a budget for the research project.

WORK PLAN

The work plan details when tasks will be accomplished and who will accomplish them. All phases from planning through implementation and dissemination need to be included in the work plan. Researchers need to be realistic in estimating the amount of time needed to accomplish the project, making sure that adequate slack is included to manage unforeseen complications. Time constraints on students or considerations of the clinic may dictate that certain events happen at certain times. When this is the case, the researchers should develop the work plan by proceeding backward from a set date to ensure that all necessary preliminary tasks are accomplished. Table 27–1 shows a work plan developed for a study required for completion of an academic degree. In this example, data collection will occur at a burn clinic held only once

a month. The work plan therefore revolves around the set dates on which the clinic is held.

APPENDICES

In the appendices, the researcher provides detailed information that may be required by reviewers of the proposal but is not required for a basic understanding of what the proposal entails. Common items include the curricula vitae of the investigators, informed consent forms, and very detailed procedures such as diagrams of equipment or specific maneuvers.

APPROVALS

Once the proposal is prepared, it requires approval, sometimes from individuals at several different levels. Student proposals require the approval of research advisors and committees. Clinical research proposals require administrative approval at one or more levels in an organization. Proposals for studies using human or animal subjects require approval by human or animal subject protection committees. The procedures for obtaining academic and administrative approval vary widely from institution to institution and are not discussed further. In contrast, the procedure for obtaining approval from human participants protection committees tends to be similar at most institutions.

■ HUMAN PARTICIPANTS PROTECTION

Researchers in physical therapy must undertake many procedures to ensure the protection of the human participants they use in their studies. Researchers who use animal subjects must submit their proposals for approval from comparable animal subjects protection committees.

To protect their participants from harm, researchers must design sound studies in which dangers to participants are minimized, secure the informed consent of participants, and implement the research with care and consideration for the participants' safety. Review committees are the

TABLE 27-1 Work Plan for a Research Project	
Submit first draft to advisor	Nov 1, 2003
Finish revisions to first draft	Nov 30, 2003
Advisor approves proposal for degree requirements	Dec 5, 2003
Submit approved proposal to burn clinic director at hospital	Dec 8, 2003
Burn clinic director reviews proposal and makes suggestions or approves	Jan 6, 2004
Make protocol revisions if necessary	Jan 15, 2004
Submit institutional review board (IRB) materials for university approval	Jan 20, 2004
University IRB holds meeting	Jan 31, 2004
Build measuring device and test with researchers	Jan 31, 2004
Submit IRB materials for hospital approval	Feb 2, 2004
Hospital IRB holds meeting	Feb 18, 2004
Reserve video equipment for pilot and test days	Feb 20, 2004
Develop data collection forms	Feb 20, 2004
Pilot test with one or two patients	Mar 1, 2004
Revise forms and photocopy for data collection	Mar 3, 2004
Collect data at burn clinic	Mar 5, 2004
Arrange for photography for presentation and publication, to be done in April	Mar 15, 2004
Collect data at burn clinic	Apr 2, 2004
Enter data into computer program	Apr 12, 2004
Analyze data	Apr 28, 2004
Submit first draft of academic paper to advisor	June 6, 2004
Submit second draft of paper to advisor	Aug 12, 2004
Develop presentation script and submit to advisor	Sept 8, 2004
Advisor approves presentation script	Oct 4, 2004
Generate presentation visuals	Oct 21, 2004
Submit abstract for presentation at conference	Nov 2, 2004
Oral presentation to faculty	Nov 11, 2004
Submit third draft of paper to advisor	Nov 27, 2004
Submit final draft of paper to advisor	Dec 1, 2004
File approved copies of paper with university	Dec 7, 2004
Revise academic paper for journal publication	Jan 31, 2005
Submit for publication	Feb 15, 2005

mechanisms by which these elements of participant safety are ensured. The generic term for these committees is *institutional review board* (IRB). Since 1971, federal regulations in the United States have specified that research conducted with government funds be subject to review by a committee concerned with the rights and welfare of participants.[4] In addition, most scientific journals today require evidence that research with animal or human subjects has undergone a review, irrespective of the funding source of the research.

Although specific committee procedures vary from institution to institution, many IRBs base their work on federal guidelines. Consequently, most of the guidelines presented here are based on the guidelines of the federal government. These guidelines, along with thoughtful discussion of ethical issues posed within the clinical research process, have been well summarized by several authors.[5-8]

Institutional Review Boards

Federal regulations specify that an IRB be composed of at least five members with varying backgrounds representative of the type of research conducted at the institution: Individuals of different genders and races should be represented, at least one member must have a nonscientific background, and one member should be unaffiliated with the institution. This composition is designed to ensure that a closely knit group of scientists does not make the decisions about their own or their colleagues' projects.

The purpose of the IRB is to review research conducted under the auspices of the institution to ensure that the rights of human participants are protected. These rights are protected when research designs minimize risks to participants, when participant selection and assignment are equitable, when researchers have made provisions for the confidentiality of information, and when participants are provided with the information they need to make an informed decision about whether to participate in the research. The IRB accomplishes its purpose through regular meetings during which it reviews written proposals submitted in a format specified by the IRB and by monitoring the progress of research that it has approved.

Levels of Review

IRBs typically have three levels of review of research projects: exempt, expedited, and full. Research that is *exempt* from review includes:

- Research that involves normal educational practices
- Survey or interview procedures that do not involve sensitive areas of behavior and in which responses are recorded in such a way that they cannot be attributed to a particular individual
- Observations of public behavior
- Study of existing data that is not protected health information

Although such research is often exempt from review by the IRB, institutions usually require researchers to submit materials (such as a proposal and questionnaires) to the IRB so that the members can confirm whether the research fits the exempt category. An exempt study in rehabilitation might involve a mailed survey of clinicians to determine their opinions about contemporary practice issues.

Expedited reviews are permitted for studies that involve minimal risks to participants. Such procedures include:

- Collection of hair, nails, or external secretions
- Recording of noninvasive data
- Study of small amounts of blood through venipuncture
- Study of the effects of moderate exercise in healthy volunteers

Expedited reviews are typically done by just a few members of the IRB and do not require a meeting of the full committee. An expedited study in rehabilitation might involve measuring range of motion in a patient group, having patients complete self-reported quality of life tools, or assessing mobility gains of normal participants following an exercise program.

The IRB conducts a *full* review of:

- Research projects that involve more risks than those identified for exempt or expedited review
- Studies of lower-risk procedures in children or others who are unable to provide meaningful consent

Examples of rehabilitation studies that would require full review include assessment of the fitness level of patients with cardiovascular disease or a trial of an oral-motor program in children with cerebral palsy.

Informed Consent

In the context of research, informed consent refers to an interaction between the researcher and potential participant.[9] The researcher provides the potential participant with the information he or she needs to make an informed decision about whether to participate in the research. The potential participant then makes his or her decision and communicates it to the researcher, usually by either signing or declining to sign a written consent form. Special consideration in the informed consent process needs to be taken with individuals, such as minors and those with dementia, who are unable to provide their own consent and rely on others to protect their interests.[10-12] A fuller discussion of the principles of informed consent was provided in Chapter 3.

Consent forms must be written in language that is understandable to the individuals who will be giving consent. The typical reading level of participants should be considered, as should visual acuity and native language. A copy of the consent form itself should be provided to the participant. Box 27–2 lists the elements of an informed consent statement, and Figure 27–1 presents a sample consent form document. Consent forms may not contain exculpatory language, that is, language that asks participants to waive any of their legal rights or releases the investigator or institution from liability for negligent acts associated with the research project. Ideally, the form is contained on a single sheet of paper, with front and back sides used as needed. If more pages are needed, they should be numbered "1 of 3," "2 of 3," and the like so that participants are assured that all the needed information has been received.

The researcher should keep the signed consent forms in a secure location, and contemporary IRBs will want to know how the researcher will secure informed consent and other documents associated with the study. The length of time the forms are retained depends on the nature and length of the research and on the latency and duration of foreseeable complications related to the research procedures. Researchers should recognize that the signed consent form is usually the only point at which each participant's name is linked to the study. Therefore, secure storage of signed consent forms is an important part of maintaining participants' confidentiality.

There are two general situations in which consent forms may not be needed or appropriate. The first is the collection of data via a mailed survey. In this case, the elements of informed consent should be contained within the cover letter written by the researcher to the potential respondent and return of the questionnaire by the

---

> ### BOX 27-2
>
> ## Elements of a Consent Form
>
> Statement that the study constitutes research
> Explanation of study's purposes
> Explanation of basis of participant selection and duration of participant involvement
> Explanation of provisions for subject confidentiality
> Description of procedures, with experimental procedures identified
> Description of risks and discomforts
> Description of potential benefits to participants and others
> Description of alternative treatments, if available
> Statement of whether compensation is available for injuries
> Name of person to contact if questions or injuries arise
> Statement emphasizing that participation is voluntary
> Statement that the participant has the right to withdraw from the study at any time
> Statement of disclosure of information gained in the study that might influence participant's willingness to continue participation
> Explanation of payment arrangements, if applicable
> Consent statement
> Date line
> Participant's signature line
> Investigator's signature line
> Investigator's institutional affiliation and telephone number

respondent is taken as evidence of consent. The second situation is a study that is of a sensitive nature and signed consent forms would be a means by which the study participants could be identified. In this situation, informed consent may be obtained verbally if approved by the IRB.

■ FUNDING

Conducting research is costly. The challenge for researchers is to find funding to support their

University of Anytown
1256 Holt Road   *Anytown, Indiana 46234*
Department of Rehabilitation   *(317) 555-4300*

CONSENT TO PARTICIPATE IN A RESEARCH STUDY

TITLE OF STUDY: Comparison of Integrated Electromyographic Activity and Strength Measures in the Supraspinatus Muscle in Two Positions.

You are invited to participate in a research study that measures the electrical activity and strength of the supraspinatus muscle, which is located in the back of the shoulder. You have been invited to participate based on the assumption that you have a shoulder which is free of injury or disability. Your participation would require attendance at a single measurement session lasting approximately one hour.

Prior to your participation, an investigator will take a brief medical history to determine whether you have had previous shoulder problems which would make you ineligible to participate. Weight, height, age, and sex will also be recorded. You will be assigned a participant number so that your name will not be associated with any of the findings of this study.

The research procedure consists of measurement of muscle electrical activity and strength in two positions. The electrical activity of your supraspinatus muscle will be measured by an experienced electromyographer. He will insert a 27-gauge sterile needle containing two fine-wire electrodes into your muscle. After positioning the wires, the needle will be removed and the wires will remain in place for testing in both positions. The wires will be removed on completion of data collection in both positions.

Strength will be measured with a handheld dynamometer, which is a stationary device held by the researcher and placed at the back of your wrist. You will be asked to use your shoulder muscles to push against the device as hard as you can. This will be repeated three times in each of the two positions.

In the first position you will be seated, with your arm straight in front of you with your thumb pointing down. In the second position you will lie on your stomach with your arm out straight in front of you and with your thumb pointing up.

PAGE 1 of 2   _____ (Participant's Initials)

FIGURE 27-1. Example of a consent form.

research interests. Funds generally come from one of four sources: institutions, corporations, foundations, or the government. This section of the chapter presents a typical budget for a research study and then discusses the peculiarities of the four funding sources.

Budget

Table 27–2 presents a budget for a descriptive study that would require data collection by two clinicians and support services from one aide and one secretary. Personnel costs are determined by

CONSENT TO PARTICIPATE IN A RESEARCH STUDY (Continued)

TITLE OF STUDY: Comparison of Integrated Electromyographic Activity and Strength Measures in the Supraspinatus Muscle in Two Positions.

The risks of participation in this study include muscle fatigue or soreness from exercise, temporary discomfort from needle insertion, infection from the needle electrode, bleeding from needle insertion, and a small risk of puncture of the chest cavity which could lead to pain, difficulty breathing, and would require medical attention. To protect from infection, sterile needles and electrodes will be used and will be disposed of after each use. To protect from the risk of chest cavity puncture, the electromyographer will use needle placement designed to minimize this risk. If muscle soreness occurs, you will be instructed in procedures to minimize discomfort. No compensation is available for injuries resulting from participation in this research.

By determining the position in which the supraspinatus muscle is most effective, the results of this research may benefit patients and athletes who wish to strengthen their shoulder muscles.

If you have questions about this research or need to report an injury related to your participation in this research, contact xxxxx at (xxx) xxx-xxxx. Your participation in this research is voluntary, and your decision whether or not to participate will not affect your standing at this institution. If you elect to participate in the study, you have the right to withdraw from the study at any time without affecting your standing at the institution. You will receive a copy of this form.

CONSENT

I, _____, voluntarily consent to participate in this research study as described above. I have had a chance to ask questions of the researcher, and have had any questions answered to my satisfaction.

_____
Participant Signature

_____
Researcher Signature

_____
Date

PAGE 2 of 2

FIGURE 27-1. *Continued*

estimating the proportion of time each individual would be involved in the study, multiplying the salary by that proportion, and adding a reasonable percentage for benefits. Equipment costs should be estimated, including service and repair costs if appropriate. Consultants are individuals who are not employed by the sponsoring institution, but are engaged on a daily or hourly basis to fulfill a special need of the research project. Statistical, computer, and engineering

TABLE 27-2 Research Project Budget

Item	Explanation	Cost
Personnel		
Joyce McWain	10% time for 1 year	$10,400
Principal investigator	Benefits 30% of salary	
	Annual salary $80,000	
Randall Myers	5% time for 1 year	$4550
Coinvestigator	Benefits 30% of salary	
	Annual salary $70,000	
Ben Riley	5% time for 6 months	$650
Rehabilitation aide	Benefits 30% of salary	
	Annual salary $20,000	
Sally Knapp	5% time for 6 months	$813
Administrative assistant	Benefits 30% of salary	
	Annual salary $25,000	
Equipment		
Handheld dynamometers	Two at $1200 each	$2400
Consultants		
Statistician	30 hours at $150/hour	$4500
Dissemination		
Photocopying	1000 pages at $.10/page	$100
Visuals	Black and white diagrams $250	$650
	Poster 4' × 8' $400	
Travel	Principal investigator and coinvestigator to	$4000
	annual conference, $2000 each	
SUBTOTAL		$28,063
Overhead	30% of $28,063	$8419
TOTAL		$36,482

consultants are examples. The cost of disseminating the results of the research includes the cost of manuscript preparation, the cost of creating photographs and graphs, the cost of platform or poster presentations, and the cost of traveling to conferences to present the research. Overhead costs for the institution sponsoring the research is often figured as a percentage of the direct costs. This percentage may be specified by the funding agency or calculated by the institution in which the research is conducted.

Institution Funding

Much of rehabilitation research is funded by the institution in which it is conducted. Department managers who believe in research as an essential element of professionalism may allow staff to conduct limited amounts of research on work time. However, because research time does not produce revenue like patient care does, even the most research-oriented managers have difficulty releasing clinicians from patient care to perform research. This is particularly true in the contemporary cost-cutting, high-productivity environment that is prevalent in rehabilitation settings in the United States.

Corporation Funding

A corporation may fund a research project directly through its operating funds or indirectly through a grant from a foundation associated with the company. When a corporation provides research funds through direct giving, it is usually to support activities directly related to the corporation's function. For example, equipment manufacturers may be willing to provide equipment for and pay the salaries of researchers who are conducting studies that showcase their products. Some manufacturers are willing to loan equipment for the duration of a project; many students, who typically conduct research on a shoestring budget, have obtained loaner equipment simply by contacting the manufacturer or a local sales representative.

Researchers who accept funds directly from corporations need to be sure they understand who has control of the data and its dissemination. A corporation may wish to retain ownership of the data so that it has the prerogative of not releasing any data that are not favorable toward its product. Researchers who contact companies for support must decide whether they are willing to accept such terms, should the company request them.

Foundation Funding

Foundations are private entities that distribute funds according to the priorities set by their donors or their boards of trustees. There are different types of foundations with unique requirements for individuals seeking funding.

TYPES OF FOUNDATIONS

Foundations that provide research grants can be broadly divided into independent, company-sponsored, and community foundations. The funds of an independent foundation usually come from a single source, such as a family, an individual, or a group of individuals. Independent foundations give grants in fields specified by the few individuals who administer the fund; giving is often limited to the local geographical region in which the fund is located. Independent foundations that support rehabilitation research in the United

States include the American Occupational Therapy Foundation, the Foundation for Physical Therapy, and the American Speech-Language-Hearing Foundation. Comparable foundations, such as the United Kingdom's Physiotherapy Research Foundation, exist in other countries.[13]

A company-sponsored foundation is an independent entity that is funded by contributions from a company. Although the foundation is independent from the corporation, it tends to give grants in fields related to the company's products or customers. Giving is often limited to the geographical region or regions in which the company is located.

Community foundations are publicly supported by funds derived from many donors. The mission of a community foundation is to meet the needs of its locale; thus the projects it funds must be directly related to the welfare of the community.

IDENTIFYING FOUNDATIONS

Large institutions supported by several grant agencies have grants administration officers who can help researchers identify appropriate funding sources. The Foundation Center, a nonprofit organization, publishes comprehensive references that can also help researchers identify foundations that fund studies in their area of interest.[14,15] These references are available in hard copy and electronic formats in many university or public libraries. The information provided for each foundation includes the size of the fund, the amount given annually, the names of agencies to whom funds were given, and the types of projects funded (e.g., scholarships, construction of new facilities, education, or research). Several specialized indexes focus on funding projects in health or health-related areas, such as aging.[16,17]

APPLYING FOR FOUNDATION FUNDS

The procedure for applying for foundation funds varies greatly from foundation to foundation. Funding decisions in independent foundations may rest with a very few individuals.

Consequently, applying for funds is relatively informal. A letter of inquiry describing the research in general terms should be sent to the foundation. Ways in which the research meets the goals of the foundation should be emphasized. The reply from the foundation will indicate whether the idea is appealing to them and will ask for additional information if it is. The additional information required is likely to be fairly brief and can be assembled in a format determined by the researcher.

Corporate-sponsored foundations often have more formalized grant application procedures. However, the letter of inquiry is still the first means by which the researcher contacts the foundations. If the general area of the research is within the scope of the foundation's activities, the foundation will respond with directions for formal application for funds.

Government Funding

The federal government is a major provider of research grants in the United States. Box 27–3 provides a partial listing of the government agencies that provide funding for health sciences research. Several references provide detailed information about the grant programs of the federal government[18-20] or about strategies for applying for government grant funds.[21]

The procedure for obtaining federal grant funding is far more formal than that for obtaining foundation funding. First, the grant funds must be made available. To do this, Congress must both authorize the grant-funding program and then, in a separate legislative step, appropriate funds for the program. Administration of appropriated funds is delegated to a large grants administration bureaucracy in Washington, D.C. When funds are appropriated for a grant program, notice is placed in *The Federal Register*, the daily federal government news publication. Once notice is placed in the register, application materials can be released to potential grant recipients. Applications are highly formalized, and grant applicants must certify that they are in

---

BOX 27–3

Partial Listing of U.S. Federal Government Funding Sources for Health Research

Department of Health and Human
  Services
Administration for Children and Families
Centers for Disease Control and
  Prevention
National Institute for Occupational Safety
  and Health
National Institutes of Health
  National Cancer Institute
  National Heart, Lung, and Blood Institute
  National Institute of Arthritis and
    Musculoskeletal and Skin Diseases
  National Institute of Child Health and
    Human Development
  National Institute of Neurological
    Disorders and Stroke
  National Institute on Aging
  National Institute for Dental Research
  National Center for Medical
    Rehabilitation Research
  National Institute of Deafness and
    Other Communication Disorders
  National Institute of Mental Health
Office of Alternative Medicine
National Science Foundation
Department of Education
  National Institute for Disability and
    Rehabilitation Research
Veterans Health Administration

---

compliance with a variety of federal regulations related to nondiscrimination and protection of human participants. Although the process is formalized, the individuals who direct the various grant programs are available to discuss the application process with grant writers.

The awarding of federal grants is usually accomplished by a peer review committee. Experienced researchers are assembled to review the submitted proposals and make recommendations about their disposition. Often only one or two reviewers read the entire proposal; the rest of the committee members read only the abstract of the study and hear the primary reviewers' descriptions and evaluations of the project. It is therefore imperative that the abstract of the grant proposal accurately reflect the scope of the project for which funding is sought.

Federal grant proposals will have one of three outcomes: approval with funding, approval without funding, or disapproval. A proposal is disapproved if the study does not meet the purpose of the grant or its design is not acceptable. Proposals that meet the technical requirements are approved and given a certain priority level. Only those with the highest priority level are funded.

After writing the research proposal, obtaining administrative and institutional review board approval, and securing the funds needed to implement a project, the researcher must contend with the substantial logistical details of implementing a project.[22,23] The second half of this chapter addresses a number of these concerns, including recruitment of participants, data collection, and data analysis.

■ OBTAINING PARTICIPANTS

The time and effort required to obtain research participants are often far greater than the researcher anticipates. For example, assume that we wish to implement a study of older adults who have undergone total knee arthroplasty. We plan to study two groups who undergo different inpatient and outpatient postoperative rehabilitation. Measurement of certain outcomes will be taken at discharge, 3 months postoperatively, and 6 months postoperatively. If we know that 100 such surgeries are performed in a 6-month period at our facility, we may assume that there will be no difficulty obtaining two study groups of 40 participants each for our study. Table 27–3 shows, however, several ways in which the number of available participants will be far fewer than the 100 patients who undergo the surgery. If the scenario in Table 27–3 was realized, we would be faced with a situation in which fewer than 20 participants were available per group

TABLE 27-3 Eventual Sample from a Potential 100 Patients		
Reason for Participation or Nonparticipation	**N**	**N Remaining**
Total knee arthroplasties performed in 6 months	100	100
Young patient with hemophilia	3	97
Patient with perioperative complications	5	92
Patient lives more than 60 miles away or has received outpatient care at another clinic	10	82
Patient's surgeon does not wish to participate	12	70
Patient does not consent to be in study	10	60
Patient does not complete outpatient care	12	48
Patient dies before 6-month visit	2	46
Patient moves or cannot be located to schedule 6-month appointment	4	42
Patient does not come to the scheduled 6-month follow-up appointment	6	36

during the 6 months in which participants were to be recruited.

Researchers need to plan their participant recruitment strategy carefully to ensure an adequate number of participants. Different strategies are appropriate when recruiting inpatients, outpatients, or the general public. In all cases, recruitment of participants should take place after an institutional review board has approved both the conduct of the study and the procedures to be used for ensuring the informed consent of participants.

Inpatient Recruitment

In the inpatient setting, the admitting physician is clearly in control of the care that the patient receives while in the hospital. Thus, securing inpatients for study requires careful work with the medical staff of the institution. In fact, the best way to secure participants for study is to invite key physicians to collaborate in the entire research endeavor. In addition, the administrative chain of command within the facility will need to be followed to secure permission to implement the project.

After securing the permission of the admitting physician, the researcher contacts participants directly to secure their informed consent. As with all participant recruitment methods, patients must be approached in a manner that conveys that regardless of whether they choose to participate, their care will not be prejudiced. Researchers and physicians should determine together the best procedure for securing patient consent: The physician may mention the study to the patients first and indicate that the researcher will visit with details; the researcher may accompany the physician on rounds so that they can jointly present the study to patients, assuring them that the different professionals are working together on the research endeavor; or the researcher may present the study first, giving patients the opportunity to discuss the study later with the physician before consenting.

Outpatient Recruitment

Outpatient recruitment is somewhat easier than inpatient recruitment because the physician is not necessarily the point of control for the research. If a descriptive, correlational, or methodological study is being conducted that does not involve any procedures contraindicated by the current condition of the patient, the researcher can feel free to proceed without obtaining referring physician consent. As is the case with inpatients, it is wise to inform the referring physicians of the ongoing project, so that they will not be alarmed if patients tell them that they have participated in a research study.

After the study, it is courteous to send the referring physicians of participants a summary of the study results, along with your assessment of how the results will allow you to serve their patients better in the future. Alternatively, collaboration with physicians may prove rewarding for both physicians and researchers while having the added benefit of providing researchers with easier access to some participants.

If the research protocol requires a departure from a physician's orders, then permission must be sought and gained from both the physician and the patient, as described under Inpatient Recruitment. Again, collaboration or communication with the physicians about the study results may make them more willing to have their patients participate in future studies.

Recruitment of patients who have completed their course of treatment requires careful consideration of the confidentiality of their medical records, particularly since the implementation of the Health Insurance Portability and Accountability Act (HIPAA) in the United States (and similar acts in other countries). Consider a case in which a university-based researcher contacts a clinic to request access to patient records to identify participants who meet certain inclusion criteria. The clinic, being interested in the project, agrees to participate in the study and provides the researcher with the names and addresses of patients with the particular diagnosis. Patients would have good reason to be concerned about breaches of confidentiality if they received a letter from an unknown researcher requesting their participation in a study based on the fact that they had had a certain surgery and were seen for treatment at a certain clinic. In today's environment, such a recruitment procedure would probably not be approved by the IRB. Alternate procedures would involve having a clinic employee—who already has access to the clinic records—write a letter to eligible patients explaining the study and asking for their permission to release their name and address to the researcher.

Recruitment of the Lay Public

When a study requires the participation of the lay public rather than patients, researchers are challenged by the need to balance their desire for convenient access to a particular group of participants with their hope that results will be generalizable beyond the particular sample studied. In the past, this balance has often been lacking: Use of health professions students as a convenient source of participants has limited the generalizability of many studies to young, healthy individuals, who make up the majority of health professions students.

Groups that consist of individuals with a wide range of educational, racial, and socioeconomic characteristics are desirable for many studies. If one works in a large organization, recruiting participants from employees at all levels—from upper administration to maintenance staff—often provides the sort of variety that is desired.

Researchers who require specific types of participants need to be creative in identifying existing groups from which to recruit. Examples of groups that may yield good participant pools for certain populations include churches, senior citizen or retirement centers, apartment complexes, health clubs, day care centers, and youth or adult sport leagues. For example, if one wished to study balance in the well elderly, participants might be found in church groups, senior bowling leagues, residential retirement centers, or senior citizen centers with daytime programs. The choice of which group to use would depend on the contact the researcher has with members of the groups and how seriously biased the group membership is in light of the particular research question. For instance, if a researcher's great aunt bowls 3 days a week in a senior league, she might be able to recruit plenty of participants for a balance study. However, if the researcher believes that the senior bowlers would be biased in the direction of better balance than most of the well elderly, the bowling league may not be a good choice, no matter how easy it would be to obtain participants from the group.

Once a researcher has determined that a particular group is suitable for study, the appropriate administrative approval is needed—be it from the director of personnel, the manager of the bowling alley, the pastor of the church, or the administrator of the retirement center. When seeking such approval, the researcher needs to prepare a brief version of the study proposal, written in terms understandable to the person whose approval is sought. A blank consent form should be included along with documentation of the IRB approval. To gain administrative approval, the researcher will need to convince the official that the study has value; that participation in the study will not greatly disrupt the facility's routine; that participants are at minimal risk of harm and will be treated with dignity and respect; and, if appropriate, that participants may enjoy the participation and interaction with others that it affords.

Once administrative approval has been given to recruit participants from a particular facility, the researcher needs to make initial contact with potential participants. This may be done by discussing the study at a group meeting, writing letters to particular potential participants, or posting flyers in areas frequented by the members of the desired group. Whatever the format, this initial information should include the purpose of the study, the actual activities in which the participant would be participating, the time commitment required to participate, and the means by which interested parties can contact the researcher.

■ DATA COLLECTION

The three major types of data collection tools used by rehabilitation researchers are biophysiological instruments, interviews, and questionnaires. Details regarding the development and administration of interviews and questionnaires are presented in Chapters 13 and 16 and are not repeated here. This section of the chapter focuses on general principles of data collection or specific data collection issues related to the use of biophysiological instruments.

Data Collection Procedures

When using existing instrumentation, the researcher must be familiar with both the manufacturer's instructions for use of the equipment and the protocols that other researchers have followed with the equipment. From this information, decisions can be made about the procedures for data collection. Although a general procedure for data collection will have been developed for the research proposal, very detailed procedural guidelines should be established and written down so that they can be implemented uniformly within the study. For example, a procedure such as height measurement seems simple and would not require detailed description in a proposal. However, before data collection is begun, the specific procedure for taking the height measurement should be developed: Will the measurement be taken with participants barefoot, stocking-footed, or in shoes? Will participants be instructed to stand comfortably or stand tall? Should the head be comfortably erect or in military axial extension? Written standardization procedures are particularly important if more than one researcher will be measuring participants.

Accuracy checks of the equipment should be conducted, if necessary. Goniometers can be checked against known angles, scales can be checked against known weights, and calibration of equipment can be accomplished according to manufacturer's instructions. In some instances, the researcher may wish to have an engineer or manufacturer's technician give the equipment a mechanical or electrical checkout to determine that it is operating properly before data are collected.

Safeguarding Data

When collecting data, the researcher needs to take steps to ensure quality and completeness. Although specific suggestions for data collection are provided in the following sections, all researchers must consider the overriding concern for the safety of data that have been collected. Briefcases get lost, cars get stolen, hard drives crash, dogs chew, and buildings can be destroyed by fires or floods. Given the many possible disasters that can threaten one's data, it makes sense to maintain backup copies of the information one has collected. If the data are collected and stored on computer disk, make a backup copy of the disk. If the data are collected on handwritten forms, either make copies of the completed forms or transfer the information to a data file soon after collecting it.

The two copies of the data should be stored in two different locations; it does no good to have two copies of the data if both are in the same file that was stored directly under the pipe that burst. If several researchers collaborate with one another, then different researchers should probably keep the data in different locations. The IRB will want to know how data storage and backup procedures protect the confidentiality of the participants, particularly if the data set includes information that could identify participants.

Protecting Participant Identity

When each participant enters the trial, he or she should be assigned a number and, if appropriate, a study group according to one of the plans developed in Chapter 8. A master list specifying each participant's name, contact information if appropriate, study identification number, and group membership should be maintained. If data recorders and participants are blind to group membership, generally only one researcher has access to the master list. This researcher should keep the master list in a secure location where other researchers will not accidentally come across the information; a second copy should be kept separately from the original copy, but still in a secured location.

Data Recording Forms

Researchers must design forms for data collection. Today, the form may be a pen-and-paper form or one that is filled out directly on a computer or even a personal digital assistant.

The form should contain space for each participant's identification number but not name. The order of items on the form should be carefully considered to coincide with the order in which the information will be collected. Adequate space should be left for a readable response to the information.

In general, the information should be collected at the highest measurement level possible. For example, adult ages should be recorded as age at last birthday. Even if the researcher plans to categorize participants into age groups, such as those younger than 60 and those 60 and older, it is wise to collect the information as actual age and then code it into groups. In this way, if a later research question requires actual age, that information is available. If just the group membership (younger than 60 or 60 and older) is recorded originally, then there is no way to later determine participants' actual ages.

If data require coding (e.g., conversion of letters into numbers and collapse of actual ages into age groups) for analysis, the form should be designed to facilitate the coding process. Figure 27–2 shows a completed data collection form with space for data coding for the hypothetical total knee arthroplasty study described in Section 6 of this text (see Tables 19–1 and 19–2). The blank spaces on the right-hand side of the form are for the pieces of information that will be entered in the computer data file. Some information such as the date and the name of the researcher collecting the data may not be relevant to the final data set, but may be useful to have if there is a question about a piece of information. For two of the deformity variables, actual angular value is reduced to a category; however, there is room on the form for both the actual value and the code that corresponds to the category in which the angular value belongs.

Pilot Study

A pilot study is crucial to the smooth running of a research trial. In a pilot study, the researchers go through a dress rehearsal of the research study, using a few volunteers similar to those who will participate in the study. The pilot study allows the researchers to take care of small glitches in the procedure and reveals the little details that need attending to: How long does it actually take to collect the data? Is the planned sequence cumbersome? Is another assistant needed for one part of the study? How much paper is used for the computer printout, and is there enough available to complete the study? Is an extension cord or extra batteries needed to power the equipment? Should office supplies be handy?

Scheduling Participants and Personnel

The pilot study allows the researcher to make educated guesses about how the data collection will proceed. Participants in the actual study should expect the researcher to provide a realistic estimate of the time it will take to complete their participation. Participants may not mind participating in a study that requires 5 hours of data collection as long as they know up-front that this is the time that will be involved. Participants will understandably be upset and may withdraw from participation if they are initially led to believe that data collection will require 1 hour and are still waiting to finish after 3 hours.

Adequate personnel need to be available for data collection. The types of tasks that need to be accomplished are greeting participants as they arrive, explaining the study and securing informed consent, telephoning participants who have not arrived as expected, gathering background information and screening participants to ensure that they meet inclusion criteria, preparing participants for data collection, collecting the actual data, spotting participants for safety, and thanking participants for their assistance. In some studies, one researcher could handle all these tasks; in others, five or six researchers might be required.

TOTAL KNEE ARTHROPLASTY REHABILITATION STUDY

BACKGROUND INFORMATION

Case Number (CN)   _1_ _5_

Clinic Attended (CL)
1 =   Community Hospital
2 =   Memorial Hospital   _2_
3 =   Religious Hospital

Patient Sex (SEX)
      0 =   Male
      1 =   Female   _1_

Patient Age in years at last birthday (AGE)   _6_ _8_

Type of Prosthesis (PRO)
      1 =   Total condylar
      2 =   Posterior stabilizer
      3 =   Flat tibial plateau   _2_

Miscellaneous Information
      Surgeon   _Bennett_
      Side of Surgery   _Ⓡ_
      Date of Surgery   _2-12-04_
      Diagnosis   _OA_

THREE WEEK POSTOPERATIVE DATA

Date   _3-5-04_

Three-week ROM, degrees (W3R)
Clinician   _60_   _0_ _7_ _6_

SIX WEEK POSTOPERATIVE DATA

Date   _3-25-04_

Clinician   _60_

Six-week ROM, degrees (W6R)   _0_ _7_ _0_

SIX MONTH POSTOPERATIVE DATA

Date   _8-15-04_

Six-month ROM, degrees (M6R)   _0_ _9_ _5_

Six-month Extension Torque, N•m (E)   _1_ _7_ _0_

FIGURE 27–2. Data collection form, with coding column.

Six-Month Flexion Torque, N•m (F)   *1* *0* *2*

Gait Velocity, cm/s (V)   *1* *6* *5*

Flexion Contracture at Six Months (DFC)

    Value   *8°*

    1 =   >15 degrees
    (2 =)   6 to 15 degrees
    3 =   0 to 5 degrees   *2*

Varus/Valgus Angulation in Stance (DVV)

    Value   *4° varus*

    1 =   >10 degrees valgus
    2 =   >5 degrees varus or 6 to 10 degrees valgus
    (3 =)   5 degrees varus to 5 degrees valgus   *3*

Mediolateral Stability (DML)
    1 =   Marked instability
    (2 =)   Moderate instability
    3 =   Stable   *2*

Anteroposterior Stability with Knee at 90° Flexion (DAP)
    1 =   Marked instability
    (2 =)   Moderate instability
    3 =   Stable   *2*

Distance Walked (ADW)
    5 =   Unlimited
    (4 =)   4 to 6 blocks
    3 =   2 to 3 blocks
    2 =   Indoors only
    1 =   Transfers only   *4*

Assistive Device (AAD)
    5 =   None
    4 =   Cane outside
    (3 =)   Cane full time
    2 =   Two canes, crutches
    1 =   Walker or unable   *3*

Stair Climbing (ASC)
    (5 =)   Reciprocal, no rail
    4 =   Reciprocal, with rail
    3 =   One at a time, with or without rail
    2 =   One at a time, with rail and assistive device
    1 =   Unable to climb stairs   *5*

Rising from Chair (ARC)
    (5 =)   No arm assistance
    4 =   Single arm assistance
    3 =   Difficult with two arm assistance
    2 =   Needs assistance of another
    1 =   Unable to rise   *5*

FIGURE 27–2. *Continued*

■ DATA ANALYSIS

The ease with which the data analysis is accomplished depends greatly on whether the researcher has (1) written a well-developed proposal with a sound plan for data analysis and (2) collected data carefully with an eye to the analysis stage. In discussing data analysis, this section presumes that a computer statistical package and a statistical consultant are available. For all but the smallest data sets, both are necessary. After a discussion of the roles of computers and consultants, suggestions are provided for the three steps of data analysis: data coding, data entry, and statistical analysis.

Many computer statistical packages are available for use on personal or mainframe computers. Three widely used statistical packages are SPSS, Statistical Analysis System (SAS), and Biomedical Data Processing (BMDP); all three are available in mainframe or personal computer versions. Many other programs are also available.[24,25] The basic procedure for all of the computer statistical packages is that the variables of interest are defined, the data are coded and entered into a data file, and then the analyses are run.

Statistical consultants can be used in several different ways. First, they can be consulted during the planning stages of a project to help determine whether the planned design can be analyzed in a way that will answer the research question. Second, they can help the researcher determine the sample size needed to obtain statistically significant results given certain assumptions about the size of differences between groups and the extent of variability within groups. Third, they can provide access to and are knowledgeable about statistical software. Fourth, they can check any analysis the researcher might have done on his or her own. Finally, they can review the written report of a research project to ensure that what the researcher has written about the statistical analysis is in fact what was done.

Before working with statistical consultants, the researcher must have a clear idea of the purposes of his or her research. A list of proposed variables and the values they may take is essential because statistical decisions will be based in part on the measurement characteristics of the data. Consultants may also wish to review published reports of studies similar to the one being planned so they can see the type of analysis that is the norm in the discipline or for a particular journal.

The researcher and consultant must be clear about who will do which tasks associated with the analysis. Will the consultant enter data, run the analysis, prepare summary tables, and summarize the results for the researcher? Or will the researcher enter the data, receive a stack of printouts, and contact the consultant only if there are any questions? Because the consultant will likely work for an hourly fee, the researcher should ask the consultant for an estimate of the number of hours that will be required for the level of involvement desired.

Data Coding

The first step of data analysis is to develop a coding scheme for the data. The coding scheme for our hypothetical total knee arthroplasty data was initially presented in Table 19–1. Figure 27–2 shows how the coding scheme is translated into a form that encourages simultaneous data collection and coding.

Responses that are letters or descriptors (A, B, C, and D on multiple-choice items; "strongly agree," "agree," "neutral," "disagree," and "strongly disagree" for Likert-type items) are generally converted into numbers for data analysis. Some statistical programs permit the researcher to enter the letter and convert it to a number; others require that numbers be entered.

The researcher needs to decide how to handle missing data points. One option is to simply leave them as blanks in the data set. In other instances, the researcher may want frequency counts of missing data or may wish to analyze a subgroup of individuals who did not respond to a certain question. In these cases, missing data need to be given their own code. The number

9 or 99 is often used as the code for missing data. For some analyses, researchers "impute" values by, for example, entering the mean value for any missing data.

Some questionnaire items may permit multiple responses. For example, a multiple-choice item may ask respondents to indicate all the choices that apply to their situation. Coding of multiple responses is often best accomplished by converting the single item into several yes/no items. Assume that in our coding system a "yes" response is coded 1 and a "no" response is coded 0. The response for a respondent who checked A, C, and E out of A through F responses for a multiple-answer item would be coded as follows: A = 1, B = 0, C = 1, D = 0, E = 1, and F = 0.

Once the coding scheme is accomplished, the researcher should go through the data and convert it to codes as necessary. Although some researchers may be able to sit in front of the computer with raw data and simultaneously code and enter it, most will have a more accurate data set, and will save time in the long run, if they perform coding and entering separately. After the data have been coded initially, the codes need to be rechecked and corrected by either the original coder or another member of the research team.

Data Entry

Once the data are coded, they need to be entered into the computer for analysis. In many instances, the data file can be created through a standard spreadsheet program and then transferred into a format that can be used by the statistical software. Although the actual procedures for data entry vary from package to package, the basic structure of a data file is that the variables are represented by columns and the participants by rows, as shown initially in Table 19–2 for the hypothetical study of patients with total knee arthroplasty.

When data have already been coded before they are entered, the researcher can enter data quickly without needing to think about what the numbers actually mean. Some researchers find that data entry goes more quickly if one person reads the numbers aloud and another enters them.

After data entry, the data set needs to be edited against the data-coding sheets. For some variables, it is possible to do "logical" tests of the data—if a variable can take values of 1 through 5, then the presence of a few 6s in the data base must be errors. Only after the data set is edited, or "cleaned," is the researcher ready to run the statistical analyses that will answer the research questions.[26,27]

Statistical Analysis

Too often, investigators test their research hypotheses without first gaining a sense of the character of the data set. The first statistical procedure done should be running frequencies and descriptive data for each variable within the data set as a whole. In doing so, the researcher can get a sense of the distribution, means and standard deviations, and frequencies of the variables overall. If there are very extreme values for some variables, the researcher should recheck them against the original data sheets for accuracy. If the person collecting the data thought there might be an irregularity, it may be noted on the original data collection sheet. Extreme values are known as *outliers* and may sometimes be deleted from a data set with justification. A statistical consultant can help the researcher decide when it is reasonable to delete outliers.

Next, the researcher should divide the total sample into groups, if appropriate to the study purposes. For example, after the descriptive information about the total knee arthroplasty sample has been examined, frequencies, means, and standard deviations for each of the clinics under study should be run. This tells the researcher whether data are normally distributed and whether there is homogeneity of variance within the subgroups of interest. This information is essential to determining whether the assumptions for parametric testing are met. If they are not, then the researcher adopts the nonparametric contingency plan for the variables that have not met parametric assumptions.

Only after the data have been examined as noted previously can the statistical tests of interest be conducted. Many of the programs have a dizzying array of options from which to choose for a given statistical test. If uncertain about which options are appropriate, the researcher should use the services of a statistical consultant.

■ SUMMARY

A research proposal is a blueprint for a study, specifying the investigators, research problem, purposes, methods, references, methods of dissemination of results, budget, and work plan. Research proposals must be approved by facility administrators, an academic committee, an IRB, or some combination of these entities. The role of the IRB is to ensure that the investigators have put into place procedures needed to safeguard the rights of their participants, including their privacy rights. Research proposals are also used to secure funding for the study. Major sources of funding include institutions, corporations, foundations, and the government. Increasing levels of formalization of the grant application and award process are exerted as the research moves from institutional funding to government funding. Many private foundations and government agencies sponsor research that is of interest to rehabilitation professionals.

Implementation of a research project requires attention to detail at every step of the process. Recruitment of participants involves consideration of physician consent, participant consent, administrative approval, and generalizability of research findings. Researchers must attend to many details related to data collection, including specific procedures, ensuring the safety of the data, protecting the identity of participants, developing data collection forms, conducting pilot studies, and scheduling participants and personnel. Data analysis for all but the smallest data sets requires the use of a computer statistical package and a statistical consultant.

REFERENCES

1. Whyte J. Building a program of outcomes research: personal reflections. *Am J Phys Med Rehabil.* 2001;80: 865-874.
2. Krathwohl DR. *How to Prepare a Research Proposal. Guidelines for Funding and Dissertations in the Social and Behavioral Sciences.* 3rd ed. Syracuse, NY: Syracuse University Press; 1988.
3. Brink P, Wood MJ. *Basic Steps in Planning Nursing Research: From Question to Proposal.* 5th ed. Boston, Mass: Jones & Bartlett; 2001.
4. US Department of Health and Human Services. *Title 45 CFR Part 46 Protection of Human Subjects.* Available at: http://ohsr.od.nih.gov/mpa/45cfr46.php3. Accessed October 30, 2003.
5. King NMP, Henderson GE, Stein J, ed. *Beyond Regulations: Ethics in Human Subjects Research.* Chapel Hill, NC: University of North Carolina Press; 1999.
6. Smith T. *Ethics in Medical Research: A Handbook of Good Practice.* New York, NY: Cambridge University Press; 1999.
7. Evans D, Evans M. *A Decent Proposal: Ethical Review of Clinical Research.* New York, NY: John Wiley & Sons; 1996.
8. Levine RJ. *Ethics and Regulation of Clinical Research.* 2nd ed. New Haven, Conn: Yale University Press; 1988.
9. Federman DD, Hanna KE, Rodriguez LL, Institute of Medicine (US) Committee on Assessing the System for Protecting Human Research Participants. *Responsible Research: A Systems Approach to Protecting Research Participants.* Washington, DC: National Academies Press; 2003.
10. Allmark. The ethics of research with children. *Nurs Res.* 2002;10:7-19.
11. Bravo G, Pâquet M, Dubois MF. Knowledge of the legislation governing proxy consent to treatment and research. *J Med Ethics.* 2003;29:44-50.
12. AGS Ethics Committee. Informed consent for research on human subjects with dementia. *J Am Geriatr Soc.* 1998;46:1308-1310.
13. Wiles R. Physiotherapy Research Foundation: review of activity 1995-2001. *Physiotherapy.* 2003;89:138-139.
14. *The Foundation Directory.* 2003 ed. New York, NY: Foundation Center; 2003.
15. *Corporate Foundation Profiles.* 12th ed. New York, NY: Foundation Center; 2002.
16. *Grants for the Physically and Mentally Disabled.* 2003/2004 ed. New York, NY: Foundation Center; 2003.
17. *National Guide to Funding in Health.* 8th ed. New York, NY: Foundation Center; 2003.
18. *Catalog of Federal Domestic Assistance.* Available at: http://www.cfda.gov. Accessed January 6, 2004.

19. *Annual Register of Grant Support 2004*. 37th ed. Chicago, Ill: RR Bowker Publishing; 2004.

20. *Directory of Research Grants 2004*. Westport, Conn: Greenwood Publishing Group; 2004.

21. Reif-Lehrer L. *Grant Application Writer's Handbook*. 4th ed. Boston, Mass: Jones & Bartlett Publishers; 2004.

22. Selby-Harrington ML, Donat PL, Hibbard HD. Guidance for managing a research grant. *Nurs Res*. 1993;42:54-58.

23. Findley TW, Daum MC, Macedo JA. Research in physical medicine and rehabilitation: VI. Research project management. *Am J Phys Med Rehabil*. 1989;68:288-299.

24. Morgan WT. A review of eight statistics software packages for general use. *Am Stat*. 1998;52:70-82.

25. The Scientific Computing and Instrumentation Internet guide to statistical software. *Sci Computing Instrumentation*. 2002;19(10):36-38.

26. Roberts BL, Anthony MK, Madigan EA, Chen Y. Data management: cleaning and checking. *Nurs Res*. 1997; 46:350-352.

27. Findley TW, Stineman MG. Research in physical medicine and rehabilitation: V. Data entry and early exploratory data analysis. *Am J Phys Med Rehabil*. 1989;68:240-251.

Publishing and Presenting Research

Publication of Research	Presentation of Research
Types of Publications	Platform Presentations
Peer Review Process	Poster Presentations
Authorship and Acknowledgment	**Summary**
Multiple Publication	
Style Issues	
Components of a Research Article	

Research can never influence practice if it remains in a file drawer. Therefore, the culmination of the research endeavor is the dissemination of results. When made public, research can fulfill its goal of adding to the body of evidence on which clinicians draw when working with patients or clients. This is not to say, however, that all research that is conducted should be disseminated. Some research is so flawed that valid conclusions cannot be drawn from the results. Given this caveat, once an investigator has obtained results that have something to add to the body of knowledge, he or she needs to find the appropriate way to disseminate the results. There are two main mechanisms for doing so: publication and presentation.

This chapter describes the publication and presentation process and presents guidelines for developing effective publications and presentations. Guidelines for manuscript preparation, a complete manuscript in two different formats, and a presentation script and visuals are provided in Appendixes D through G, respectively.

■ PUBLICATION OF RESEARCH

The main vehicle for publication of research results is the journal article. This section differentiates between types of publications and journals; discusses the peer review process, authorship, and acknowledgment issues in publication; and presents a variety of language and usage issues that arise when writing about research.

Types of Publications

Professional publications usually fall into one of three categories: journals, magazines, and newsletters. Newsletters present news of interest to subscribers or members. They may occasionally highlight important research findings but do not report original research. Many state chapters of professional associations publish newsletters regularly.

Magazines are publications with full-length articles about general topics of interest to professionals. Some magazine articles may refer to

463

original research, but they do not ordinarily report original research. Articles on practice management, overviews of patient care for certain groups, and discussions of professional issues are appropriate topics for professional magazines.

In general, journals have as their primary purpose the reporting of original research findings in a defined area, although some journals have as their mission the publication of review articles. When publication of original research is the primary focus of a journal, this does not preclude publication of review articles, editorials, or other features such as book reviews or the news of a professional association. There are two types of journals: peer reviewed or non–peer reviewed. In considering a manuscript submitted for publication, editors of peer-reviewed, or *refereed*, journals contact professionals who are knowledgeable about the content area of a manuscript to determine whether the manuscript has scientific rigor and significantly adds to knowledge in the discipline. The final decision about whether a paper is published is made by an editor who is a scholar within the discipline. Publication decisions for non–peer-reviewed, or *nonrefereed*, journals may be made by individuals who are professional editors rather than scholars within the discipline. A journal's peer review status may be mentioned in its instructions to authors and can be found in directories of serials that are in the reference section of the library.[1,2]

Peer Review Process

The personnel involved in the peer review process typically include the journal editor, an editorial board chaired by the editor, and manuscript reviewers. All of these individuals are scholars or practitioners in the discipline or related areas. The journal editor is appointed by the managing body that publishes the journal; the editorial board is usually appointed by the editor, with the consent of the managing body that publishes the journal; and the editorial board establishes qualifications for being a manuscript reviewer and accepts applications from interested professionals. For many journals, all these positions are voluntary; however, the editors of larger journals may receive a stipend or honorarium.

When a manuscript is submitted to a peer-reviewed journal for consideration for publication, a chain of events is triggered. The editor or staff reviews the manuscript to determine whether it meets technical requirements (e.g., length, reference style) and whether it fits the general mission of the journal. If either of these conditions is not met, the manuscript is returned to the authors without further review. If the manuscript meets the technical and mission criteria, then it is retained for further review.

The manuscript is usually assigned for review to one editorial board member and one or more manuscript reviewers. The board and manuscript reviewers are selected on the basis of their area of expertise in the profession or their knowledge of the research methods used by the authors. The board member and reviewers critique the manuscript to determine the soundness of the research design, the importance and usefulness of the research in light of other literature and the needs of practitioners, and the clarity and readability of the manuscript.

The manuscript reviewers summarize their opinions of the manuscript to the editorial board member and indicate whether they believe it merits publication. The editorial board member synthesizes his or her opinion with the input from the various reviewers and renders an opinion about the paper to the editor.

Based on the information from the editorial board member and reviewers, the editor makes a decision about publication of the manuscript. A manuscript generally has one of four fates: acceptance, provisional acceptance pending revision, rejection with suggestion to rewrite, or rejection without suggestion to rewrite. Very few manuscripts are accepted for publication without revisions. A manuscript may be accepted provisionally pending revisions when the content and structure of the study seem sound and useful, but the article format needs to be polished. A rejection with a suggestion to rewrite usually means that the topic is important to the profession, but the article as written is too incomplete or disorganized to permit judgment about the credibility of the research. A rejection without a suggestion to rewrite usually means that the topic is simply not a high priority for the journal or that the research methods are too flawed to permit valid conclusions.

As might be inferred by the process just described, peer review is time-consuming. Several months may elapse between submission and a first decision about the manuscript. Author revisions may take several more months, as will final editing of the manuscript by the journal staff. Moreover, because many journals have a backlog of articles waiting to be published, publication of an accepted paper may be delayed several more months. It is not uncommon for more than a year to elapse between submission of a manuscript and its eventual publication.

Authorship and Acknowledgment

Today, many journal articles are cowritten by multiple researchers. In addition to the authors, there are often individuals who have contributed to the study and deserve acknowledgment at the conclusion of the article. Because authorship and acknowledgment involve prestige and recognition, there are often controversies about who should be an author, in what order the authors should be presented, and who should be acknowledged.

Various groups provide guidelines to help researchers make authorship and acknowledgment decisions.[3-5] The International Committee of Medical Editors, whose guidelines are followed by many biomedical journals, specifies that for an investigator to be listed as an author of a journal article, substantial contributions should be made in each of the following areas:

- Conception and design, or analysis and interpretation of data
- Drafting the article or revising it critically for important intellectual content

- Final approval of the version to be published[3(p928)]

The American Psychological Association, whose guidelines are followed by many social science and education journals, specifies that authorship "is reserved for people who make a primary contribution to and hold primary responsibility for the data, concepts, and interpretation of results for a published work. Authorship encompasses not only those who do the actual writing but also those who have made substantial scientific contributions to a study."[5(p6)] Mere collection of the data does not meet the requirements of either group, nor does holding an administrative post at the facility at which the research was conducted or simply editing the final manuscript for grammar and style. The central criterion is that those who are listed as authors must have made important intellectual contributions to the work.

The order in which the authors' names are listed should reflect the relative strength of the contributions they have made to the project, with the first author contributing the most and the last author contributing the least. This order should be discussed when tasks are being divided among the researchers in the early stages of a project. The order may change somewhat as the project progresses; before submission of the paper for publication, the authors should negotiate among themselves what the final order will be.

Authors should acknowledge individuals who have made contributions to the project that do not qualify them as authors. Such contributors may include those who collected or analyzed some of the data, colleagues who loaned facilities or fabricated equipment, or peers who provided critical review of early drafts of the manuscript. All acknowledged individuals should receive a copy of the manuscript and give their permission to be named.

Multiple Publication

Journals hold the copyright to materials they publish, requiring that authors transfer the copyright of a work to them in the event it is published. Therefore, journals require authors to disclose prior publication and do not typically accept for consideration papers that have been published in full elsewhere. In addition, journals do not typically permit multiple submission of articles. That is, authors cannot submit the same article for consideration by more than one journal at a time. Therefore, authors identify the journal they think is a best fit for their work, submit the article to that journal for consideration, and wait for a decision from that journal. If the first journal to which an article is submitted rejects the article, the authors are then free submit it to another journal.

Style Issues

The research article is a specialized form of writing. Its hallmarks are precision, conciseness, and consistency. The novelist uses words to paint pictures and uses different words to convey similar meanings in different contexts. Whereas creative use of language makes novels enjoyable, it makes research articles infuriating if different terms are used to represent the same construct.

Each journal publishes its own instructions for authors. These instructions typically specify the types of articles accepted for review, the editorial process, the format that the manuscript should take, the reference style to use, procedures for manuscript submission, and the style manual that should be used to prepare the paper. These instructions can be found in selected issues of the journal or on the journal website.

A style manual is a document of technical information for authors. Most journals that publish rehabilitation research have adopted the style, or a variant of the style, described in the *American Medical Association Manual of Style*[6] or the *Publication Manual of the American Psychological Association*.[5] The major difference between the two styles is the way that references are cited in the text and the format of the reference list. Table 28–1 shows the two different styles for in-text citations and reference lists.

Style manuals specify such things as when numbers are presented as numerals (e.g., 227) and when they are written out (e.g., two hundred twenty-seven), what levels of headings and subheadings to use, how to present mathematical symbols, how to set up tables, how to cite literature in the text of an article, and what format to follow for the reference list at the end of the article. They also present useful writing style and grammar suggestions, including how to differentiate among confusing terms (e.g., *affect* and *effect*), when to use certain punctuation marks, and how to avoid exclusionary language. Table 28–2 presents several style problems that commonly appear in the papers of novice authors. This table can help writers eliminate these mistakes from their papers, but it is no substitute for frequent reference to a style manual. In addition to style manuals, several excellent references provide general guidelines for scientific and medical writing.[7-9]

A set of style guidelines that should be of particular importance to rehabilitation professionals relates to references about people with disabilities. Authors (and clinicians) should pay close attention to the implications of the words they use to refer to this population. Table 28–3 presents a set of guidelines for writing about people with disabilities.[10]

Components of a Research Article

The components of a research article are as follows:

1. Title and title page
2. Abstract
3. Introduction
4. Methods
5. Results
6. Discussion
7. Conclusions
8. Acknowledgments
9. References
10. Tables
11. Figures

TABLE 28-1	Comparison of American Medical Association and American Psychological Association Styles for In-Text Citation and Reference Lists

American Medical Association Manual of Style[6]:

Like Basso and Knapp[1] in the 1980s, Chen and colleagues[2] concluded that use of continuous passive motion after total knee arthroplasty did not have an effect on postoperative edema.

References

1. Basso DM, Knapp L. Comparison of two continuous passive motion protocols for patients with total knee implants. Phys Ther. 1987;67:360-363.
2. Chen B, Zimmerman JR, Soulen L, DeLisa JA. Continuous passive motion after total knee arthroplasty: a prospective study. Am J Phys Med Rehabil. 2000;79:421-426.

Publication Manual of the American Psychological Association[5]:

Like Basso and Knapp (1987), Chen, Zimmerman, Soulen, and Delisa (2000) concluded that use of continuous passive motion after total knee arthroplasty did not have an effect on postoperative edema.

References

Basso, D. M., Knapp, L. (1987). Comparison of two continuous passive motion protocols for patients with total knee implants. *Physical Therapy, 67,* 360-363.

Chen, B., Zimmerman, J. R., Soulen, L., & DeLisa, J. A. (2000). Continuous passive motion after total knee arthroplasty: A prospective study. *American Journal of Physical Medicine and Rehabilitation, 79,* 421-426.

Appendix D provides a numbered list of guidelines for the preparation of each section; Appendix E and Appendix F present the same hypothetical manuscript in AMA and APA style, respectively. Each hypothetical manuscript is annotated with numbers that correspond to the items in Appendix D. Writers should consult the appropriate style manual for additional guidance. In addition, those who expect to present a great deal of graphical data may benefit from consulting detailed texts for guidance.[11,12]

■ PRESENTATION OF RESEARCH

Presentation is the second major format by which research results are disseminated. Many professional associations hold meetings at which research presentations are made. The process of selecting a paper for presentation usually involves submission of an abstract of the study, generally many months in advance of the conference. Some associations use peer review to select abstracts for presentation; others accept any abstracts that meet the technical guidelines and can be accommodated within the conference schedule. Some associations specify that abstracts must be of studies that have not been presented previously. However, because conference presentations are less permanent and less accessible than publications, some conference organizers permit presentation of studies that have been presented elsewhere, particularly if they target a different audience. Thus, as long as it is permitted by the conference organizer, researchers may feel comfortable presenting the results of a study at both a local and national meeting or at meetings for different professional groups. For example, a study related to the roles

TABLE 28-2 Common Style Problems in Manuscripts of Novice Authors

Problem	Example of Problem	Corrected Text
Abbreviation is used without being identified at the first use.	Many children with CP experience communication difficulties. The type of CP has an impact on…	Many children with cerebral palsy (CP) experience communication difficulties. The type of CP has an impact on…
Sentence begins with a numeral.	224 responses were received.	Two hundred twenty-four responses were received. OR We received 224 responses.
Abbreviation of units of measurement is inconsistent or nonstandard (standard units do not have to be spelled out the first time they are used).	Velocity was measured in centimeters per second, with the younger group walking at a rate of 180 cm/sec.	Velocity was measured in cm/s, with the younger group walking at a rate of 180 cm/s.
Language includes jargon or informal terms understood by a small group of professionals.	The participants completed 20 reps of quad sets.	The participants completed 20 repetitions of isometric quadriceps femoris muscle contractions.
Punctuation after quotation marks is incorrect.	Boswell stated that "complacency rules in many professions."	Boswell stated that "complacency rules in many professions."
Author refers to himself or herself in the third person. First person language is preferred today, even in scientific writing.	This author believes that Mayberry overstated his findings.	I believe that Mayberry overstated his findings.
Comparative terms are used, but no comparison is made.	Johnson found an increase in strength of the middle deltoid muscle.	Johnson found an increase in strength of the middle deltoid muscle after completion of the exercise program.
Exclusionary terms are used or awkward constructions are made.	The therapist should not let his emotions cloud his judgment. OR The therapist should not let his/her emotions cloud his/her judgment.	Therapists should not let their emotions cloud their judgment. OR Emotions should not cloud the therapist's judgment.
Male or female is used as a noun rather than an adjective.	We studied 50 females.	We studied 50 women.
Author unnecessarily hyphenates prefixed words.	The post-test scores for the non-injured hand were…	The posttest scores for the noninjured hand were…

of physical therapists and athletic trainers in the clinical setting might be appropriate for presentation at a conference of physical therapists and at a conference for athletic trainers, as long as the conference organizer for the later conference is willing to accept previously presented work.

There are two major formats for conference presentations: platform presentations and poster presentations. Guidelines are available to help individuals plan effective research presentations.[8,12-14] Each presentation format is described and illustrated in the following sections.

TABLE 28-3 Guidelines for Writing about People with Disabilities	
Sensational or Negative Portrayal	*Straightforward, Positive Portrayal*
Traumatic brain injury patient [focuses on the injury rather than the person]	*Individual with a traumatic brain injury* [focuses on the person rather than the injury; use *patient* only if the person is, in fact, undergoing health care]
Physically challenged [euphemisms imply that disabilities cannot be dealt with in a straightforward manner]	*Person with a disability* [puts the person first, then the disability; acknowledges the disability directly]
Special children [attempts to glorify differences]	*Children with disabilities* [straightforward portrayal]
Wheelchair-bound [evokes a confined image contrary to the active role of many people who use wheelchairs]	*Uses a wheelchair* [describes the wheelchair as the tool that it is]
Suffers from multiple sclerosis [sensationalizes the disease]	*Has multiple sclerosis* [states the disease matter-of-factly]

Modified from *Guidelines for Reporting and Writing about People with Disabilities.* The Life Span Institute, Research and Training Center on Independent Living, University of Kansas. Available at: http://www.lsi.ku.edu/lsi/internal/guidelines.html. Accessed January 9, 2004.

Platform Presentations

A platform presentation is made by a researcher to an audience of peers attending the conference. The presentation time is usually short—anywhere from 10 to 20 minutes is common. High-quality visuals are expected to accompany the presentation and most major conferences today use digital projection systems, enabling researchers to incorporate text, tables and graphs, clip art, still photography, and digital video as appropriate to the presentation. A suggested sequence for development of a research presentation is presented here. Appendix G provides a script and visuals for a presentation of the manuscript presented in Appendixes E and F.

1. Complete a draft of the manuscript. A manuscript provides the complete picture of the study to be described in the presentation. However, because most presentations precede submission of the work for publication, the author does not often have a final version of the manuscript available to guide the development of the presentation. However, a draft of the manuscript can help the presenter decide which elements are essential and which can be deleted

for the presentation. In addition, because most research presentations follow the same sequence as a journal article, a draft manuscript provides a ready-made outline for the presentation.

2. Determine which manuscript content is essential for the presentation. Because conference research presentations are brief, presenters need to be selective about the information they include in the presentation. Examine each paragraph of the draft manuscript to determine whether it is essential to an understanding of the project. A guideline for developing the presentation is to spend approximately:

- 10% of the allotted time establishing the problem and context of the study
- 20% of the time describing the methods
- 30% of the time presenting the results
- 30% of the time discussing the results
- 10% of the time summarizing the conclusions

The introduction section of the paper can be shortened by deleting many specific references to the related literature and developing the problem conceptually. The methods section can be shortened by eliminating detail about measurement procedures and minimizing technical information about the instruments used. Remember that a presentation audience just needs to understand the methods and does not need enough detail to replicate them in a future study.

Whereas research papers often include separate instrumentation and procedures sections, a presentation may flow more smoothly if the two are combined. Similarly, some repetition may be eliminated if the data analysis, results, and some parts of the discussion sections of the presentation are integrated. Conclusions should be clear and concise, providing the audience with a few memorable "take-home" points.

3. Divide the manuscript into segments. A general guideline for preparation of a conference presentation is to have each visual displayed for between 10 and 20 seconds, for an average of 4 visuals per minute. A 10-minute presentation might therefore have 40 visuals. This requires that the researcher divide the essential content into small "sound bites" that can each be illustrated with a visual. Varying the length of the segments helps maintain audience interest.

4. Design the visuals. For each text segment, decide whether it is best illustrated with text, a table, a photograph, a drawing, or a graph. Most conferences are set up for horizontal projection, so the presenter should design visuals in a horizontal format. Presentation software is widely available within standard integrated office software packages.

Slides of text should generally contain no more than 10 lines of text and no more than six words per line. The style should be telegraphic, using phrases rather than complete sentences. Text should not exactly repeat the script of the presentation; audiences do not like to have visuals read to them. Use of uppercase and lowercase letters is thought to be more readable than using all capital letters; simple sans serif typefaces are preferred.

Tables of information should contain no more than three columns and no more than seven rows. Use of data tables as they appear in the manuscript is rarely suitable, because they contain far more information than can be absorbed in 10 to 20 seconds. Graphs are often more effective than tables in a presentation.

Photographs should be clear enough that the audience can locate the item of interest quickly. Photographers should strive for an uncluttered background that contrasts well with the subject. Sometimes photographs are simply not the best way to get a visual message across. For example, a line diagram of a particular piece of equipment may be able to focus attention on the relevant portion of the instrument; an illustration of an anatomical part may be more effective than a photograph.

Graphs should be used to illustrate the relationships between different numbers within the data set. Pie charts show proportions well, bar graphs effectively illustrate differences in quantities between groups, and line graphs are ideal for illustrating change across time. Because the visual will be displayed for a limited time, the graph should be as simple and clear as possible. Labels should be large enough to read; words should be kept to a minimum.

5. Draft the visuals. Most large conferences use electronic data projection systems to display presentation graphics directly from the presenter's laptop computer. Presentation software, such as PowerPoint, is a common component of integrated software packages that include word processing, spreadsheet, and presentation capabilities, enabling researchers or their support staff to create their own presentations. Smaller conferences may still rely on slide projection; in this case, researchers can use hospital or university media services departments to assist in producing slides from their graphics program or commercial slide production services, which are available in most large cities.

6. Integrate text and visuals. Once the visuals have been produced, the researcher needs to practice delivering the text and visuals together. Manuscript text is often too sterile for presentation purposes and needs to be redrafted into a more conversational tone. In addition, the text that goes with each visual should help integrate the visuals with the text, without repeating exactly the same information. Integrating the text and visuals is an iterative process that may require a couple rounds of revision of visuals and text until they match well and tell the research story effectively. Figure 28–1 shows a sample graph with presentation text that highlights its important points. Session moderators will cut off presenters who run beyond their allotted time, so it is important to time the practice run-throughs and make adjustments as needed to meet the time limits of the conference.

Presenters need to decide if they want to use a script, notes, or just their visuals to guide the presentation. While some experienced presenters do not use any prompts other than their visuals, most novice presenters benefit from written materials to guide their talk. Even in a high-tech environment, some presenters like to use 3- × 5-inch cards on which a script or notes for each visual is written. Others like to use standard-sized paper on which the script or notes for each visual are written in paragraph form, with marks inserted to indicate when to change the visual. Still others like to use the "notes" feature of their graphics program to print out hard copies of the visuals with accompanying text. Appendix G shows the text and visuals

for a presentation of the hypothetical paper provided in Appendixes E and F.

Poster Presentations

Poster presentations are a common feature at conferences and are becoming increasingly accepted as a means of disseminating scientific information. A poster session consists of a collection of large posters describing research studies. The posters are generally displayed for several hours, and presenters are required to be with their posters for a certain portion of the display time. The advantages of a poster session over a platform presentation are (1) conference attendees can view the posters when they have time and (2) the researcher has more opportunity to interact with interested colleagues.

The space available for the posters is generally about 4 × 8 feet. At most large conferences, the norm is now an attractive single-panel poster that is unrolled from a tube and tacked up onto the board. Although these posters are often designed by professional graphic artists working with the researcher through the media services department of a hospital or university, it is

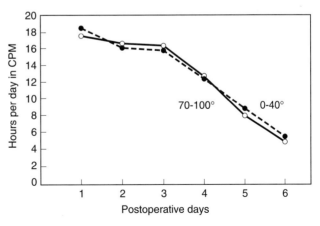

FIGURE 28–1. Example of visual and text for a platform presentation. Text highlights important features of the graph shown in the visual. *CPM,* Continuous passive motion]

The two CPM groups received nearly identical hours per day in CPM, as shown by the two lines on this graph. Observe the gradual reduction in hours of CPM per day, starting at about 18 hours per day and ending up at less than 6 hours per day by the sixth postoperative day.

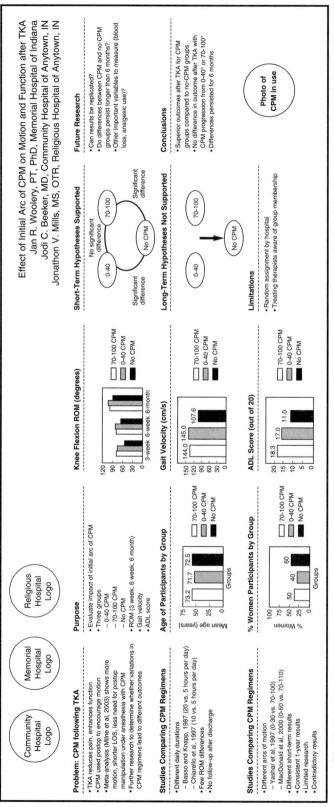

FIGURE 28–2. Schematic diagram for a poster presentation. *ADL*, Activities of daily living; *CPM*, continuous passive motion; *ROM*, range of motion. (From Woolery JR, Beeker JC, Mills JV. Effect of initial arc of CPM on motion and function after TKA [hypothetical article presented in appendices E-G].)

possible for researchers without access to these resources to design attractive posters in standard graphics packages and send them to a commercial printer for production. It is, however, still acceptable to create a multiple-panel poster by designing a series of mini-posters that are easily printed on a standard color printer and mounted and laminated at a local copy shop. Researchers who prepare posters should ensure that the type is readable from a distance of 2 to 3 feet and that the sequence in which the poster should be examined is clear. Figure 28–2 shows a schematic diagram of a poster.

■ SUMMARY

Research results are disseminated through either publication or presentation. Publication of research results in journals is a formal process guided by peer review. Journal articles usually follow a standard sequence: introduction, methods, results, discussion, and conclusions. Presentation of research usually occurs at conferences through a platform talk with accompanying visuals or through a poster session in which the researcher can interact with conference attendees less formally than in the platform format. Presentations usually follow the same sequence as journal articles.

REFERENCES

1. *The Serials Directory*. Birmingham, Ala: EBSCO Industries, Inc.; 2003.
2. *Ulrich's Periodicals Directory*. 42nd ed. New Providence, NJ: RR Bowker; 2003.
3. International Committee of Medical Journal Editors. *Uniform requirements for manuscripts submitted to biomedical journals: writing and editing for biomedical publication*. Available at: http://www.icjme.org. Accessed January 9, 2004.
4. Friedman PJ. *A new standard for authorship*. Available at: http://www.councilscienceeditors.org/services/friedman_ article.cfm. Accessed January 9, 2004.
5. *Publication Manual of the American Psychological Association*. 5th ed. Washington, DC: American Psychological Association; 2001.
6. *American Medical Association Manual of Style*. 9th ed. Baltimore, Md: Williams & Wilkins; 1998.
7. Day RA. *How to Write and Publish a Scientific Paper*. 5th ed. Phoenix, Ariz: Oryx Press; 1998.
8. Browner WS. *Publishing and Presenting Clinical Research*. Baltimore, Md: Lippincott Williams & Wilkins; 1999.
9. Knight KL, Ingersoll CD. Structure of a scholarly manuscript: 66 tips for what goes where. *J Ath Train*. 1996;31:201-206.
10. Life Span Institute, Research and Training Center on Independent Living, University of Kansas. *Guidelines for Reporting and Writing about People with Disabilities*. Available at: http://www.lsi.ku.edu/lsi/internal/guidlines.html. Accessed January 9, 2004.
11. Cleveland WS. *The Elements of Graphing Data*. Revised. Murray Hill, NJ: AT&T Bell Laboratories; 1994.
12. Nicol AA, Pexman PM. *Displaying Your Findings: A Practical Guide for Creating Figures, Posters, and Presentations*. Washington, DC: American Psychological Association; 2003.
13. Anholt RRH. *Dazzle 'em with Style: The Art of Oral Scientific Presentation*. New York, NY: WH Freeman; 1994.
14. Alley M. *The Craft of Scientific Presentations: Critical Steps to Succeed and Critical Errors to Avoid*. New York, NY: Springer Verlag; 2002.

Random Numbers Table

Table of 14,000 Random Units

Line/Col.	(1)	(2)	(3)	(4)	(5)	(6)	(7)	(8)	(9)	(10)	(11)	(12)	(13)	(14)
1	10480	15011	01536	02011	81647	91646	69179	14194	62590	36207	20969	99570	91291	90700
2	22368	46573	25595	85393	30995	89198	27982	53402	93965	34095	52666	19174	39615	99505
3	24130	48360	22527	97265	76393	64809	15179	24830	49340	32081	30680	19655	63348	58629
4	42167	93093	06243	61680	07856	16376	39440	53537	71341	57004	00849	74917	97758	16379
5	37570	39975	81837	16656	06121	91782	60468	81305	49684	60672	14110	06927	01263	54613
6	77921	06907	11008	42751	27756	53498	18602	70659	90655	15053	21916	81825	44394	42880
7	99562	72905	56420	69994	98872	31016	71194	18738	44013	48840	63213	21069	10634	12952
8	96301	91977	05463	07972	18876	20922	94595	56869	69014	60045	18425	84903	42508	32307
9	89579	14342	63661	10281	17453	18103	57740	84378	25331	12566	58678	44947	05585	56941
10	85475	36857	43342	53988	53060	59533	38867	62300	08158	17983	16439	11458	18593	64952
11	28918	69578	88231	33276	70997	79936	56865	05859	90106	31595	01547	85590	91610	78188
12	63553	40961	48235	03427	49626	69445	18663	72695	52180	20847	12234	90511	33703	90322
13	09429	93969	52636	92737	88974	33488	36320	17617	30015	08272	84115	27156	30613	74952
14	10365	61129	87529	85689	48237	52267	67689	93394	01511	26358	85104	20285	29975	89868
15	07119	97336	71048	08178	77233	13916	47564	81056	97735	85977	29372	74461	28551	90707
16	51085	12765	51821	51259	77452	16308	60756	92144	49442	53900	70960	63990	75601	40719
17	02368	21382	53404	60268	89368	19885	55322	44819	01188	65255	64835	44919	05944	55157
18	01011	54092	33362	94904	31273	04146	18594	29852	71585	85030	51132	01915	92747	64951
19	52162	53916	46369	58586	23216	14513	83149	98736	23495	64350	94738	17752	35156	35749
20	07056	97628	33787	09998	42698	06691	76988	13602	51851	46104	88916	19509	25625	58104
21	48663	91245	85828	14346	09172	30168	90229	04734	59193	22178	30421	61666	99904	32812
22	54164	58492	22421	74103	47070	25306	76468	26384	58151	06646	21524	15227	96909	44592
23	32639	32363	05597	24200	13363	38005	94342	28728	35806	06912	17012	64161	18296	22851
24	29334	27001	87637	87308	58731	00256	45834	15398	46557	41135	10367	07684	36188	18510
25	02488	33062	28834	07351	19731	92420	60952	61280	50001	67658	32586	86679	50720	94953
26	81525	72295	04839	96423	24878	82651	66566	14778	76797	14780	13300	87074	79666	95725
27	29676	20591	68086	26432	46901	20849	89768	81536	86645	12659	92259	57102	80428	25280
28	00742	57392	39064	66432	84673	40027	32832	61362	98947	96067	64760	64584	96096	98253
29	05366	04213	25669	26422	44407	44048	37937	63904	45766	66134	75470	66520	34693	90449
30	91921	26418	64117	94305	26766	25940	39972	22209	71500	64568	91402	42416	07844	69618
31	00582	04711	87917	77341	42206	35126	74087	99547	81817	42607	43808	76655	62028	76690
32	00725	69884	62797	56170	86324	88072	76222	36086	84637	93161	76038	65855	77919	88006
33	69011	65797	95876	55293	18988	27354	26575	08625	40801	59920	29841	80150	12777	48501
34	25976	57948	29888	88604	67917	48708	18912	82271	65424	69774	33611	54262	85963	03547
35	09763	83473	73577	12908	30883	18317	28290	35797	05998	41688	34952	37888	38917	88050
36	91567	42595	27958	30134	04024	86385	29880	99730	55536	84855	29080	09250	79656	73211
37	17955	56349	90999	49127	20044	59931	06115	20542	18059	02008	73708	83517	36103	42791
38	46503	18584	18845	49618	02304	51038	20655	58727	28168	15475	56942	53389	20562	87338
39	92157	89634	94824	78171	84610	82834	09922	25417	44137	48413	25555	21246	35509	20468
40	14577	62765	35605	81263	39667	47358	56873	56307	61607	49518	89656	20103	77490	18062
41	98427	07523	33362	64270	01638	92477	66969	98420	04880	45585	46565	04102	46880	45709
42	34914	63976	88720	82765	34476	17032	87589	40836	32427	70002	70663	88863	77775	69348
43	70060	28277	39475	46473	23219	53416	94970	25832	69975	94884	19661	72828	00102	66794
44	53976	54914	06990	67245	68350	82948	11398	42878	80287	88267	47363	46634	06541	97809
45	76072	29515	40980	07391	58745	25774	22987	80059	39911	96189	41151	14222	60697	59583
46	90725	52210	83974	29992	65831	38857	50490	83765	55657	14361	31720	57375	56228	41546
47	64364	67412	33339	31926	14883	24413	59744	92351	97473	89286	35931	04110	23726	51900
48	08962	00358	31662	25388	61642	34072	81249	35648	56891	69352	48373	45578	78547	81788
49	95012	68379	93526	70765	10593	04542	76463	54328	02349	17247	28865	14777	62730	92277
50	15664	10493	20492	38391	91132	21999	59516	81652	27195	48223	46751	22923	32261	85653
51	16408	81899	04153	53381	79401	21438	83035	92350	36693	31238	59649	91754	72772	02338
52	18629	81953	05520	91962	04739	13092	97662	24822	94730	06496	35090	04822	86772	98289
53	73115	35101	47498	87637	99016	71060	88824	71013	18735	20286	23153	72924	35165	43040
54	57491	16703	23167	49323	45021	33132	12544	41035	80780	45393	44812	12515	98931	91202
55	30405	83946	23792	14422	15059	45799	22716	19792	09983	74353	68668	30429	70735	25499
56	16631	35006	85900	98275	32388	52390	16815	69298	82732	38480	73817	32523	41961	44437
57	96773	20206	42559	78985	05300	22164	24369	54224	35083	19687	11052	91491	60383	19746
58	38935	64202	14349	82674	66523	44133	00697	35552	35970	19124	63318	29686	03387	59846

Table of 14,000 Random Units—cont'd

Line/Col.	(1)	(2)	(3)	(4)	(5)	(6)	(7)	(8)	(9)	(10)	(11)	(12)	(13)	(14)
59	31624	76384	17403	53363	44167	64486	64758	75366	76554	31601	12614	33072	60332	92325
60	78919	19474	23632	27889	47914	02584	37680	20801	72152	39339	34806	08930	85001	87820
61	03931	33309	57047	74211	63445	17361	62825	39908	05607	91284	68833	25570	38818	46920
62	74426	33278	43972	10119	89917	15665	52872	73823	73144	88662	88970	74492	51805	99378
63	09066	00903	20795	95452	92648	45454	09552	88815	16553	51125	79375	97596	16296	66092
64	42238	12426	87025	14267	20979	04508	64535	31355	88064	29472	47689	05974	52468	16834
65	16153	08002	26504	41744	81959	65642	74240	56302	00033	67107	77510	70625	28725	34191
66	21457	40742	29820	96783	29400	21840	15035	34537	33310	06116	95240	15957	16572	06004
67	21581	57802	02050	89728	17937	37621	47075	42080	97403	48626	68995	43805	33386	21597
68	55612	78095	83197	33732	05810	24813	86902	60397	16489	03264	88525	42786	05269	92532
69	44657	66999	99324	51281	84463	60563	79312	93454	68876	25471	93911	25650	12682	73572
70	91340	84979	46949	81973	37949	61023	43997	15263	80644	43942	89203	71795	99533	50501
71	91227	21199	31935	27022	84067	05462	35216	14486	29891	68607	41867	14951	91696	85065
72	50001	38140	66321	19924	72163	09538	12151	06878	91903	18749	34405	56087	82790	70925
73	65390	05224	72958	28609	81406	39147	25549	48542	42627	45233	57202	94617	23772	07896
74	27504	96131	83944	41575	10573	08619	64482	73923	36152	05184	94142	25299	84387	34925
75	37169	94851	39117	89632	00959	16487	65536	49071	39782	17095	02330	74301	00275	48280
76	11508	70225	51111	38351	19444	66499	71945	05422	13442	78675	84081	66938	93654	59894
77	37449	30362	06694	54690	04052	53115	62757	95348	78662	11163	81651	50245	34971	52924
78	46515	70331	85922	38329	57015	15765	97161	17869	45349	61796	66345	81073	46106	79860
79	30986	81223	42416	58353	21532	30502	32305	86482	05174	07901	54339	58861	74818	46942
80	63798	64995	46583	09765	44160	78128	83991	42865	92520	83531	80377	35909	81250	54238
81	82486	84846	99254	67632	43218	50076	21361	64816	51202	88124	41870	52689	51275	83556
82	21885	32906	92431	09060	64297	51674	64126	62570	26123	05155	59194	52799	28225	85762
83	60336	98782	07408	53458	13564	59089	26445	29789	85205	41001	12535	12133	14645	23541
84	43937	46891	24010	25560	86355	33941	25786	54990	71899	15475	95434	98227	21824	19585
85	97656	63175	89303	16275	07100	92063	21942	18611	47348	20203	18534	03862	78095	50136
86	03299	01221	05418	38982	55758	92237	26759	86367	21216	98442	08303	56613	91511	75928
87	79626	06486	03574	17668	07785	76020	79924	25651	83325	88428	85076	72811	22717	50585
88	85636	68335	47539	03129	65651	11977	02510	26113	99447	68645	34327	15152	55230	93448
89	18039	14367	61337	06177	12143	46609	32989	74014	64708	00533	35398	58408	13261	47908
90	08362	15656	60627	36478	65648	16764	53412	09013	07832	41574	17639	82163	60859	75567
91	79556	29068	04142	16268	15387	12856	66227	38358	22478	73373	88732	09443	82558	05250
92	92608	82674	27072	32534	17075	27698	98204	63863	11951	34648	88022	56148	34925	57031
93	23982	25835	40055	67006	12293	02753	14827	22235	35071	99704	37543	11601	35503	85171
94	09915	96306	05908	97901	28395	14186	00821	80703	70426	75647	76310	88717	37890	40129
95	50937	33300	26695	62247	69927	76123	50842	43834	86654	70959	79725	93872	28117	19233
96	42488	78077	69882	61657	34136	79180	97526	43092	04098	73571	80799	76536	71255	64239
97	46764	86273	63003	93017	31204	36692	40202	35275	57306	55543	53203	18098	47625	88684
98	03237	45430	55417	63282	90816	17349	88298	90183	36600	78406	06216	95787	42579	90730
99	86591	81482	52667	61583	14972	90053	89534	76036	49199	43716	97548	04379	46370	28672
100	38534	01715	94964	87288	65680	43772	39560	12918	86537	62738	19636	51132	25739	56947
101	13284	16834	74151	92027	24670	36665	00770	22878	02179	51602	07270	76517	97275	45960
102	21224	00370	30420	03883	96648	89428	41583	17564	27395	63904	41548	49197	82277	24120
103	99052	47887	81085	64933	66279	80432	65793	83287	34142	13241	30590	97760	35848	91983
104	00199	50993	98603	38452	87890	94624	69721	57484	67501	77638	44331	11257	71131	11059
105	60578	06483	28733	37867	07936	98710	98539	27186	31237	80612	44488	97819	70401	95419
106	91240	18312	17441	01929	18163	69201	31211	54288	39296	37318	65724	90401	79017	62077
107	97458	14229	12063	59611	32249	90466	33216	19358	02591	54263	88449	01912	07436	50813
108	35249	38646	34475	72417	60514	69257	12489	51924	86871	92446	36607	11458	30440	52639
109	38980	46600	11759	11900	46743	27860	77940	39298	97838	95145	32378	68038	89351	37005
110	10750	52745	38749	87365	58959	53731	89295	59062	39404	13198	59960	70408	29812	83126
111	36247	27850	73958	20673	37800	63835	71051	84724	52492	22342	78071	17456	96104	18327
112	70994	66986	99744	72438	01174	42159	11392	20724	54322	36923	70009	23233	65438	59685
113	99638	94702	11463	18148	81386	80431	90628	52506	02016	85151	88598	47821	00265	82525
114	72055	15774	43857	99805	10419	76939	25993	03544	21560	83471	43989	90770	22965	44247
115	24038	65541	85788	55835	38835	59399	13790	35112	01324	39520	76210	22467	83275	32286
116	74976	14631	35908	28221	39470	91548	12854	30166	09073	75887	36782	00268	97121	57676

Continued

Table of 14,000 Random Units—cont'd

Line/Col.	(1)	(2)	(3)	(4)	(5)	(6)	(7)	(8)	(9)	(10)	(11)	(12)	(13)	(14)
117	35553	71628	70189	26436	63407	91178	90348	55359	80392	41012	36270	77786	89578	21059
118	35676	12797	51434	82976	42010	26344	92920	92155	58807	54644	58581	95331	78629	73344
119	74815	67523	72985	23183	02446	63594	98924	20633	58842	85961	07648	70164	34994	67662
120	45246	88048	65173	50989	91060	89894	36063	32819	68559	99221	49475	50558	34698	71800
121	76509	47069	86378	41797	11910	49672	88575	97966	32466	10083	54728	81972	58975	30761
122	19689	90332	04315	21358	97428	11188	39062	63312	52496	07349	79178	33692	57352	72862
123	42751	35318	97513	61537	54955	08159	00337	80778	27507	95478	21252	12746	37554	97775
124	11946	22681	45045	13964	57517	59419	58045	44067	58716	58840	45557	96345	33271	53464
125	96518	48688	20996	11090	48396	57177	83867	86464	14342	21545	46717	72364	86954	55580
126	35726	58643	76869	84622	39098	36083	72505	92265	23107	60278	05822	46760	44294	07672
127	39737	42750	48968	70536	84864	64952	38404	94317	65402	13589	01055	79044	19308	83623
128	97025	66492	56177	04049	80312	48028	26408	43591	75528	65341	49044	95495	81256	53214
129	62814	08075	09788	56350	76787	51591	54509	49295	85830	59860	30883	89660	96142	18354
130	25578	22950	15227	83291	41737	79599	96191	71845	86899	70694	24290	01551	80092	82118
131	68763	69576	88991	49662	46704	63362	56625	00481	73323	91427	15264	06969	57048	54149
132	17900	00813	64361	60725	88974	61005	99709	30666	26451	11528	44323	34778	60342	60388
133	71944	60227	63551	71109	05624	43836	58254	26160	32116	63403	35404	57146	10909	07346
134	54684	93691	85132	64399	29182	44324	14491	55226	78793	34107	30374	48429	51376	09559
135	25946	27623	11258	65204	52832	50880	22273	05554	99521	73791	85744	29276	70326	60251
136	01353	39318	44961	44972	91766	90262	56073	06606	51826	18893	83448	31915	97764	75091
137	99083	88191	27662	99113	57174	35571	99884	13951	71057	53961	61448	74909	07322	80960
138	52021	45406	37945	75234	24327	86978	22644	87779	23753	99926	63898	54886	18051	96314
139	78755	47744	43776	83098	03225	14281	83637	55984	13300	52212	58781	14905	46502	04472
140	25282	69106	59180	16257	22810	43609	12224	25643	89884	31149	85423	32581	34374	70873
141	11959	94202	02743	86847	79725	51811	12998	76844	05320	54236	53891	70226	38632	84776
142	11644	13792	98190	01424	30078	28197	55583	05197	47714	68440	22016	79204	06862	94451
143	06307	97912	68110	59812	95448	43244	31262	88880	13040	16458	43813	89416	42482	33939
144	76285	75714	89585	99296	52640	46518	55486	90754	88932	19937	57119	23251	55619	23679
145	55322	07589	39600	60866	63007	20007	66819	84164	61131	81429	60676	42807	78286	29015
146	78017	90928	90220	92503	83375	26986	74399	30885	88567	29169	72816	53357	15428	86932
147	44768	43342	20696	26331	43140	69744	82928	24988	94237	46138	77426	39039	55596	12655
148	25100	19336	14605	86603	51680	97678	24261	02464	86563	74812	60069	71674	15478	47642
149	83612	46623	62876	85197	07824	91392	58317	37726	84628	42221	10268	20692	15699	29167
150	41347	81666	82961	60413	71020	83658	02415	33322	66036	98712	46795	16308	28413	05417
151	38128	51178	75096	13609	16110	73533	42564	59870	29399	67834	91055	89917	51096	89011
152	60950	00455	73254	96067	50717	13878	03216	78274	65863	37011	91283	33914	91303	49326
153	90524	17320	29832	96118	75792	25326	22940	24904	80523	38928	91374	55597	97567	38914
154	49897	18278	67160	39408	97056	43517	84426	59650	20247	19293	02019	14790	02852	05819
155	18494	99209	81060	19488	65596	59787	47939	91225	98768	43688	00438	05548	09443	82897
156	65373	72984	30171	37741	70203	94094	87261	30056	58124	70133	18936	02138	59372	09075
157	40653	12843	04213	70925	95360	55774	76439	61768	52817	81151	52188	31940	54273	49032
158	51638	22238	56344	44587	83231	50317	74541	07719	25472	41602	77318	15145	57515	07633
159	69742	99303	62578	83575	30337	07488	51941	84316	42067	49692	28616	29101	03013	73449
160	58012	74072	67488	74580	47992	69482	58624	17106	47538	13452	22620	24260	40155	74716
161	18348	19855	42887	08279	43206	47077	42637	45606	00011	20662	14642	49984	94509	56380
162	59614	09193	58064	29086	44385	45740	70752	05663	49081	26960	57454	99264	24142	74648
163	75688	28630	39210	52897	62748	72658	98059	67202	72789	01869	13496	14663	87645	89713
164	13941	77802	69101	70061	35460	34576	15412	81304	58757	35498	94830	75521	00603	97701
165	96656	86420	96475	86458	54463	96419	55417	41375	76886	19008	66877	35934	59801	00497
166	03363	82042	15942	14549	38324	87094	19069	67590	11087	68570	22591	65232	85915	91499
167	70366	08390	69155	25496	13240	57407	91407	49160	07379	34444	94567	66035	38918	65708
168	47870	36605	12927	16043	53257	93796	52721	73120	48025	76074	95605	67422	41646	14557
169	76504	77606	22761	30518	28373	73898	30550	76684	77366	32276	04990	61667	64798	66276
170	46967	74841	50923	15339	37755	98995	40162	89561	69199	42257	11647	47603	48779	97907
171	14558	50769	35444	59030	87516	48193	02945	00922	48189	04724	21263	20892	92955	90251
172	12440	25057	01132	38611	28135	68089	10954	10097	54243	06460	50856	65435	79377	53890
173	32293	29938	68653	10497	98919	46587	77701	99119	93165	67788	17638	23097	21468	36992
174	10640	21875	72462	77981	56550	55999	87310	69643	45124	00349	25748	00844	96831	30651

Table of 14,000 Random Units—cont'd

Line/Col.	(1)	(2)	(3)	(4)	(5)	(6)	(7)	(8)	(9)	(10)	(11)	(12)	(13)	(14)
175	47615	23169	39571	56972	20628	21788	51736	33133	72696	32605	41569	76148	91544	21121
176	16948	11128	71624	72754	49084	96303	27830	45817	67867	18062	87453	17226	72904	71474
177	21258	61092	66634	70335	92448	17354	83432	49608	66520	06442	59664	20420	39201	69549
178	15072	48853	15178	30730	47481	48490	41436	25015	49932	20474	53821	51015	79841	32405
179	99154	57412	09858	65671	70655	71479	63520	31357	56968	06729	34465	70685	04184	25250
180	08759	61089	23706	32994	35426	36666	63988	98844	37533	08269	27021	45886	22835	78451
181	67323	57839	61114	62192	47547	58023	64630	34886	98777	75442	95592	06141	45096	73117
182	09255	13986	84834	20764	72206	89393	34548	93438	88730	61805	78955	18952	46436	58740
183	36304	74712	00374	10107	85061	69228	81969	92216	03568	39630	81869	52824	50937	27954
184	15884	67429	86612	47367	10242	44880	12060	44309	46629	55105	66793	93173	00480	13311
185	18745	32031	35303	08134	33925	03044	59929	95418	04917	57596	24878	61733	92834	64454
186	72934	40086	88292	65728	38300	42323	64068	98373	48971	09049	59943	36538	05976	82118
187	17626	02944	20910	57662	80181	38579	24580	90529	52303	50436	29401	57824	86039	81062
188	27117	61399	50967	41399	81636	16663	15634	79717	94696	59240	25543	97989	63306	90946
189	93995	18678	90012	63645	85701	85269	62263	68331	00389	72571	15210	20769	44686	96176
190	67392	89421	09623	80725	62620	84162	87368	29560	00519	84545	08004	24526	41252	14521
191	04910	12261	37566	80016	21245	69377	50420	85658	55263	68667	78770	04533	14513	18099
192	81453	20283	79929	59839	23875	13245	46808	74124	74703	35769	95588	21014	37078	39170
193	19480	75790	48539	23703	15537	48885	02861	86587	74539	65227	90799	58789	96257	02708
194	21456	13162	74608	81011	55512	07481	93551	72189	76261	91206	89941	15132	37738	59284
195	89406	20912	46189	76376	25538	87212	20748	12831	57166	35026	16817	79121	18929	40628
196	09866	07414	55977	16419	01101	69343	13305	94302	80703	57910	36933	57771	42546	03003
197	86541	24681	23421	13521	28000	94917	07423	57523	97234	63951	42876	46829	09781	58160
198	10414	96941	06205	72222	57167	83902	07460	69507	10600	08858	07685	44472	64220	27040
199	49942	06683	41479	58982	56288	42853	92196	20632	62045	78812	35895	51851	83534	10689
200	23995	68882	42291	23374	24299	27024	67460	94783	40937	16961	26053	78749	46704	21983

From Beyer WH, ed. *Standard Mathematical Tables*. Boca Raton, Fla: CRC Press; 1984:555-558.

Areas in One Tail of the Standard Normal Curve

This table shows the shaded area

Z	.00	.01	.02	.03	.04	.05	.06	.07	.08	.09
0.0	.500	.496	.492	.488	.484	.480	.476	.472	.468	.464
0.1	.460	.456	.452	.448	.444	.440	.436	.433	.429	.425
0.2	.421	.417	.413	.409	.405	.401	.397	.394	.390	.386
0.3	.382	.378	.374	.371	.367	.363	.359	.356	.352	.348
0.4	.345	.341	.337	.334	.330	.326	.323	.319	.316	.312
0.5	.309	.305	.302	.298	.295	.291	.288	.284	.281	.278
0.6	.274	.271	.268	.264	.261	.258	.255	.251	.248	.245
0.7	.242	.239	.236	.233	.230	.227	.224	.221	.218	.215
0.8	.212	.209	.206	.203	.200	.198	.195	.192	.189	.187
0.9	.184	.181	.179	.176	.174	.171	.169	.166	.164	.161
1.0	.159	.156	.154	.152	.149	.147	.145	.142	.140	.138
1.1	.136	.133	.131	.129	.127	.125	.123	.121	.119	.117
1.2	.115	.113	.111	.109	.107	.106	.104	.102	.100	.099
1.3	.097	.095	.093	.092	.090	.089	.087	.085	.084	.082
1.4	.081	.079	.078	.076	.075	.074	.072	.071	.069	.068
1.5	.067	.066	.064	.063	.062	.061	.059	.058	.057	.056
1.6	.055	.054	.053	.052	.051	.049	.048	.048	.046	.046
1.7	.045	.044	.043	.042	.041	.040	.039	.038	.038	.037
1.8	.036	.035	.034	.034	.033	.032	.031	.031	.030	.029
1.9	.029	.028	.027	.027	.026	.026	.025	.024	.024	.023
2.0	.023	.022	.022	.021	.021	.020	.020	.019	.019	.018
2.1	.018	.017	.017	.017	.016	.016	.015	.015	.015	.014
2.2	.014	.014	.013	.013	.013	.012	.012	.012	.011	.011
2.3	.011	.010	.010	.010	.010	.009	.009	.009	.009	.008
2.4	.008	.008	.008	.008	.007	.007	.007	.007	.007	.006
2.5	.006	.006	.006	.006	.006	.005	.005	.005	.005	.005
2.6	.005	.005	.004	.004	.004	.004	.004	.004	.004	.004
2.7	.003	.003	.003	.003	.003	.003	.003	.003	.003	.003
2.8	.003	.002	.002	.002	.002	.002	.002	.002	.002	.002
2.9	.002	.002	.002	.002	.002	.002	.002	.001	.001	.001
3.0	.001									

Reprinted with permission from Colton T. *Statistics in Medicine.* Boston, Mass: Little, Brown & Co; 1974.

Questions for Narrative Evaluation of a Research Article

STEP ONE
Classification of Research and Variables

❍ Was data collection prospective or retrospective? (Chapter 6)

❍ Was the purpose of the research description, relationship analysis, difference analysis, or some combination? (Chapter 6)

❍ Was the study experimental or nonexperimental? (Chapter 6)

❍ Was the study conducted according to the assumptions and methods of the quantitative, qualitative, or single-system paradigms? (Chapter 5)

❍ What were the independent variables? (Chapter 6)

❍ What were the dependent variables? (Chapter 6)

STEP TWO
Analysis of Purposes and Conclusions

❍ Is there a conclusion for every purpose?

❍ Is there a purpose for every conclusion?

❍ Are there significant results that should be evaluated for possible alternative explanations and clinical importance? (Chapter 19)

❍ Are there nonsignificant results that should be evaluated for power and clinical importance? (Chapter 19)

STEP THREE
Analysis of Design and Control Elements

❍ What was the design of the study? (Chapters 9 through 11)

❍ Was the independent variable implemented in a laboratory-like or clinic-like setting? (Chapter 6)

❍ Was selection of subjects done randomly, by cluster, by convenience, or purposively? (Chapter 8)

❍ Were subjects assigned to groups through individual random assignment, block assignment, systematic assignment, matched assignment, or consecutive assignment? (Chapter 8)

❍ Were extraneous experimental-setting variables under tight laboratory-like control or loose, clinic-like control? (Chapter 6)

❍ Were extraneous subject variables under laboratory-like or clinic-like control? (Chapter 6)

❍ What was the level of control over measurement techniques? (Chapters 6, 17, and 18)

❍ Was information controlled through incomplete information, participant masking, or researcher masking? (Chapter 6)

STEP FOUR
Validity Questions

❍ Construct Validity (Chapter 7)

Were the variables in the study defined and implemented in meaningful ways?

Construct Underrepresentation

Were variables well developed and defined?

Were there enough levels of the independent variable? Was treatment administered as an all-or-none phenomenon or in varying levels?

Do the dependent variables provide information in all areas important to the phenomenon under study?

Was the independent variable administered at a lower intensity or in a different manner than would be typical in a clinical setting?

Experimenter Expectancies

Were the experimenter's expectations transparently obvious to participants?

Were there differences between the construct as labeled and the construct as implemented, based on the influence of the experimenter?

Interaction of Different Treatments

What uncontrolled treatments might have interacted with the independent variable?

Interaction of Testing and Treatment

Could any of the measurements used in the study have contributed to a treatment effect?

○ Internal Validity (Chapter 7)

Was the independent variable the probable cause of differences in the dependent variables?

History and Interaction of History and Assignment

What events other than implementation of the independent variable occurred during the study that might have plausibly caused changes in the dependent variable?

If any historical events took place, did the events have an equal impact on treatment and control groups?

Maturation and Interaction of Maturation and Assignment

Could changes in the dependent variable have been the result of the passage of time, rather than the implementation of the independent variable?

If a control group was present, were the same maturational influences at work for them as for the treatment group?

Testing

Is familiarity with testing procedures a likely explanation for differences in the dependent variable?

Were tests conducted with equal frequency for treatment and control groups so that any testing effects were consistent for all groups within the study?

Instrumentation and Interaction of Instrumentation and Assignment

Were instruments calibrated appropriately?

Were measurements taken under controlled environmental conditions such as temperature or humidity?

If the instrument was a human observer, what measures were taken to ensure consistency of observations?

Were instruments expected to be equally sensitive across the values expected for both the treatment and control groups?

Statistical Regression to the Mean

Were participants selected for the study based on an extreme score on a single administration of a test?

Can improvements or declines in performance be attributed to statistical regression rather than true change?

Assignment

Were participants assigned to groups randomly?

If not assigned randomly, what factors other than the one of interest might have influenced their assignment?

Mortality

What proportions of participants were lost from the treatment and control groups?

Were the proportions of participants lost equal for the treatment and control groups?

What are possible explanations for differential loss of participants from the groups?

Diffusion or Imitation of Treatments

Were treatment and control group members able to share information about their respective routines?

Was either the treatment or control regimen likely to have been perceived as more desirable by participants in the other group?

Compensatory Equalization of Treatments

Were researchers aware of which participants were in which group?

Were those implementing the treatments likely to have paid extra attention to control group members because of the presumed inferiority of care they received?

Compensatory Rivalry or Resentful Demoralization

Did participants know whether they were in the treatment or control group?

Were control-group members likely to have either tried harder or withdrawn their efforts because they knew they were in the control group and perceived it to be a less desirable alternative than being in the treatment group?

○ Statistical Conclusion Validity (Chapter 19)

Were statistical tools used appropriately?

Low Power

Are statistically insignificant results related to small sample size, high within-group variability, or small between-groups differences?

Do statistically insignificant differences seem clinically important?

Lack of Clinical Importance

Are statistically significant results clinically important?

Error Rate Problems

If multiple statistical tests were performed, did the researcher set a conservative alpha level to compensate for alpha level inflation?

Are identified significant differences isolated and difficult to explain, or is there a pattern of significant differences that suggests true differences rather than Type I errors?

Violated Assumptions

Were tests used appropriately for independent and dependent samples?

Were assumptions about normal distribution of data and homogeneity of variance satisfied?

Failure to Use Intention-to-Treat Analysis

Was everyone who was entered into the study included in the final data analysis according to the treatment they were intended to have, whether or not he or she completed the study?

If not, did the authors present a sound rationale for using a completer analysis instead of an intention-to-treat analysis?

○ External Validity (Chapter 7)

To whom and under what conditions can the research results be generalized?

Selection

Were volunteers used for study? In what ways do these volunteers differ from clinical populations?

Are results from normal participants generalized to patient populations?

Do the authors limit their conclusions to participants similar to those studied?

Setting

To what extent did the experimental setting differ from the setting to which the researchers wish to generalize the results?

Were control elements implemented fastidiously, as in a laboratory, or pragmatically, as in a clinic?

Time

How much time elapsed between the collection of the data in the study and the present time?

Do differences in overall clinical management of patients make the studied procedures less appropriate today than when the study was implemented?

STEP FIVE
Place Study into Literature Context

O Do results confirm or contradict the findings of others?

O Does this study correct some of the deficiencies identified in other studies?

O Does the study examine constructs or variables unstudied by others?

O How do the sample size and composition compare with those of other studies?

O How does the validity of this study compare with that of related studies?

STEP SIX
Personal Utility Questions

O Are your setting and the research setting similar enough to warrant application of the results of the research to your clinical practice?

O Does the study cause you to question some of the assumptions under which you have managed patients?

O Do the methods of this study suggest ways in which you can improve on the design of a study that you are planning?

Basic Guidelines for Preparing a Journal Article Manuscript

This appendix contains basic guidelines for preparing a journal article manuscript in either American Medical Association (AMA)[1] or American Psychological Association (APA)[2] style. Additional suggestions about general scientific writing have been included as well, based on the work of Day[3] and Browner.[4] These guidelines can help jump-start the writing process or answer some questions when other resources are not available. They are not, however, a substitute for regular consultation of more detailed and authoritative references: the style manual specified by a journal, the instructions for authors for specific journals, and general books and articles about scientific writing.

1. General Guidelines

   1.1 Double-space everything, including block quotes, tables, and references.

   1.2 Margins should be a minimum 1 inch; some journals request more generous margins.

   1.3 Do not right-justify the text or hyphenate words at the ends of lines. These adjustments may make an attractive document but hinder the editing process.

   1.4 Generally plan for about 15 pages of text, plus title page, abstract page, tables, references, and figures. Consult journal instructions to authors for more specific length guidelines. Note that articles describing qualitative research may be longer than typical and follow a somewhat different outline; refer to examples in the literature for guidance.

   1.5 Manuscript pagination is as follows: Title page is page 1 but may or may not include the page number; abstract page is page 2; text begins on page 3. Tables follow the references. Each table begins on a new page, and table pages are numbered consecutively with the manuscript. The final numbered manuscript page is the one on which the figure legends are written; it starts on a separate page following the tables. APA style requires numbering in the top right corner of the page, beginning with the title page. AMA style does not specify; refer to specific journal guidelines.

   1.6 Determine formats for headings and subheadings and use them consistently. APA style requires the following for papers with three heading levels:

Method

Participants

Facility A

   AMA style does not specify, but indicates that the format for headings needs to be consistent throughout the paper and follow any guidelines set by the specific journal. A sample set of headings is given:

Method

Participants

Facility A.

2. Title and Title Page

   2.1 Title should be concise, yet specific. Include important variables under study.

"Knee Function after Total Knee Arthroplasty" is too concise if the study is really one of "Effect of Two Continuous Passive Motion Regimens on Knee Function Six Months after Total Knee Arthroplasty."

2.2 Titles are generally descriptive (such as "Effect of Continuous Passive Motion on Knee Range of Motion after Total Knee Arthroplasty"), but may be assertive (such as "Continuous Passive Motion Does Not Improve Knee Range of Motion after Total Knee Arthroplasty"). Some believe that assertive titles place too much emphasis on the conclusion without considering the context that the full article provides.

2.3 Consider using terms that are indexed in the databases interested readers are likely to search; for example, use "total knee arthroplasty" rather than "total knee replacement" because "arthroplasty" is indexed and "replacement" is not.

2.4 Title in APA style is in uppercase and lowercase letters, centered on the page. AMA style does not specify and refers authors to specific journal guidelines.

2.5 APA style specifies a two-part byline including the author's name without titles and degrees and the institutional affiliation of the author, centered on separate lines beneath the title. More detailed information about authors goes in an author note at the end of the paper, or on the title page if the manuscript is undergoing a masked review. AMA style includes highest degrees and refers authors to specific journal guidelines for additional details.

3. Abstract

3.1 Limit the abstract to 120 (APA) or 250 (AMA) words.

3.2 Summarize the study's purpose, procedures, results, and major conclusions. For reports of original research, AMA style requires use of a structured abstract with headings: "Context," "Objective," "Design," "Setting," "Participants," "Intervention," "Outcome Measures," "Results," "Conclusions."

3.3 Use major indexing terms within the abstract because users of electronic bibliographic databases often search abstracts as well as titles.

3.4 Do not cite references or provide p values because these are meaningful only in the context of the study.

4. Introduction

4.1 No heading is used for the introduction. Repeat the title and then begin the first paragraph (APA) or just begin the first paragraph (AMA).

4.2 In a paper of 15 pages, the introduction section is typically 2 to 3 pages.

4.3 Cite only the most relevant citations about the topic area. A journal article does not contain an exhaustive review of the literature, rather, it places the problem into the context of the literature.

4.4 In-text citation of references is very different in AMA and APA styles (see Table 28–1 for a side-by-side comparison of the two citation styles).

4.4.1 AMA style uses numerical citations with superscripts, numbered in the order in which they are cited. If superscripts are unavailable, then the number should be enclosed in parentheses.

If the text refers to an author's name, the numeral follows the name directly. If the author's name is not mentioned and the entire sentence is related to the citation, the numeral goes at the end of the sentence. If the citation refers to only part of the sentence, the numeral is placed at the conclusion of that part of the sentence.

If there are two authors, always include both surnames when citing names in the text. For citations with three or more authors, use the first author's surname with "et al," "and colleagues," "and coworkers," or "and associates." When using a numbered reference style like the AMA, writers often cite references with the author name and publication date in parentheses in early drafts of the paper. This prevents repeated renumbering of references as the paper is edited. For the final draft, the names and parentheses are removed and the correct numbers inserted. Alternately, many authors use bibliographic management software to manage references and prevent the need for repeated renumbering of citations as a paper evolves. Note that in AMA style, "et al" is used without punctuation, consistent with other AMA conventions that minimize punctuation for abbreviations and initials.

  4.4.2 APA style uses author-date citation style in which author surnames and publication dates are entered at the appropriate point in the manuscript. If the text refers to the author's name, then only the publication date needs to be included in parentheses following the use of the author's name. If the author's name is not mentioned in the text, then the author surname and date are included in parentheses at the appropriate point in the text. When there are two authors, include both surnames in the parenthetical citation (Brown & Preston, 2003). When there are three to five authors include all names at first reference (Brown, Preston, & Glass, 2003) and shorten with et al. in subsequent citations (Brown et al., 2003). With six or more authors use "et al." at first reference. Note that in APA style, "et al." is used with punctuation, consistent with other APA conventions for abbreviations and punctuation.

4.5 Suggested first paragraph: Broadly state the problem, with documentation as needed.

4.6 Suggested second through fourth paragraphs, as needed: Summarize what is known about the problem, that is, what others have found out about the problem in their own research.

4.7 Suggested last paragraph: Identify the gap in the literature that needs to be filled, and then state the purpose of your research. State research hypotheses if appropriate. Identify major variables, using the names that you will use throughout the rest of the paper. If you have several purposes, place them in order of importance or in the order that they will be discussed in the rest of the paper.

5. Methods

5.1 The methods section is usually subdivided into "Participants," "Instruments," "Procedures," and "Data Analysis" or similar subheadings.

5.2 In a paper of 15 pages, the methods section is typically 3 to 5 pages long.

5.3 Cite literature needed to justify the methods you used, or cite others' procedures if they are too lengthy to be repeated in your article.

5.4 The participants subsection should describe inclusion and exclusion criteria, sampling and assignment methods, and source of the participants.

5.5 The instruments subsection should describe each instrument used in data collection.

  5.5.1 Present instruments in the order that you will eventually present the rest of your methods and results. For example, if you have taken range of motion, strength, and functional measures and plan to discuss them in that order, describe the goniometers first, the dynamometers second, and the functional scale last.

  5.5.2 If you developed the instrument, provide details about the instrument development process.

  5.5.3 If you performed reliability or validity testing with the instruments but this was not the primary purpose of the research, present reliability or validity information here. If the research is methodological, then reliability or validity information belongs in the results section.

5.6 The procedures subsection should describe what you did in enough detail that others can replicate the study. Refer to other authors if necessary to justify your procedures.

5.7 Consider combining the instrument subsection with the procedures subsection if the equipment used is nontechnical and familiar to most professionals to whom the article would be of interest.

5.8 The data analysis subsection should include data reduction procedures and statistical testing for each variable.

5.8.1 If possible, present information about the data analysis in the order of variables presented earlier in the paper.

5.8.2 State the statistical package used and alpha level if appropriate.

5.8.3 If necessary, justify or clarify your use of statistical procedures with references.

6. Results

6.1 Sometimes the results section is subdivided by variables or classes of variables.

6.2 Text is often short, with much of the information presented in tables and figures. Tables and figures should substitute for information in the text, not repeat it. Tables and figures are numbered separately in order of their appearance in the text (see Sections 11 and 12).

6.3 Present variables in previously established order.

6.4 Do not discuss the implications of the results here; just present the appropriate descriptive and statistical information.

6.5 In a paper of 15 pages, the results section is typically only 1 to 2 pages long, supplemented by figures and tables.

7. Discussion

7.1 The discussion is the heart of the paper, the place for interpretation of the results.

7.2 In a paper of 15 pages, the discussion is typically 3 to 4 pages long.

7.3 Additional references are often cited to place the results into a broader context.

7.4 Suggested first section: Interpret the major results in terms of your original hypotheses.

7.5 Suggested second section: Examine the results that were as predicted by your hypothesis, reinforcing the theory that led you to the hypothesis.

7.6 Suggested third section: Examine the results that were not as predicted, speculating about the meaning of the inconsistent results.

7.7 Suggested fourth section: Discuss the limitations of the study.

7.8 Suggested fifth section: Discuss the clinical implications of the findings.

7.9 Suggested sixth section: Discuss directions for future research.

8. Conclusions

8.1 Not all articles have a conclusions section. APA style manuscripts do not typically have a separate conclusions section. If the conclusions are not a separate section, they are integrated into the discussion.

8.2 In a paper of 15 pages, the conclusions are typically less than a page long. The conclusions are stated concisely, in the order in which the questions were posed in the purpose section of the study.

8.3 Avoid making sweeping conclusions that are not grounded in your results.

9. Author Note and Acknowledgments

9.1 In AMA style author information is on the title page and acknowledgments are placed on a separate page between the end of the text and the references. In APA style, author notes, including acknowledgments, are placed between the references and the tables, unless the paper will be undergoing masked review, in which case they are placed on the title page.

9.2 Each person acknowledged should have given permission to be acknowledged.

9.3 Be specific about the contribution of each person, for example: "critical review," "manuscript preparation," or "data collection."

10. References

10.1 Begin references on a separate page.

10.2 Double-space references.

10.3 List only references cited in the study.

10.4 AMA style numbers references in the reference list in the order they are cited in text. APA style puts references in order alphabetically by the surname of the first author and does not number the references.

10.5 Place references into proper format. Pay attention to punctuation, capitalization, and italicization in the various elements of the reference (see Table 28–1 for a side-by-side comparison of the two styles).

10.5.1 AMA formats for the different elements of a journal article citation are as follows:

Authors: Smith DL, Riley JW, Anderson MD. (There is no internal punctuation within each name; names are separated by commas; a period follows the final name).

Journal article title: Effects of prolonged sitting on attention span: a study of rehabilitation professionals. (Only the first word is capitalized unless there is a proper name within the title; the first word after a colon starts with a lower-case letter; a period follows the title.)

Journal name: Arch Phys Med Rehabil. (Use the MEDLINE abbreviation for the journal name or abbreviate according to MEDLINE conventions if the journal is not indexed in MEDLINE. The journal abbreviation or name is italicized or underlined if an italicized font is not available, and a period follows.)

Year, volume, issue, and pages: 2001;79:3002-3007. (The year comes first, followed by a semicolon; the volume number comes next, followed by a

colon; an issue number is given only if each issue begins with page 1 (if the issue number is necessary, it is enclosed in parentheses); the page numbers are last, followed by a period. Inclusive page numbers are listed and the full page number is repeated on each side of the hyphen.)

10.5.2 APA reference listings use a hanging indent (the first line of each reference is flush with the left margin and the remaining lines are indented). Formats for the different elements of a journal article citation are as follows:

Authors: Smith, D.L., Riley, J.W., & Anderson, M.D. (Use internal punctuation within each name; names are separated by commas; use an ampersand before the last author; a period follows the final name.)

Publication date: (2001). (The year of publication is given in parentheses after the author names, followed by a period.)

Journal article title: Effects of prolonged sitting on attention span: A study of rehabilitation professionals. (The first word of both the title and subtitle are capitalized, as are proper names within the title; a period follows the title.)

Journal name and publication information: Archives of Physical Medicine and Rehabilitation, 79, 3002-3007. (Use the full name of the journal in italics; add volume number, also in italics; an issue number is used only if each issue begins with page 1. If the issue number is necessary, it is enclosed in parentheses. The page numbers are last, not in italics, followed by a period.

Inclusive page numbers are listed and the full page number is repeated on each side of the hyphen.)

10.6 Consult the appropriate style manual for detailed directions on specific formats for other types of references (e.g., book, chapter in a book, dissertation).

11. Tables

11.1 Tables consist of rows and columns of numbers or text.

11.2 Vertical lines are not used in tables; use horizontal lines only.

11.3 Tables should not repeat information in the text. If a table can be summarized in a sentence or two, then it should probably not be a table.

11.4 Number tables (e.g., Table 1, Table 2, Table 3) according to their order in the paper. Refer to each table in the text, highlighting the most important information. If there is only one table, it is not numbered.

11.5 Table titles should describe the specific information contained within the table; for example, "Data" is too general a title; "Mean Knee Function Variables by Clinic" is more specific.

11.6 Each table begins on a separate page placed after the references. Tables may be continued onto additional pages.

12. Figures

12.1 Figures are illustrative materials such as graphs, diagrams, or photographs.

12.2 Figures should not repeat information in text or tables. They should be used only when visual information is more effective than tabular or text information.

12.3 Figures are numbered (e.g., Figure 1, Figure 2, Figure 3) in order of their appearance in the paper. If there is only one figure, it is not numbered.

12.4 Figure legends are listed on a separate sheet following the tables. The legend should make the figure meaningful on its own by explaining any abbreviations and describing concisely the important points being illustrated. The figure legend page is the last numbered page of the manuscript.

12.5 The figure itself is not labeled or numbered on its face. Figures are identified outside the figure area or on the back of the figure; be careful not to damage the figure by labeling it.

12.6 Identification of figures in theses or dissertations will deviate from this format. Because they are used in the format prepared by the author, rather than being typeset in a journal, figure numbers and legends must accompany the figures themselves and figure pages are numbered.

REFERENCES

1. *American Medical Association Manual of Style*. 9th ed. Baltimore, Md: Williams & Wilkins; 1998.
2. *Publication Manual of the American Psychological Association*. 5th ed. Washington, DC: American Psychological Association; 2001.
3. Day RA. *How to Write and Publish a Scientific Paper*. 5th ed. Phoenix, Ariz: Oryx Press; 1998.
4. Browner WS. *Publishing and Presenting Clinical Research*. Baltimore, Md: Lippincott Williams & Wilkins; 1999.

American Medical Association Style: Sample Manuscript for a Hypothetical Study

The following short, hypothetical manuscript on continuous passive motion following total knee arthroplasty is based, with a few changes in the demographic variables, on the hypothetical data set presented in Chapter 19 in Tables 19–1 and 19–2. The circled numbers in the manuscript correspond to guidelines listed in Appendix D.

Effect of Initial Arc of Continuous Passive Motion on Motion
and Function Following Total Knee Arthroplasty   ←(2.1)

Jan R. Woolery, PhD;

Jodi C. Beeker, MD;   ←(2.5)

Jonathon V. Mills, MS

JR Woolery is Research Therapist, Department of Physical Therapy,
Memorial Hospital of Indiana, 555 Main Street, Anytown, IN 46234
(USA). Address all correspondence to Dr. Woolery. E-mail:
jrwoolery@memorialindiana.org   ←(9.1)

JC Beeker is Orthopedic Surgeon, Department of Orthopedic
Surgery, Community Hospital of Anytown, Anytown, IN.

JV Mills is Staff Therapist, Occupational Therapy Department,
Religious Hospital of Anytown, Anytown, IN.

Presented at the 2004 Annual Conference of the Association of
Hip and Knee Surgeons, New Orleans, La, February 20-24, 2004.

This study was approved by the institutional review boards of
Memorial Hospital of Indiana, Community Hospital of Anytown,
and Religious Hospital of Anytown.

ABSTRACT

(3.2)→ **Context:** Optimal progression of range of motion (ROM) in continuous passive motion (CPM) devices following total knee arthroplasty (TKA) is not well established, despite their use for over 20 years. **Objective:** To compare the effects of two CPM regimens with different initial arcs of motion to no CPM on knee motion and function up to 6 months after TKA. One CPM regimen began with motion set at 70° to 100° of knee flexion and progressed toward full extension; the other began with motion set at 0° to 40° of knee flexion and progressed toward full flexion. **Design:** Controlled trial with 6-month follow-up. **Setting:** Three community hospitals in the Midwestern region of the United States. **Participants:** Ten consecutive patients over the age of 50 years following unilateral TKA at each of three different hospitals. **Interventions:** Patients were assigned by hospital to receive 6 days of CPM starting at 70° to 100° of flexion, CPM starting at 0° to 40° of flexion, or no CPM. **Outcome Measures:** Knee flexion ROM 3 and 6 weeks postoperatively and knee flexion ROM, gait velocity, and activities of daily living (ADL) score 6 months postoperatively. **Results:** Significant differences among groups were identified for all dependent variables, with higher scores for CPM groups. There were no significant differences between the CPM groups. **Conclusions:** CPM groups had better outcomes than the no-CPM group, regardless of the initial arc of motion.

3

(4.1)→   Total knee arthroplasty is a common surgical procedure used
to reduce pain and enhance function for individuals with knee
impairment secondary to osteoarthritis. Continuous passive
motion (CPM) is used to encourage early motion of the knee
joint after total knee arthroplasty (TKA). Milne and colleagues[1] ←(4.4.1)
conducted a meta-analysis of 14 randomized controlled trials of
CPM following TKA, showing that CPM combined with PT resulted
in more active knee flexion at discharge, a shorter length of
stay, and less need for postoperative manipulation than PT
alone. They recommended further research to determine whether
there are differences in CPM effectiveness with different CPM
protocols or with different patient or diagnostic groups.   ←(4.5)

Studies comparing different CPM regimens have identified few
short-term differences among groups and no long-term differences.
Groups receiving different daily durations of CPM were compared
by Basso and Knapp[2] and Chiarello and colleagues[3]; in both cases
no ROM differences between groups were identified at discharge.
(4.6)→ Pope and colleagues[4] found no ROM differences between groups
receiving CPM with different initial arcs of motion (0° to 40°
versus 0° to 70° of knee flexion). Finally, Yashar and associates[5]
and MacDonald and colleagues[6] compared groups receiving CPM with
an initial flexion arc of motion from 0° to up to 50° to those

receiving CPM with an accelerated initial flexion arc of motion from 70° to up to 110°. Yashar and colleagues[5] identified a short-term advantage for the accelerated group on knee flexion ROM, but no long-term differences. MacDonald and colleagues[6] found no short-term or long-term differences between CPM groups or a control group receiving usual care without CPM. Thus, on one potentially important CPM variable, initial arc of motion, the research is limited and the results are contradictory.

Therefore, we designed a study to further evaluate the impact of the initial arc of motion of CPM on short-term and long-terms outcomes after TKA. Specifically, the purpose of this study was to determine whether there were differences between two CPM protocols (initial arc of motion of 0° to 40° versus 70° to 100°) ←(4.7) and no CPM on knee flexion ROM at 3 and 6 weeks postoperatively and on knee flexion ROM, gait velocity, and ADL score at 6 months postoperatively. We hypothesized that there would be no differences between CPM groups at any time, that there would be differences between the no-CPM group and both CPM groups at 3 and 6 weeks postoperatively, and that there would be no differences among groups at 6 months postoperatively.

METHODS

Participants   ←(5.1)

Participants were patients who were at least 50 years old, had a diagnosis of osteoarthritis, and underwent TKA in 2003 at one of three hospitals in Anytown, Indiana: Community Hospital, Memorial Hospital, and Religious Hospital. Before beginning this study, the characteristics of patients undergoing TKA was compared across the three participating hospitals and found to be similar for age, sex, diagnosis, and type of prosthesis   ←(5.4) implanted. Because of the similarity of patients at the three hospitals, we assigned the CPM protocol randomly to hospitals rather than individually to patients. Patients at Community Hospital received an initial arc of 70° to 100° of CPM, patients at Religious Hospital received an initial arc of 0° to 40°, and patients at Memorial Hospital received no CPM. The first 10 patients in 2003 who met the inclusion criteria and consented to participate were entered into the trial at each hospital. Twelve eligible patients (three at Community, five at Religious, and four at Memorial) did not consent to participate in the study.

For the 30 patients who entered the trial, half were women and the mean (SD) age was 72.5 (4.7) years. The sex distribution and mean age across groups was similar: 50% women, 73.2 (5.6) years for the 70° to 100° CPM group; 40% women, 71.7 (6.5) years for the 0° to 40° CPM group; and 60% women, 72.5 (4.7) years for the no-CPM group. All 30 patients completed the trial.

Instruments   ←(1.6)

CPM Units. ACME CPM (ACME Orthopedics, Roadrunner, Ariz) units were used to deliver the CPM treatment at all three facilities.

(5.5)→ **Goniometers.** ROM measurements were taken with the 12-inch, full-circle, plastic universal goniometers available at each facility.

(11.4)→ **ADL Scale.** We modified the Brigham and Women's Knee Rating Scale[7] to assess ADL (Table 1). The values for each of the four subscales (distance walked, assistive device, stair climbing, and rising from a chair) were added for each person to give a single ADL score that could range from a low of 4 to a high of 20.

Procedure

Patients underwent the assigned postoperative rehabilitation protocol. For the two CPM groups the units were applied in the recovery room and used for 20 hours on the first postoperative day. On subsequent days the ROM was advanced 10° (toward more   ←(5.6) flexion for the 0° to 40° group and toward extension for the

70° to 100° group) per day and the time in the unit was reduced by about 2 hours per day. Each day the time spent in CPM was recorded for each patient. Knee flexion ROM measurements were taken with patients supine according to the procedures described by Norkin and White,[8] with values recorded to the nearest degree. ←(5.3) The 3-week and 6-week measures were taken by the treating therapists at each hospital when patients came for their routine outpatient physical therapy visits. The 6-month measures were all taken in the physical therapy department at Community Hospital by an independent investigator (JVM) who was unaware of group assignment. Velocity was measured by having the participant walk at a comfortable pace across a 20-m measured distance. Each participant was timed with a stopwatch during the center 10 m of the walk and time was converted to cm/s for analysis. Within the modified Brigham and Women's Knee Rating Scale, use of an assistive device, rising from a chair, and stair climbing were actually observed and rated; distance walked was a self-reported measure.

Data Analysis

Analysis of variance (ANOVA) was used to test for differences between groups for each of the following dependent variables: 3-week ROM, 6-week ROM, and 6-month ROM; gait

velocity; and ADL score. The Newman-Keuls procedure was used for

(5.8)→ post hoc analysis. Alpha was set at .05 for each analysis. SPSS

for Windows 10.02 was used for the data analysis (SPSS Inc,

(5.8.2)→ Chicago, Ill).

RESULTS

Average time spent in CPM per day was similar for the two CPM

(6.2)→ groups (Figure). There were significant differences between groups

for all variables (Table 2). For all variables, post hoc analysis

showed that the CPM groups were not statistically different from

one another, but that both were significantly different from the

no-CPM group.

DISCUSSION

Of our three hypotheses, two were supported: (1) that there

would be no differences between the CPM groups at any time and

(2) that there would be 3- and 6-week differences between the   ←(7.4)

no-CPM group and both the CPM groups. The significant differences

between the no-CPM and CPM groups is consistent with the

meta-analysis findings of Milne and colleagues,[1] strengthening

the case for using CPM to improve short-term postoperative ROM after TKA. In addition, our findings suggest that the benefits extend beyond ROM to include gait and other functional outcomes.

The lack of differences between the CPM groups is consistent with the work of Yashar and colleagues[5] and MacDonald and associates[6] who also found no difference in ROM outcomes between groups receiving different initial arcs of motion. Further, the ←(7.5) addition of gait velocity and ADL measures in our study provides evidence that both impairment and disability level outcomes are similar regardless of the direction in which ROM is progressed with CPM.

Our final hypothesis, that differences between the no-CPM group and the CPM groups would not be present at 6 months, was not supported. We plan to continue the study to determine ←(7.6) if differences in all variables disappear by 1 year postoperatively, as has been found by others.[4-6] ←(7.3)

The functional importance of our gait and ADL findings is apparent if one looks at the mean values for the different groups. The no-CPM group had an average gait velocity of only 107.6 cm/s, well below the averages of the two CPM groups (144.0 and 145.6 cm/s). The ADL scores of the CPM groups were approximately 18 and 17 of 20, respectively. This indicates minor impairment on two of the components or moderate impairment on one. In contrast, the average ADL score for the no-CPM group was 11, indicating moderate to severe impairment in one or more of the ADL components.

In interpreting these results, several limitations or alternative explanations must be considered. First, because the treatments were assigned by hospital and not by patient, systematic differences between the hospitals could explain the   ←(7.7) difference in results. Second, because the treating therapists could not be masked to the group membership of the participants, their expectations may have influenced subject performance. Despite these limitations, the results have clinical implications for facilities using CPM for patients after TKA. Our results seem to indicate that patients who receive CPM—regardless of the initial arc of motion—do better on important outcome measures until at least 6 months after surgery compared with patients who do not receive CPM.

(7.9)→ Further research must be done to see if these results can be replicated, to see whether differences between CPM and no-CPM groups persist longer than 6 months, and to determine whether there are other important differences among CPM groups (e.g., blood loss or analgesic use) that would suggest an optimal direction for increasing motion after surgery.

11

CONCLUSIONS

Patients who underwent TKA and received CPM with different initial
arcs of motion (starting at 70° to 100° of flexion or starting at
(8.2)→ 0° to 40° of flexion) had significantly better knee flexion ROM at
3 weeks and 6 weeks and significantly better knee flexion ROM,
gait velocity, and ADL scores at 6 months postoperatively than
did those who did not receive CPM.

12

ACKNOWLEDGMENTS   ←(9.1)

We thank Ben Counter, PhD, for assistance with the statistical analysis of the study and Ellen Redline, PT, PhD, for her critical review of an earlier draft of the manuscript.   ←(9.3)

13

REFERENCES ←(10.1)

(10.4)→ 1. Milne S, Brosseau L, Robinson V, Noel MJ, Davis J, Drouin H, et al. Continuous passive motion following total knee arthro-
(10.2)→ plasty (Cochrane Review). In: *The Cochrane Library*. Chichester, UK: John Wiley & Sons; 2003: Issue 4.

2. Basso DM, Knapp L. Comparison of two continuous passive motion protocols for patients with total knee implants. *Phys Ther*. 1987;67:360-363.

3. Chiarello CM, Gundersen L, O'Halloran T. The effect of continuous passive motion duration and increment on range of motion in total knee arthroplasty patients. *J Orthop Sports Phys Ther*. 1997;25:119-127.

4. Pope RO, Corcoran S, McCaul K, Howie DW. Continuous passive motion after primary total knee arthroplasty: does it offer any benefits? *J Bone Joint Surg Br*. 1997;79:914-917.

5. Yashar AA, Venn-Watson E, Welsh T, Colwell CW, Lotke P. Continuous passive motion with accelerated flexion after total knee arthroplasty. *Clin Orthop*. 1997;345:38-43.

6. MacDonald SJ, Bourne RB, Rorabeck CH, McCalden RW, Kramer J, Vaz M. Prospective randomized clinical trial of continuous passive motion after total knee arthroplasty. *Clin Orthop*. 2000;380:30-35.

14

7. Ewald FC, Jacobs MA, Miegel RE, Walker PS, Poss R, Sledge CB. Kinematic total knee replacement. *J Bone Joint Surg Am*. 1984;66:1032-1040.

8. Norkin CC, White DJ. *Measurement of Joint Motion: A Guide to Goniometry*. Philadelphia, Pa: FA Davis Co; 1995:142-143.

15

Table 1. Modified Brigham and Women's Knee Rating Scale[7] ←(11.5)

Variable ←(11.1)	Scoring Criteria	←(11.2)
Distance walked	5 = Unlimited	
	4 = 4 to 6 blocks	
	3 = 2 to 3 blocks	
	2 = Indoors only	
	1 = Transfers only	
Assistive device	5 = None	
	4 = Cane outside	
	3 = Cane full time	
	2 = Two canes or crutches	
	1 = Walker or unable	
Stair climbing	5 = Reciprocal, no rail	
	4 = Reciprocal, rail	
	3 = One at a time, with or without rail	
	2 = One at a time, with rail and assistive device	
	1 = Unable	

(11.6)→ Table 1 (continued). Modified Brigham and Women's Knee Rating Scale[7]

Variable	Scoring Criteria
Rising from a chair	5 = No arm assistance
	4 = Single arm assistance
	3 = Difficult with two arm assistance
	2 = Needs assistance of another
	1 = Unable

17

Table 2. Outcomes for 70° to 100° CPM, 0° to 40° CPM, and No-CPM Groups

| Outcomes | Group Means (SD) | | | ANOVA | |
	70°-100° CPM (n=10)	0°-40° CPM (n=10)	No CPM (n=10)	F	P
3-week flex- ion ROM (°)	77.6 (19.8)	72.6 (18.9)	49.1 (14.6)	7.21	.003
6-week flex- ion ROM (°)	78.9 (17.1)	82.8 (12.3)	58.6 (12.3)	8.53	.003
6-month flex- ion ROM (°)	100.0 (7.1)	103.3 (4.1)	85.8 (10.0)	15.63	<.001
Gait velocity (cm/s)	144.0 (19.6)	145.6 (20.7)	107.6 (29.4)	8.25	.002
ADL score	18.3 (2.2)	17.0 (2.4)	11.0 (4.1)	16.24	<.001

CPM = continuous passive motion; ROM = range of motion;

ADL= activities of daily living.

(12.4)→ **FIGURE LEGEND**

Figure. Mean daily time in continuous passive motion (CPM) for patients in each CPM group.   ←(12.5)

19

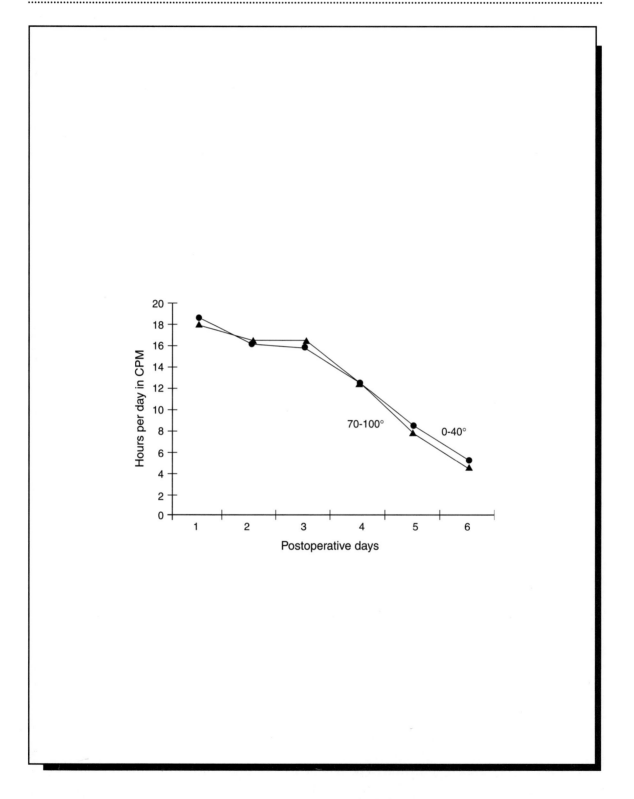

American Psychological Association Style: Sample Manuscript for a Hypothetical Study

The following short, hypothetical manuscript on continuous passive motion following total knee arthroplasty is based, with a few changes in the demographic variables, on the hypothetical data set presented in Chapter 19 in Tables 19–1 and 19–2. The circled numbers in the manuscript correspond to guidelines listed in Appendix D.

Running head: INITIAL ARC OF MOTION FOR CPM

Effect of Initial Arc of Continuous Passive Motion on Motion   ←2.1

and Function Following Total Knee Arthroplasty

Jan R. Woolery

Memorial Hospital of Indiana, Anytown, IN   ←2.5

Jodi C. Beeker

Community Hospital of Anytown (IN)

Jonathon V. Mills

Religious Hospital of Anytown (IN)

2   Initial Arc of Motion

Abstract

(3.1)→ Two continuous passive motion (CPM) regimens with different initial arcs of motion (70° to 100° and 0° to 40° of knee flexion) were compared to no CPM on knee motion and function up to 6 months after total knee arthroplasty (TKA). Ten consecutive patients over the age of 50 years following unilateral TKA were studied at each of three different community hospitals. Group assignments were made randomly by hospital. CPM groups scored higher on all measures, including knee range of motion, gait velocity, and function. There were no significant differences between the CPM groups. The findings are consistent with past research supporting the use of CPM following TKA, with little differentiation between groups receiving different CPM regimens.

Effect of Initial Arc of Continuous Passive Motion on
(4.1)→   Motion and Function Following Total
Knee Arthroplasty

Total knee arthroplasty is a common surgical procedure used
to reduce pain and enhance function for individuals with knee
impairment secondary to osteoarthritis. Continuous passive
motion (CPM) is used to encourage early motion of the knee
joint after total knee arthroplasty (TKA). Milne et al. (2003) ←(4.4.2)
conducted a meta-analysis of 14 randomized controlled trials of
CPM following TKA, showing that CPM combined with PT resulted
in more active knee flexion at discharge, a shorter length of
stay, and less need for postoperative manipulation than PT
alone. They recommended further research to determine whether
there are differences in CPM effectiveness with different CPM
protocols or with different patient or diagnostic groups.

Studies comparing different CPM regimens have identified few
short-term differences among groups and no long-term
(4.6)→ differences. Groups receiving different daily durations of CPM
were compared by Basso and Knapp (1987) and Chiarello,
Gundersen, and O'Halloran (2000); in both cases no ROM
differences between groups were identified at discharge. Pope,
Corcoran, McCaul, and Howie (1997) found no ROM differences
between groups receiving CPM with different initial arcs of

4   Initial Arc of Motion

motion (0° to 40° versus 0° to 70° of knee flexion). Finally, Yashar, Venn-Watson, Welsh, Colwell, and Lotke (1997) and MacDonald et al. (2000) compared groups receiving CPM with an initial flexion arc of motion from 0° to up to 50° to those receiving CPM with an accelerated initial flexion arc of motion from 70° to up to 110°. Yashar et al. (1997) identified a short-term advantage for the accelerated group on knee flexion ROM, but no long-term differences. MacDonald et al. (2000) found no short-term or long-term differences between CPM groups or a control group receiving usual care without CPM. Thus, on one potentially important CPM variable, initial arc of motion, the research is limited and the results are contradictory.

Therefore, we designed a study to further evaluate the

(4.7)→ impact of the initial arc of motion of CPM on short-term and long-terms outcomes after TKA. Specifically, the purpose of this study was to determine whether there were differences between two CPM protocols (initial arc of motion of 0° to 40° versus 70° to 100°) and no CPM on knee flexion ROM at 3 and 6 weeks postoperatively and on knee flexion ROM, gait velocity, and ADL score at 6 months postoperatively. We hypothesized that there would be no differences between CPM groups at any time, that there would be differences between the no-CPM group and both CPM groups at 3 and 6 weeks postoperatively, and that

there would be no differences among groups at 6 months
postoperatively.

Methods

Participants   ←(5.1)

Participants were patients who were at least 50 years old, had a
diagnosis of osteoarthritis, and underwent TKA in 2003 at one of
three hospitals in Anytown, Indiana: Community Hospital,
Memorial Hospital, and Religious Hospital. Before beginning this
study, the characteristics of patients undergoing TKA was
(5.4)→ compared across the three participating hospitals and found to
be similar for age, sex, diagnosis, and type of prosthesis
implanted. Because of the similarity of patients at the three
hospitals, we assigned the CPM protocol randomly to hospitals
rather than individually to patients. Patients at Community
Hospital received an initial arc of 70° to 100° of CPM, patients
at Religious Hospital received an initial arc of 0° to 40°, and
patients at Memorial Hospital received no CPM. The first
10 patients in 2003 who met the inclusion criteria and
consented to participate were entered into the trial at each
hospital. Twelve eligible patients (three at Community, five at
Religious, and four at Memorial) did not consent to participate
in the study.

6   Initial Arc of Motion

For the 30 patients who entered the trial, half were women and the mean (SD) age was 72.5 (4.7) years. The sex distribution and mean age across groups was similar: 50% women, 73.2 (5.6) years for the 70° to 100° CPM group; 40% women, 71.7 (6.5) years for the 0° to 40° CPM group; and 60% women, 72.5 (4.7) years for the no-CPM group. All 30 patients completed the trial.

Instruments

(1.6)→   *CPM units.* ACME CPM (ACME Orthopedics, Roadrunner, Ariz) units were used to deliver the CPM treatment at all three facilities.

Goniometers. ROM measurements were taken with the 12-inch, (5.5)→ full-circle, plastic universal goniometers available at each facility.

ADL scale. We modified the Brigham and Women's Knee Rating (11.4)→ Scale (Ewald, et al., 1984) to assess ADL (Table 1). The values for each of the four subscales (distance walked, assistive device, stair climbing, and rising from a chair) were added for each person to give a single ADL score that could range from a low of 4 to a high of 20.

Procedure

Patients underwent the assigned postoperative rehabilitation protocol. For the two CPM groups the units were applied in the recovery room and used for 20 hours on the first postoperative   ←(5.6)

day. On subsequent days the ROM was advanced 10° (toward more

flexion for the 0° to 40° group and toward extension for the 70°

to 100° group) per day and the time in the unit was reduced by

about 2 hours per day. Each day the time spent in CPM was

recorded for each patient. Knee flexion ROM measurements were

taken with patients supine according to the procedures

described by Norkin and White (1995) with values recorded to   ←(5.3)

the nearest degree. The 3-week and 6-week measures were taken

by the treating therapists at each hospital when patients came

for their routine outpatient physical therapy visits. The

6-month measures were all taken in the physical therapy

department at Community Hospital by an independent investigator

(JVM) who was unaware of group assignment. Velocity was

measured by having the participant walk at a comfortable pace

across a 20-m measured distance. Each participant was timed

with a stopwatch during the center 10 m of the walk and time

was converted to cm/s for analysis. Within the modified

Brigham and Women's Knee Rating Scale (1984), use of an assis-

tive device, rising from a chair, and stair climbing were actu-

ally observed and rated; distance walked was a self-reported

measure.

8   Initial Arc of Motion

Data Analysis

Analysis of variance (ANOVA) was used to test for differences between groups for each of the following dependent variables: (5.8)→ 3-week ROM, 6-week ROM, and 6-month ROM; gait velocity; and ADL score. The Newman-Keuls procedure was used for post hoc analysis. Alpha was set at .05 for each analysis. SPSS for Windows 10.02 was used for the data analysis (SPSS Inc, Chicago, Ill).   ←(5.8.2)

Results

Average time spent in CPM per day was similar for the two CPM groups (Figure 1). There were significant differences between groups for all variables (Table 2). For all variables,   ←(6.2) post hoc analysis showed that the CPM groups were not statistically different from one another, but that both were significantly different from the no-CPM group.

Discussion

Of our three hypotheses, two were supported: (1) that there would be no differences between the CPM groups at any time and (7.4)→ (2) that there would be 3- and 6-week differences between the no-CPM group and both the CPM groups. The significant differences between the no-CPM and CPM groups is consistent with the meta-analysis findings of Milne et al. (2003) strengthening the case for using CPM to improve short-term postoperative ROM after TKA. In addition, our findings suggest that the benefits extend beyond ROM to include gait and other functional outcomes.

The lack of differences between the CPM groups is consistent
(7.5)→ with the work of others (Yashar et al., 1997; MacDonald et al., 2000) who also found no difference in ROM outcomes between groups receiving different initial arcs of motion. Further, the addition of gait velocity and ADL measures in our study provides evidence that both impairment and disability level outcomes are similar regardless of the direction in which ROM is progressed with CPM.

Our final hypothesis, that differences between the no-CPM
(7.6)→ group and the CPM groups would not be present at 6 months, was not supported. We plan to continue the study to determine if differences in all variables disappear by 1 year postopera-tively, as has been found by others (Yashar et al., 1997; Pope
(7.3)→ et al., 1997; MacDonald et al., 2000).

The functional importance of our gait and ADL findings is apparent if one looks at the mean values for the different groups. The no-CPM group had an average gait velocity of only 107.6 cm/s, well below the averages of the two CPM groups (144.0 and 145.6 cm/s). The ADL scores of the CPM groups were approximately 18 and 17 of 20, respectively. This indicates

10   Initial Arc of Motion

minor impairment on two of the components or moderate impair-

ment on one. In contrast, the average ADL score for the no-CPM

group was 11, indicating moderate to severe impairment in one

or more of the ADL components.

In interpreting these results, several limitations or

alternative explanations must be considered. First, because the

treatments were assigned by hospital and not by patient,   ←(7.7)

systematic differences between the hospitals could explain the

difference in results. Second, because the treating therapists

could not be masked to the group membership of the partici-

pants, their expectations may have influenced subject perform-

ance. Despite these limitations, the results have clinical

implications for facilities using CPM for patients after TKA.

Our results seem to indicate that patients who receive CPM—

regardless of the initial arc of motion—do better on important

outcome measures until at least 6 months after surgery compared

with patients who do not receive CPM.

Further research must be done to see if these results can be

replicated, to see whether differences between CPM and no-CPM

(7.9)→ groups persist longer than 6 months, and to determine whether

there are other important differences among CPM groups (e.g.,

blood loss or analgesic use) that would suggest an optimal

direction for increasing motion after surgery.

(8.1)→   In summary, patients who underwent unilateral TKA and

received CPM with different initial arcs of motion (starting at

Initial Arc of Motion   11

70° to 100° of flexion or starting at 0° to 40° of flexion) had

significantly better knee flexion ROM at 3 weeks and 6 weeks

and significantly better knee flexion ROM, gait velocity, and

ADL scores at 6 months postoperatively than did those who did

not receive CPM.

References   ←(10.1)

Basso, D. M., Knapp, L. (1987). Comparison of two continuous

(10.4)→ passive motion protocols for patients with total knee

implants. *Physical Therapy, 67,* 360-363.   ←(10.2)

Chiarello, C. M., Gundersen, L., & O'Halloran, T. (1997). The

effect of continuous passive motion duration and increment on

range of motion in total knee arthroplasty patients. *Journal

of Orthopaedic and Sports Physical Therapy, 25,* 119-127.

Ewald, F. C., Jacobs, M. A., Miegel, R. E., Walker, P. S.,

Poss, R., & Sledge, C. B. (1984). Kinematic total knee

replacement. *Journal of Bone and Joint Surgery American,

66,* 1032-1040.

MacDonald, S. J., Bourne, R. B., Rorabeck, C. H., McCalden,

R.W., Kramer, J., & Vaz, M. (2000). Prospective randomized

clinical trial of continuous passive motion after total knee

arthroplasty. *Clinical Orthopedics and Related Research,

380,* 30-35.

12   Initial Arc of Motion

Milne, S., Brosseau, L., Robinson, V., Noel, M. J., Davis, J., Drouin, H., et al. (2003). Continuous passive motion following total knee arthroplasty (Cochrane Review). In: *The Cochrane Library* (Issue 4). Chichester, UK: John Wiley & Sons.

Norkin, C. C., & White, D.J. (1995). *Measurement of joint motion: A guide to goniometry* (pp. 142-143). Philadelphia, PA: FA Davis.

Pope, R. O., Corcoran, S., McCaul, K., & Howie, D.W. (1997) Continuous passive motion after primary total knee arthroplasty: does it offer any benefits? *Journal of Bone and Joint Surgery British, 79,* 914-917.

Yashar, A.A., Venn-Watson, E., Welsh, T., Colwell, C. W., & Lotke, P. (1997) Continuous passive motion with accelerated flexion after total knee arthroplasty. *Clinical Orthopedics and Related Research, 345,* 38-43.

(9.1)→ **Author Note**

Jan Woolery, Department of Physical Therapy, Memorial Hospital of Indiana; Jodi Beeker, Department of Orthopedic Surgery, Community Hospital of Anytown, Anytown, IN; Jonathon Mills, Occupational Therapy Department, Religious Hospital of Anytown, Anytown, IN.

We thank Ben Counter, PhD, for assistance with the statistical analysis of the study, and Ellen Redline, PT, PhD, for her (9.3)→ critical review of an earlier draft of the manuscript.

Correspondence concerning this article should be addressed to Jan Woolery, Department of Physical Therapy, Memorial Hospital of Indiana, 555 Main Street, Anytown, Indiana 46234 (USA). E-mail: *jrwoolery@memorialindiana.org*

14   Initial Arc of Motion

(11.6)→ Table 1
Modified Brigham and Women's Knee Rating Scale[a]   ←(11.5)

(11.1)→ Variable   Scoring Criteria   ←(11.2)

Variable	Scoring Criteria
Distance walked	5 = Unlimited
	4 = 4 to 6 blocks
	3 = 2 to 3 blocks
	2 = Indoors only
	1 = Transfers only
Assistive device	5 = None
	4 = Cane outside
	3 = Cane full time
	2 = Two canes or crutches
	1 = Walker or unable
Stair climbing	5 = Reciprocal, no rail
	4 = Reciprocal, rail
	3 = One at a time, with or without rail
	2 = One at a time, with rail and assistive device
	1 = Unable

Table 1(continued)

Modified Brigham and Women's Knee Rating Scale[a]

Variable	Scoring Criteria
Rising from a chair	5 = No arm assistance
	4 = Single arm assistance
	3 = Difficult with two arm assistance
	2 = Needs assistance of another
	1 = Unable

[a]See Ewald, et al. (1984).

16   Initial Arc of Motion

Table 2

Outcomes for 70° to 100° CPM, 0° to 40° CPM, and No-CPM Groups

| | Group Means (SD) | | | ANOVA | |
Outcomes	70°–100° CPM (n=10)	0°–40° CPM (n=10)	No CPM (n=10)	*F*	*P*
3-week flexion ROM (°)	77.6 (19.8)	72.6 (18.9)	49.1 (14.6)	7.21	.003
6-week flexion ROM (°)	78.9 (17.1)	82.8 (12.3)	58.6 (12.3)	8.53	.003
6-month flexion ROM (°)	100.0 (7.1)	103.3 (4.1)	85.8 (10.0)	15.63	<.001
Gait velocity (cm/s)	144.0 (19.6)	145.6 (20.7)	107.6 (29.4)	8.25	.002
ADL score	18.3 (2.2)	17.0 (2.4)	11.0 (4.1)	16.24	<.001

CPM = continuous passive motion; ROM = range of motion;

ADL = activities of daily living.

(12.4)→   Figure Caption

Figure 1. Mean daily time in continuous passive motion (CPM) for

patients in each CPM group.

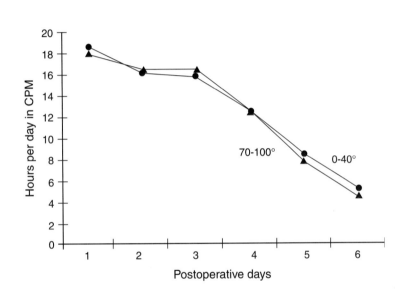

Sample Platform Presentation Script with Slides

1. Good afternoon. I'm pleased to be here in New Orleans to present the results of our study of the effect of the initial arc of continuous passive motion on knee motion and function following total knee arthroplasty.

Effect of Initial Arc of CPM on Motion and Function Following TKA

Jan R. Woolery, PT, PhD
Jodi C. Beeker, MD
Jonathon V. Mills, MS, OTR

Memorial Hospital of Indiana, Anytown, IN
Community Hospital of Anytown, IN
Religious Hospital of Anytown, IN

2. As we all know, total knee arthroplasty is a common surgical procedure used to reduce pain and enhance function for individuals with knee impairment secondary to osteoarthritis. Continuous passive motion (CPM) is used to encourage early motion of the knee joint after total knee arthroplasty (TKA). Recently Milne and colleagues published a Cochrane Review of 14 randomized controlled trials of CPM following TKA. They found small but significant benefits of CPM combined with PT—it resulted in more active knee flexion at discharge, a shorter length of stay, and less need for postoperative manipulation than PT alone. However, they recommended further research to determine whether there are differences in CPM effectiveness with different CPM protocols or with different patient or diagnostic groups.

Problem: CPM following TKA

- TKA reduces pain, enhances function
- CPM used postop to encourage motion
- Meta-analysis (Milne et al, 2003) shows more motion, shorter LOS, less need for postop manipulation under anesthesia with CPM
- Further research to determine whether variations in CPM regimens lead to different outcomes

---

Studies Comparing CPM Regimens

- Different daily durations
  - Basso and Knapp, 1987 (20 vs 5 hours per day)
  - Chiarello et al, 1997 (10 vs 5 hours per day)

- Few ROM differences

- No follow-up after discharge

---

3. There are only a few studies out there that examine differences between CPM regimens. Groups receiving different daily durations of CPM were compared by Basso and Knapp and Chiarello and colleagues; in both cases few ROM differences between groups were identified at discharge, and there was no follow-up to see what happened after discharge.

Studies Comparing CPM Regimens

- Different arcs of motion
  - Yashar et al, 1997 (0-30 vs 70-100)
  - MacDonald et al, 2000 (0-50 vs 70-110)

- Different short-term results

- Consistent 1-year results

- Limited research

- Contradictory results

---

4. Two studies compared CPM using different arcs of motion. Yashar and associates and MacDonald and colleagues both compared groups receiving CPM with an initial flexion arc of motion from 0° to up to 50° to those receiving CPM with an accelerated initial flexion arc of motion from 70° to up to 110°. Yashar identified a short-term advantage for the accelerated group on knee flexion ROM, but MacDonald did not. Neither study found differences at 1 year postop. Thus, on this potentially important CPM variable, initial arc of motion, the research is limited and the results are contradictory.

Outcomes in CPM Literature

- Impairment and Cost Outcomes
  - Reported often
  - Range of motion
  - Length of stay

- Disability Outcomes
  - Reported rarely
  - Gait velocity
  - Activities of daily living

---

5. Another aspect of the CPM literature is that authors have often reported on impairment and cost outcomes such as range of motion and length of hospital stay. Disability level outcomes such as gait velocity or activities of daily living have rarely been reported.

6. Therefore, we designed a study to evaluate the impact of the initial arc of motion of CPM on short-term and long-terms outcomes in CPM protocol. Specifically, the purpose of this study was to determine whether there were differences between a CPM protocol starting at 0 to 40 degrees, a CPM protocol starting at 70 to 100 degrees, and no CPM. The dependent variables we looked at were ROM at 3 weeks, 6 weeks, and 6 months; gait velocity, and ADL score.

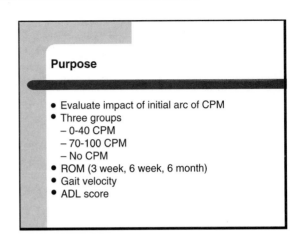

7. We hypothesized that in the short term there would be differences between the no-CPM group and both CPM groups at 3 and 6 weeks postoperatively, but no difference between the two CPM groups.

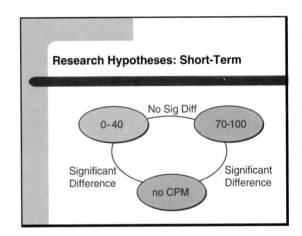

8. For the long term, we hypothesized that there would be no differences among groups at 6 months postoperatively.

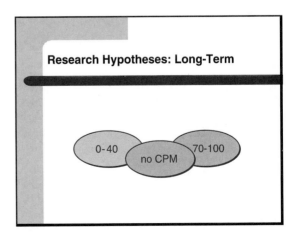

Inclusion Criteria

- At least 50 years old
- Diagnosis of OA
- Unilateral TKA
- One of 3 hospitals

9. Participants were patients who were at least 50 years old, had a diagnosis of osteoarthritis, and underwent a unilateral TKA in 2003 at one of three hospitals in Anytown, Indiana: Community Hospital, Memorial Hospital, and Religious Hospital.

Random Allocation by Hospital

- Patient demographics, disease characteristics,
- postoperative management, surgical outcomes similar across three hospitals
- 70-100 CPM: Community Hospital
- 0-40 CPM: Religious Hospital
- No CPM: Memorial Hospital

10. Before beginning this study, the characteristics of patients undergoing TKA was compared across the three participating hospitals and found to be similar for age, sex, diagnosis, type of prosthesis implanted and so forth. Because of the similarity of patients at the three hospitals, we assigned the CPM protocol randomly to hospitals rather than individually to patients. Patients at Community Hospital received an initial arc of 70 to 100° of CPM, patients at Religious Hospital received an initial arc of 0 to 40°, and patients at Memorial Hospital received no CPM.

Participants

- Enrolled first 10 in 2003 who met criteria and consented at each hospital

- 12 individuals did not consent
  - 3 at Community
  - 5 at Religious
  - 4 at Memorial

- All 30 completed all measurement sessions

11. The first 10 patients in 2003 who met the inclusion criteria and consented to participate were entered into the trial at each hospital. Twelve eligible patients did not consent to participate in the study. Our patients really came through for us, and all 30 who were entered into the study completed all the measurement sessions.

12. The average age of participants in the three groups was very similar, as shown in the graph.

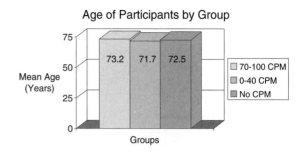

Age of Participants by Group

Mean Age (Years)

73.2 71.7 72.5

□ 70-100 CPM
□ 0-40 CPM
■ No CPM

Groups

13. In addition, the proportion of men and women was fairly evenly distributed across the groups as shown.

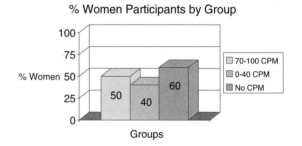

% Women Participants by Group

% Women

50 40 60

□ 70-100 CPM
□ 0-40 CPM
■ No CPM

Groups

14. For the two CPM groups the units were applied in the recovery room and used for 20 hours on the first postoperative day. On subsequent days the ROM was advanced 10° (toward more flexion for the 0° to 40° group and toward extension for the 70° to 100° group) per day and the time in the unit was reduced by about 2 hours per day. Each day the time spent in CPM was recorded for each patient.

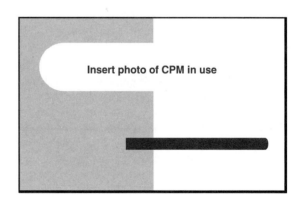

Insert photo of CPM in use

15. The two CPM groups received nearly identical hours per day in CPM, as shown by the two lines on this graph. You can observe the gradual reduction in hours of CPM per day, starting at about 18 hours per day and ending up at less than 6 hours per day by the sixth postoperative day.

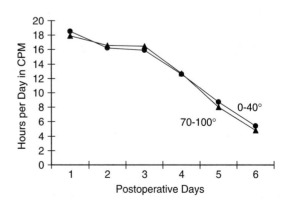

Hours per Day in CPM

0-40°

70-100°

Postoperative Days

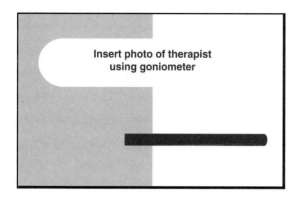

16. We took knee flexion measures as shown in the slide. We used a 12-inch, full-circle goniometer according the procedures outlined by Norkin and White.

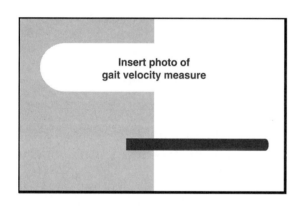

17. Gait velocity measures were taken 6 months after surgery as shown, by timing the participant with a stopwatch during the middle 10 meters of a 20-meter walkway. The data were converted to centimeters per second.

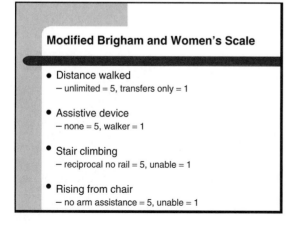

18. The Modified Brigham and Women's knee function scale was administered 6 months after surgery. The distance each participant was able to walk was a self-reported measure, but we directly observed assistive device use, stair climbing, and rising from a chair. The four activity scores are summed to create a single ADL score with the highest level of function scored as 20.

19. We used an analysis of variance to test for differences between groups for each of the dependent variables. The Newman-Keuls procedure was used for post-hoc analysis. Alpha was set at .05 for each analysis.

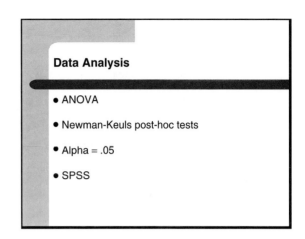

20. Mean knee flexion range of motion at 3 weeks, 6 weeks, and 6 months after surgery can be seen to increase across time for all groups. The CPM groups both achieved better than an average of 90 degrees of flexion by 6 months but the group that did not receive CPM had an average of slightly less than 90 degrees of flexion by then.

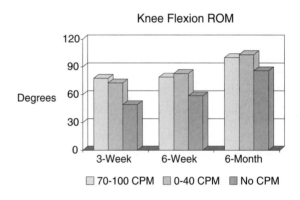

21. Mean gait velocity for both CPM groups was more than 140 centimeters per second; for the no-CPM group it was less than 110 centimeters per second.

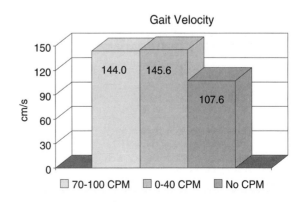

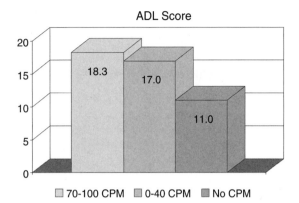

ADL Score

22. The mean ADL scores for the two CPM groups were 18 and 17 out of 20; the mean score for the no-CPM group was 11.

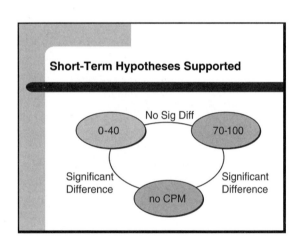

23. Our short-term hypotheses were supported, as the two CPM groups were better than the no-CPM group on all variables, but there were no differences between the two CPM groups.

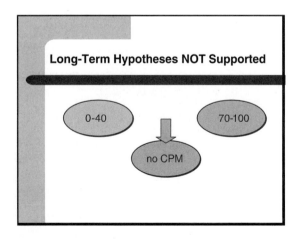

24. Our long-term hypotheses were not supported. We had thought that all three groups would have similar outcomes by 6 months postoperatively. We were surprised to find that the no-CPM group was still lagging behind both CPM groups on all variables after 6 months.

25. The functional importance of our gait and ADL findings is apparent if we looks again at the mean values for the different groups. The no-CPM group had an average gait velocity of less than 110 cm/s, well below the averages of the two CPM groups. Gait velocity may be important for community ambulation safety and it may affect how much community ambulation an individual chooses to do.

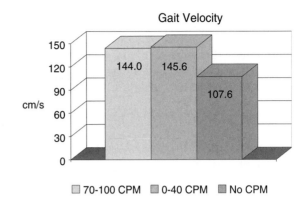

26. The ADL scores of the CPM groups were approximately 18 and 17 of 20, respectively. This indicates minor impairment on two of the components or moderate impairment on one. In contrast, the average ADL score for the no-CPM group was 11, indicating moderate to severe impairment in one or more of the ADL components. If, for example, stair climbing and distance walked are limited, this can reduce community ambulation, important life activities such as grocery shopping, and recreational activities such as travel.

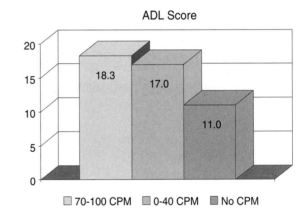

27. There are two main limitations of our research design. First, because the treatments were assigned by hospital and not by patient, there may have been systematic differences between care at the hospitals that could explain the differences in results. Second, because the treating therapists were aware of group membership of the participants, their expectations may have influenced patient performance.

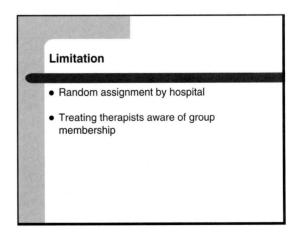

Future Research

- Can results be replicated?

- Do differences between CPM and no-CPM groups persist longer than 6 months?

- Other important variables to measure (blood loss, analgesic use)?

28. Future research in the area should focus on replicating these results, studying whether differences between the CPM and no-CPM groups persist longer than 6 months, and determining whether other important variables—such as postoperative blood loss or analgesic use—are affected by differences in CPM regimens.

Conclusions

- Superior outcomes after TKA for CPM groups compared to no-CPM groups

- No difference in outcome after TKA with CPM progression from 0-40° or 70-100°

- Differences persisted for 6 months

29. There are really three messages that I hope you take home from this presentation today. First, there were superior outcomes after total knee arthroplasty for both CPM groups compared to no-CPM. Second, there was no difference in outcome after total knee arthroplasty based on the arc of motion at which the CPM was started. And third, these differences persisted for 6 months after surgery. Based on this work, we plan to continue to use CPM on a routine basis at our facilities, but will leave the initial arc of motion to the discretion of the physician and therapist.

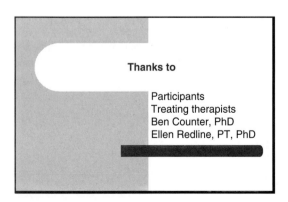

Thanks to

Participants
Treating therapists
Ben Counter, PhD
Ellen Redline, PT, PhD

30. I'd like to publicly than the study participants, who all showed up for all the measurement sessions; the treating therapists at all three hospitals who do such a great job day in and day out; Dr. Ben Counter, our statistics whiz; and Dr. Ellen Redline, who helped us design this presentation.

31. I'd be happy to take any questions at this time.

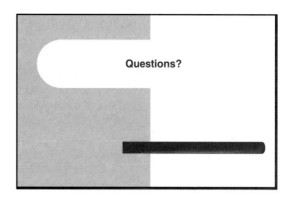

Glossary

A priori theory. Theory that is articulated before conducting research to test elements of the theory.

A-B designs. A family of single-system designs in which baseline (A) and intervention (B) phases are alternated. Common forms are A-B, A-B-A, B-A-B, A-B-A-B.

Absolute frequency. The number of times that a given score is obtained in a frequency distribution. Contrast with *relative frequency*.

Absolute reliability. The extent to which a score varies on repeated measurements; it is quantified by the standard error of measurement.

Accessible population. The subset of the target population who are actually available for a given study.

Active control group. A group within a study that receives a standard treatment. Often used when it is unethical to withhold treatment. Contrast with *passive control group.*

Ad hoc theory. Descriptive theory in which a nonexhaustive list of characteristics is used to describe a phenomenon.

Adjusted frequency. A method of correcting the relative frequency of a given score in a frequency distribution when data points are missing. Calculated by dividing the number of observations for each score by the number of valid scores for each variable.

Adjusted rates. Rates that enable valid comparisons across populations with different proportions of various subgroups; calculated by adjusting the rates for one population based on the composition of the population to which it is being compared; contrast with *crude rates.*

Alpha level inflation. A phenomenon that occurs when researchers conduct many statistical tests within a given study, leading to an increased probability of obtaining chance significant differences.

Alpha level. The probability of concluding that the null hypothesis is false, when in fact it is true. The alpha level is set by the researcher before data analysis; contrast this with *probability level,* which is generated by the data analysis.

Alternate hypothesis. The statistical hypothesis that there is a difference between levels of the independent variable. Contrast with *null hypothesis.*

Alternating-treatment design. A single-system design including the use of different treatments, each administered independently of the other.

Analysis of covariance (ANCOVA). A form of analysis of variance in which the effect of an intervening variable is mathematically removed from the analysis.

Analysis of variance (ANOVA). A family of statistical tests used to analyze differences between two or more groups; based on partitioning the sum of squares into that attributable to between-group differences and that attributable to within-group differences.

Archival data. Records or documents of the activities of individuals, institutions, or governments found in sources such as medical records, voter registration rosters, newspapers and magazines, and meeting minutes.

Artifacts. Physical evidence, particularly within a qualitative research design, which contributes to the understanding of the research question.

Assignment threat. An internal validity threat that is realized when subjects are assigned to groups in ways that do not ensure their equivalence.

Attribute variable. A variable created not by manipulation, but through division of subjects into groups based on an existing attribute such as sex or age; also called *classification variable*.

Autonomy. The moral principle that individuals should be permitted to be self-determining.

Backward regression strategy. A multiple regression strategy in which a researcher begins with all possible variables of interest in the equation and deletes them one at a time if their presence does not contribute enough to the equation.

Beneficence. The moral principle that people should act to promote the welfare of others.

Beta. The probability of making a Type II error; inversely related to alpha.

Beta-weight. Used to interpret multiple-regression equations by standardizing the slopes associated with each independent variable within the equation.

Between-groups difference. One of the determinants of statistical differences; the magnitude of the mean difference between groups.

Between-groups independent variable. An independent variable with independent levels. Typically, this means that the comparison groups within a study are populated by different research participants, each of whom is exposed to only one level of the independent variable.

Between-groups sum of squares. The sum of the squared deviations of the group means from the grand mean, with each deviation weighted according to sample size.

Between-subjects design. An experimental design in which all of the independent variables are between-subjects factors.

Between-subjects factor. An independent variable whose different levels are administered to different groups of participants.

Bimodal distribution. A frequency distribution in which there are two modes, or most frequently occurring scores.

Blinding. A form of research control wherein information about group membership is withheld from subjects, clinicians, data collectors or statisticians involved in the study. Studies are described as single-, double-, triple-, or quadruple-blind studies based on the number of parties who are unaware of group assignment. Also referred to as *masking*.

Block. A grouping of subjects based on a classification or attribute variable, such as age, sex, or diagnosis.

Bonferroni adjustment. Divides the total alpha level for an experiment by the number of statistical tests conducted to control for alpha level inflation.

Boolean operators. The terms "AND," "OR," and "NOT" used during an electronic database search of literature to expand or narrow the search of a specific topic.

C statistic. An analysis method for single-system research designs; the sum of squared deviation scores related to the treatment effect are divided by the sum of squared deviation scores related to the baseline.

Canonical correlation. A correlation used when assessing the relationship between two sets of variables.

Case mix adjustments. Data analysis techniques used to equalize groups on important variables when the researcher is not able to control how participants are placed into groups.

Case report. Systematic, nonexperimental description of clinical practice; contrast with *case study* and *single-system design*.

Case study. Method of structuring a qualitative research project by detailed analysis of a well-defined unit or case; contrast with *case report* and *single-system design*.

Case-control design. An epidemiological research design in which groups of patients with and without a desired effect are compared to determine whether they have different proportions of presumed causes; contrast with *cohort design*, which proceeds from cause to effect.

Case-to-case generalizability. An alternate notion of generalizability wherein results generated from single case experiments are thought to be applicable to different individuals with similar characteristics as the original cases. Contrast with *sample-to-population generalizability*.

Categorical theory. Descriptive theory in which the characteristics that describe a phenomenon are exhaustive.

Causal conclusion. A conclusion that an effect was caused by a factor being studied; generally justified only in the presence of controlled manipulation of the variable under study.

Causal-comparative research. Nonexperimental research in which assignment to groups is based on preexisting characteristics, or attributes, of subjects; also called *ex post facto research*.

Ceiling effect. A measurement phenomenon in which an instrument cannot register gains in scores for the participants of interest.

Celeration line. Method of analyzing single-system research by determining a trend line

in one phase, extrapolating the trend into the next phase, and determining whether the data in the second phase differ significantly from the extrapolated trend line.

Change score. One way to express changes in status; simply the difference between the post-treatment and pretreatment scores. Contrast with *effect size* and *standardized response mean*.

Chi-square distribution. A distribution of squared z scores; it forms the basis for chi-square tests of differences between groups when the dependent variable is in the form of a frequency or percentage.

Classical measurement theory. An approach to measurement that assumes that every measurement or obtained score consist of a true component and an error component.

Classification variable. A variable created not by manipulation, but through division of subjects into groups based on an existing attribute such as sex or age; also called *attribute variable*.

Closed-format item. Questionnaire items that require a specific type of response, such as a "yes or no" question; contrast with *open-format item*.

Cluster sampling. A type of probability sampling using naturally occurring groups as the sampling units. Often used when an appropriate sampling frame does not exist or when logistical constraints to travel are present.

Coefficient of determination. The square of the correlation coefficient; indicates the percentage of variance shared by the variables.

Cohort design. An epidemiological research design that works forward from cause to effect; contrast with *case-control design*, which works from effect to cause.

Cohort. In general, any group. More specifically, groups that follow one another in time, as in subsequent school-year classes.

Compensatory equalization of treatments. A threat to internal validity that is realized when a researcher who has preconceived notions about which treatment is more desirable showers attention on subjects receiving the treatment perceived to be less desirable.

Compensatory rivalry. This threat to internal validity is realized when members of one group react competitively to the perception that they are receiving a less desirable treatment than the other groups.

Competence. A component of the informed consent process requiring prospective patients or research participants to be physically and mentally capable of making participation decisions for themselves.

Completely randomized design. A study design in which all independent variables are manipulable and participants are assigned randomly to each of these variables during the study. Contrast with *randomized block design*.

Completer analysis. A statistical analysis approach in which only those participants who complete the entire study are included in the data analysis. Contrast with *intention-to-treat analysis*.

Comprehension. A component of the informed consent process requiring that information about the project be communicated in ways that are understandable to prospective patients or research participants.

Concept. A phenomenon expressed in words; sometimes used as a more concrete term than *construct*.

Conceptual framework. Theory that specifies relationships between variables but does not have a deductive component; used interchangeably with *model*.

Concurrent validity. The extent to which a developing measure is comparable to a measurement standard.

Condition-specific outcome tools. Measurement tools designed to document the status of individuals having a specific diagnosis or condition.

Confidence interval. A range of scores around a statistic; represents a specified probability that the true value is within the range.

Confounding variable. A factor other than the independent variable that may influence the research outcomes. Synonym of *extraneous variable*.

Consecutive sampling. A form of convenience sampling in which all participants who meet the inclusion criteria are placed into the study as they are identified. Typically used when a sampling frame does not exist at the beginning of the study.

Constant comparative method. Qualitative research method in which theory is continually tested and evaluated as additional data becomes available.

Construct underrepresentation. A threat to construct validity that is realized when the independent or dependent variables are poorly developed.

Construct validity. Threats to construct validity are realized when the independent or dependent variables within a study are not well developed or are incorrectly labeled.

Construct. A property that is invented for a specific purpose; sometimes used as a more abstract term than *concept*.

Content analysis. A process by which the text of archival records is reduced to quantifiable information.

Content validity. The extent to which a measurement is a complete representation of the concept of interest.

Contingency table. An array of data organized into a column variable and a row variable, showing how each individual in the data set scored on both variables.

Continuous variable. A variable that theoretically can be measured to finer and finer degrees.

Contrast. Comparison of two means; specifically, multiple-comparison tests conducted as part of complex analysis of variance tests.

Control. The minimization of extraneous factors that may influence the outcomes of a research study.

Correlation coefficient. Mathematical expression of the degree of relationship between two or more variables; several different forms exist.

Correlational research. Research conducted for the purpose of determining the interrelationships among variables.

Counterbalancing. Randomizing the order of presentation of the experimental conditions in a repeated treatment design in which participants are exposed to more than one of the experimental conditions.

Covariate. An intervening or extraneous variable; often adjusted mathematically.

Cramer's V. A correlation used when there are two categorical variables.

Criterion validity. The extent to which one measure is systematically related to other measures or outcomes; subdivided into concurrent and predictive validity.

Criterion-referenced measure. A measurement framework in which each individual's performance is evaluated with respect to some absolute level of achievement.

Cross-over design. A study design in which participants receive all interventions in a randomized order.

Cross-sectional design. A study design in which measurement and description of a sample is accomplished at a single point in time.

Crude rates. Rates calculated using the entire population at risk; contrast with *specific* and *adjusted rates.*

Cumulative frequency. The sum of relative frequencies of scores in a frequency distribution, up to and including the score of interest.

Deductive reasoning. Reasoning that proceeds from the general to the specific.

Degrees of freedom. The number of items that are free to vary. For example, the degrees of freedom for the mean is $n - 1$, meaning that if a certain mean score is desired, $n - 1$ of the values are free to fluctuate as long as one can control the final value.

Delphi technique. A survey design in which several rounds of a questionnaire are administered, each round building on information collected in previous rounds.

Dependent variable. The measured variable; used to determine the effects of the independent variable.

Descriptive theory. The least restrictive form of theory, simply describing the phenomenon of interest.

Developmental research. A type of nonexperimental research that studies participants at more than one point in time to document the effects of the passage of time.

Deviation score. Calculated by subtracting the mean of a data set from each raw score.

Dichotomous variable. A variable that can take only two values, such as male/female or present/absent.

Diffusion of treatments. This threat to internal validity is realized when participants in treatment and control groups share information about their respective treatments.

Directional hypothesis. A specific type of alternate hypothesis in which the researcher specifies which mean is expected to be greater than the other.

Disclosure. A component of the informed consent process requiring the provision of information regarding risks and benefits of treatment or research.

Discrete variable. A variable that can assume only distinct values. An example is a ligamentous laxity scale, which can assume values of hypomobile, normal, and hypermobile.

Discriminant analysis. An analysis technique in which multiple predictor variables are used to place individuals into groups.

Dummy coding. The process of assigning arbitrary numbers to nominal independent variables (e.g., male = 0, female = 1).

Effect size. One way to express changes in status; the mean change score divided by the standard deviation of the pretreatment score; standardizes the magnitude of change across many different variables. Contrast with *change score* and *standardized response mean*.

Effectiveness. Usefulness of a particular treatment to the individuals receiving it under typical clinical conditions, usually determined by nonexperimental methods in outcomes research; contrast with *efficacy*.

Efficacy. Biological effect of treatment delivered under carefully controlled conditions, usually determined by randomized controlled trial; contrast with *effectiveness*.

Eigenvalue. Values generated within a factor analysis that are used to assist in determining the number of factors in the final solution. Eigenvalues are related to the percentage of variability within the data set that can be accounted for by each factor.

Empiricism. Reliance on observation and experimentation to determine the nature of reality.

Epidemiology. The study of disease, injury, and health in a population. Epidemiological research documents the incidence of a disease or injury, determines causes for the disease or injury, and develops mechanisms to control the disease or injury.

Ethnographic research. Research whose purpose is to develop an in-depth picture of the culture of a particular group or unit.

Evaluation research. Research conducted to determine the effectiveness of a program or policy.

Evidence-based practice. Clinical practice that integrates the results of sound scientific research with clinical experience and patient values.

Ex post facto research. Nonexperimental analysis of differences in which the independent variable is not manipulated. An example is research that examines differences between men and women on various dependent variables. Also called *causal-comparative research*.

Exclusion characteristics. Specific criteria that, if present, will eliminate an individual from participation in a research study.

Experimental research. Research in which at least one independent variable is subjected to controlled manipulation by the researcher.

Experimenter expectancy. A threat to construct validity that is realized when the participants are able to guess the ways in which the experimenter wishes them to respond.

Explanatory theory. Theory that examines the *why* and *how* questions that undergird a problem.

External criticism. Concerns about the authenticity of archival records.

External validity. Concerns the issue of to whom, in what settings, and at what times the results of research can be generalized.

Extraneous variable. A factor other than the independent variable that may influence the research outcomes. Synonym of *confounding variable*.

***F* distribution.** A distribution of squared t statistics; the basis of analysis of variance.

Facets. The factors of interest within a generalizability study; examples of facets might be raters, days, and times of measurement.

Factor. The presumed cause of a measured effect. In experimental research, at least one factor is manipulated by the researcher. A synonym for *independent variable.*

Factor analysis. A multivariate correlational technique used to reduce a large number of variables into a smaller number of factors by clustering related variables.

Factorial design. A design in which there are at least two independent variables, and all levels of each independent variable are crossed with all other independent variables.

False negative. Classified as not having a condition when, in fact, one does have the condition.

False positive. Classified as having a condition when, in fact, one does not have the condition.

Fastidious research. The practice of employing precise control of all aspects of research implementation; may result in limited ability to generalized findings to the clinical setting.

Fisher's exact test. A modified chi-square statistic that is sometimes used if the dependent variable consists of only two categories.

Floor effect. A measurement phenomenon in which an instrument of cannot register greater declines in scores for the participants of interest.

Forward regression strategy. A multiple regression strategy in which a researcher adds one variable at a time to the equation until additional variables do not contribute enough to the final equation.

Frequency distribution. A tally of the number of times each individual score is represented in a data set; can be presented visually as a histogram or a stem-and-leaf plot.

Friedman's ANOVA. The nonparametric version of the repeated measures analysis of variance.

General theory. A form of theory focusing on basic frameworks for practice or action. Also known as *middle-range theory.*

Generalizability theory. An extension of classical measurement theory that quantifies the extent of variability on repeated measures that can be attributed to different facets of interest.

Generic outcome tools. Measures of health-related quality of life designed for use with individuals who have a wide variety of health conditions.

Grand mean. The mean of all scores across all groups.

Grand theory. A form of theory focusing on broad conceptualizations of phenomena addressing large ideas such as human functioning or entire professions.

Grounded theory. A qualitative research approach that starts from an atheoretical perspective and develops theory that is grounded in the information gathered.

Health-related quality of life (HRQL). Quality of life concept that includes elements related to physical, psychosocial, and social functioning; measured by generic tools such as the Short Form-36, Sickness Impact Profile, and Functional Status Questionnaire.

Heuristic. Discovering or revealing relationships that may lead to further development of a particular line of research.

Histogram. A graphical presentation of a grouped frequency distribution using a bar graph.

Historical research. Research in which past events are documented because they are of inherent interest or because they provide a perspective that can guide decision making in the present.

History. This threat to internal validity is realized when events unrelated to the treatment of interest occur during the course of the study and cause changes in the dependent variable.

Homoscedasticity. One of the assumptions that should be met before calculating a correlation coefficient. Homoscedasticity means that for each value of one variable, the other variable has equal variability.

Hypothesis. A conjectural statement of the relationship between variables. Sometimes used interchangeably with *proposition*.

Idiographic. Pertaining to a particular case in a particular time and context; the opposite of *nomothetic*.

Incidence. The rate of new cases of a condition that develop during a specified period of time; the formula is *new cases during a time period/ population at risk during a time period*.

Inclusion characteristics. Specific criteria that, if present, will allow an individual to be considered for participation in a research study.

Independent *t* test. A parametric test of differences between two independent samples.

Independent variable. The presumed cause of a measured effect. In experimental research, at least one independent variable is manipulated by the researcher. A synonym for *factor*.

Inferential statistics. The branch of statistics used to determine whether there are significant differences between groups, based on inferring population parameters from sample statistics.

Informant. Term used by qualitative researchers to describe the research participants for the study.

Informed consent. A process by which health care practitioners or investigators provide potential participants with the information they need to make informed decisions about treatment or participation within a study. Four components are required for autonomy in making such decisions: disclosure, comprehension, voluntariness, and competence.

Institutional review board. A review committee within an organization that ensures that the rights of human research participants are protected by reviewing written research proposals and monitoring the progress of research it has approved.

Instrumentation. This threat to internal validity is realized when changes in measuring tools themselves are responsible for observed changes in the dependent variable.

Intention-to-treat analysis. A statistical analysis approach in which each participant who was entered in the study is included in the final data analysis according to the treatment they were intended to have, whether or not they completed the study.

Interaction. A research question in which the effect of one variable is assessed to determine whether it is consistent across the different levels of a second independent variable.

Interaction design. A single-system design used to evaluate the effect of different combinations of treatments.

Interaction of different treatments. A threat to construct validity that may be realized when treatments other than the one of interest are administered to participants.

Internal criticism. Concerns about the neutrality of the interpretation of information found in archival records.

Internal validity. Concerns whether the independent variable is the probable cause of changes in the dependent variable.

Interrater reliability. The consistency among different judges' ratings of the same participant or response. In its purest form, interrater reliability is determined by having the judges perform the ratings of one group of participants at the same point in time.

Interval scale. Has the real-number system properties of order and distance, but lacks a meaningful origin.

Intraclass correlation coefficient (ICC). A family of correlation coefficients that allows comparison of two or more repeated measures; used to analyze measurement reliability.

Intrarater reliability. The consistency with which one rater assigns scores to a single set of responses on two or more occasions.

Jadad scale. A quality scoring system for randomized controlled trials, based on a 5-point scale, with points given for appropriate randomization, masking, and descriptions of withdrawals and drop outs.

Kappa (κ). A reliability coefficient used with two or more nominal variables with two or more categories; corrects agreement percentages to account for chance agreements.

Kendall's tau (τ). A correlation used when both variables are ranked.

Keyword search. A literature search technique using any words that are found in the database.

Kruskal-Wallis test. The nonparametric version of the one-way analysis of variance.

Level. A value of the independent variable; for example, a design in which the independent variable consists of a treatment group and a control group is said to have two levels of the independent variable.

Level analysis. An analysis method for single-system research designs; the determination of the difference between the end of the celeration line in one phase and beginning of the celeration line in the subsequent phase.

Levels of evidence. An approach to the critical evaluation of research articles that rates the quality of evidence based on the research design of the study. In brief, the top rating is given to randomized control trials, followed by cohort designs, case-control studies, case series, and expert opinion without critical appraisal, respectively.

Likelihood ratio. A ratio that provides information regarding the usefulness of a positive diagnostic test result for ruling in a condition or of a negative diagnostic test result for ruling out a condition.

Likert-type items. Used to assess the strength of response to a declarative statement. The most typical set of responses is "strongly agree," "agree," "undecided," "disagree," and "strongly disagree."

Linear regression. Analysis technique used to predict scores on one variable from scores on one or more other variables.

Logistic regression. Regression technique used to predict dichotomous outcomes from numerical independent variables.

Longitudinal design. A study design in which measurement and description of a sample is accomplished several times over an extended period of time.

Main effect. The effect of one independent variable across all levels of another independent variables. Contrast with *simple main effect*.

Manipulation. A characteristic of experimental research requiring the researcher to expose participants to experimental procedures under controlled conditions.

Mann-Whitney test. The nonparametric version of the independent *t* test.

Masking. A form of research control wherein information about group membership is withheld from subjects, clinicians, data collectors or statisticians involved in the study. Studies are described as single-, double-, triple-, or quadruple-masked studies based on the number of parties who are unaware of group assignment. Also referred to as *blinding*.

Maturation. This threat to internal validity is realized when changes within a participant resulting from the passage of time occur during the course of a study and cause changes in the dependent variable.

McNemar test. A statistical test that analyzes frequency or percentage data collected on repeated occasions.

Mean. The sum of observations divided by the number of observations.

Median. The middle score of a ranked distribution.

Member checking. Method of verification in qualitative research by which informants review results generated by the researcher to correct technical errors or challenge the researcher's interpretation of their situation.

Meta-analysis. A form of systematic review of the literature, based on the statistical pooling of results across studies. Literally, the analysis of analyses.

Metatheory. An abstract form of theory focusing on how knowledge is created and organized, literally "theorizing about theory."

Methodological research. Research conducted to determine the reliability and validity or clinical and research measures.

Middle-range theory. A form of theory focusing on basic frameworks for practice or action. Also known as *general theory*.

Mixed design. A design in which some of the independent variables are between-subjects factors and some of the independent variables are within-subject factors; also called a *split-plot design*.

Mode. The most frequently occurring score within a distribution; if there are two modes, the distribution is called *bimodal*.

Model. A theory that specifies relationships between variables but does not have a deductive component; used interchangeably with *conceptual framework*.

Mortality. This threat to internal validity is realized when participants are lost from the different study groups at different rates or for different reasons.

Multiple baseline design. A single-system design in which several participants are studied after baselines of varying lengths.

Multiple correlation. A correlation used to assess the variability shared by more than two variables.

Multiple regression. Extension of simple correlation and regression techniques to use multiple independent variables to predict a numerical dependent variable.

Multivariate analyses. Statistical tools designed for simultaneous analysis of multiple dependent variables.

Multivariate analysis of variance (MANOVA). A form of analysis of variance that uses an omnibus test to determine whether there are significant differences on the factor of interest when the dependent variables of interest are combined mathematically; the analysis of several dependent variables simultaneously.

Narrative review. A form of literature review that provides readers with broad-based summaries of published information regarding the topic of interest. Contrast with *systematic review*.

Naturalistic. One term for qualitative research; refers specifically to the philosophy that qualitative researchers should study subjects in their natural setting.

Negative predictive value. The percentage of individuals identified by a test as negative who actually do not have the diagnosis.

Nested design. A design in which there are at least two independent variables, but not all levels of the independent variables are crossed.

Newman-Keuls test. A multiple-comparison procedure.

Nominal scale. Has none of the properties of a real-number system; provides classification without placing any value on the categories within the classification.

Nomothetic. Relating to general or universal principles; opposite of *idiographic*.

Nondirectional. A *t*-test hypothesis in which the researcher is open to the possibility that one mean is either greater than or less than the other mean.

Nonexperimental research. Research in which there is no manipulation of an independent variable.

Nonmaleficence. The moral principle of doing no harm.

Nonparametric tests. Statistical tests that do not rest on assumptions related to the distribution of the populations from which the samples are drawn.

Nonprobability sample. A sample that is created without random selection from a larger population of interest.

Nonrefereed journal. A journal that does not require peer review of a submitted manuscript before publication.

Norm-referenced measure. A measure that judges individual performance in relation to group norms.

Normal curve. A symmetric, bell-shaped frequency distribution that can be defined in terms of the mean and standard deviation of a set of data.

Normative research. Research that uses large, representative samples to generate norms on measure of interest.

Null hypothesis. The statistical hypothesis that there is no difference between groups; contrast with *research hypothesis*.

Number. A numeral that has been assigned quantitative meaning.

Numeral. A symbol that does not necessarily have quantitative meaning; it is a form of naming.

Odds ratio. Method of estimating relative risk by calculating the ratio of the odds that each of two groups will possess a certain characteristic.

Omnibus test. An overall test of a hypothesis within an analysis of variance; if the omnibus test identifies a significant difference between groups, then multiple-comparison procedures are needed to determine the location of the differences.

Open-format item. An interview or survey item allowing respondents freedom to structure

their responses as desired; contrast with *closed-format item.*

Operational definition. A specific description of the way in which a construct is presented or measured within a study.

Ordinal scale. Has only one of the properties of a real number system: order. Ordinal scales do not ensure that there are equal intervals between categories or ranks.

Outcomes research. Analysis of clinical practice as it actually occurs for the purpose of determining effectiveness of clinical methods.

Outlier. An extreme value or data point that is sometimes eliminated from a data set, with appropriate justification.

Paired-*t* test. A statistical test that determines the difference between two paired measures.

Paradigm. A belief system researchers use to organize their discipline.

Parallel group design. A study design in which each group receives only one of the levels of the independent variable. For example, one group receives a treatment and the other group receives a placebo.

Parameter. A characteristic of a population; estimated by sample statistics.

Parametric tests. Statistical tests that rest on assumptions related to the distribution of the populations from which the samples are drawn.

Partial correlation. A correlation used to assess the relationship between two variables with the effect of the third variable eliminated.

Participant-observation. Qualitative, ethnographical research method in which the researcher participates in and experiences a new culture, describing observations from within the reality of the culture.

Passive control group. A group within a study that receives either no treatment or a sham or placebo treatment. Contrast with *active control group.*

Pathokinesiology. The application of anatomy and physiology to the study of abnormal human movement.

Patient-specific outcome tools. Measurement tools designed to identify individualized goals and detect individual changes in status related to those goals.

Pearson correlation coefficient. Analysis of the relationship between two variables; ranges in value from +1.0 to −1.0; calculated by determining the average of the crossproducts of the *z* scores of both variables.

PEDro scale. A quality scoring system for randomized controlled trials, based on a 10-point scale, with points given for randomization and allocation, baseline similarity of groups, masking, participant retention, and use of appropriate statistical tools.

Percentile rank. Standardization of a raw score to a percentile ranking based on the distribution.

Period prevalence. The prevalence within a time-frame established by the researcher. For example, the proportion of individuals reporting a given condition within a year of the study interview. Contrast with *point prevalence*.

Phenomenology. A qualitative research approach whose purpose is to describe some aspect of life as it is lived by the participants.

Phi (ϕ). A shortcut version of the Pearson *r* correlation applicable when both variables are dichotomous; a correlation for use with nominal data.

Platform presentation. A short presentation of research results to an audience attending a professional conference.

Point prevalence. The prevalence at the exact time of measurement. For example, the proportion of individuals reporting a given condition on the day they are interviewed for a study. Contrast with *period prevalence*.

Policy research. Research conducted to inform policy making and implementation.

Population. The entire group of interest from which a sample may be taken and to which the research results may be generalized.

Population variance. A measure of variability; the sum of the squared deviations from the mean divided by the number within the sample (N). Contrast with *sample variance*.

Positive predictive value. The percentage of individuals identified by the test as positive who actually have the diagnosis.

Positivism. A research tradition that rests on the objective measurement of reality; the traditional method of science.

Post hoc comparisons. Tests that are used to make pair-wise comparisons of means after an omnibus test has identified significant differences between more than two means.

Poster presentation. A display of research results at a professional conference. The poster is typically displayed for hours or days, with the researcher present for a required period of time to answer questions from individual attendees interested in the work.

Postpositivist. The qualitative research tradition, resting on the assumption of multiple constructed realities.

Power. The likelihood that a statistical test will detect a difference when one exists. Power is calculated by 1 − beta.

Practice theory. A form of theory focusing on particular applications of grand or general theories. Also known as *specific theory*.

Pragmatic research. The practice of closely simulating the clinical setting in research implementation; may result in the presence of numerous extraneous variables and limited ability to draw causal conclusions.

Predictive theory. A theory that is used to make predictions based on the relationships between variables.

Predictive validity. The ability of a measurement made at one point in time to predict future status.

Pretest probability. A percentage estimate, generated by the researcher or clinician, of the participant or patient having the condition of interest.

Prevalence. The proportion of a population who exhibit a certain condition at a given point in time; the formula is *existing cases/ population examined at a given point in time.*

Primary sources. Scholarly works that constitute the first documentation of the results of a study; the traditional primary source in the health sciences is the journal article, which reports the findings of original research.

Probability (*p*) level. The probability of obtaining a certain test statistic if the null hypothesis is true; the probability level is generated by the data analysis itself. Contrast with *alpha level,* which is set by the researcher.

Probability sample. A sample that is created with some level of random selection from a larger population of interest.

Proportion. A fraction in which the numerator is a subset of the denominator; the formula is *a/a + b.*

Proposition. A statement of the relationship between concepts. Sometimes used interchangeably with *hypothesis.*

Prospective research. A research approach in which the researcher completes data collection after the research question is developed. Also used by epidemiologists as a synonym for *cohort design.*

Proxy. The authority to act for another; in the informed consent process "proxy consent" may be required from parents or legal guardians of individuals who are too young or too incapacitated to make participation decisions for themselves.

Purposive sampling. A specialized type of nonprobability sampling, typically used for qualitative research, in which researchers have specific reasons for selecting particular participants for a study.

Q-sort. A survey research technique in which respondents generate a forced-choice ranking of many alternatives.

Qualitative paradigm. A research framework acknowledging the presence of multiple constructed realities, the interdependence of the investigator and subject, the time- and context-dependent nature of knowledge, the indistinguishability of cause and effect, and the impact of researcher values on the investigation. Contrast with *quantitative paradigm.*

Qualitative research. A research paradigm based, in part, on assumptions of multiple constructed realities, interdependence of investigator and participant, and time- and context-dependency of information.

Quantitative paradigm. The traditional method of science, emphasizing measurement, control, and reproducibility. Contrast with *qualitative paradigm.*

Quasiexperimental research. A form of experimental research characterized by nonrandom assignment of subjects to groups or repeated treatments to the same group.

Questionnaire. A written self-report instrument used in survey research.

Randomized block design. A study design in which one of the factors of interest is not manipulable. Participants are placed into blocks based on the nonmanipulable factor (such as sex or disease status) and then randomized into treatment groups.

Randomized clinical trial. The name often given to clinical research in which participants are randomly assigned to treatment and control groups.

Rate. A proportion expressed over a particular unit of time, often multiplied by a constant to obtain whole number values.

Ratio. Expresses the relationship between two numbers by dividing the numerator by the denominator; the simple formula is *a/b*.

Ratio scale. Exhibits all three components of a real-number system: order, distance, and origin. All the arithmetic functions of addition, subtraction, multiplication, and division can be applied to ratio scales.

Real-number system. A system using numerical values having the characteristics of order, distance, and origin.

Receiver-operator curve (ROC). Method of graphing test data to determine cutoff points that balance *sensitivity* and *specificity*.

Refereed journal. A journal that requires peer review of a submitted manuscript before publication.

Relative frequency. The percentage of individuals with a given score in a frequency distribution. Contrast with *absolute frequency* and *adjusted frequency*.

Relative reliability. Exists when individual measurements within a group maintain their position within the group on repeated measurement; quantified by correlation coefficients.

Relative risk. Comparison of the probability that different groups with different characteristics will be affected by disease or injury in some way.

Reliability. The extent to which measurements are repeatable.

Repeated measures analysis of variance. One of a family of analysis of variance techniques; used to determine differences between two or more dependent samples.

Research hypothesis. A statement that makes predictions about the expected outcome of the study; contrast with *null hypothesis*.

Resentful demoralization. This threat to internal validity is realized when members of one group react negatively to the perception that they are receiving a less desirable treatment than the other groups.

Residual. The amount of variability left unexplained after a data analysis; part of some analysis of variance and linear regression procedures.

Retrospective research. A research approach in which data are collected before the research question is developed. Also used by epidemiologists as a synonym for *case-control design*.

Reversed treatment design. A design in which the subjects or groups receive treatments that are expected to cause changes in opposite directions. This is in contrast to typical control-group designs, in which the control group is not expected to change.

Risk ratio. Method of calculating relative risk by creating a ratio of the incidence rate for one subgroup and the incidence rate for another subgroup; contrast with *odds ratio*.

Robust. Describes statistical procedures that tolerate violation of their assumptions without distortion of the probability of making a Type I error.

Sample variance. A measure of variability; the sum of the squared deviations from the mean divided by the degrees of freedom for the mean $(N - 1)$. Contrast with *population variance*.

Sample. The subgroup of the population of interest that is available for study.

Samples of convenience. A type of nonprobability sampling that uses readily available participants.

Sample-to-population generalizability. The traditional notion of generalizability, wherein results generated from a sample are thought to be applicable to the larger population of interest. Contrast with *case-to-case generalizability*.

Sampling distribution. A distribution of sample means formed by drawing repeated samples from the same population. Ordinarily, the sample distribution is a theoretical distribution with a standard deviation estimated by dividing a single sample standard deviation by the square root of the number within the sample.

Sampling error. The chance process that results in samples with different characteristics even when the same random process is used to select the samples from the same population.

Sampling frame. A listing of potential participants in the accessible population that fit the inclusion criteria.

Scheffé test. A multiple-comparison procedure.

Scree method. A factor analysis method that uses graphical examination of patterns of eigenvalues to assist in determining the number of factors in the final solution.

Secondary analysis. Research that reanalyzes data collected for one purpose to answer new research questions.

Secondary sources. Scholarly works, such as book chapters or literature reviews, that are interpretations of original sources such as journal article reports of original research.

Selection. This threat to external validity is realized when the selection process is biased because it yields participants who are in some manner different from the population to whom researchers hope to generalize their results.

Self-report measures. These measures are the foundation of survey research; it is assumed that meaningful information can be obtained by asking the parties of interest what they know, what they believe, and how they behave.

Semantic differential items. A type of closed-format item that uses adjective pairs, such as "invigorating–dull" to represent different ends of a continuum.

Semistructured interview. An interview technique based on predeveloped questions, but with latitude for the interviewer to clarify questions as needed for the interviewee, thereby obtaining more information for the study.

Sensitivity. The percentage of individuals with a particular diagnosis who are correctly identified as positive by a test.

Serial dependency. A phenomenon in a data series that is associated with the ability to predict the next point from the previous point.

Setting. This threat to external validity is realized when peculiarities of the setting in which the research was conducted make it difficult to generalize results to other settings.

Significant difference. The statistical judgment that a difference between levels of the independent variable is unlikely to be due to sampling error or chance.

Simple main effect. The effect of one independent variable at each level of another independent variable. Contrast with *main effect*.

Simple random sampling. A type of probability sampling in which each member of the population has an equal chance of being selected for the sample and selection of each participant is independent of selection of other participants.

Single-system design. Experimental research designs in which the unit of interest is a single person or setting, studied over time under baseline and treatment conditions.

Single-system paradigm. A research framework focusing on the effects of treatment on individuals rather than larger groups of patients or participants.

Skewed. A distribution that is not symmetric, that is, one with a long tail at its upper or lower end.

Slope. A characteristic of a line; the ratio of the change in Y that accompanies a change of one unit of X.

Snowball sampling. A type of nonprobability sampling in which current participants in a study are asked to identify other potential members of the sample. Typically used when potential members of a sample are difficult to identify.

Spearman's rho (ρ). A shortcut version of the Pearson *r* correlation used when both variables are ranked.

Specific rates. Rates calculated for specific subgroups of the population; contrast with *crude rates*.

Specific theory. A form of theory focusing on particular applications of grand or general theories. Also known as *practice theory*.

Specificity. The percentage of individuals without a particular diagnosis who are correctly identified as negative by a test.

Split-plot design. A design in which some of the independent variables are between-subjects factors and some are within-subject factors; also called a *mixed design*.

Standard deviation. The square root of the variance; expressed in the units of the original measure.

Standard error of measurement. A measure of absolute reliability; represents the standard deviation of measurement errors.

Standard error of the estimate. The standard deviation of the difference between individual data points and the regression line through them.

Standard error of the mean. The standard deviation of the sampling distribution.

Standard distribution. A distribution with a mean of 0.0 and a standard deviation of 1.0.

Standardized response mean. One way to express changes in status; the mean change score divided by the standard deviation of the change scores. Contrast with *change score* and *effect size*.

Statistic. A characteristic of a sample; used to estimate population parameters.

Statistical conclusion validity. Concerns whether statistical tools have been used and their results interpreted properly within a study.

Statistical regression to the mean. This threat to internal validity may be realized when participants are selected based on extreme scores on a single administration of a test.

Status quo. The existing state of affairs.

Stem-and-leaf plot. A method of data presentation in which each individual score is divided into a "stem" (i.e., the digit 3 in the number 34) and "leaf" (i.e., the digits 5 and 9, respectively, in the numbers 35 and 39).

Stepwise regression strategy. A multiple regression strategy in which both forward and backward regression strategies are used to generate the regression equation.

Stratified sampling. A type of probability sampling used when certain subgroups must be represented in adequate numbers within the sample or when preserving the proportions of subgroups in the population within the sample is important. In stratified sampling the accessible population is stratified according to the variable of interest and then participants are selected from within each stratum.

Structured interview. Oral administration of a written questionnaire without deviation from the wording of the questionnaire.

Subject-heading search. A literature search technique using particular words or phrases that are used as indexing terms within the database.

Survey research. Research in which the data are collected by having participants complete questionnaires or respond to interview questions.

Survival analysis. A mathematical tool that analyzes the changing proportion of individuals who have or have not experienced a certain outcome (e.g., death) across time after an event (e.g., stroke); accounts for the declining number of individuals who remain in the analysis across time. Now used for many outcomes other than the survival and death outcomes that gave the analysis its name.

Systematic review. A form of literature review that requires a documented search strategy and explicit inclusion and exclusion criteria for studies reviewed, reducing author bias toward or against particular methods or outcomes. Contrast with *narrative review*.

Systematic sampling. A type of probability sampling in which every *n*th person on a list is chosen for participation.

***t* distribution.** A flattened standard curve; the basis for *t* tests, which are used to assess the differences between two groups or between paired data.

Target population. The group of individuals to whom the researchers hope to generalize their findings.

Tentativeness. The idea that theory is not a permanent explanation of phenomena, but continually evolving as more knowledge is acquired.

Testability. The characteristic of a theory that requires it to be formulated in ways that allow the theory to be tested.

Testing. This threat to internal validity is realized when repeated testing itself is likely to result in changes in the dependent variable.

Test-retest reliability. The ability of a measurement to be repeated from one test occasion to another.

Theory. A body of interrelated principles that present a systematic view of phenomena; a theory is testable and tentative.

Time. This threat to external validity is realized when the results of a study are applicable to limited time frames.

Total sum of squares. The sum of the squared deviations of all individual scores from the grand mean.

Transform. Mathematical manipulation of data, usually to make it fit a distribution.

Trend. Related to data analysis of single-system research designs; describes whether the direction of change during a study phase is upward or downward.

Triangulation. A method of establishing reliability in qualitative research; consists of comparing responses across several different sources.

T-score. Standardization of a raw score based on a mean of 50 and a standard deviation of 10, eliminating negative scores.

Tukey test. A multiple-comparison procedure.

Two standard deviation band analysis. A method of analyzing single-system data by calculating a two standard deviation band around the baseline data and observing the pattern of intervention data that fall within and outside the band.

Type I error. A statistical error in which it is determined that a difference between groups exists when, in fact, there is no difference. The probability of making a Type I error is alpha.

Type II error. A statistical error in which it is concluded that there is a no difference between groups when, in fact, there is a difference. The probability of making a Type II error is beta.

Unstructured interview. An interview technique wherein the order and way in which the topics are covered are left to the interviewer as he or she interacts with participants.

Utility. The moral principle that we should act to bring about the greatest benefit and the least harm.

Validity. The meaningfulness of test scores as they are used for specific purposes.

Variance. Conceptually, the average of the squared deviations about the mean. The *population variance* is found by dividing the sum of the squared deviations by the number within the sample; the *sample variance* is found by dividing the sum of the squared deviations by n–1.

Voluntariness. A component of the informed consent process requiring that prospective research participants or patients be free from coercion with regard to the decision to participate in treatment or research.

Wilcoxon rank sum test. The nonparametric version of the independent t test; synonymous with *Mann-Whitney test.*

Wilcoxon signed rank test. The nonparametric version of the paired-t test.

Withdrawal design. A family of single-system designs characterized by implementation and withdrawal of treatment over the course of the study; known generically as A-B-A designs.

Within-group independent variable. An independent variable with dependent levels. Typically, this means that the comparisons within a study are made within a single group that is exposed to all levels of the independent variable at different points in the study.

Within-group sum of squares. The sum of the squared deviations of all individual scores from their respective group means.

Within-group variability. One of the determinants of statistical differences; the magnitude of the variance of individuals within the comparison groups.

Within-subject design. A design in which all of the factors are within-subject factors.

Within-subject factor. An independent variable whose different levels are administered to the same group of participants. The comparison of interest is within the participant group.

Yates' correction. A correction factor sometimes used with chi-square tests in which the expected frequency in several cells is very small.

z score. A deviation score divided by the standard deviation; indicates how many standard deviations the raw score is above or below the mean.

Mathematical and Statistical Symbols

Descriptive Statistics

Σ (capital sigma)	The sum of what follows
N	Number of observations or number of participants
μ (mu)	The population mean
$\overline{X}$	Sample mean
x	The deviation score
σ^2 (sigma squared)	The population variance
s^2	The sample variance
σ (sigma)	The population standard deviation
s	The sample standard deviation

Inferential Statistics

H_0	The null hypothesis of no difference between levels of the independent variable on the dependent variable of interest.
H_1	The alternate hypothesis of a difference between levels of the independent variable of the dependent variable of interest.
p	The probability of the given test statistic if the null hypothesis is true; a statistical difference is identified if the probability is less than the α set by the researcher.

α (alpha)	The probability of making a Type I error; set by the researcher.
β (beta)	The probability of making a Type II error; inversely related to α.
t	Test statistic for use with mean differences between two groups.
F	Test statistic for use with mean differences between two or more groups.
χ^2 (chi squared)	Test statistic for use with nominal data.

Correlational Statistics

r	Pearson product moment correlation.
r^2	Coefficient of determination.
R	Multiple regression correlation coefficient.
R^2	Proportion of variability accounted for by a multiple regression correlation coefficient.
ρ (rho)	Spearman's rho. Correlation coefficient used with ranked variables.
τ (tau)	Kendall's tau. Correlation coefficient used with ranked variables.
ϕ (phi)	Correlation coefficient used with nominal data.
κ (kappa)	Reliability coefficient used with nominal data.

Index

Note: Page numbers followed by "t" denote tables; page numbers followed by
"b" denote boxes. Italic page numbers indicate illustrations.